I0004414

167031

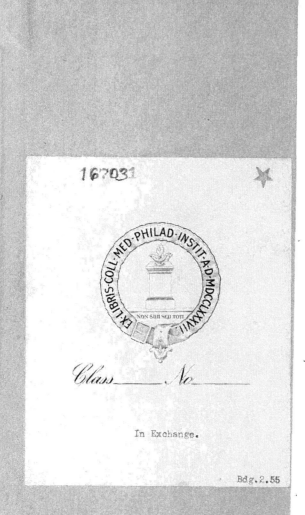

EX·LIBRIS·COLL·MED·PHILAD·INSTIT·A·D·MDCCLXXXVII·

NON SIBI SED TOTI

Class _____ No _____

In Exchange.

Bdg. 2. 55

LIBRARY OF THE
COLLEGE OF PHYSICIANS
OF PHILADELPHIA

Digitized by the Internet Archive
in 2016

ttps://archive.org/details/iournalofoklahom3919okla

VOL. XXXIX

NUMBER 1

January, 1946

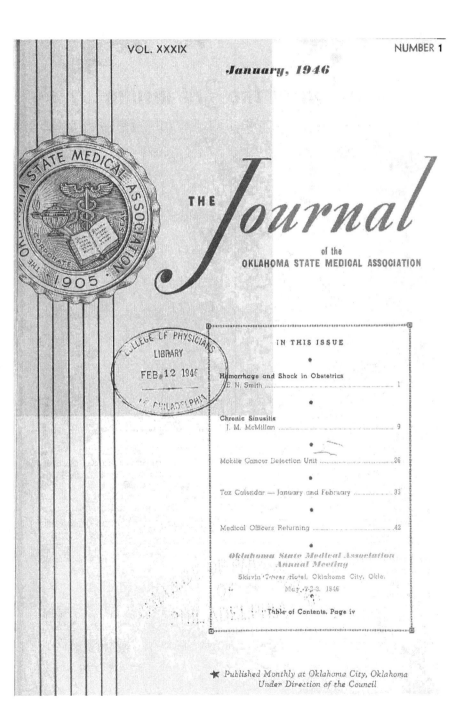

THE *Journal*

of the
OKLAHOMA STATE MEDICAL ASSOCIATION

COLLEGE OF PHYSICIANS
LIBRARY

FEB 12 1946

OF PHILADELPHIA

★ *Published Monthly at Oklahoma City, Oklahoma
Under Direction of the Council*

Evolution of the 3rd insulin...

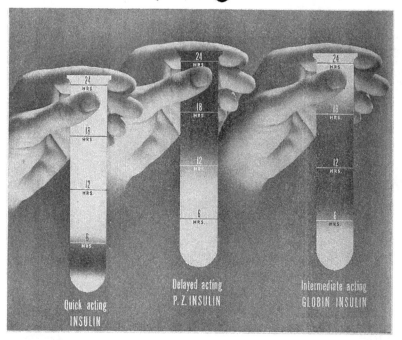

Quick acting
INSULIN

Delayed acting
P. Z. INSULIN

Intermediate acting
GLOBIN INSULIN

A NEW type of insulin is available for the diabetic —Globin Insulin. First there was a quick-acting but short-lived form. Next came a slow-acting but prolonged type. Now there is the intermediate-acting 'Wellcome' Globin Insulin with Zinc. Activity begins with moderate promptness yet it continues for sixteen or more hours, sufficient to cover the periods of maximum carbohydrate intake. Activity diminishes by night so that nocturnal reactions are minimal.

A single injection daily of 'Wellcome' Globin Insulin with Zinc controls the hyperglycemia of many patients. Physicians are rapidly learning to take advantage of this new third form of insulin when prescribing for their patients.

'Wellcome' Globin Insulin with Zinc is a clear solution, comparable to regular insulin in its freedom from allergenic properties.

Accepted by the Council on Pharmacy and Chemistry, American Medical Association. Developed in the Wellcome Research Laboratories, Tuckahoe, New York. U. S. Patent No. 2,161,198. Available in vials of 10 cc., 80 units in 1 cc. and vials of 10 cc., 40 units in 1 cc. Literature on request. 'Wellcome' trademark registered.

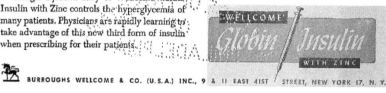

WELLCOME
Globin Insulin
WITH ZINC

BURROUGHS WELLCOME & CO. (U.S.A.) INC., 9 & II EAST 41ST STREET, NEW YORK 17, N. Y.

THE JOURNAL
of the
OKLAHOMA STATE MEDICAL ASSOCIATION

| VOLUME XXXIX | OKLAHOMA CITY, OKLAHOMA, JANUARY, 1946 | NUMBER 1 |

Hemorrhage and Shock in Obstetrics

EDWARD N. SMITH, M.D.
OKLAHOMA CITY, OKLAHOMA

An analysis of the maternal–mortality statistics in the State of Oklahoma reveals that 34 per cent died as a result of hemorrhage and shock . (See Fig. 1). This is not the

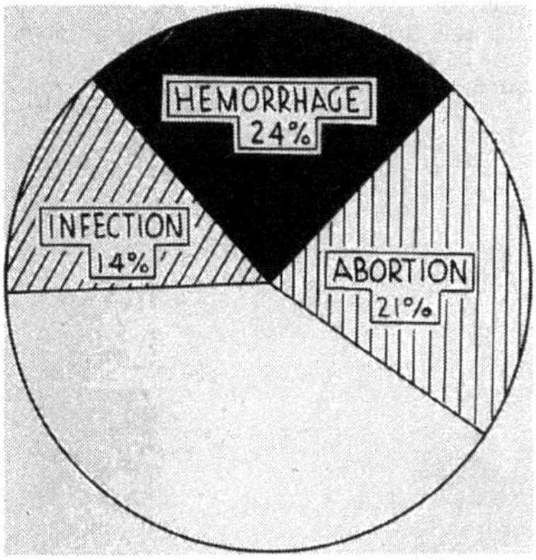

Figure 1   Oklahoma statistics on maternity mortality

complete picture however, since an additional 21 per cent die following abortion, and one-half of all abortion deaths are due to hemorrhage.

Pastore and others have shown a remarkable parallel between the degree of blood loss and the frequency of infection which follows later in the puerperium. They were able to predict, with considerable accuracy, the patient who later was to become infected, by carefully measuring the amount of blood loss sustained at delivery. Since one-

half of the 21 per cent of abortion deaths die from infection, the conclusion is inescapable that foregoing hemorrhage in many of these cases had set the stage for the lethal infection.

An additional 14 per cent of maternal deaths (excluding abortion deaths) occurred as a result of puerperal infection, which again, no doubt, was influenced by blood loss. (See Fig. 2). Thus, we see that blood loss,

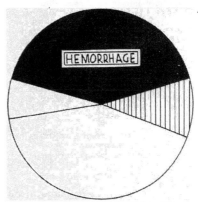

Figure 2   Corrected to show true role of hemorrhage

shock, or the combination, is known to account for at least 34 per cent of maternal deaths in this State, and almost certainly is the secondary cause of many additional deaths from infection.

To the minds of most doctors who attend childbirth, a death from hemorrhage is en-

167031
OCT 15 1947

visoned as a sudden, spectacular, overwhelming, and terrifying gush of blood coming from the vagina, without previous warning, causing the death of the patient in the space of ten or fifteen minutes. We usually think of this type of hemorrhage as being associated with placenta previa, or post partum bleeding. While such deaths do occur, in circumstances as sudden and catastrophic as indicated, they are relatively rare. If these were the *only* women dying of hemorrhage, the death rate from blood loss would be negligible.

A fact which should be emblazoned in the mind of every obstetrician, is that on the average, the length of time elapsing between the first recognized hemorrhagic tendency and the death of the patient is at least seven hours. If only we realized that we had seven hours in which to control a hemorrhage, we could transport a patient from anywhere in Oklahoma to almost any other location in Oklahoma. Seven hours is time enough to collect and sterilize any equipment we might need. Seven hours is sufficient time to round up and cross-match any number of donors. Consultation or skilled assistance is available to any Oklahoma physician no matter where he practices, in less than seven hours.

Prevention of death from hemorrhage, can be simplified into three phases. First, teach the patient to report any abnormality which might predict excessive blood loss. Second, "take alarm early." Third, take prompt and efficient action. The action taken depends of course on the type of bleding, the gestational state of the patient, and modifying circumstances.

We must realize the danger inherent in a long continued, even though small or moderate, rate of blood loss. Everyone takes alarm at the hemorrhage which gushes forth, but all too seldom do we give proper attention to the slow, steady flow, or to the large amount of blood absorbed in sponges and packs.

In order to prevent these deaths from hemorrhage, it is necessary to understand some of the fundamental factors involved. These may be listed as:

a. Circulatory changes in the maternal organism.
b. Physiological factors associated with hemorrhage.
c. Hemorrhagic Shock.
d. Therapeutic measures to combat hemorrhage and shock.

CIRCULATORY CHANGES IN THE MATERNAL ORGANISM

As gestation continues, the pelvic veins enlarge remarkably, as do also the veins and arteries of the uterus. Toward the end of pregnancy, the placental sinuses are filled with blood, all of these changes necessitating an increased bulk of blood. Part of this increased bulk is supplied by contraction of the spleen, which in pregnancy is usually smaller than normal. The rest of the increase is made up by the production of more blood. This amounts to about a 25 per cent increase, due largely to an increase in the plasma content. Thus, the volume is made larger by the addition of the "cell-less elements." The blood itself shows further changes, in that there is about a 30 per cent increase in the fibrinogen content and an increase in the viscosity.

The heart rate is not much increased in normal pregnancy, but the minute volume is greatly increased. In the last months, this increase may amount to 35 per cent or 50 per cent. This enormously increases the strain on the maternal heart, but allows up to two times the blood output, without increase in the cardiac rate.

Eight per cent of the body weight is made up of blood. This amounts to approximately 40 cc. per pound of body weight, and for a 150 pound woman, the total quantity of blood would be approximately 6,000 cc. or about six quarts of blood. (See Fig. 3). Physiologists

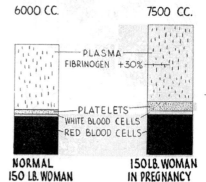

Figure 3　Comparison of normal and pregnancy blood volumes

are agreed that a loss of 30 per cent blood volume in the space of a few hours causes a drain on the system which probably cannot be met by the natural methods of compensation. Unless additional aid is provided, death from hemorrhage will ensue. Thirty per cent of 6,000 cc. is 1800 cc. of blood. Obstetricians almost never *measure* blood loss and are accustomed to seeing considerable blood after a normal delivery. We would be startled to find how close to this possibly fatal limit the blood loss approaches in many of our cases.

Nature has wisely provided several mechanisms by which the pregnant patient is better equipped to meet sudden blood loss. There occurs in normal pregnancy in the latter months, a constant seepage of "blood," (the fluid element) out of the capillaries and into the cells. This is not the pitting edema commonly seen, although if carried to extremes such edema would result. Instead, it is a somewhat water-logged condition of individual cells. While this mass of fluid might be unfavorable to the patient exhibiting toxemia, it is nevertheless a safety factor in blood loss, since fluid replacement can begin almost immediately back into the blood stream from this vast storehouse. We may call this the "extra-capillary reserve." Another factor concerns the increased excitability of the muscular coats of the arteries, permitting them to clamp down more vigorously than usual. This, also, may have implications of harm in toxemias. Other factors operating to minimize blood loss in labor would include the slight temperature rise, the concentration of blood elements from fluid loss, the slight increase in acidity, and the increased level of adrenalin during the emotions of labor. While some of these factors may be a detriment to the patient's welfare in other ways, they are at least changes affording quicker blood clotting during labor and after delivery.

PHYSIOLOGICAL FACTORS ASSOCIATED WITH HEMORRHAGE

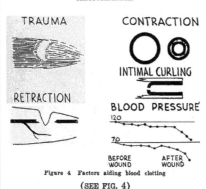

Figure 4   Factors aiding blood clotting

(SEE FIG. 4)

Blood Clotting

Clotting may be hastened by several factors in addition to the natural coagulation of blood. These factors include: trauma to the tissues, releasing the mechanism which precipitates the clotting; contraction of the

muscular coat of the artery itself, thereby narrowing its lumen; curling inward of the intimal layer of the artery; a fall in blood pressure after a certain degree of hemorrhage has occurred; and retraction of the severed artery so that it lies underneath a layer of muscle or fascia. The fall in blood

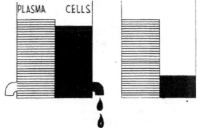

Figure 5   Anaemia

pressure will be discussed at some length later. All of these factors combined may be sufficient to stop profound hemorrhage even from an artery as large as the popliteal.

Because we use the red cell count, or the level of the hemoglobin, as an index to diagnosis or therapy on so many occasions, we are apt to think that these elements of blood are the most important constituents. The fluid and colorless portion of the blood is usually far more important than the number of red cells or hemoglobin level. The body can withstand a loss of red blood cells easier than it can withstand the loss of an equal volume of plasma or serum. (Many pernicious anemia patients are comfortable with a red cell count not over 1,000,000 per cubic millimeter if kept in bed.)

Anemia and Hemorrhage

(See Fig. 5)

Anemia represents the loss of red cellular elements of the blood, and progressive anemia may be noted by observing the hemoglobin level in the blood. It is unfortunate that we think of hemorrhage in the same way. (See Fig. 6). Sudden hemorrhage represents a loss of *both* cellular and blood elements, and until fluid replacement and other reparative measures have begun to operate, the hemoglobin is unchanged from its original level. The patient may bleed to death, but the last drop of blood lost might be just as rich as the first. It is discouraging to note how many physicians still rely on the hemoglobin level, or the red blood cell count to warn them of the

HEMORRHAGE

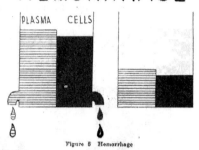

Figure 8 Hemorrhage

degree of their patient's blood loss. These same laboratory aids, taken two days later, would be more nearly accurate.

(See Fig. 7).

The mechanism by which the body is able to maintain the approximate volume of circulating blood at all times is extremely complex. This mechanism not only attempts to keep in relative balance the amounts of fluid versus cells, but at the same time it provides for the nourishment of tissue cells and for the disposal of waste products which are manufactured by those cells. Fluid may be supplied artificially to the body through several avenues, such as the subcutaneous, intravenous, and proctoclysis routes in addi-

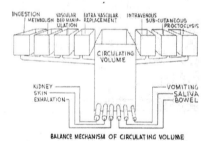

BALANCE MECHANISM OF CIRCULATING VOLUME

Figure 7 Balance of circulating volume

tion to which there are four natural sources of fluid intake. The first of these natural sources is through ingested fluids. Secondly, in the process of digestion of the food elements, protein and carbohydrates, an amount

of water nearly equal to that of food, is produced in the metabolism. A third method which is constantly being utilized by the normal patient concerns a rearrangement of the huge vascular bed including the rearrangement of capillary spaces. The central nervous system automatically and almost instantly may divert blood from some unimportant organ such as the skin, to protect an important or vital organ. In pregnancy, this system may not work too well, and leg cramps, numbness of the extremities, fainting or nausea and vomiting are all too common. The patient is said to have an "unstable vasomotor system." The fourth method of replacement is by means of seepage from the huge volume of tissue spaces, back into the vascular stream. In this manner, considerable replacement can take place utilizing the fluid and lymph contained in the lymph spaces.

Fluid is constantly being eliminated by the body through several channels, any one of which may be forced to accelerate its capacity for fluid disposal. The most active mechanism of elimination is through the kidney. The second most active moisture loss occurs through the skin. A third source of moisture loss in the expired lung air. Another constant source of fluid loss occurs by means of the moisture present in defecated material. The loss of fluid by saliva is negligible under usual circumstances, but in ptyalism, spitting habit, or mouth breathing, may become important. The fluid and body juices lost by vomiting represent a serious loss to the body since they are rich in chemical necessities as well as water, which makes it extremely important to guard the food and fluid intake of the vomiting patient. Fortunately, however, vomiting is an uncommon and intermittent process.

The effects of hemorrhage are modified by external circumstances, such as; the original blood volume and cell count before hemorrhage, the youth or senescence of the vascular walls, especially to surrounding vital centers, and more particularly by the rate/volume of blood loss. The results may be divided into immediate and remote.

EARLY DEFENSE AGAINST HEMORRHAGE

a. The loss of a considerable amount of blood (See Fig. 8) sets in motion a train of defense reactions calculated to allow the subject to continue life. The first and most easily discernible has to do with the clotting of the blood. This one property is the most important single phenomenon connected with hemorrhage, and were it not for this, a trivial wound would result in death.

b. Increase in the speed of circulation, which may or *may not* be accompanied by a rising pulse rate. The increased speed of circulation expresses an effort on the part of the body to deliver as much blood as formerly to the vital centers despite a minimized circulating volume.

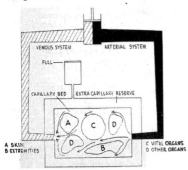

Figure 8 Normal vascular system

c. Contraction of the spleen. It is now thought that the reduced blood volume is met, at least in part, in obstetrical cases, by contraction of the spleen, with the subsequent discharge into the circulation of a quantity of fluid which is more than usually rich in blood cells.

d. Increased respiration. With a decreased amount of circulating volume there is a beginning disparity between the oxygen need and the oxygen supply. This is met by increasing the depth of respirations, which in severe cases are sighing or gasping and which may occasionally resemble the Cheyne-Stokes type.

e. Restlessness. The anxiety phase of hemorrhage is a constant finding in the later stages and one which seems an anachronism to continued existence. It is doubtless the result of insufficient blood supply to cortical centers.

f. Rearrangement of blood disposition. This phenomenon is extremely important, ordinarily allowing marked adjustment to the demands of hemorrhage. Depending on vasomotor phenomena, it will be less prompt in a sclerotic arterial system, and less dependable if there is additional injury or narcosis from anaesthesia, toxemias, drugs, etc. To effect this arrangement, the arterioles which serve relatively unimportant organs, are contracted. The skin, mucous membranes, inestines, etc., are deprived of circulation, becoming cold and pallid. This vasoconstriction is accomplished by stimulation of the sympathetic nervous system, and by these means, life can continue with certain unimportant functions rendered dormant. The sympathetic nervous system, is its vigorous attempts to constrict the vascular bed, stimulates the secretory system of the skin, with resultant sweat production and clamminess. Sufficient constriction may actually *raise* the blood pressure at this point. Thus, we note that the fall in blood pressure which we see all too often in hemorrhage, represents a failure of the compensatory mechanisms to keep up with the loss of blood. It is a late and dangerous sign, and should always cause the physician to act at once to combat the blood loss. The second part of the mechanism will be mentioned as a delayed effect, although it probably begins early in the course of hemorrhage.

Delayed Effects

a. Replacement of lost fluid. This is mentioned as a late finding, mainly because it make take several hours for completion. As soon as blood volume is decreased from hemorrhage, there is a beginning transfer of fluid from the lymph spaces around the cells, through the capillary membranes, back into the closed vascular system. The immediate effect of this is to deprive the tissues of their usual moisture, thus explaining the early, constant, and pronounced symptom of thirst, which is the universal cry of the wounded.

b. Replacement of red and white cells. This is the final item of repair and taken from a few days to several weks, depending on the individual.

HEMORRHAGIC SHOCK

The term "shock" first appeared in the literature about 1795. Since then despite many attempts and much research, no definition entirely satisfactory has been proposed, mainly because there are several different types of shock, respective to several different inciting causes.

Shock may follow:

1. Mechanical trauma: operative, accidental, or intestinal.
2. Thermal trauma: burns, freezing, peritoneal cooling.
3. Hemorrhage: internal, external and into tissues.
4. Pain.
5. Asphyxia: constrictive, narcotic, anesthetic.
6. Miscellaneous: infection, eclampsia, peritonitis, etc.

This discussion is limited to hemorrhagic shock.

One constant physical fact common to all types of shock regardless of the inciting cause, is the loss, temporary or permanent, of circulating volume within the closed vascular system. When this loss is sudden, the shock is apt to be sudden and severe. When the loss is gradual, the state of shock begins imperceptibly, and all too often catches us therapeutically off guard.

Beginning with a loss of circulating volume, (See Fig. 9) there is a reduction in cardiac filling, and therefore, a reduction in

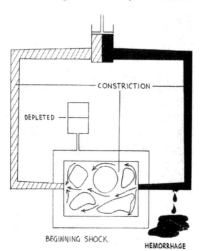

Figure 9   Beginning hemorrhagic shock

cardiac output. The pulse rate generally begins to increase at this point, but it may , remain steady, or even *slow* somewhat. Thus, pulse rate is not a dependable sign of impending or early shock. If the blood loss has been sudden there will be little or no changes in the hemoglobin or hemotocrit reading, (as before noted — Refer to Fig. 6), and these tests are equally unreliable.

With the reduced cardiac output, the sympathetic nervous system goes into vigorous action. The blood is shunted away from unimportant organs, such as the skin, mucous membranes, extremities, viscera, etc., thus conserving the blood to bathe the vital centers. The muscular activity is decidedly curtailed, and with the skin and extremities oligemic, the radiation of heat is curtailed and conserved. The patient is lethargic, and cold.

At this point, the sympathetics cause a constriction of the arteries and veins, thereby lessening the blood spaces which need to be filled. Also, the volume of the capillary bed is reduced by constriction. This entire mechanism is an exceedingly valuable one, and as a result of arterial constriction, the blood pressure remains relatively level, or even rises. Thus, we see the fallacy of trying to diagnose early shock, or to judge the degree of shock, by observing the blood pressure. The intense activity of the sympathetics carries over to activation of the sweat glands,

and the patient is cold and clammy.

Not until after approximately 20 per cent of the total circulating blood volume has been lost does this mechanism of defense begin to fail. It is only here, in well advanced shock when the arterial, venous, and capillary bed can constrict no more, that the blood pressure begins to fall. Remember then, *any* patient so far advanced in shock as to have a failing blood pressure, needs at least 1,000 cc. of fluid replacement and often much more. And promptly. Furthermore, *do not be fooled* by the fact that the fluid replaced has brought the blood pressure up, e.g., 90/60. That is only because the patient's body is using every mechanism of defense. Too many tragedies have followed complacency at this point. *Replace until the blood pressure is normal, the pulse is normal, and the skin no longer cold and clammy.* One thousand cc. is just a start all too often. For permanent benefit these fluids must contain colloids. Patients have been drowned in glucose or saline solution, trying to combat shock.

Another practical point concerns the use of stimulants and adrenalin. The patient is already making a last ditch stand, and adrenalin or other stimulants are useless or worse, causing certain organs to work (metabolism) which the body has purposely rendered dormant for conservation purposes.

Should the fluid be incompletely replaced (See Fig. 10) or not at all, the progressive

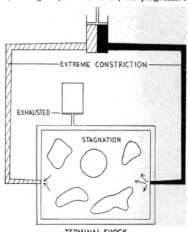

TERMINAL SHOCK
Figure 10   Terminal shock

fall in blood pressure, circulating volume, and cardiac filling would result in a definite lack of oxygen in the tissues. This is the terribly dangerous "shock pitch," for with anoxia, the vital centers in the brain and spinal cord, adrenals, etc., begin to fail, and the capillary bed begins to dilate and stagnate. This is the beginning of the end. While morphine may minimize pain which in turn causes some types of shock, morphine is worse than useless at this point because it adds to the oxygen lack.

Oxygen is now used in nearly every severe case of pneumonia. Belatedly, we are learning to use it early in eclampsia. When will we learn to use it early in shock? We would, if the patient were cyanotic, but there is little cyanosis because there is so little blood going through the skin. Any anaesthetic should long ago have been discontinued, because of the additional anoxia. By this time an anesthetic is superfluous.

Further progression of the shock causes under activity of the adrenal cortex, failure of renal and hepatic function, and a general break down of all metabolism. Potent adrenal extracts may in the future save these patients but they are not yet available.

There are then, briefly, three stages of hemorrhagic shock. In the earliest stage, the fluid loss may be compensated by simple measures such as cessation of further fluid loss, hot coffee, warm blankets, body rest, relief of pain, and simple stimulants. The second stage demands more vigorous therapy, and recovery will not occur unless the circulating volume is replaced by intravenous fluid. At this point, as mentioned above, conservation of every defense measure. The third stage is the break down of defense and unless vigorously and correctly treated soon reaches an irreversible stage beyond which no amount of any known therapy will save the patient.

These three stages may pass from one to the other rapidly and imperceptibly or worse yet the wonderful system of defense may lull us in to fancied security. The hemoglobin blood pressure and red cell count are useless or actually misleading. The over all clinical picture is the only safe criterion.

THERAPY

Beyond all doubt, the best therapeutic agent in hemorrhagic shock is the replacement of whole blood, carefully cross-matched and with compatible Rh factors. Because, however, we seldom take over 500 cc. from one donor, all too often we think 500 cc. is sufficient for the patient. If in clinical shock she should certainly have 1,000 cc. and all too often twice that or more.

Unfortunately, even in well equipped hospitals, the shortest time that is necessary to type and match and collect donors blood may be over two hours. Too often, especially in rural practice, whole blood is simply not available.

A very effective substitute is available, in amost every drug store in almost every town, and it should be in every physician's automobile. The dried plasma commercially available is a precious life saver, if used early and adequately. The quantity used however, should be as great or greater than whole blood. It has the decided advantages of availability, stability, and will not spoil from time or heat. It need not be warmed, matched, typed, tested for Rh or syphilis. There is only rare anaphylaxis.

Glucose or saline are the next most valuable, and often keep the patient alive until plasma or whole blood is available. While these crystalized solutions cannot be given in huge quantities without caution (in cases of low serum protein) nevertheless, any fluid is better than no fluid. The use of atrophine, adrenal cortex, metrazol, etc., are beyond the scope of this essay.

TREATMENT OF GRAVE EMERGENCIES

Even though the patient may be near death from blood loss, many lives can be saved by prompt and efficient action. More than one pair of hands are needed and the more trained help available the better.

1. Lower the head. This conserves the blood supply to vital centers and facilitates venous return and cardiac filling.

2. Insulate from chilling with a blanket.

3. Supply oxygen if possible and artificial resuscitation if necessary.

4. As rapidly as possible replace the intravenous fluid. In a grave emergency the veins are usually collapsed making it difficult to puncture them with a large needle and even if punctured, the fluid may run so slowly that the patient dies under treatment. This is particularly true of blood or plasma. Do not hesitate to cut down on a vein and the best vein for rapid therapy runs just anterior to the internal malleous. A longitudinal incision about two inches in length extending through the skin and subcutaneous fat will expose the vein. It should be elevated by passing a probe or hemostat underneath. Cut across the vein or insert without cutting, the largest available needle and secure the needle in the vein with the needle and vein grasped in a hemostat or by tieing in place with a suture. For this reason a canula is better than a needle. It is advisable and often imperative that the fluids be administered by positive pressure, and one of the best methods is by means of large syringes. Have an assistant fill one syringe while the operator pumps blood or plasma with the second syringe. A bowl of normal saline is useful for rinsing and for supplementary injections if there is any delay. Do not be afraid to give the fluid rapidly. Since over 1,000 cc. pass

through the heart per minute you will not overload the heart by rapid transfusion. In addition to opening a vein, there are other avenues available for fluid administration. A stout, large needle may be pushed through the outer layer of the sternum about two inches below the junction with the clavicles until the point of the needle rests within the marrow cavity. (When properly inserted the oily marrow can be withdrawn into a syringe as a test.) Even whole blood will absorb at a fairly rapid rate through this portal.

Corpora cavernosa of the penis can be utilized in males. In grave emergencies it is sometimes necessary to sacrifice the finer details of sterile technique in favor of the more urgent need for fluid replacement. I feel it is better later to face the treatment of infection in a living patient since we now have the sulfonamides, Penicillin, and other antibiotics, than to let the patient die from shock.

In any form of rapid fluid replacement there is a note of caution. As soon as possible the bleeding point must be secured if only temporarily. If fluid is replaced (as it should be) to the point where the blood pressure recovers, any life saving clot may be blown out. Many an ectopic pregnancy death attests this tragedy. Replace the fluids as rapidly as possible but be prepared to block any further fluid loss.

Morphine should be used cautiously and only for severe pain or restlesness. In a real emergency it is not needed and may be decidedly harmful.

Moving the patient causes pain, anxiety, chilling, greater demand for oxygen and may dislodge the clot — all unfortunate factors. Move her as little as possible until the bleeding has been scotched and the fluid has been replaced. Insulation against drafts or chilling is valuable but heat therapy is detrimental. Only dry blankets should be used. The shock patient may easily be burned by a hot water bag which seems only comfortable to the attendant. The use of one or two blankets is enough.

CONCLUSION

1. Take alarm early. Very few hemorrhages are overwhelming. It is the steady, drip, drip, drip, which is misleading, and the patient all too often hits the "shock pitch" before we are organized to act. By actual investigation, an average of seven hours elapses in obstetrical deaths, between the first sign of bleeding and death.

2. Do not depend on pulse rate, laboratory reports or blood pressure readings. They do not reflect the patient's proximity to death.

3. Treat adequately. The patient in shock needs at least 1,000 cc. of blood or plasma.

There is no satisfactory substitute, although there are several temporary ones. Plasma in your car will save a life sometime, if you carry it long enough, and use it early enough.

4. Severe blood loss, even if not sufficient to result in shock, is often the precursor of a lethal infection.

SUMMARY

The real evaluation of deaths from hemorrhage in obstetrics is composed of deaths from frank hemorrhage, deaths from abortion (hemorrhage and infection) and deaths from infection (preceded by hemorrhage). Viewed in this perspective it becomes the most important single cause of maternal mortality.

By actual investigation in nine out of ten deaths from hemorrhage in Oklahoma, the blood loss began during or just after delivery or abortion. The physician who accepts obstetrical cases must accept the responsibility for those deaths, and must in the future be prepared to prevent them.

What A Galaxy

On Dr. Welch's pathological staff were William T. Councilman, who had worked earlier in Vienna, Strasbourg, Leipzig, and Prague, Alexander C. Abbott, hygienist and bacteriologist, George H. F. Nuttall, bacteriologist, and Simon Flexner, Fellow in Pathology. Walter Reed (later of yellow fever fame), Dr. A. W. Clement (veterinarian), and J. Whitridge Williams (later obstetrician), William T. Howard, Jr., and J. Homer Wright were doing research work in the laboratory though they did not live in the Hospital. On Dr. Osler's medical staff were Henry A. Lafleur, Resident Physician, Harry Toulmin, Assistant, D. M. Reese and J. A. Scott, interns. William Sydney Thayer acted as Differentiating Physician for the Out-Patient Department, and John Hewetson, August Hoch, and later Harold Parsons and Frank R. Smith were Assistant Resident Physicians. Another member of the staff who became a close friend of mine was Rupert Norton (son of Charles Eliot Norton). Dr. Lafleur was in charge of the courses in the Clinical Laboratory. He resigned as Resident Physician late in 1891 and was succeeded by Dr. Thayer.—*Time and the Physician. The Autobiography of Lewellys F. Barker. p. 42. G. P. Putnam's Sons. New York. 1942.*

What's In A Name?

Many have wondered about the origin of my name, Lewellys Franklin. It seems that my father wished to have me called something more distinctive than James, William or any other common family name. He had been a great admirer of Benjamin Franklin, having read his *Autobiography* and *Poor Richard's Almanack*, so he decided upon Franklin as my middle name. In a letter to John Alleyn, Franklin wrote: "Be studious and you will be learned. Be industrial and frugal and you will be rich. Be sober and temperate and you will be healthy. Ben in general virtuous, and you will be happy. At least you will, by such conduct, stand the best chances for such consequences." Whether or not my father ever read this particular passage, the ideas expressed agreed closely with his own views of a well-ordered life.—*Time and the Physician. The Autobiography of Lewellys F. Barker. Page 4. G. P. Putnam's Sons. New York. 1942.*

Chronic Sinusitis - A Safe Management and Treatment

JAMES M. MCMILLAN, M.D.

VINITA, OKLAHOMA

At the time of the first visit, a case of chronic sinusitis, the etiology must be determined if possible. A listing of the many causes of chronic sinusitis with a discussion of each would fill a good sized volume. I will merely list a few of them with short comments:

1. Predisposing factors:
   a. Allergies — from food, pollens, smoke, dusts, chemical and bacteria.
   b. Fatigue—overwork, and loss of sleep are factors especially during wartime.
   c. Malnutrition — deficiencies of vitamin and minerals, especially vitamins A, C and D.
   d. Glandular Diseases — especially the climateric of male and female.
   e. Climate — in either wet or dusty climates or where there are rapid changes of temperature.
   f. Hereditary — narrowed or constricted air channels.
2. Local Factors
   a. Malformations — traumas and anomalies of the nasal structures.
   b. Foreign Bodies and Tumors causing obstructions.
   c. Chronic Rhinitis — this is probably due to chronic allergies, or the so-called old-fashioned catarrah.
3. Exciting factors:
   a. Bacterial invasion of devitalized mucous membranes with extension into the sinus cavities through the ostei.
   b. Para apical tooth abscesses with extension into sinuses especially to the maxillary.
   c. Osteomyelitis.
   d. Transfers by blood and lymphatics of infected material.
   e. Following acute infectious diseases.

Symptoms are many and varied, but the most common for chronic sinusitis, are headache, dizziness, pressure pains, fullness in the affected sinuses, point pains in top of head and back of neck, pains in various parts of the body or muscular rheumatism, neuritis and neuralgia pains in neck, arm and shoulders and accompanied by nasal stuffiness. Many complain of an eyestrain, and a feeling of pinching pressure through the bridge of the nose. There is a chronic secretion from the nose which may be purulent, blood streaked or clear. There are acute exacerbations in which the symptoms of acute sinusitis occur with extreme pain and fever, but in chronic sinusitis the temperature is abnormally subnormal. In the latter case the patient appears to be chronically ill in general and a fever produced by vaccine, or by any foreign protein parenterally is of value in the treatment. Many complain of a "clicking" sensation and sound after blowing the nose.

The diagnosis is made by the chief complaints of the patient. The routine nose and throat examination with transillumination of the maxillary and frontal sinuses and x-ray examination are the main factors in the diagnosis. A chronic nasal secretion with pain on pressure over the sinuses affected are important diagnostic signs. Transillumination of a painful sinus at times is negative though the pain may be due to a vacuum caused by closure of the sinus opening and absorption of the air within the sinus.

The treatment is important and some of the "don't" should come first. Do not probe the chronic sinus unless absolutely necessary for drainage. The treatment lasts from six to eight weeks, and if you probe or irritate the sinuses three times weekly for that time the course of treatment will be prolonged. Most of the patients have been treated before and many women are in tears on the first attempt at probing. Irrigation of the sinuses is of little value and tends to aggravate the disease. Refrain from surgery which will leave scarification around the sinus opening or leave a strictured sinus opening. Don't allow prolonged use of ephedrine compounds and inhalers of various sorts. The ephedrine compounds may make the patient extremely nervous and cause loss of sleep and in this way injure the health of the patient. Don't overtreat with any drug ,especially the sulfonamides. Always explain to the patient that he is to be treated from six to eight weeks, that the treatment will not be painful and that he is not to start the treatment if he is to be away for even a weeks interval.

The objectives of treatment are: 1. establishment of natural sinus drainage; 2. riddance of the infection or irritating factor; 3. restoration of normal sinus function; 4. restoration of the health of the patient.

Establishment of natural sinus drainage is accomplished by removal or shrinkage of obstructions. If there is a hypertrophic rhinitis present shrinkage with ephedrines in the form of Rhinazine by Lederle is preferred unless hypertension or exopthalmic goiter is present. In the latter cases, neosynaphrine, one-fourth per cent, with sulfathiazole is preferable.

Always ask the patient if he is sensitive to iodine and if not, use potassium iodide, saturated solution, by mouth in the dosage of 15 drops 3 times daily in water until there is liquifaction of secretions from the nose and eyes.

Two cc Iodolake — stronger, by Lakeside Laboratories, given parenterally in the subdeltoid region on alternate days until drainage of the sinuses is established is preferable. This treatment should require only one week. All necessary probing and dilation of the sinuses should be done during this time. Removal of polyps or similar obstructions should be accomplished during the drainage period. Negative pressure helps establish drainage and leaves the positive pressure which can be treated by Tyrothricin spray. This aids in killing the infection within the sinus. The patient should be placed on a wholesome diet of fruits and vegetables, milk, cream, butter and eggs. The administration of vitamins and minerals is left to the discretion of the doctor. It is preferable to give 100 milligram tablets of ascorbic acid three times daily throughout the treatment or longer for its revitalizing influence.

Riddance of the infection is accomplished by the use of the Lilly's Streptococcus-Staphylococcus Vaccine No. 4, and the continuance of the vasoconstrictors mixed with the sulfonamides sprayed into the nose. Negative pressure is produced to be followed by the Tyrothricin spray. The vaccine dosage is given as two to four minims, but the heavy dosage of one cubic centimeter increased to two cubic centimeters on the last two inoculations is well tolerated by most patients.

Penicillin is ineffective unless drainage is established. Even so, the symptoms reoccur in a very short time in most patients. Penicillin must be given continuously in 20,000 unit inoculations every four hours, and the patient should be hospitalized, for continuous treatment, in order to maintain adequate amounts of this drug in the system. Most chronic sinusitis patients do not desire hospitalization. They are ambulatory and able to follow ordinary pursuits. Penicillin is therefore not recommended as a general treatment for chronic sinusitis. Instillation of Penicillin solution into the antrum is recommended in chronic purulent sinusitis if other methods fail.

Restoration of normal sinus function is accomplished by intravenous administration of Sodium Ascorbate, 1 to 500 solution three times weekly. Ascorbic Acid 100 milligram tablets are continuously given three times daily as in the beginning of the treatment.

The nasal shrinkage sprays are continued if hypertrophic Rhinitis is present. The tyrcthrician sprays are used as usual at each visit of the patient three times weekly, after producing negative pressure. Twelve to fifteen treatments are given using the sodium ascorbate intravenously. Gradually the pale edematous mucous membrane will return to normal and show a revitalization. If there have been some blood streaks these gradually disappear, likewise the granular appearance of the mucous membranes. In the bleeding type of mucous membrane the vitamin C is certainly indicated.

The restoration of health to the patient has practically become accomplished at the end of the six to eight week treatment. The side reactions noted are all good under this management except in a few patients who are hypersensitive to the vaccine and show a sensitivity to the iodides.

As for glandular therapy the estrogens and testosterone should be administered when indicated in the climacteric. In the series of approximately 35 cases all claimed much improvement and approximately two-thirds claimed to be cured.

What Is Hopkins?

Toward the end of our internship, I told my friend, Dr. Cullen, that I thought I should like to do some postgraduate work at the Johns Hopkins Hospital. He said, "Lew, what is Hopkins?" I showed him an issue of the *Johns Hopkins Hospital Bulletin* that contained a photograph of the hospital, and Cullen said, "If you go, I'm going with you."

The house staff was much excited when it was learned that Dr. Howard A. Kelly, the gynecologist of the Johns Hopkins Hospital, had been invited to perform an operation in the hospital. Several surgeons of the Visiting Staff were on hand. I gave the anesthetic and Tom Cullen acted as surgical assistant, handing the instruments to Dr. Kelly as he called for them. Everyone was greatly impressed with the speed and skill of Dr. Kelly's surgical technique. After the operation, Cullen said to me: "That settles it; I want to go to Johns Hopkins and work with Dr. Kelly." Having heard much of the brilliance of the work of Dr. William Osler, who was Physician-in-Chief at Johns Hopkins, my reply to Cullen was: "Well, if you choose Kelly, I'll go to Osler if he'll have me." (Cullen followed Kelly and Barker followed Osler).—*Time and the Physician. The Autobiography of Lewellys F. Barker.* pp. 34-35. G. P. Putnam's Sons. New York. 1942.

CLINICAL PATHOLOGIC CONFERENCE

University of Oklahoma School of Medicine

Presented by the Departments of Pathology and Urology

ROBERT H. AKIN, M.D.—HOWARD C. HOPPS, M.D.

DOCTOR HOPPS: Our case for this morning presents a difficult diagnostic problem. Although the patient's initial symptoms were readily and accurately evaluated something happened during his hospital course which was quite out of the ordinary and which terminated in an unexplained death. Dr. Akin will discuss the clinical aspects.

PROTOCOL

Patient: T. T., white male, age 58; admitted May 14, 1945; died June 16, 1945.

Chief Complaint: Incontinence of urine, burning on urination, and left hemiplegia.

Present Illness: This man was well until three years ago, when he awoke one morning at 5:00 a. m. unable to move his left arm or leg. In the course of succeeding months there was gradual improvement, but a residual partial paralysis of the left arm and leg persisted. About one month prior to admission he became incontinent of urine and had to wear a bag to hold urine so that he could get about. There was no history of previous urinary trouble. Approximately one week prior to admission the patient suddenly lost consciousness and fell to the ground. He recovered after a few moments and suffered no residual effects.

Past and Family History: Noncontributory.

Physical Examination: Revealed a well developed, well nourished, white male apparently not acutely ill. There was partial paralysis of the left arm and leg. Pupils were small and did not react to light or accommodation. The chest was normal; no rales were heard. The heart was not enlarged to percussion and no murmurs were heard. Blood pressure was 130/60. No masses or tenderness were noted in the abdomen. Reflexes were hyperactive in the left extremities. There was four plus pitting edema of both feet and legs.

Laboratory Data: On admission the urine was blood red and cloudy. Reaction was acid. Specific gravity was 1.010, there was a trace of albumin, no glucose. There were 200-300 red blood cells per h.p.f., occasional white blood cells, but no casts. On June 7, 1945, the urine was of amber color and there was no protein. There were 20-22 red blood cells and innumerable white blood cells per h.p.f. Urinalysis on June 14, 1945, revealed three plus proteinuria with innumerable red blood cells and white blood cells seen microscopically. On admission hemoglobin measured 10 Gm. and red blood cells 3 59/cu.mm., white blood cells numbered 7,450/cu.mm., with 67 per cent neutrophils, 28 per cent lymphocytes and 5 per cent eosinophils. Four weeks later (6-15) hemoglobin had dropped to 7.5 Gm. and red blood cells to 2.42. There was a leukocytosis of 16,450/cu.mm. with 88 per cent neutrophils and 12 per cent lymphocytes. The blood N.P.N. was 35 on May 14, 1945, phosphorus 3.2 and acid phosphates 2.1 B. U. on June 1, 1945, the N.P.N. was 60 mg. per cent. The Mazzini and Wassermann reactions were both four plus. X-ray examination on May 15, 1945, revealed no abnormality of the bony pelvis.

Clinical Course: The patient was prepared for cystoscopy on May 15, 1945, but the bladder was so irritable that detailed examination could not be made. All edema of the legs and feet had disappeared. On May 19, 1945, cystoscopy revealed considerable prostatic inflammation of the bladder mucosa with areas of sloughing. This was treated with sulfathiazole and mandelic acid. On June 1, 1945, the patients temperature spiked to 103.6 degrees F. Sulfathiazole was begun again and the patient received penicillin for seven days but the fever continued, septic in type, with peaks at 103 degrees — 105 degrees F. On June 7, 1945, bubbling rales were noted in both lungs. He failed to respond to stimulants and died on June 16, 1945.

DOCTOR AKINS: To evaluate this case properly we must go a little further back than the immediate present illness. The paralytic stroke described three years prior to hospitalization here is pretty definite evidence of a cerebro-vascular accident and suggest rather strongly marked arterosclerosis as a predisposing cause. This is one of the degenerative lesions which so often characterizes old age or senility as you know. Although this man was but 58, an age that many of us are strongly opposed to consider as the onset of senility, yet we must think of various other associated "senile" changes that may have existed and contributed to this clinical picture. Lest you misunderstand my reference to age and senility, I hasten to add that there is no absolute direct relationship between the two and that whereas in some, senility may begin at 45 years, there are many notable examples of men in their seventies who are far from senile.

At any rate this man did have cerebral signs and symptoms presumable related to arteriosclerosis. Examination revealed also considerable prostatic hyperplasia, another manifestation of senility and one responsible for many difficulties in patients of this age group. A third manifestation of old age in a patient of this sort which we must keep in the back of our mind even though there was no obvious indication in this patient, is arteriosclerotic heart disease.

The first urinary difficulty was experienced one month before admission. With the history of a previous cerebro-vascular accident one would first think of some casual relationship there, since occasionally urinary retention, with incontinence on the basis of overflow, does develop following a stroke. The interval of almost three years between these to occurrences is adequate basis to dismiss the thought.

Urinalysis promptly established the fact that this patient had a serious infection of the urinary tract. This together with the prostatic hyperplasia (enlargement of the prostate is suddenly and greatly aggravated by inflammatory edema and hyperemia) seem adequate explanation of the patient's illness. Cystoscopy revealed a marked ulcerative cystitis and treatment was begun using sulfathiazole and mandelic acid. An indwelling catheter was inserted.

Treatment in patients such as these, and we see a great many, is always a serious problem. So often the general condition of the patient is such that we have to be on constant guard again cardiac failure and/or pneumonia; we have to try to combat the effects of renal failure; we have also the problem of an infection which, in addition to doing extensive local damage, may become generalized. This man might have done better if a retention catheter had not been introduced. On the other hand the majority of patients do better with a catheter. Without knowing the exact extent of the infection in the prostatic gland, and we can't find out during these acute episodes, we can't be certain which is the better procedure. We're

inclined to establish drainage however because this, in addition to helping the infection in the majority of cases, also prepares the patient for prostatic resection and gives him a chance for complete recovery. As you have read in the "clinical course" this patient was getting along satisfactorily until, two weeks before his death, he developed a septic fever and other evidences of serious infection which did not respond to sulfathiazole or penicillin. I suspect that this represented a spread of the prostatic infection. The manner and extent of spread however is not apparent from the clinical data.

DISCUSSION

CLINICAL

QUESTION: What was the basis for the edema of the feet and legs?

DOCTOR AKIN: There was no evidence of cardiac failure and I think it must have been due to an obstructive lesion in the vessels going to the legs.

QUESTION: Did you consider the possibility of carcinoma of the prostate.

DOCTOR AKIN: The gland was smooth and not hard. X-rays revealed no metastatic lesions in the pelvis and acid phosphatase was not elevated.

QUESTION: Was the urinary infection related to catheterization?

DOCTOR AKIN: We do not know whether or not this patient was catheterized before we saw him and because of that lack of knowledge we do not know how much urinary retention might have been present. The considerable amount of blood in the urine suggests that catheterization, with considerable trauma, might have been done. In this case it might have spread an infection in the prostate. There is also the possibility that the catheter itself might have introduced pathogenic organisms.

QUESTION: How much renal damage was there?

DOCTOR AKIN: The initial N.P.N. determination did not indicate any serious degree of impairment (there may be considerable renal dysfunction before nitrogeneus retention begins). Later the N.P.N. was elevated. This could mean a renal infection or again it might mean an inflammatory destruction of the ureteral orifices. I believe that he did have pyelonephritis.

ANATOMICAL DIAGNOSIS

DOCTOR HOPPS: Several points of teaching value in this case deserve special emphasis. For one thing this case illustrates the need for constant attention and though even in those patients who have a well established diagnosis and have been in the hospital several weeks and have survived one or more changes in service. Even the case of an old man with benign prostatic hyperplasia there are, as Dr. Akin pointed out, many hazards to be on guard against and it requires frequent reevaluation to pick these up at a time when treatment is most effective.

At necropsy, from external examination, the most striking change was the definite enlargement of the left leg as compared with the right. At mid-thigh, the circumference of the legs measured 50 cm. and 33 cm. respectively. On the basis of this finding alone, plus the history, we made a tentative diagnosis of thrombophlebitis and, perhaps pulmonary embolism. The left iliac vein was found to be converted into an abscess cavity. Its lumen, for approximately eight cm., was filled with thin grayish pus, i.e., pyothrombosis. Proximally and distally to this, a solid thrombus completely obstructed, extending into the femoral and hypogastric veins below, and to the bijurcation of the vena cava above. A seven c. thrombatic embolus was found lodged in the pulmonary artery and probably acted as the precipitating cause of death.

The major disease from which this man was suffering during his last two weeks of life was pyemia. There were perhaps 30-40 septic infarcts in the lungs, several of which had been converted into frank abscesses. The pancreas contained 10 abscesses from 3 to 10 mm. in diameter and there were multiple tiny suppurative foci in the kidney.

For the proper evaluation of a septic state such as this we should consider the effects or changes under their major headings.

1. Direct effects of the organisms per se:

This includes focal abscess as were described above or perhaps the lesions will be non suppurative as they most often are in subacute bacterial endocarditis. Not infrequently there will be acute vegetative endocarditis, a manifestation which this particular patient did not show.

2. *Degenerative changes related to toxemia:*

The findings in this case are illustrative. The liver and kidneys were each considerably increased in weight and appeared swollen. Capsular surfaces were more opaque than usual and the organs appeared almost as though parboiled. Cut surfaces bulged considerably, additional evidence of parenchymay swelling with increased intracapsular tension. The heart exhibited moderate pallor and was flabby. Microscopically, in addition to the changes characteristic of "cloudy swelling," there was fatty change (degeneration) of these organs. Probably all tissues of the body undergo qualitatively similar changes in an infection of this sort, but it is in the liver, kidney and heart that they are most apparent.

3. *Changes related to defensive mechanisms:*

Here are included the so-called septic hyperplasia of the spleen (in this case it was enlarged 100 per cent and quite flabby) and hyperplasia of the lymph nodes (here enlarged 2-3 times). The von Kupffer cells of the liver, an element of the reticulo-endothelial system, and the bone marrow are also subject to hyperplasia.

On the basis of our findings we were able to reconstruct the sequence of events in this case as follows:

1. Prostatic hyperplasia led to urinary retention and predisposed to a suppurative, ulcerative cystitis which was responsible in large part for the urinary findings described and for the initial fever.

2. In addition to the prostatic hyperplasia there was focal prostatitis and seminal visiculitis which caused thrombosis and infection of periprostatic veins.

3. Extension of infection through the periprostatic veins ultimately reached the larger pelvic veins and the left iliac vein, giving rise to thrombosis and infection there.

4. Continuation of the infection in the left iliac vein lead to suppuration and embolic seeding of the blood stream, i.e. pyemia. This resulted in multiple abscesses, various degenerative changes of toxic origin and hyperplasia of spleen, lymph nodes, bone marrow, etc.

5. A larger fragment of the thrombus became dislodged and finally reached the pulmonary artery, being the immediate cause of death.

One other finding of interest was syphilitic aoritis and aortic valvulitis with aortic insufficiency. This explains the unusual pulse pressure which this patient had, 70 mm.

We were not permitted to examine the brain in this case but the evidence is quite certain of a previous cerebro-vascular accident.

DISCUSSION

QUESTION: Was there evidence of marked renal damage?

DOCTOR HOPPS: The most important lesion was, as Dr. Akin suggested, an inflammatory narrowing of the vesico-ureteral orifices causing early hydroureter and hydronephrosis. The suppurative foci were pretty recent and were not as yet extensive.

QUESTION: How old was the syphilitic aoritis?

DOCTOR HOPPS: It's difficult to say, but this was probably from 15 to 40 years old.

QUESTION: Why wasn't a heart murmur heard if there was aortic insufficiency?

DOCTOR HOPPS: Probably because it was not carefully listened for. This case illustrates the fact that many persons who have had syphilis for many years and who have not had specific therapy suffer no obvious ill effects. This man's heart was approximately 30 per cent over weight, and the left ventricle was moderately dilated, the aortic valve orifice measured 10.5 cm. in circumference as contrasted with a normal of about 7.5 cm. There was definite aortic regurgitation but not such much that he could not compensate for it.

SPECIAL ARTICLE

Further Observation on Manpower and Disease

LEWIS J. MOORMAN, M.D.
OKLAHOMA CITY, OKLAHOMA

Those who question the theory of stimulation of the mind through the toxemia of disease, tuberculosis the outstanding example, still face the fact that aside from the seeming strange psychic stimulus often associated with the toxic effects of tuberculosis there is the obvious response to environment. In other words a disease which puts one down for months creates a mental problem which must be recognized. It is well known that tuberculosis may give rise to two distinct manifestations: the depletion of physical energy and, directly or indirectly, the stimulation of mental activity. The human organism's response to environment is materially influenced by these two factors. In those who are endowed with exceptional mental qualities, and are at the same time suffering from tuberculosis, there often seems to be a strange psychic stimulus bent on creative accomplishment. Dr. Charles H. Mayo once said, "The years spent in voluntary obedience to the rules of treatment may have a lasting influence and remove the one great obstacle to success in life." Certainly, during the silent watches accompanying the course of tuberculosis, many a sufferer has discovered the saving presence of a creative instinct.

Doctors know that in the course of a long illness the essential elements of personality must be revealed. Erich Ebstein in *Tuberculose als Schiecksal* referred to the fact that biographers and critics have long recognized progressive tuberculosis in geniuses as a possible factor contributing to their individual greatness. He does not admit that the disease causes genius but agrees that it may fan into flame an otherwise dormant spark. While it is true that the Capadocian physician referred to this strange phenomenon in the 2nd Century A. D., we cite more recent observers.

Erick Stern, the poet Norvalis and Klabund wrote about the stimulating influence of the tubercle bacillus. The physician MacLeod Munro impressed with this stimulating influence said, "The patient has an insatiable craving for a full and active life. He lives in an atmosphere of feverish eagerness to seize the fleeting moments before they pass. These characteristics are particularly noticeable in those of naturally artistic or literary tastes."

Dr. Lawrence F. Flick said, "the tuberculous may make life more pleasant and make the individual more profitable to society than he otherwise would be." Havelock Ellis in *A Study of British Genius* points out the predominance of genius among tuberculous personages. Dr. J. A. Hyers in *Fighters of Fate* considers the probability of mental exaltation under the influence of the tubercle bacillus and attributes some of Chopin's great masterpieces to this motivating factor in disease. Dr. Arthur C. Jacobson in *Genius Social Revelations* believes that "the tuberculous by-products are capable of profoundly affecting the mechanism of creative minds in such a way as to influence markedly their creations." He goes on to say, "Were the present writer to give an almost sure recipe for producing the highest type of creative mind, he would postulate an initial spark of genius plus tuberculosis."

One of the critics of John Millington Synge, after referring to his supersensitive temperament said, "he naturally clutched at extremes with all the hectic greediness of a consumptive." J. Middleton Murry said of Katherine Mansfeld, "When the full tide of inspiration came, she wrote till she dropped with fatigue—sometimes all through the night, in defiance of her illness." Matthew Arnold said of Maurice de Guerin, "The temperament, the talent itself is deeply influenced by the mysterious malady; the temperament is devouring; it uses vital power too hard and too fast." Munro said of Hood: "As his health declined his poetical fire seemed to burn more brightly, and the 'Song of the Shirt,' as he pathetically put it, came from a man on his death-bed. 'The Bridge of Sighs' soon followed this, and these two poems, written within a few months of his death, set the seal upon his greatness as a poet." Munro also attributed to John Addington Symonds, "that nervous, fretful, and fitful energy which is so characteristic a feature of the artistic or intellectual phthisical patient."

Lincon Lorenz said of Sidney Lanier, "His bodily fever heightened the temperature of his spiritual passion." Dr. Vere Pearson discussing the psychology of the consumptive referred to the restless agitation of the mind and "the feeling of apprehension lest life should be shortened."

Dr. Robert L. Pitfield and Sidney Calvin wrote about John Keats' psychological response to his disease. Quoting Jeanette Marks in Genius and Disaster: "It has been said that a man is what his microbes make him, and in nothing, it would seem, is this more true than with the man of genius."

John B. Huber in his work on Consumption and Civilization made the following statement: "It appears to me that the quality of the genius of a great man, if he be consumptive, may be, in some cases at least, affected by his disease."

Dr. John Brown of Edinburgh, author of Rab and His Friends, observed a certain mental exuberance as he studied the psychology of his tuberculosis patients. Discussing the case of his young friend, Dr. William Henry Scott, he made this significant comment, "He died of consumption and had that sad malady, in which the body and soul, as if knowing their time here was short — burn as in oxygen gas — and have 'hope, the Charmer' with them to the last — putting into these twenty years the energy, the enjoyment, the mental capital and rapture of a long life." Nevinson has said of Schiller: "It is possible that the disease served in some way to increase his eager activity, and fan his intellect into keener flame."

In Tuberculosis and Genius, University of Chicago Press, 1940, the sufferers speak for themselves in no uncertain terms. In addition to this brief summary of opinions expressed in popular writings, attention is called to the fact that medical textbooks recognize the profound influence of tuberculosis of the nervous system.

Finally we must admit that the present evidence of a specific psychic stimulus from disease is founded wholly on the clinical manifestations which in some cases seem to warrant a belief in a toxic factor with psychic selection. But while we await the proof of such a stimulus we must recognize the obvious influence of environment and the compensatory efforts on the part of the patient to meet the insistent demands of a dread disease, to defeat the annulling vision of approaching death, and, in some, to disguise a consciousness of the dismal truth.

No doubt the late Robert Tuttle Morris was struggling with the uncertain origin of this psychic stimulus when in Microbes and Men he said, "great men are inspired to their finest efforts either because of, or in spite of, the stimulus of a germ disease." There is nothing original in this observation. While it must be admitted that tuberculosis holds the spotlight, it is only fair to assume that if other diseases, not affecting the mind, were of similar duration, we might expect a similar compensatory response. Finally, we may say that the manifestations of genius, whether attributed directly to the toxemia of a germ disease of the indirect influence of compensatory reactions, implies the innate possession of exceptional mental qualities.

The Medicine Man

While at work in the drugstore I was impressed by the large number of persons who bought patent medicine without any knowledge of what they contained and solely because of their virtues as vaunted in advertisements. That the sale of such proprietary medicines must be very profitable to their manufacturers became clear to me when I studied the analyses that had been made of some of them and found that mixtures that cost the makers only a few cents were sold even at wholesale for sixty cents or more. Some latent business instinct was aroused in me, and I sugested to Mr. Gibbard that our store might do well to make a "tonic" and to advertise it for sale. He agreed to this, and I was given a free hand to devise a formula and to give it a name. I remembered that most tonics prescribed by physicians were bitter and that they were made up of several ingredients. Accordingly, it was decided that the mixture should contain some gentian root and cinchona bark, as these are both bitter substances, harmless in small doses, and might well be provocative of appetite. It seemed desirable to add a little of some harmless drug that was not well known to the public at large in order that a distinctive name could be applied to the tonic. I chose blue flag (Iris versicolor) and named the mixture Franklin's Extract of Blue Flag. What good fairy influenced me to use my second name, Franklin, rather than my family name I am sure I don't know; it was, however, fortunate, for it would not have been helpful to my future medical career to have it known that I had been responsible for the origin of this proprietary medicine. For some years it had a considerable sale, helped by advertising sign boards nailed on fences in the adjacent country. I still have some qualms of conscience when I think of this rather unethical venture, but my uneasiness is salved somewhat by the fact that none of the profit from the sale of "Franklin's Extract of Blue Flag" accrued to me; it wen wholly to the drugstore in which I worked.—Time and the Physician. The Autobiography of Lewellys F. Barker, pp. 23-24. G. P. Putnam's Sons. New York. 1942.

THE PRESIDENT'S PAGE

For American Medicine 1945 was the year for decision, 1946 the year for action. In 1945 the 14 point constructive program for medical care was proposed by the Council on Medical Service and Public Relations and approved by the Board of Trustees and sanctioned by the House of Delegates of the A.M.A.

1. The immediate organization and incorporation of a National Health Congress representative of the medical and allied professions.

2. Development of a specific national health program, with emphasis on the nationwide organization of locally administered prepayment medical plans sponsored by medical societies.

But in the year 1945 the decision was made — a program presented that is realistic, fair, just and workable. The success of the proposed program will only be measured by the efforts put forth, by every individual of the profession working as a unit and thoroughly acquainting themselves with the overall program even to the minutest detail. Indifference, criticism and substitute plans will not suffice. We must develop the local and state volunteer prepayment plans and disseminate the services of the same to every section of the most remote rural communities and enlist the support of all allied professions, namely the dental, hospital, nursing and pharmaceutical professions.

We, the medical profession, will and should assume the responsibility of a just and fair distribution of medical services to the people. The 14 point program set out by the A.M.A. embodies an overall plan that will, if properly executed, leave with the people free choice of medical and hospital services, a free and democratic competitive program that meets the aims of our constitution. Never has our profession been called upon to assume such momentous problems involving such weighty decisions as in the year 1946.

Education of the public must play a major role regarding our plan and program and when this is accomplished we shall expect and will receive the support of the people we serve.

President.

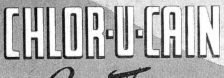

CHLOR-U-CAIN

Burn Therapy

Greatly Shortens Healing Time

CHLOROPHYLL 1%

Accelerates burn healing, shortens time by as much as 50%.*. Minimizes scar formation and speeds regeneration of tissue.

UREA 33.2%

Exerts a solvent action that aids in removing necrotic tissue debris. Tends to minimize foul odors and prevent infection.

BENZOCAINE 10%

Because only slowly absorbed, remains localized at burn site to give sustained anesthetic action.

OINTMENT BASE

Vanishing, greaseless, washable, absorbent.

WARREN-TEED

Medicaments of Exacting Quality Since 1920

THE WARREN-TEED PRODUCTS COMPANY, COLUMBUS 8, OHIO

*"Chlorophyll Urea Ointment in the Treatment of Burns and Chronic Ulcers." Industrial Medicine, 14:9, 730, Sept., 1945.

REPRINT AVAILABLE
ON REQUEST

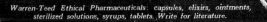

Warren-Teed Ethical Pharmaceuticals: capsules, elixirs, ointments, sterilized solutions, syrups, tablets. Write for literature.

The JOURNAL Of The
O'KLAHOMA STATE MEDICAL ASSOCIATION

EDITORIAL BOARD
L. J. MOORMAN, Oklahoma City, Editor-in-Chief
E. EUGENE RICE, Shawnee — BEN H. NICHOLSON, Oklahoma City
MR. DICK GRAHAM, Oklahoma City, Business Manager
JANE FIRRELL TUCKER, Editorial Assistant

CONTRIBUTIONS: Articles accepted by this Journal for publication including those read at the annual meetings of the State Association are the sole property of this Journal.

The Editorial Department is not responsible for the opinions expressed in the original articles of contributors.

Manuscripts may be withdrawn by authors for publication elsewhere only upon the approval of the Editorial Board.

MANUSCRIPTS: Manuscripts should be typewritten, double-spaced, on white paper 8½ x 11 inches. The original copy, not the carbon copy, should be submitted.

Footnotes, bibliographies and legends for cuts should be typed on separate sheets in double space. Bibliography listing should follow this order: Name of author, title of article, name of periodical with volume, page and date of publication.

Manuscripts are accepted subject to the usual editorial revisions and with the understanding that they have not been published elsewhere.

NEWS: Local news of interest to the medical profession, changes of address, births, deaths and weddings will be gratefully received.

ADVERTISING: Advertising of articles, drugs or compounds unapproved by the Council on Pharmacy of the A.M.A. will not be accepted. Advertising rates will be supplied on application.

It is suggested that members of the State Association patronize our advertisers in preference to others.

SUBSCRIPTIONS: Failure to receive The Journal should call for immediate notification.

REPRINTS: Reprints of original articles will be supplied at actual cost provided request for them is attached to manuscripts or made in sufficient time before publication. Checks for reprints should be made payable to Industrial Printing Company, Oklahoma City.

Address all communications to THE JOURNAL OF THE OKLAHOMA STATE MEDICAL ASSOCIATION, 210 Plaza Court, Oklahoma City 3

OFFICIAL PUBLICATION OF THE OKLAHOMA STATE MEDICAL ASSOCIATION
Copyrighted January, 1946

EDITORIALS

OKLAHOMA PHYSICIANS SERVICE
The month of January is usually a period when inventories are taken. It seems appropriate at this time that we members of the Oklahoma State Medical Association should pause in our busy lives, and take inventory of our Association's Surgical and Obstetrical prepaid service — namely the Oklahoma Physicians Service Corporation.

1. The first group was enrolled effective June 1, 1945.
2. To date including January there are 24 groups enrolled, representing 1,508 contracts totalling 3,981 people, when adding the wives and children.
3. Fourteen (14) counties, to date, have approved the plan for sale in their respective areas.
4. So far, groups have been limited to employed groups.
5. The breakdown of the finances shows all bills paid to date including $2,185.00 paid to Oklahoma physicians for services rendered. Also a good start has been made in the accumulation of funds to retire foundation notes.

In summary we would say that the corporation's seven months of existence has been fruitful, and clearly shows to the critics of organized medicine that the profession is alert to social changes and is concerning itself with constructive plans for the future.—J.F.B., M.D.

WHAT IS SECURITY?
In the December 29, 1945 Saturday Review of Literature, Arthur E. Morgan discusses *Beyond Utopia*. After pointing out the fact that Utopia may not mean felicity and that happiness is far more elusive than we have realized, he says, "Utopia will not answer the more profound problems of life. It will only release men from immediate preoccupation with material want so that they can be aware of deeper issues. For every hundred men who can stand adversity, there may be only ten, or only one, who can stand Utopia. Shakespeare has Hecate say in Macbeth:

'And you all know security
Is mortals' chiefest enemy.'

"Terrible as world conditions are, the great problem of mankind today is not to achieve Utopia, but to be prepared to survive it."

No doubt the author would readily admit that he is not advancing a new philosophy but only relating a part of the sum of human experience. Aristophnes, in his Plutus, shows that there can be no progress without wholesome rivalry between wealth and poverty. An equal distribution would stop the wheels of progress. Full realization of the vaunted four freedoms immediately would beget a fifth, freedom from work — the sum of the five equals starvation.

The politicians and law makers who would open the road to Utopia through regimented medicine should read history and give their minds time to mature. They should have about eight years formal education in statesmanship to help them realize that high human destiny should be fostered, not hindered by the course of government. Our government should always have a legislative conscience guided by knowledge and reason and an administrative head endowed with wisdom and integrity.

A WAGNERIAN SQUINT AT THOMAS JEFFERSON AND BENJAMiN FRANKLIN

Jefferson drafted the Constitution of the United States and Franklin swayed the constitutional convention at will. Jefferson pursued medical science throughout the land because of his general interest in the subject, and Franklin lacked only a medical degree of being one of the best doctors in the United States. It seems strange that these proponents of medicine and good government could have been so short sighted as to have overlooked social security including compulsory health insurance. Since the founders of our government failed so utterly in this respect it is remarkable that the American people did not fill the breach rather than let the opportunity pass to certain government officials. But, seeing that Bismarck with his social security program set the stage for Hitler and since the German people have achieved such a high place in the history of civilization, perhaps we should have a great American Bismarck even at the cost of a few billion bucks and personal liberty. The Teutonic philosophy which has helped to put the German people where they are today may be just what the people of the United States need. If so, why worry about a little small change and the loss of individual freedom.

If we want to move on toward the goal the German people have attained we should accept the Wagner proposal without delay. But we should make up our minds and let Congress know. Its time to decide what are the eternal pillars of Society. Strange to say, in spite of the failure of Jefferson and Franklin and their associates, we have grown stronger and lived longer and have whipped the devil out of our undemocratic enemies. Why not make up our minds to keep the devil out of our democracy.

MEN WITHOUT GUNS
A Moving Story

The Editorial Office has just received a copy of the remarkable book, *Men Without Guns*[1] by Dewitt Mackenzie. Neither men with the brush nor men with the pen can truly portray the heroic spirit, the brave deeds and the remarkable skill of our medical men at war. Yet, it must be agreed that the twelve outstanding contemporary artists contributing the 118 colorful illustrations around which Dewitt Mackenzie has built his interesting pen pictures, present the comprehensive story with a vivid sense of reality.

Competing with the painters canvas are the trenchant words from the pen of Major General Norman T. Kirk, the Surgeon General of the United States Army. In the foreword he says:

"Unequivocally and without fear of contradiction, I say with pride and reverence that one of the greatest contributions to victory has been made by the doctors, nurses and enlisted men of the Army Medical Department. Without their tireless devotion to duty, their courage and complete disregard for self-safety, the Medical Department would not be able to point today to a record of achievement unmatched in the long history of warfare.

"Because of the heroism and skill of the men and women portrayed between the covers of this book, countless thousands of our fighting men have survived wounds that would have meant certain death in the last war. Their deeds on the battlefields, in front-line medical units and in the great general hospitals, have done much to frustrate and discourage a murderous enemy intent upon destroying us with every diabolically ingenious instrument of war he could devise.

"This volume is titled 'Men Without Guns.'" It is a fitting name for a book that tells the story of men and women who fight with surgical instruments and drugs — penicillin, sulfa, plasma, atabrine and other life-saving medical agents."   This remarkable book in addition to the graphic gallery representing the tragic episodes of modern warfare as seen through the eyes of gallant artists who accompanied the men without guns, presents the following chapters: "Introducing the Corpsman; Doctor to The Army; Southwest Pacific; Saipan; Italy; D-Day in Normandy; Burma Road; the Warrior Comes Home.

The text and the paintings make a striking saga, saturated with the savory spirit of Weelum MacLure "A Doctor of the Old School."

Men Without Guns should be on the reception room table in every doctor's office.

1 Men Without Guns. Dewitt Mackenzie. 177 Drawings, including 118 plates in full color by famous contemporary

artists. A dozen American artists braved the hardships and perils of war to make the notable series of historical paintings reproduced from the Abbot Collection of Paintings, now the property of the U. S. Government.

APROPOS THE PRESENT AGITATION ABOUT REST AND EXERCISE

Recent studies by Starr Maycock and Battles University of Pennsylvania are timely and it is to be hoped that further investigations may throw additional light upon the unknown factors and serve as a guide for the clinician who should be able to find the happy mean and stabilize the pendulum which is swinging high.

In the following original articles, the authors bring out the facts briefly noted below: "Convalescence from Surgical Procedures. Studies of the Circulation Lying and Standing, of Tremor, and of a Program of Bed Exercises and Early Rising. By Isaac Starr, M.D. and Robert L. Maycock, M.D. Convalescence from Surgical Procedures. Studies of Various Physiological Responses to a Mild Exercise Test. By Isaac Starr, M.D., Robert L. Maycock, M.D. and Marjorie G. Battles."

While these reports seem to be rather significant the authors modestly suggest that some hints for future studies of convalescence may be drawn from their studies.

Under No. 1, the following facts appear in the Summary:

"Forty-four patients have been studied before and repeatedly after surgical operations. The test used consisted of estimates of pulse rate, blood pressure, and cardiac output (ballistocardiogram) under standard conditions in both the horizontal and vertical positions. The results have been subjected to statistical analysis.

"The average of results obtained in 25 cases operated upon for hernia disclosed that the following significant changes occurred during postoperative convalescence:

"In the horizontal position cardiac output was diminished soon after operation, and blood presure was diminished later. In the vertical position pulse rate was increased, cardiac output tended to be increased and systolic blood pressure to be diminished.

"The difference between the lying and standing pulse rates, and the ratio between lying and standing cardiac outputs increased after operation. There was more tremor on standing, and occasionally subjects were unable to remain standing after operation."

"The scatter of the data was great enough to prevent the development of a simple test for the duration of convalescence which could be applied to single individuals. Nevertheless significant comparisons could easily be made between small series of cases.

"Ten cases of hernia were given a program of exercises in bed and early rising beginning with the second or third day after op-

eration. Comparison with a group not so treated showed that the exercised group tolerated the upright position better than the controls when the latter were first allowed out of bed. This advantage lasted only for a day, however, so we doubt whether anything important was gained by the exercise program."

In No. II we find the following Summary and Conclusions:

"By means of a standard mild exercise test we have sought for abnormalities during convalescence from surgical procedures.

"Oxygen consumption, and volume, and rate of respiration have been determined before, during, and after standard exercise. Cardiac output (ballistocardiogram) and pulse rate were estimated before, just after, and five minutes after the same standard exercise.

"Measurement of the magnitude of the changes induced by the exercise, revealed no significant differences which could be attributed to convalescence. However, when attention was given to the duration of the changes induced by the exercise, the averages showed significant differences, the increased oxygen consumption, respiration, and pulse rate declining to the resting level more slowly during convalescence than before operation.

"The respiration and oxygen consumption of subjects at rest were not significantly changed during convalescence.

"The variability in the physiologic response to exercise was so large that a test of the type used gives no promise of providing a satisfactory measure of the duration of convalescence in individual cases. However, the slow return to normal of pulse rate, respiration, and oxygen consumption after exercise is over may have some value as an indication of persisting abnormality in certain individuals and will provide significant differences when data obtained from a series of 10 or more cases are averaged."

That such studies are under way is encouraging but so far definite criteria for the guidance of the clinician or surgeon are still wanting. The average doctor may well wonder what control studies on unoperated individuals might reveal.

1. The work described in this paper was done under a contract, recommended by the Committee on Medical Research, between the Office of Scientific Research and Development and the University of Pennsylvania

PRIMARY ATYPICAL PNEUMONIA AND SUSPECTED IMMUNITY

Lembcke and Young,[1] following a suggestion that those who had primary atypical pneumonia in 1942 seemed to be relatively free from respiratory infections in 1943-1944 initiated a followup study to ascertain the facts and report the same. The authors were in position to successfully pursue such a study as one of them had reported the 1942 cases which were to be followed.

Their interest was stimulated by Kneeland and Smetana[3] who discussed this possibility in 1940. After a careful study, Lembcke and Young reported as follows: "It is concluded that primary atypical pneumonia neither confers immunity against nor predisposes to the subsequent development of other common types of respiratory illness."

1. Incidence of Respiratory Infections following Attack by Primary Atypical Pneumonia is Unchanged. Paul A. Lembcke and Lawrence E. Young The American Journal of the Medical Sciences. Vol. 210, No. 6, No. 885, 1945.

2. Young, L. E., Story, M., and Redmond, A. J.: American Journal Medical Science, Vol. 206, No. 756, 1943.

3. Kneeland, Y., and Smetana, H. F.: Bull. Johns Hopkins Hosp., Vol. 67, No. 229, 1940.

Propinquity

I took up residence in the Johns Hopkins Hospital in 1891 to live there practically continuously for the next nine years. hTe hospital superintendent assigned me to a room on the third floor of the Administration Building, which I found to be next to the bedroom occupied by Dr. Osler himself, who at that time was unmarried. In his spare time he was busily engaged in writing, with the aid of his secretary, Miss Blanche O. Humptom, his *Principles and Practice of Medicine*, the textbook that was to become the most popular medical volume of its time, undergoing a long series of revisions by the author during his lifetime, and revised and translated by others and used widely after his death. Through this proximity to Dr. Osler's room, I learned how systematically he ordered his life, rising nearly always at the same hour, arriving at the medical wards punctually at nine each morning, eating and exercising at regular times, and working at the writing of his textbook for a definite number of hours each day. Except on evenings when he was unavoidably kept out by social functions, it was jokingly said that one could safely set one's watch at ten o'clock precisely each night when one heard him drop his boots on the floor just outside his bedroom.—*Time and Physician. The Autobiography of Lewellys F. Barker. pp.* 40-41. *G. P. Putnam's Sons. New York.* 1942.

Ben Franklin On Exercise

He had spells of gout and recurrent colds. It was hard to find time for the exercise he knew he needed. Thinking about it, he concluded that the amount of exercise was to be measured "not by time or by distance but by the degree of warmth it produces in the body," he wrote to his son on 19 August 1772. "Using round numbers without regard to exactness but merely to make a great difference . . . there is more exercise in one mile's riding on horsback than in five in a coach; and more in one mile's walking on foot than in five on horseback; to which I am yadd, that there is more in walking one mile up and down stairs than in five on a level floor. The two latter exercises may be had within doors when the weather discourages going abroad; and the last may be had when one is pinched for time, as containing a great quantity of exercise in a handful of minutes. The dumb-bell is another exercise of the latter compendious kind. By the use of it I have in forty swings quickened my pulse from sixty to one hundreds beats in a minute, counted by a second watch; and I suppose the warmth generally increases with quickness of pulse."— *Benjamin Franklin by Carl Van Doren, pp.* 405-406. *The Viking Press. New York.* 1938.

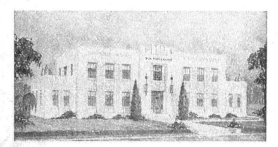

VON WEDEL CLINIC

PLASTIC and GENERAL SURGERY
Dr. Curt von Wedel

INTERNAL MEDICINE and DIAGNOSIS
Dr. Harry A. Daniels

Special attention to cardiac and gastro intestinal diseases

TRAUMATIC and INDUSTRIAL SURGERY
Dr. Clarence A. Gallagher

Complete laboratory and X-ray facilities. Electrocardiograph.

610 Northwest Ninth Street
Opposite St. Anthony's Hospital
Oklahoma City

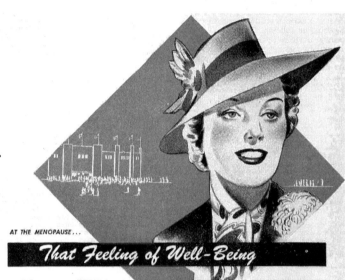

AT THE MENOPAUSE...

That Feeling of Well-Being

Patients on "Premarin" therapy usually experience a general feeling of well-being in addition to relief of symptoms; this is confirmed by most of the many clinical reports. Rendering the patient symptom-free is, of course, the **prime consideration of treatment; many physicians, however, feel that the restoration of a brighter mental outlook is also an important consideration when instituting therapy.** "Premarin" will be found to exhibit the desirable characteristics of both the natural estrogens and the synthetic substances. Although highly potent, "Premarin" is derived exclusively from natural sources; it is exceptionally well tolerated, and unpleasant side effects are seldom noted.

HIGHLY POTENT
ORALLY ACTIVE
NATURALLY OCCURRING
ESSENTIALLY SAFE
WATER SOLUBLE
WELL TOLERATED

"Premarin"
Reg. U. S. Pat. Off.

TABLETS

CONJUGATED ESTROGENS (equine)

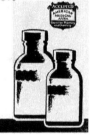

Available in 2 potencies:

No. 866 (the YELLOW tablet), in bottles of 20, 100 and 1.000 tablets
No. 867 HALF-STRENGTH (the RED tablet), in bottles of 100 and 1,000 tablets

AYERST, McKENNA & HARRISON LTD.,
22 E. 40th St., New York 16, N. Y.

ASSOCIATION ACTIVITIES

IMPORTANT NOTICE

The following Section 20, Chapter 24, Article 12 of the Medical Practice Act of Oklahoma, Oklahoma Statutes, 1931, is quoted in order to bring to mind the fact that all licenses to practice medicine in the State of Oklahoma must be *registered in the county in which the physician intends to practice.* If a physician moves from one county to another he must register his license in the county to which he moves and establishes practice.

"Section 20. *Recordation of License; Penalty.* It shall be the duty of every person holding license or certificate authorizing him to practice medicine and surgery in this State, to have it recorded in the office of the county clerk of the county wherein his office is to be located. Every such person, on the change of residence to another county, must have his certificate recorded, in like manner, in the county to which he shall move his residence; and said certificate shall be displayed in his office as evidence of his having complied with the law. The absence of such record in the office of the county clerk shall be prima facie evidence of the want of possession of such license or certificate and every such physician and surgeon holding such license or certificate, who shall practice medicine and surgery, in any county of this State, without first having complied with the terms of this section, as herein provided, shall be deemed guilty of a misdemeanor, and, upon conviction thereof, shall be fined in any sum not less than Twenty-five ($25.00) Dollars, and not more than One Hundred ($100.00) Dollars."

PLANS FOR ANNUAL MEETING MOVING RAPIDLY

Dr. J. H. Robinson, Chairman of the Scientific Work Committee, announces that work is progressing rapidly on the Annual Meeting. Several Distinguished Speakers have been contacted and acceptances have been received from a number. The Chairman and Secretaries of the various Scientific Sections are working out the Section Programs and announcement will be made shortly of the Scientific Programs that have been lined up.

The Annual Meeting is to be held in Oklahoma City, May 1, 2 and 3, at the Skirvin Tower Hotel. The commercial exhibit booths will be on the Mezzanine of the Silver Glade Room. All booths have been sold.

OKLAHOMA DIVISION OF AMERICAN CANCER SOCIETY OPENS NEW OFFICE

The Oklahoma Division of the American Cancer Society, under the direction of the Executive Director, Mr. Hugh Payne, has opened new offices in the Braniff Building in Oklahoma City. Extensive plans are under way for the proposed Mobile Detection Clinic. An outline of these plans appear elsewhere in this issue.

FURTHER CRITERIA REDUCTIONS FOR MEDICAL OFFICERS ANNOUNCED

Further criteria reductions to make additional doctors available for civilian practice were announced on December 31, 1945 by Major General Norman T. Kirk, the Surgeon General of the Army.

While the number of professional men affected by this action will not be more than a thousand, the Surgeon General's Office has ordered this revision of criteria in line with the Medical Department's policy of doing everything possible to expedite the return of doctors, dentists, and veterinarians to private life.

Under the new separation plan which becomes effective January 1, 1946, (with the exception of a comparatively small number in scarce categories) dentists, and veterinarians will be released with a critical score of 65 instead of the 70 points previously required. This same group will also be able to get out of the service, if the age of 45 has been reached instead of the former age limit of 48.

The time factor of 42 months service, which will make any of this group eligible for separation, remains the same.

The following specialists in scarce categories will be released with a critical score of 80, continuous service since Pearl Harbor, or if the age of 45 has been reached; eye, ear, nose specialists; orthopedic surgeons; and internal medicine specialists.

A requirement of 70 points, 45 months service, or 45 years age limit will make the following eligible for separation; gastroenterologists, cardiologists, urologists, dermatologists, anaesthetists, psychiatrists, general surgeons, physical therapy officers, radiologists, and pathologists.

Plastic surgeons will be eligible for release if they have a critical score of 80, or service since Pearl Harbor, or if they are 48 years of age.

WILLIAM E. EASTLAND, M.D.

F. A. C. R.

RADIUM AND X-RAY THERAPY
DERMATOLOGY

405 Medical Arts Bldg.

Oklahoma City, Oklahoma   Phone 3-1446

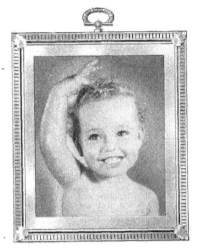

DOCTOR, MEET THE DARICRAFT BABY

Perhaps you are "meeting" the Daricraft Baby every day in your own practice. If not, may we call to your attention the following significant points of interest about Vitamin D increased Daricraft:

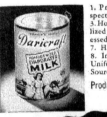

1. Produced from inspected herds; 2. Clarified; 3. Homogenized; 4. Sterilized; 5. Specially Processed; 6. Easily Digested; 7. High in Food Value; 8. Improved Flavor; 9. Uniform; 10. Dependable Source of Supply.

Producers Creamery Co.
Springfield, Mo.

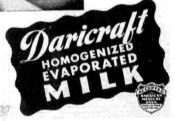

Daricraft
HOMOGENIZED
EVAPORATED
MILK

REFRESHER TRAINING FOR DOCTORS LEAVING SERVICE

Refresher training of 12 weeks' duration will be given Army doctors leaving the service who desire to brush up on latest developments in fields of medicine, surgery, or neuropsychiatry in which they may not have been actively practicing during the past year, Major General Norman T. Kirk, Surgeon General of the Army, announced.

This training, which will prepare retiring Army doctors for return to private practice with latest knowledge of medical advances made during the way, will be given at Army hospitals until June 30, 1946. Reserve Corps, National Guard, and AUS Medical Corps officers who are to be separated will be eligible for this schooling.

The election of the period of refresher training is entirely voluntary, and applications may be made through channels to The Surgeon General in the case of medical officers assigned to the Army Service Forces, Army Ground Forces and Army Air Forces. Medical officers returning from overseas may make application for refresher training from the Reception Stations or Separation Centers through the ASF Liaison Officer directly to The Surgeon General. *It is pointed out that medical officers cannot be recalled to active duty from terminal leave for the purpose of accepting a professional assignment for refresher training.*

Numerous requests have been received by The Surgeon General from Reserve Corps, National Guard, and AUS Medical officers who are about to be separated and who desire to remain in service for a short period of professional duty prior to return to civilian life. These officers are anxious to return to their civilian practices with the advantages of the latest medical knowledge. Due to the tremendous demand for refresher training placed upon civilian medical teaching centers, many of these medical officers have been unable to arrange for refresher training.

The Surgeon General emphasizes the fact that the refresher training is accomplished by a 12-week temporary duty assignment in the professional field of interest at an Army hospital without per diem. Such an assignment will afford the medical officer a period of clinical work under supervision, and excellent opportunities for collateral study of recent advances in medicine, surgery, and neuropsychiatry.

GENERAL GEORGE LULL BECOMES SECRETARY AND GENERAL MANAGER OF A.M.A.

Major General George F. Lull, Deputy Surgeon General of the Army, whose notable record in that capacity won him the Distinguished Service Medal, the highest non-combatant award, has retired from the Army after 33 years of service with the Medical Corps.

General and Mrs. Lull will move to Chicago, where General Lull will become Secretary and General Manager of the American Medical Association. He will take up his new duties officially in July, when the retirement of Dr. Olin West, the present Secretary and General Manager, becomes effective, but he will immediately join the staff of the American Medical Association to familiarize himself with the work of the organization.

The citation for the Distinguished Service Medal stated that, in his capacity as Chief of the Personnel Service, General Lull was largely responsible for the development of policies and studies which resulted in outstanding achievements in the Army's medical program.

Early in World War I he commanded a base hospital at Camp Beauregard, Louisiana and later organized and commanded Base Hospital No. 35 of the A.E.F. From 1922 until 1926 General Lull was Director of the Department of Preventive Medicine at the Army Medical Center. In 1929 he was appointed Medical Adviser to the Governor General of the Philippine Islands, where he served for three years. He had charge of the Vital

by way of contrast

Reliable interpretation of gallbladder films
and more accurate diagnosis are achieved readily
by the vivid contrast obtained with

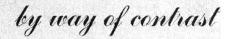

PRIODAX

PRIODAX shadows are homogeneous, of optimum
density and are not obscured by overlying
opaque material.

Vomiting or severe diarrhea are almost
eliminated since PRIODAX is not related to
phenolphthalein or any of its derivatives and is excreted almost entirely through the urine.

PRIODAX beta-(4-hydroxy-3,5-diiodophenyl)-alpha-
phenyl-propionic acid. Available in 0.5 Gm. tablets in economy boxes of 100 envelopes and in boxes of 1, 5 and 25
envelopes. Each envelope contains six easily swallowed
tablets constituting the usual dose. Instructions for the
patient accompany each envelope.

TRADE-MARK PRIODAX—REG. U. S. PAT. OFF.

Schering CORPORATION • BLOOMFIELD, N. J.
IN CANADA, SCHERING CORPORATION LIMITED, MONTREAL

Effective
Convenient
Economical

T HE effectiveness of Mercurochrome has been demonstrated by more than twenty years of extensive clinical use. For professional convenience Mercurochrome is supplied in four forms—Aqueous Solution in Applicator Bottles for the treatment of minor wounds, Surgical Solution for preoperative skin disinfection, Tablets and Powder from which solutions of any desired concentration may readily be prepared.

Mercurochrome

(H. W. & D. brand of merbromin, dibromoxymercurifluorescein-sodium)

is economical because stock solutions may be dispensed quickly and at low cost. Stock solutions keep indefinitely.

Mercurochrome is antiseptic and relatively non-irritating and non-toxic in wounds.

Complete literature will be furnished on request.

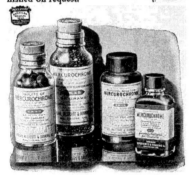

HYNSON, WESTCOTT
& DUNNING, INC.
BALTIMORE, MARYLAND

Records Division of the Surgeon General's Office from 1932 to 1936.

The following four years he was Director of the Department of Sanitation at the Medical Field Service School, Carlisle Barracks, Pennsylvania. In 1940 he returned to the Surgeon General's Office as Chief of Personnel Service until May 31, 1943, when he was appointed Deputy Surgeon General.

Born in Pennsylvania March 10, 1887, General Lull received his M. D. degree from Jefferson Medical College in 1909, a Certificate of Public Health from Harvard Technology School of Public Health in 1921, and his degree of Doctor of Public Health from the University of Pennsylvania in 1922. He is an honor graduate of the 1913 class of Army Medical School.

ACCIDENT POLICY AS APPROVED BY COUNCIL MEETS WITH GREAT SUCCESS

Two years ago Dr. V. K. Allen, Tulsa, Dr. LeRoy Long, Oklahoma City and Dr. Malcolm Phelps, El Reno, were appointed on the Insurance Committee and were given the task of working out a broad coverage, low cost accident insurance for the members of the Association. After obtaining figures from several companies, a program offered by the North American Accident Insurance Company was decided upon and presented to the Council on October 7. The Council endorsed the program whereby immediate action was taken in offering the policy to the members over the state.

The first county contacted was Beckham which went 99 per cent. Units have been installed in Greer, Harmon, Kiowa and Jackson counties, participation running nearly 100 per cent in each of the counties. At the present time the program is being installed in Tulsa County and is progressing nicely. At an early date the remaining counties will be covered.

This accident coverage is underwritten by the North American Accident Insurance Company, an old line company originating in 1886 with home offices in Chicago. Since 1902 the company has operated in Oklahoma. Mr. C. W. Cameron is the state manager and Mr. Joe H. Jones the Tulsa manager. The service work for the doctors in the state is being handled by Mr. Jones. Every effort is being made to handle all claims on the policy within 24 hours after completed proofs are received in the Oklahoma City office.

MOBILE DETECTION CLINIC ADOPTED BY OKLAHOMA DIVISION OF AMERICAN CANCER SOCIETY

At its meeting on January 6 the Medical Committee of the Oklahoma Division of the American Cancer Society unanimously adopted the following outline in relation to policy, planning, procedure and operation of Mobile Detection Clinics:

Policy

1. No county or community in this State will be serviced by the Detection Clinic except by invitation of the local County Medical Society.

2. Mobile (traveling) Detection Clinics shall be conducted only for those persons who cannot afford to pay for special examination. The designation "who cannot afford to pay for special examination" is defined as "those persons who may be in position to take care of family or individual subsistence on meager basis, yet who cannot afford additional expenses in connection with special examination."

3. *Duties of Local Physician.*

a. The local physician shall determine who is eligible for examination under the above definition.

b. All persons who present themselves for examination must be referred by local physician. The local County Medical Society shall have a designated member present to determine eligibility for

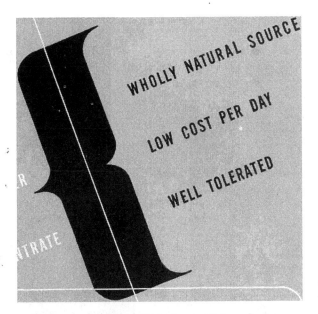

WHOLLY NATURAL SOURCE

LOW COST PER DAY

WELL TOLERATED

These are advantages which, for many years, have fixed White's Cod Liver Oil Concentrate in the minds of physicians everywhere as their first thought in prescribing.

TO THESE ADVANTAGES ADD

Cost to the patient has *not* increased. Average "infant antirachitic" prophylactic dosage costs *still* less than a penny a day.

Three palatable, convenient dosage forms — LIQUID (for drop dosage to infants), TABLETS AND CAPSULES.

Ethically promoted — not advertised to the laity.

WHITE'S COD LIVER OIL CONCENTRATE

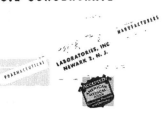

LABORATORIES, INC
NEWARK 2, N. J.

examination of those who have no family physician.

c. The local physician shall be present at time patient is examined. If local physician is unable to be present because of an emergency, a written report of the examination shall go to patient's physician only.

4. *History Requirements*

The history of each patient examined shall be executed in advance of Detection Clinic date by referring physician. The forms for this purpose shall be furnished by the Oklahoma Division, American Cancer Society.

5. *Biopsy*

Biopsy shall be left to the discretion of the local physician and staff members of the Mobile Detection Clinic.

If tissue is taken, it shall be examined free of charge when properly prepared and sent to any member of the Oklahoma Pathologist Association. A written report, on prepared form furnished by the Oklahoma Division of American Cancer Society, will be returned promptly to the local referring physician. A copy of the report and slide shall be kept in a central depository as agreed upon by the Oklahoma Division of the American Cancer Society and the Oklahoma Pathologist Association.

Personnel of Detection Clinic Staff

The personnel of each Detection Clinic Staff shall be composed of qualified specialists selected by the Medical Committee of the Oklahoma Division of the American Cancer Society and the Cancer Committee of the Oklahoma State Medical Association.

Method of Procedure of Service

1. The Detection Clinic will visit those places in the State, previously determined upon by the Sub-Committee on Policy, Planning, Procedure and Operation, and then only upon invitation by the local County Medical Society.

2. The Executive Director of the Oklahoma Division, American Cancer Society, upon direction of Chairman of Sub-Committee on Policy, Planning Procedure and Operation, will visit any local County Medical Society to explain the workings of the Detection Clinic, and shall also make all arrangements for a Detection Clinic visit when so desired.

3. Such items as to the time of day the clinic will start, the place, the advisability of a public meeting,

NEUROLOGICAL HOSPITAL

Twenty-Seventh and The Paseo
Kansas City, Missouri

Modern Hospitalization of Nervous and Mental Illnesses, Alcoholism and Drug Addiction.

THE ROBINSON CLINIC
G. WILSE ROBINSON, M.D.
G. WILSE ROBINSON, Jr., M.D.

DIAGNOSTIC CLINIC OF INTERNAL MEDICINE AND ALLERGY

Philip M. McNeill, M. D., F. A. C. P.

General Diagnosis

CONSULTATION BY APPOINTMENT

Special Attention to Cardiac, Pulmonary and Allergic Diseases

Electrocardiograph, X-Ray, Laboratory and Complete Allergic Surveys Available.

1107 Medical Arts Bldg.
Oklahoma City, Okla.

Phone 2-0277

Not for just a year

Recognition of rickets in 46.5% of children between the ages of two and 14 years[1] has demonstrated the necessity for vitamin D supplementation, not for just a year, or for infancy alone, but throughout childhood and adolescence—as long as growth persists.

Upjohn makes available convenient, palatable, high potency vitamin preparations derived from natural sources, in forms to meet the varied clinical requirements of earliest infancy through late childhood.

1. Am. J. Dis. Child. 66:1 (July) 1943.

Upjohn Vitamins

FIGHT INFANTILE PARALYSIS
JANUARY 14-31

FINE PHARMACEUTICALS SINCE 1886

Kalamazoo 99, Michigan

shall be determined by the Secretary of the local County Medical Society, the Executive Director of the Oklahoma Division, American Cancer Society and the Local Commander of the Field Army.

4. In each instance there will be a meeting of the Local County Medical Society following the Detection Clinic, at which time there shall be a scientific program on cancer.

Operation of Detection Clinic

1. All patients to be examined will be notified by family physician to be present at set time and place in advance of Detection Clinic visit.

2. Usually the staff members can keep in operation four examination tables. In order to examine as many patients as possible there should be at least one nurse for each table in operation.

3. *Nursing Personnel*
It will be the responsibility of the Oklahoma Division, American Cancer Society to provide sufficient nurses for the purpose. In this connection, the President of the State Nurses Association has assumed responsibility for providing nurses in any area in the State, provided her office is notified in advance.

4. *Secretarial Aid*
It will be the responsibility of the Oklahoma Division of the American Cancer Society to provide sufficient secretarial help.

5. *Equipment*
All equipment necessary for the operation of the Detection Clinics will be supplied and transported to and from the site of operation by the Oklahoma Division, American Cancer Society.

General Information

Publicity
All publicity relative to the Detection Clinic's visit shall have the approval of the officers of the Local County Medical Society.

Expenses
The Oklahoma Division of the American Cancer Society will bear all expenses in relation to the actual operation of the Detection Clinic. The medical personnel of the Detection Clinic Staff shall receive no compensation for services or expenses.

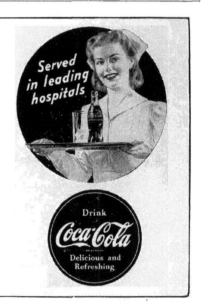

Pure.. Wholesome.. Refreshing

Safeguarded constantly by scientific tests, Coca-Cola is famous for its purity and wholesomeness. It's famous, too, for the thrill of its taste and for the happy after-sense of complete refreshment it always brings. Get a Coca-Cola, and get the feel of refreshment.

Served in leading hospitals. Drink Coca-Cola. Delicious and Refreshing.

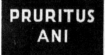 **PRURITUS ANI**

The itching of pruritus ani may often be relieved by dilatation, especially when caused by a tight or spastic sphincter muscle which prevents bulky or dry stool from being expelled regularly and smoothly.

YOUNG'S RECTAL DILATORS have been found very effective in breaking the impulse of rectal muscle to keep itself locked. Sold only by prescription. Obtainable at your surgical supply house; available for patients at ethical drug stores. In sets of 4 graduated sizes, adult $4.75, children's set $4.50. Write for Brochure.

F. E. YOUNG & COMPANY, 424 E. 75th St., Chicago 19, Illinois

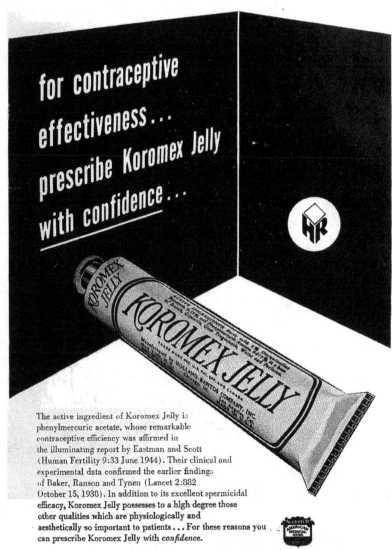

for contraceptive
effectiveness...
prescribe Koromex Jelly
with confidence...

The active ingredient of Koromex Jelly is
phenylmercuric acetate, whose remarkable
contraceptive efficiency was affirmed in
the illuminating report by Eastman and Scott
(Human Fertility 9:33 June 1944). Their clinical and
experimental data confirmed the earlier findings
of Baker, Ranson and Tynen (Lancet 2:882
October 15, 1938). In addition to its excellent spermicidal
efficacy, Koromex Jelly possesses to a high degree those
other qualities which are physiologically and
aesthetically so important to patients ... For these reasons you
can prescribe Koromex Jelly with *confidence*.

Write for literature.

Holland-Rantos Co., Inc.

551 Fifth Avenue, New York 17, N. Y.

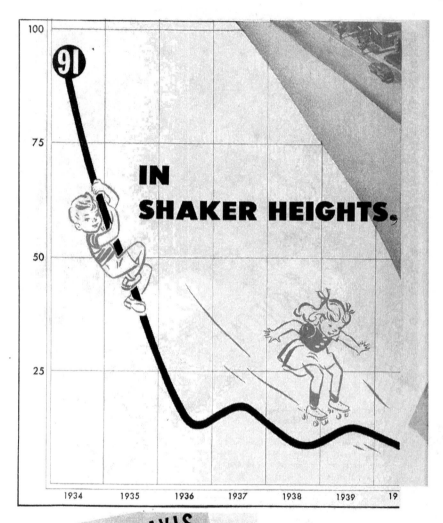

IN SHAKER HEIGHTS.

PARKE, DAVIS & COMPANY
DETROIT 32, MICHIGAN
Sole producers of

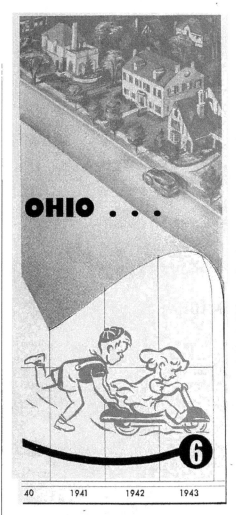

OHIO . . .

Nine years' routine immunization of Shaker Heights children of pre-school age against whooping cough, using Sauer's vaccine, has cut the annual incidence of pertussis in this age group from 91 to a yearly average of 6 during a 4-year period . . . and the six who contracted the disease in 1943 were children *who had not been immunized.*[1]

[1] Garvin, J. A., Ohio State M. J. 41:229, 1945.

...PERTUSSIS VACCINE IMMUNIZING (SAUER)

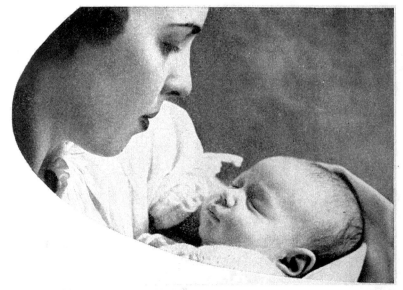

Sleep insurance for doctors

To the harassed doctor, 'Dexin' brand High Dextrin Carbohydrate helps provide "sleep insurance"—nights made peaceful by fewer frantic calls from worried mothers. His 'Dexin' babies sleep more soundly, and are less subject to disturbances that interrupt slumber. The high dextrin content of 'Dexin' (1) diminishes intestinal fermentation and the tendency to colic and diarrhea, and (2) promotes the formation of soft, flocculent, easily digested curds.

'Dexin', palatable but not too sweet, is readily soluble in hot or cold milk or other bland fluids. 'Dexin' does make a difference.

'Dexin' Reg. Trademark

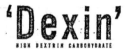

HIGH DEXTRIN CARBOHYDRATE

Composition—Dextrins 75% • Maltose 24% • Mineral Ash 0.25% • Moisture 0.75% • Available carbohydrate 99% • 115 calories per ounce • 6 level packed tablespoonfuls equal 1 ounce • Containers of twelve ounces and three pounds • Accepted by the Council on Foods and Nutrition, American Medical Association.

Literature on request

 BURROUGHS WELLCOME & CO. (U.S.A.) INC. 9 & 11 E. 41st St., New York 17, N.Y.

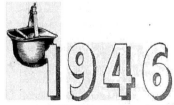

ARMOR AND ARMAMENTARIUM

Guns are silent and grass grows in the foxholes, but there can be no peace treaty in the endless war on mankind's immortal enemy—Disease. Home comes the physician from his lifesaving on the battlefields of man-made death abroad to march again beside his colleagues who have so valiantly held the casemates of health at home.

Battle front and home front, boulevard and dirt road, the mighty facilities of the medical center and the challenge of practice in the lonely farmhouse—all are the front line trenches in humanity's continuing crusade to tame cannibal protoplasm. There is no discharge in that war.

The first cry of pain in the world was the first call for a physician. It has been answered as it echoed down the centuries; it will be answered in the unrolling years of the future.

As this questioning year of 1946 opens with the world convalescing from malignant political disease, we would like to claim the privilege of welcoming the thousands of physicians returning from unparalleled service on war fronts—of saluting those who shouldered such heavy burdens at home—of expressing the confidence that the traditional unity of the profession armed with new and potent weapons will drive the front lines of the war on disease ever forward.

We know that we are joined in this expression by all organizations which seek to play their roles, large and humble, as institutions of supply to those "bound by the covenant and oath, according to the law of medicine." S. H. CAMP AND COMPANY, Jackson, Mich.

CONFERENCE OF STATE PRESIDENTS AND OFFICERS OF STATE MEDICAL ASSOCIATIONS

Dick Graham Elected To Executive Board

The Michigan and California State Medical Association are to be complimented for their initiative in bringing about an Annual Conference of Presidents and Officers of State Medical Associations.

The first Conference held in Chicago at the time of the meeting of the House of Delegates of the American Medical Association presented an excellent program on adequate Health Service for all of the people.

The Conference met with such outstanding success that its future activities were assured by the action of those in attendance in creating a permanent organization. Dr. A. S. Brunk of Michigan was elected President for the coming year and Dick Graham was elected to the Executive Committee for a three year term.

Tax Calendar

JANUARY — FEBRUARY

H. E. Cole Company
Plaza Court
Oklahoma City

General

Delinquent advalorem taxes carry penalty of one per cent per month.

Fiscal Year Income Tax Returns are due on the 15th day of the third month following the close of the taxable year.

State Inheritance Tax or Estate Tax Returns due twelve months after date of death; tax due and payable fifteen months after death. Federal tax return due and tax payable fifteen months after death.

State and federal Gift Tax Returns must be filed by both donors and donees on or before March 15.

January

Day	Nature of Report or Payment	To Whom Made
1	1946 Advalorem Tax Returns Due —Personal, Intangible and Real Estate — Property Owned This Day Basis for 1946 Assessment	Co. Assessor
1	Applications due for Homestead Exemption	Co. Assessor
1	Return of Federal Income Tax for Calendar Year 1945 Due	Col. of Int. Rev.
15	Last Day to File Original 1945 Declaration of Estimate and Pay Federal Income Tax for Taxpayers Meeting Requirements after September 1, 1945, and Individuals Classed as Farmers. If Final 1945 income tax return is completed and filed by January 15, it will not be necessary to file an estimate.	Col. of Int. Rev.
15	Last Day to File Amended 1945 Declaration of Estimated of Individuals and Pay Fourth Quarterly Installment of Federal Income ax. If Final 1945 income tax return is completed and filed by January 15, it will not be necessary to file an estimate.	Col. of Int. Rev.
15	Last Day to File Return and Pay State Sales Tax for December, 1945	Ok'a. Tax Com.
20	Last Day to File Return and Pay State Motor Fuel Tax for December, 1945.	Ok'a. Tax Com.
20	Last Day to File Return and Pay State Use Tax for December, 1945.	Okla. Tax Com.
20	Last Day to File Return and Pay State Special Fuel Use Tax for December, 1945.	Okla. Tax Com.
31	Last Day to File Quarterly Withholding Tax Return Form W-2 Fourth Quarter 1945 and Pay Tax; Attach Form W-2 Receipt for Tax Withheld in 1945 for Each Employee and Form W-3 Reconciliation of Quarterly Returns, 1945.	Col. of Int. Rev.
31	Last Day to File Return and Pay State Gross Production Tax for December 1945.	Okla. Tax Com.
31	Last Day to File Return and Pay State Proration Excise Tax for December, 1945.	Okla. Tax Com.
31	Last Day to File Return and Pay State Unemployment Compensation for last Quarter, 1945.	Okla. Employment Security Com.
31	Last Day to File Return and Pay Social Security Tax (O.A.B.) for Last Quarter 1945.	Col. of Int. Rev.
31	Last Day to File 1945 Return and Pay First Quarter Excise Tax Form 940, Title IX under Social Security Act. (This Tax, known as federal unemployment insurance tax, amounts to three per cent of the 1945 payroll, less amount paid to State Unemployment Compensation Funds.	Col. of Int. Rev.
31	Last Day to File Return and Pay Federal Excise and Miscellaneous Taxes for December, 1945.	Col. of Int. Rev.
31	Last Day to File Employer's Application for Termination of Coverage Under the Oklahoma Employment Security Law.	Okla. Employment Security Com.

February

1	Last Day to Register Motor Vehicles	Co. Tag Agent
1	Third Quarter 1945 Ad valorem Tax Due	Co. Treas.
10	Last Day to Pay January Withholding Tax paid to Depository	

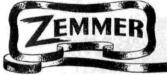

Prescribe or Dispense

Zemmer Pharmaceuticals

A complete line of laboratory controlled ethical pharmaceuticals.   OK 1-46

Chemists to the Medical Profession for 44 years.

The Zemmer Company   Oakland Station Pittsburgh 13, Pa.

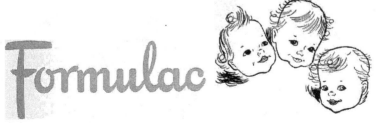

for adequate infant nutrition

FORMULAC, newly introduced on the market, is the
trade name for a fortified infant food which makes
supplementary vitamin administration unnecessary.

FORMULAC (a reduced milk in liquid form) was developed
by E. V. McCollum. It is sufficiently supplemented with
vitamins and minerals to render it an adequate food for
babies. Incorporation of the vitamins *into the milk itself*
eliminates the risk of maternal error or carelessness.

FORMULAC presents a flexible basis for formula preparation.
Supplemented by carbohydrates at your discretion, it may
readily be adjusted to fit each individual child's needs.

FORMULAC has been tested clinically, and found satisfactory
in promoting infant growth and development.

FORMULAC is inexpensive—within price range
of even low income groups. It is on sale at
most grocery and drug stores.

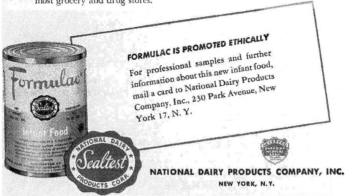

FORMULAC IS PROMOTED ETHICALLY

For professional samples and further
information about this new infant food,
mail a card to National Dairy Products
Company, Inc., 230 Park Avenue, New
York 17, N. Y.

NATIONAL DAIRY PRODUCTS COMPANY, INC.
NEW YORK, N.Y.

Banks by the 10th of the month is applicable only to those employers whose withholding tax is in excess of $100.00 monthly.		Depository Bank
15	Last Day to File Return and Pay State Sales Tax for January, 1946.	Okla. Tax Com.
15	Last Day to File State Income Tax Information Return for 1945 (Form 500-501).	Okla. Tax Com.
15	Last Day to File Federal Income Tax Information Return for 1945 (Form 1906-1909). This applies to fixed or determinable income of $500.00 or more not reported on Withholding Receipt.	Col. of Int. Rev. Sorting Division, Washington, D. C.
20	Last Day to File Return and Pay State Motor Fuel Tax for January, 1946.	Okla. Tax Com.
20	Last Day to File Return and Pay State Use Tax for January, 1946.	Okla. Tax Com.
20	Last Day to File Return and Pay State Use Tax for January, 1946.	Okla. Tax Com.
20	Last Day to File Return and Pay State Special Fuel Use Tax for January, 1946.	Okla. Tax Com.
28	Last Day to File Return and Pay State Gross Production Tax for January, 1946.	Okla. Tax Com.
28	Last Day to File Return and Pay State Proration Excise Tax for January, 1946.	Okla. Tax Com.
28	Last Day to File Return and Pay Federal Excise and Miscellaneous Taxes for January, 1946.	Col. of Int. Rev.
28	Last Day to Pay Third Quarter 1945 Ad valorem Tax.	Co. Treas.

Urology Award

The American Urological Association offers an annual award 'not to exceed $300' for an essay (or essays) on the result of some specific clinical or laboratory research in Urology. The amount of the prize is based on the merits of the work presented, and if the Committee on Scientific Research deem none of the offerings worthy, no award will be made. Competitors shall be limited to residents in urology in recognized hospitals and to urologists who have been in such specific practice for not more than five years. All interested should write the Secretary, for full particulars.

The selected essay (or essays) will appear on the program of the forthcoming meeting of the American Urological Association, to be held at the Netherland Plaza, Cincinnati, Ohio, July 22-25, 1946.

Essays must be in the hands of the Secretary, Dr. Thomas D. Moore, 899 Madison Avenue, Memphis, Tennessee, on or before July 1, 1946.

WOMAN'S AUXILIARY

"Starving Amidst Plenty" was the topic of the November meeting of the Auxiliary to the Tulsa County Medical Society.

With good health an important factor in the nation's welfare and sufficient food necessary for good health, it is appalling to find that malnutrition is widespread in spite of the adequate supply of food available today. This can be eliminated to a great extent by learning facts of good nutrition.

Mrs. Carl Hotz, former president, and an experienced gardener, gave an interesting talk on Garden Soil in relation to food.

The luncheon demonstrated food values necessary to the buoyant health, strength and vitality needed for the busy lives we lead today.

The meeting on December 4th will be at Philbrook, where colored slides on flower arrangements will be shown through the courtesy of the Tulsa Garden Club. Mrs. N. M. Hulings will give a talk featuring Christmas Suggestions. Mrs. D. W. LeMaster will be in charge, assisted by members of the Flower Arrangement Committee of the Tulsa Garden Club.

Hostesses will be Mrs. J. W. Rogers, Mrs. Walter Larragee, Mrs. David Shapiro, Mrs. Allen Kramer and Mrs. E. W. Reynolds.

Members are allowed to bring a guest to this meeting.

Tulsa County News

Dr. and Mrs. C. G. Stuard have chosen the name of James Charles for their son, born November 15th at St. John's Hospital. Grandparents are Mr. and Mrs. James A. Taylor, Stillwater, and Mrs. C. G. Stuard, Sr., Waurika.

Dr. J. E. McDonald has been discharged from the army and is busy getting his office opened.

The family of Dr. Frank A. Stuart have returned to Tulsa and Dr. Stuart is expecting to be discharged from the army around the first of the year.

RADIUM
(Including Radium Applicators)

FOR ALL MEDICAL PURPOSES

Est. 1919

Quincy X-Ray and Radium Laboratories
(Owned and directed by a Physician-Radiologist)

HAROLD SWANBERG, B.S., M.D., Director

W.C.U. Bldg.   Quincy, Illinois

THE WILLIE CLINIC AND HOSPITAL

A private hospital for the diagnosis, study and treatment of all types of neurological and psychiatric cases. Equipped to give all forms of recognized therapy, including hyperpyrexia, insulin and metrazol treatments, when indicated. Consultation by appointment.

JAMES A. WILLIE, B.A., M.D.
Attending Neuro-psychiatrist

218 N. W. 7th St.—Okla. City, Okla.   Telephones: 2-6944 and 3-6071

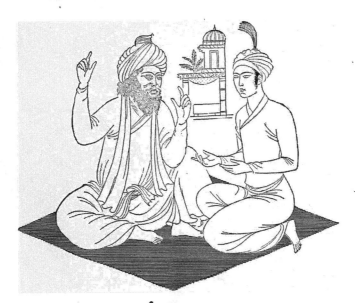

In the City of Bagdad lived Hakeem, the Wise One,

and many people went to him for counsel, which he gave freely to all, asking nothing in return.

There came to him a young man, who had spent much but got little, and said: "Tell me, Wise One, what shall I do to receive the most for that which I spend?"

Hakeem answered: "A thing that is bought or sold has no value unless it contains that which cannot be bought or sold. Look for the Priceless Ingredient."

"But what is this Priceless Ingredient?" asked the young man.

Spoke then the Wise One: "My son, the Priceless Ingredient of every product in the market-place is the Honor and Integrity of him who makes it. Consider his name before you buy."

Copyright, 1922, 1945, E. R. Squibb & Sons

E·R·SQUIBB & SONS

MANUFACTURING CHEMISTS TO THE MEDICAL PROFESSION SINCE 1858

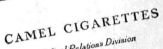

CAMEL CIGARETTES

Medical Relations Division

ONE PERSHING SQUARE
NEW YORK 17, N.Y.

Dear Doctor:

You may recall having been asked the question:
"What cigarette do you yourself smoke, Doctor?"

In the past few months every physician in private
practice in the United States has been asked that
same question...asked solely and clearly on the
basis of _personal preference as a smoker._

Three nationally known independent research groups
did the asking in what we believe is one of the
most impartial and most comprehensive surveys of
physician preference ever conducted.

You may or may not be a cigarette smoker, but we
believe you will be interested not only in the
results of these surveys, but in the methods by
which these results were obtained.

Yours very truly,

A. G. Clarke

A. G. Clarke
Director
Medical Relations Division

CALEDONIA 5-1910

A physician asked <u>us</u> the question first —

A smoker himself, he asked: "What cigarette do most doctors smoke?"

We know that many physicians smoke, that many of them prefer Camels; but we couldn't answer the doctor's query.

We turned the question over to three nationally known independent survey groups. For months these three groups worked . . . separately . . . each one employing the latest scientific fact-finding methods.

This was no mere "feeling the pulse" poll. No mere study of "trends." This was a nationwide survey to discover the actual fact . . . and from the statements of physicians themselves.

To the best of our knowledge and belief, every physician in private practice in the United States was asked: "What cigarette do you smoke?"

The findings, based on the statements of thousands and thousands of physicians, were checked and re-checked.

ACCORDING TO THIS RECENT NATIONWIDE SURVEY:

More doctors smoke Camels than any other cigarette

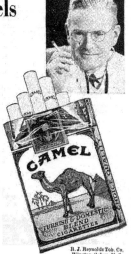

And by a very convincing margin!

Naturally, as the makers of Camels, we are gratified to learn of this preference. We know that no one is more deserving of a few moments to himself than the busy physician . . . of a few moments of relaxation with a cigarette if he likes. And we are glad to know that so many more physicians find in Camels the same added smoking pleasure that has made Camels such an outstanding favorite among *all* smokers.

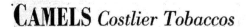

CAMELS *Costlier Tobaccos*

R. J. Reynolds Tob. Co.
Winston-Salem, N. C.

MEDICAL CORPS OFFICERS RELEASED FROM SERVICE

Adams, Felix ....Vinita
Aisenstadt, E. A. ......66 Jamison Place, Kansas City, Mo.
Akins, Jack O. ....Medical Arts Building, Tulsa
Alexander, Robert L..................................Okmulgee
Allgood, J. M. ....721 E. Cypress, Altus
Anderson, Paul S. ....Walker Building, Claremore
Appleton, M. M. ....400 N. W. 10th, Okla. City
Baker, A. T. ....618 N. Fifth, Durant
Baker, Roscoe C. ....711 W. Oak Avenue, Enid
Ballantine, Henry T. ....Muskogee
Barkett, N. F. V. ......Medical Arts Bldg., Okla. City
Bartheld, Floyd ....114½ N. First, McAlester
Batchelor, John J. ....Medical Arts Bldg., Okla. City
Battenfield, John Y. ....Ellison Infirmary, Norman
Bednar, Gerald ....Medical Arts Bldg., Okla. City
Bell, A. H. ....301 N. W. 12, Okla. City
Bennett, Henry G. ....Medical Arts Bldg., Okla. City
Bigler, Earl E. ....Claremore
Birge, Jackson P. ....724 E. 17, Okla. City
Blue, Johnny ....Hales Building, Okla. City
Boatright, Lloyd C. ....1216 N. W. 36, Okla. City
Bolton, V. L. ....Strong Mem. Hosp., Rochester, N. Y.
Boone, Wilmot B. ....2112 W. 41, Tulsa
Bond, Ira T. ....810½ Main, Duncan
Border, C. L. ....Hightower Bldg., Okla. City
Bradley, Frank L. ....Talihina
Brown, Gerster W. ....Medical Arts Bldg., Okla. City
Brown, Spencer ....Muskogee
Buchan, William H. ....1531 S. St. Louis, Tulsa
Buford, Elvin L. ....Guymon
Buttermore, Ralph M. ......447 S. Pittsburg Ave., Tulsa
Campbell, Wm. J. ....301 N. W. 19, Okla. City
Carlock, John H. ....Gilbert Building, Ardmore
Cheatwood, Wm. R. ....Box 1139, Santa Fe, N. M.
Choice, R. W. ....Wakita
Clark, John V. ....1706 S. E. 29, Okla. City
Coates, R. R. ....Chickasha
Coker, B. B. ....145½ Main, Durant
Coley, Joe H. ....Hightower Bldg., Okla. City
Cook, Edward T., Jr. ......503 W. Alabama, Anadarko
Cowart, O. Hiram ....Bristow
Cox, Arlo K. ....1011 N. Noble, Watonga
Craig, Paul E. ....Daniels Building, Tulsa
Cunningham, Donald ....Ardmore
Curry, J. F. ....Sapulpa
Curry, John R. ....952 Stuart Bldg., Lincoln, Neb.
Darnell, Elmer E. ....Colony
Davidson, Wallace N. ....Cushing
Davis, Thomas H. ....Medical Arts Bldg., Tulsa
Davis, Wesley W. ....Chickasha
Devanney, Louis ....Sayre
Devanney, Phil J. ....113 N. Fourth, Sayre
Dew, H. A. ....Marlow
Donovan, Mark ....1213 N. W. 38, Okla. City
Dorwart, F. G. ....Muskogee
Doyle, Wm. H. ....Third and Wall Streets, Muskogee
Dube, Paul H. ....Lakewood, Ohio
Dunnington, Wm. G. ....305 S. Grand, Cherokee
Elkins, M. G., Jr. ....320 E. Wade, El Reno
Ellison, Gayfree ....Clinton
Emenhiser, Lee K. ....Medical Arts Bldg., Okla. City
Ensey, J. E. ....Altus
Etter, Forest S. ....Bartlesville
Evans, A. M. ....Perry
Foerster, Hervey ....Medical Arts Bldg., Okla. City
Fowler, Arthur ....Sulphur
Fried, David N. ....Jones
Gearhart, Elmer ....Box 32, Kaw
Gibbens, Murray ....Muskogee
Gibbs, Allen G. ....521 N.W. 11, Okla. City
Glasgow, J. G. ....Bethany
Godfrey, James T. ....Ardmore

Geen, Rayburn W. ....447 S. Pittsburg, Tulsa
Gordon, D. M. ....300 Masonic Bldg., Ponca City
Gordon, James M. ....1466 Bixby Bldg., Ardmore
Green, Charles E. ....Lawton
Greenberger, Edward ....McAlester
Hamm, Leslie T. ....319 Koehler Bldg., Lawton
Hazel, Onis G. ....Medical Arts Bldg., Okla. City
Hemphill, Paul H. ....Pawhuska
Henry, Millard ....McAlester
Herrmann, Jess D. ....1147 N. W. 38, Okla. City
Hinshaw, J. R. ....McAlester
Holcomb, Mark D. ....402 E. Summit, Lawton
Holcombe, R. N. ....Muskogee
Hood, Frederick R. ....Osler Building, Okla. City
Hood, James O. ....420 E. Keith, Norman
Howard, Walter Alonzo ....Box 386, Chelsea
Hubbard, John Clarence ....1501 N. E. 11, Okla. City
Hubbard, John R. ....1501 N. E. 11, Okla. City
Hubbard, Ralph ....1501 N. E. 11, Okla. City
Hubbard, Wm. ....1501 N. E. 11, Okla. City
Hucherson, D. C. ....800 N. E. 13, Okla. City
Huff, T. J., Jr. ....Walters
Huggins, James Richard ..Medical Arts Bldg., Okla. City
Hughes, Horton E. ....14 E. 9, Shawnee
Ingle, John D. ....93rd & Euclid, Cleveland, Ohio
Ishmael, Wm. K. ....605 N. W. 10, Okla. City
Jacobs, Raymond G. ....Enid
Johnston, L. A. S. ....Holdenville
Jones, William A. ....Elk City, Kansas
Kahn, Robert W. ....605 Euclid, Lawton
Kaiser, George L. ....Manhattan Bldg., Muskogee
Kendall, Robert L. ....220 S. Mortum, Okmulgee
Kern, Clyde V. ....1228 S. Florence, Tulsa
Kernek, Clyde ....Holdenville
Kimball, George H. ....Medical Arts Bldg., Okla. City
King, Everett J. ....Duncan
Klotz, Wm. F. ....20 Comm-Little Bldg., Memphis, Tenn.
Knight, Claude R. ....Wewoka
Lawson, Pat ....Marietta
LeHew, Elton ....Pawnee
Lemon, Cecil W. ....Medical Arts Bldg., Okla. City
Levick, Julius E. ....Elk City
Lindsey, Ray H. ....Pauls Valley
Lingenfelter, Paul B. ....Clinton
Little, Aaron C. ....Minco
Lively, C. E. ....McAlester
Livingston, L. G. ....Cordell
Love, Albert J. ....11 Dewey, Sapulpa
Lowrey, R. W. ....Atoka
Loy, Mm. A. ....215 Almeda Street, Norman
Lyons, Mason Russell ....Carnegie
Mansur, Harl D. ....Ardmore
Matthews, Newman S. ....400 N. W. 10, Okla. City
McClellan, C. W. ....305 Fifth Street, Claremore
McCollum, Wiley T. ....Waynoka
McDonald, Glen W. ....State Health Dept., Okla. City
McDonald, John E. ....Natl. Mutual Bldg., Tulsa
Mercer, Wendell J. ....Enid
Messinger, R. P. ....807 N. W. 23, Okla. City
Miles, John B. ....Anadarko
Miller, J. E. ....1616 N. W. 33, Okla. City
Miller, Nesbit L. ....Medical Arts Bldg., Okla. City
Mills, Charles K. ....602 E. Creek, McAlester
Mitchell, Joseph N. ....Koehler Building, Lawton
Mohler, Eldon O. ....Ponca City
Morey, John ....1314 S. Johnston, Ada
Morgan, Louis S. ....310 Community Bldg., Ponca City
Mulvey, Bert ....Medical Arts Bldg., Okla. City
Munding, I. A. ....Medical Arts Bldg., Tulsa
Murdoch, Raymond L. ....Medical Arts Bldg., Okla. City
Nagle, Patrick S. ....Schuler Clinic, Carlsbad, N. M.
Neal, Laile G. ....Ponca City
Neff, Everett B. ....Osler Bldg., Okla. City

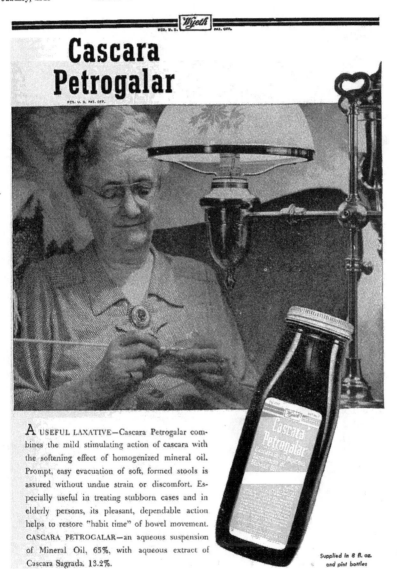

Cascara Petrogalar

REG. U. S. PAT. OFF.

A USEFUL LAXATIVE—Cascara Petrogalar combines the mild stimulating action of cascara with the softening effect of homogenized mineral oil. Prompt, easy evacuation of soft, formed stools is assured without undue strain or discomfort. Especially useful in treating stubborn cases and in elderly persons, its pleasant, dependable action helps to restore "habit time" of bowel movement. CASCARA PETROGALAR—an aqueous suspension of Mineral Oil, 65%, with aqueous extract of Cascara Sagrada, 13.2%.

Supplied in 8 fl. oz. and pint bottles

WYETH INCORPORATED • PHILADELPHIA 3 • PA.

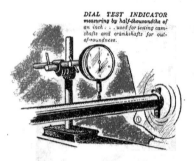

DIAL TEST INDICATOR measuring by half-thousandths of an inch . . . used for testing camshafts and crankshafts for out-of-roundness.

WHEN IT'S *Precision*

YOU REQUIRE . . .

FOR the treatment of pernicious anemia, medical science has found a specific in liver therapy.

But like the highly sensitive dial test indicator which measures within .0005 inch, liver extract—to give precise results—must be manufactured with the utmost care.

. . . *And nothing less than precision will meet the requirements of the competent physician.*

For these requirements, Purified Solution of Liver, Smith-Dorsey, deserves your confidence.

Its uniform purity and potency are traceable to the conditions under which it is produced—to the capably staffed laboratories, the modern facilities, the rigidly standardized testing procedure.

You may be assured of *precision* in liver therapy when you use

PURIFIED SOLUTION OF

Liver

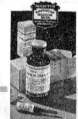

Supplied in the following dosage forms: 1 cc. ampoules and 10 cc. and 30 cc. ampoule vials, each containing 10 U.S.P. Injectable Units per cc.

THE SMITH-DORSEY COMPANY
Lincoln, Nebraska

Manufacturers of Pharmaceuticals to the Medical Profession Since 1908

Neilson, W. P. ....Enid
Noell, Robert ....Medical Arts Bldg., Okla. City
Oglesbee, Carson L. ....305 Manhattan Bldg., Muskogee
Parker, E. R. ....112 S. 13, Frederick
Parker, W. E. ....Sebeka, Minnesota
Parsons, Jack F. ....Main and Kansas, Cherokee
Perry, Fred T. ....Okeene
Petty, James S. ....113½ W. Oklahoma, Guthrie
Phelan, Ralph S. ....East D. Avenue, Waurika
Pigford, Charles A. ....Medical Arts Bldg., Tulsa
Pittman, Cole D. ....Bartlesville
Points, Blair ....Madill
Poole, Warren E. ....2117 Somerset, Okla. City
Porter, H. H. ....Medical Arts Bldg., Tulsa
Prather, Frank W. ....Veterans Hosp., Sulphur
Price, Neal J. ....2528 N. W. 27, Okla. City
Raff, J. S. ....Madill
Ragan, Tillman A. ....619 W. Boyd, Norman
Rayburn, Charles R. ....Box 151, Norman
Records, J. W. ....301 N. W. 12, Okla. City
Reichert, R. J. ....Box 96, Moore
Reiff, William H. ....234 West St., Stillwater
Ridgeway, Elmer Jr. ....1315 Broadway Place, Okla. City
Ritzhaupt, Louis ....Guthrie
Roberts, R. E. ....1720 College, Stillwater
Royer, C. A. ....Medical Arts Bldg., Okla. City
Rubin, H. J. ....Albany Hotel, Tulsa
Rucker, R. W. ....Bartlesville
Rucks, W. W., Jr. ....301 N. W. 12, Okla. City
Rutherford, V. M. ....217 W. Ercoupe, Midwest, City
Sanger, Fenton A. ....Perrine Bldg., Okla. City
Sanger, W. W. ....301 N. W. 12, Okla. City
Sayles, W. J. ....20 E. Street, Miami
Schaff, H. V. ....Holdenville
Schnitman, Jacob ....Gould
Sellers, Fred M. ....Mangum
Shadid, Alexander ....Elk City
Shields, H. B. ....1702 Cherokee, Enid
Shircliff, E. E. ....128 N. W. 14, Okla. City
Shorbe, Howard ....605 N. W. 10, Okla. City
Simon, John F. ....Alva
Sisler, Frank H., Jr. ....Bristow
Smith, Carlton E. ....305 N. Fifth, Henryetta
Smith, L. P. ....Vet. Hospital, Muskogee
Smith, Raymond O. ....3242½ N. E. 11, Tulsa
Starkey, Wayne O. ....Altus
Stevens, James W. ....1126 W. Vinita, Sulphur
Stone, Samuel N., Jr. ....Edmond
Stotts, Charles S. ....Fairfax
Stowers, Aubrey E. ....Sentinel
Stuard, Charles G. ....Medical Arts Bldg., Tulsa
Talley, Evans E. ....114 E. Broadway, Enid
Taylor, Jim M. ....Medical Arts Bldg., Okla. City
Taylor, L. C. ....5417 N. W. 56, Okla. City
Taylor, Lloyd W. ....514 E. Brown, Hugo
Tisdal, W. C. ....709 Frisco, Clinton
Tool, Charles D. ....800 N. E. 13, Okla. City
Tracy, G. W. ....1501 E. Park, Okla. City
Turnbow, W. R. ....1040 S. Yukon, Tulsa
Vahleberg, Ernest R. ....First Natl. Bldg., Okla. City
Wainwright, Tom L. ....Medical Arts Bldg., Okla. City
Waltrip, Jesse R. ....110 W. Main St., Yale
Waters, Floyd Leo ....Hugo
Weaver, Wm. N. ....Muskogee
Wheeler, Homer C. ....McAlester
Wildman, S. F. ....Medical Arts Bldg., Okla. City
Wilhite, L. R. ....Perkins
Wilson, Charles H. ....Medical Arts Bldg., Okla. City
Wilson, Jewell R. ....202 W. Oak, Seminole
Witt, Richard E. ....2700 N. Walker, Okla. City
Witten, Harold B. ....Valley View Hospital, Ada
Wolfe, I. C. ....Muskogee
Wolff, John Powers ....Osler Bldg., Okla. City
Wolohon, H. C. ....2345 N. W. 32, Okla. City
Wood, Jason G. ....701 N. Bradley, Weatherford
Woodburn, J. T. ....Muskogee
Yandell, H. R. ....Medical Arts Bldg., Tulsa
Yeakel, Earl L. ....Savings Bldg., Okla. City
Zampetti, H. A. ....Santa Monica, California

The Preference
is Overwhelming

A comprehensive report published in *Human Fertility*[1] shows an overwhelming preference by experienced clinicians for the "Diaphragm and Jelly" method of conception control.

The report covering 36,955 new cases shows that the diaphragm and jelly method was prescribed for 34,314, or 93%.

On the evidence supplied by competent clinicians we continue to suggest that for the optimum in protection the physician should prescribe the combined use of a vaginal diaphragm and spermatocidal jelly.

When you specify "RAMSES"[*] a product of highest quality is assured.

Gynecological Division
JULIUS SCHMID, INC.
Established 1883
423 West 55th Street   New York 19, N. Y.

1. Human Fertility, 10:25, March, 1945.

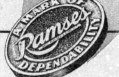

[*]The word "RAMSES" is a registered trademark of Julius Schmid, Inc.

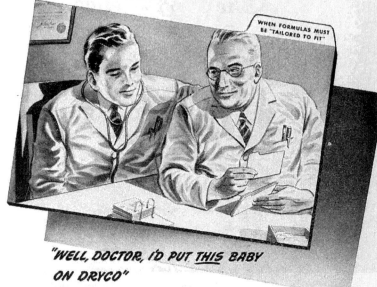

"WELL, DOCTOR, I'D PUT *THIS* BABY ON DRYCO"

"His condition requires careful dietary supervision — with Dryco you can easily adjust the formula to meet his requirements."

Because Dryco offers the physician wide limits of formula flexibility, it is ideally suited to *special* feeding... besides being perfectly suited to *normal* cases. It may be prescribed with or without added carbohydrate... and may be employed in *concentrated* form also when indicated.

The high-protein, low-fat ratio of Dryco (2.7 to 1) assures optimum protein intake and minimal gastro-intestinal upsets from fat indigestion. In addition, Dryco contains adequate vitamins A, B_1, B_2, and D, plus essential milk minerals.

BORDEN'S PRESCRIPTION PRODUCTS DIVISION
350 MADISON AVENUE, NEW YORK 17, N. Y.

In Canada Write The Borden Company, Limited, Spadina Crescent, Toronto

DRYCO *is made from spray-dried, pasteurized, superior quality whole milk and skim milk. Provides 2500 U.S.P. units vitamin A and 400 U.S.P. units vitamin D per reconstituted quart. Supplies 31½ calories per tablespoon. Available at all drug stores in 1 and 2½ lb. cans.*

USE
DRYCO
THE "CUSTOM FORMULA"
INFANT FOOD

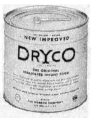

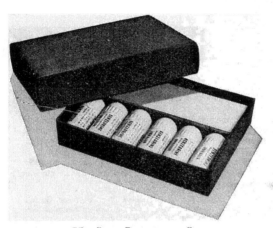

a clinical supply

If you would like a supply of sample-size Benzedrine Inhalers—*free of charge and without obligation*—just write "Six Inhalers" on your prescription blank and mail to *Smith, Kline & French Laboratories, Dept. 25, 429 Arch St., Phila. 5, Pa.*

free!

sample size

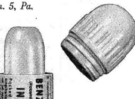

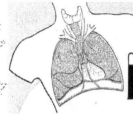

In the Pneumonias

DURING the recent past, numerous investigations have shown that penicillin is the treatment of choice in the pneumonias (pneumococcic, streptococcic, staphylococcic).* Penicillin is virtually nontoxic, even in the massive dosages at times required. Its efficacy apparently is the same against sulfonamide-resistant and nonresistant organisms of the groups named. Even in advanced stages of the disease, in the presence of serious complications, penicillin usually proves a life-saving measure.

Since penicillin has become available in quantities that may well be adequate for all needs, it merits being the physician's first thought with every pneumonia patient.

*Stainsby, W. J.; Foss, H. L., and Drumheller, J. F.: Clinical Experiences with Penicillin, Pennsylvania M. J. 48:119 (Nov.) 1944.

McBryde, A.: Hemolytic Staphylococcus Pneumonia in Early Infancy; Response to Penicillin Therapy, Am. J. Dis. Child. 68:271 (Oct.) 1944.

Stainsby, W. J., Chairman, Commission for the Study of Pneumonia Control of the Medical Society of the State of Pennsylvania: Up-to-Date Facts on Pneumonia, Pennsylvania M. J. 48:266 (Dec.) 1944.

Larsen, N. P.: Observations with Penicillin, Hawaii M. J. 3:272 (July-Aug.) 1944.

PENICILLIN-C.S.C.

Penicillin-C.S.C. deserves the physician's preference not only in the pneumonias, but whenever penicillin therapy is indicated. Rigid laboratory control in its manufacture, and bacteriologic and biologic assays, safeguard its potency, sterility, nontoxicity, and freedom from pyrogens. The state of purification reached in Penicillin-C.S.C. is indicated by the notably small amount of substance required to present 100,000 Oxford Units. Because of this purity, incidence of the undesirable reactions, attributed by many investigators to inadequate purification, is greatly reduced.

PHARMACEUTICAL DIVISION

COMMERCIAL SOLVENTS CORPORATION

17 East 42nd Street   New York 17, N. Y.

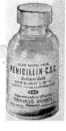

Penicillin-C.S.C. stands accepted by the Council on Pharmacy and Chemistry of the American Medical Association.

MEDICAL ABSTRACTS

THE GLUCOSE TOLERANCE TEST IN DIAGNOSIS OF DIABETES AND HYPERINSULINISM. Elmer L. Severinghaus, M.D., Department of Medicine, University of Wisconsin, Madison, Wisconsin.

In this the author calls attention to the four features, namely: 1. the initial level; 2. the peak of the curve; 3. the rate of decline; 4. the occurrence of a phase lower than the initial level sometimes in the third or fourth hours. These are used in connection with the diagnosis of not only diabetes, but other conditions.

The rate of decline is the most important factor in connection with diabetes, the slow rate being characteristic. Of course, if the initial rate is much above the upper limit of 120, these two factors are essentially all that is necessary in the diagnosis of diabetes. The only exception he mentions are chronic nephritis or a temporary emotional episode.

The peak has no particular significance in the diagnosis of diabetes, or hyperinsulinism. In cases where the initial blood sugar level was within normal limits, the occurrence of a distinctly high peak, that is, one above 180, it is usually associated with either thyrotoxicosis or some other factor disturbing the autonomic nervous system.

Those who two to four hours after the intake of glucose show blood sugar levels which are significantly lower than the initial level of the curve, are pointed out as being helpful in other conditions giving rise to hypoglycemia such as those rare types with an adenemo of the pancreas.

Important factors influencing the blood levels during the sugar tolerance test are recognized as being complex and worthy of consideration. Insulin hormone, from the anterior pituitary, the thyroid, adrenal cortex, and the adrenal medulla all tend to an elevation of the blood sugar level. However, the author indicates that an attempt to make diagnoses of pituitary thyroid adrenal or other endocrine disorders on the basis of the tolerance tests should not be considered satisfactory.

The paper was discussed by Dr. Seale Harris of Birmingham, Alabama, who stated that if the test is not extended to the fifth or sixth hour, a case of hypoglycemia may be overlooked. He also implied that a single tolerance test may not be sufficient for diagnosis. He says many cases of neurosis will show hypoglycemia if the six hour tolerance test is done.

Dr. Edward H. Rynearson of Rochester, Minnesota, made some pertinent remarks which implied that he had no great amount of confidence in the sugar tolerance test, particularly as it applies to hyperinsulinism.

Dr. Elliott P. Joslin of Boston, Massachusetts, implied in his discussion that he considered peak blood sugar as it goes up to high, very significant.

Dr. Samuel Soskin of Chicago, Illinois, was very frank with his discussion as follows: "Dr. Severinghaus has confined his remarks to the oral form of the glucose tolerance test, and I agree with him and with Dr. Harris as to its clinical value or rather its lack of value. In outspoken cases of diabetes or of hyperinsulinism it is not needed for diagnosis. In borderline cases it is not a reliable diagnostic aid. As a matter of fact, anyone who has performed repeated oral dextrose tolerance tests on apparently normal individuals will agree that one can get about as much variation in the test in the same normal person at different times as Dr. Sevringhaus has shown in his slides of abnormal individuals. It is just as question of repeating the test often enough. I must say I find it rather surprising that members of a specialized society such as this still waste time and energy performing the oral test and still spend serious thought on its significance. As Dr. Hynearson has rightly said, it has caused many people to be labelled as diabetics who are not diabetic at all; and it has failed to pick up many

potential or early diabetics." He says there is a better way of doing the test, namely, the intravenous administration of dextrose.

Dr. I. Arthur Mirsky, of Cincinnati, Ohio, has among other things said as follows: "The inaccuracies of the data obtained by means of the oral dextrose tolerance curve cannot be overemphasized. A recent experience may illustrate my point. In a patient with obstructive jaundice, a flat curve was obtained after the administration of sugar by mouth, while a normal curve was obtained when the sugar was given by vein. Obviously, the flat curve was due to faulty absorption. There is a great variability in rate of absorption of sugar from the intestinal tract from time to time which in turn may be responsible for variations in the character of the oral tolerance curve."

Dr. Otto Porges of Chicago, Ill., made this significant remark: "Dr. Sevringhaus mentioned that fasting before performing the glucose tolerance test has an influence on the blood sugar curve. I want to point out that not only fasting, but even the character of meal of the preceding evening has an effect. If that meal contained carbohydrates, there is a great difference in the blood sugar curve."

Dr. Herman O. Mosenthal of New York City said, "There is one point with which I absolutely agree, but I believe it should be confirmed, namely, that the height of the blood sugar curve is of no significance. I think it was McLane of England who first called such curves 'lag' curves. We found the same thing true, namely, that they did not signify diabetes. Lawrence of England at a meeting here once, accentuated that fact."

COMMENT: This is a very significant publication inasmuch as it is both presented and discussed by outstanding specialists on the subject and also at a meeting of specialists all of whom at the meeting seemed to concur with those who discussed the subject.

The fact remains that the glucose tolerance test is not a highly dependable clinical aid. Personally, I prefer repeated blood sugar's over a period of time both fasting and postprandial not only for the diagnosis of diabetes but for the diagnosis of associated conditions. Diagnosis is in these conditions much like that in many other conditions, in that observation, therapy and the influence of therapy and careful followup are more important than the initial tests.—H.J., M.D.

BRITTAIN ISCHIOFERMORAL ARTHRODESIS. Robert A. Knight and Michael M. Bluhm, Jr., Bone and Joint Surgery. Vol. 27, No. 4, October, 1945.

In 1941 Brittain described a method of arthrodesis of the hip, in which a large tibial graft is inserted into a cleft in the ischium, through an oblique osteotomy. The shaft of the femur is then displaced medially toward the ischium, supporting the graft and "short-circuiting" the diseased hip joint. This operation was done for tuberculosis of the hip and other diseases of the hip joint requiring arthrodesis.

The authors have used this operation since March, 1943 and in the present article reports the results of nine cases of tuberculosis of the hip, with a total of 12 hips operated upon, since three were cases of bilateral hip tuberculosis.

They find the method successful and more reliable than the extra-articular methods previously described. There is an oblique osteotomy performed across the upper third of the femur and the bone graft is driven into the ischium after making a hole for it with the osteotome. This graft is passed through the osteotomy wound into the ischium in a line upward and inward and parallel the neck of the femur. This permits an ankylosis to take place above the upper end of the distal fragment, throwing the weight of the leg on the ischium below the head of the femur. This is more advantageous than where the arthrodesis is done above the head of the femur. The work is all extra-capsular. E.D.M., M.D.

RECURRENT DISLOCATION OF ANKLE DUE TO RUPTURE OF EXTERNAL LATERAL LIGAMENT. E. Hambly. British Medical Jr., Vol. 1, 413. 1945.

An operation for recurrent dislocation of the ankle due to rupture of the external lateral ligament is reported. The ligament is repaired by splitting the peroneus longus tendon from above downward. The detached end is threaded through the lateral malleolus and through the os calcis, and back again on itself. This reconstitutes the ligament.

A case report is given in which the operation was successful. The patient has had no further trouble. E.D.M., M.D.

INTERNAL FIXATION OF FRACTURES OF THE NECK OF THE FEMUR. Duncan W. Boucher. The Canadian Med. Ass'n. Jr. Vol. 50, No. 31. 1945.

The author reports the use of the three-flanged, centrally cannalized nail, in the internal fixation of forty-seven fractures of the neck of the femur. Subcapital fracture occurred in 16.2 per cent, transcervical fracture in 41.8 per cent, and basilar fractures, either interfrochanteric or pertrochanteric, in 41.8 per cent. The ages ranged from 54 to 89 years, with most in the eighth decade. The fractures were more common in women than in men, 83.2 per cent, as compared with 16.7 per cent. Nineteen patients, or 40 per cent had complications on admission, which affected the end result.

Anesthesia was induced, in most cases, with nitrous oxide and oxygen; in some, with a spinal anesthetic; and in one, by local infiltration. Roentgenograms guided the procedure, before, during and after the operation. Extra-articular technique was followed in the introduction of the three-flanged nail, with the thigh in a position of abduction, hyperextension, and in internal rotation, and with the knee preferably fully extended. The guide wire was inserted well into the head of the femur, and the nail was threaded over the wire, and hammered home. Vigorous movements were then carried out by the surgeon to test the thoroughness of the operative procedure. Smooth movement, without recurring deformity, indicated solid impaction.

Patients were up on about the fourth day, and were bearing weight on the injured limb by the ninth week or sooner.

The end results were good in 72.3 per cent, fair in 8.3 and 10.6 per cent died. No nails were extracted, except in those patients who died while in the hospital, and in one case of absorption of the neck of the femur. —E.D.M., M.D.

A HIGH FLUID INTAKE IN THE MANAGEMENT OF EDEMA, ESPECIALLY CARDIAC EDEMA. CLINICAL OBSERVATIONS AND DATA. F. R. Schemm. M.D., F.A.C.P., Great Falls, Montant.

F. R. Schemm,—in a little over 8 years, treated 402 cases of edema with a regime of high fluid intake and low sodium intake. The theory behind his regime appears to be physiologically sound. In edema there is an increase of extracellular fluid while the cells themselves are actually dehydrated. The extracellular fluid

is held by an increase in the concentration of the sodium ion. Forcing fluids causes an excretion of the excess sodium and salts in the extracellular spaces and a reduction in the amount of edema.

High fluid intake, sharp restriction of sodium in the diet, and a mild acid ash diet was in general the regime followed by Schemm. In many instances high fluid intake alone was used with success. In other instances it was necessary to restrict the sodium intake sharply to bring about a reduction in edema. The loss of edema was often so rapid that oppressive degrees of hydrothorax and ascites rarely required aspiration. So called "water intoxication" was not encountered although syndromes answering this description were seen which were found to be due to loss of body-fluid volume or disturbances of electrolyte pattern, or to "true" dehydration.

In 393 periods of observation or cases with gross edema, the edema cleared entirely in 94% or 369 instances. In 25 instances, or 6% the regime failed and the patient died unrelieved of edema. These were all cases of advanced disease with the uremic syndrome present in most and with the oral intake negligible because of vomiting or semi-stupor. Obviously in many of the 369 instances in which edema cleared completely, the result could be properly attributed, in whole or in part, to change in such factors, as the amount of rest, digitalis, oxygen, or diuretic drugs. But in 102 instances of treatment of gross edema, no change was made that might effect the clearing of edema except to institute the high fluid regime.

The high fluid intake regime was used in all cases of edema regardless of the etiological cause. The cases used included cardiac decompensation due to all types of cardiac disease, all types of renal disease, eclampsia, lymphoblastoma, pernicious anemia, diabetes mellitus, and myxedema.

SPINAL FLUID PROTEIN AND COLLODIOL MASTIC TESTS. E. A. Fennel, M.D., The Clinic, Honolulu, T. H.

E. A. Fennel reviewed the standard texts on the subject of spinal fluid protein and collodial mastic tests. In them he found considerable disagreement and confusion of thought on the subject.

He reviewed a number of his own cases in which total protein, albumin and globulin determinations, colloidal mastics, and Wassermanns were recorded. He found very little correlation between the amount of albumin and globulin (and their ratio) in the spinal fluid and the colloidal mastic. From his results he drew the following conclusions:

1. The only laboratory test that is diagnostic or pathognomonic of syphilis of the central nervous system is the properly applied complement fixation test. (Wassermann) or precipitation test (there are 57 varieties) for the detection of luetic "reagin" and the "syphilitic body". No other test serves this purpose.

2. The "colloidal curves", popularly called paretic, tabetic, and meningitic should be called prezone, midzone, and endzone since they do not indicate these three diseases and are quite non-specific.

3. These curves probably depend on the "protein pattern" of the spinal fluid and are equally useful— or useless—in other diseases of the central nervous system, as in syphilis.

FREE SAMPLE

DR. _____
ADDRESS _____
CITY _____
STATE _____

chap cream

AR-EX COSMETICS, INC.,

ROUGH HANDS
FROM TOO MUCH SCRUBBING?
Soften dry skin with AR-EX CHAP CREAM! Contains carbonyl diamide, shown in hospital test to make skin softer, smoother, and even whiter! Archives of Derm. and S., July, 1943. FREE SAMPLE.

AR-EX CHAP CREAM

1036 W. VAN BUREN ST., CHICAGO 7, ILL.

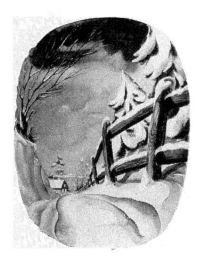

OPEN SEASON *for* COLDS

During these winter months, colds can well hit a new high in morbidity among a hard working population long on rationed foods.

Relief of exhausting cough is effectively accomplished by administration of LIQUID PEPTONOIDS* WITH CREOSOTE, a palatable bronchial sedative that quiets the cough, promotes expectoration and helps check extension of the inflammatory processes. In the early treatment of respiratory symptoms arising from the common cold, prescribe

LIQUID PEPTONOIDS
REG. U S. PAT. OFF

WITH CREOSOTE

Each tablespoonful contains 2 minims of pure beechwood creosote and 1 minim of guaiacol combined with peptones and carbohydrates—a unique formula that tends to prevent gastric irritation and eructations.

DOSAGE: For adults, one teaspoonful hourly.

SUPPLIED. 6 and 12 ounce bottles.

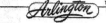

THE ARLINGTON CHEMICAL COMPANY · YONKERS 1, NEW YORK
*The word "Peptonoids" is a registered trademark of The Arlington Chemical Company.

4. The "protein pattern" involves a consideration of (a) the total protein concentration, (b) the albumin content, (c) the globulin content, (d) the ratio of globulin to albumin, and (e) the quality of the globulins.

5. The proper interpretation of the protein content of the spinal fluid needs much further physiologic and clinical study.

6. Practical (i.e., cheap in time, money, and spinal fluid, though accurate) chemical methods for determining the protein content and partitioning of albumins and globulins are not yet ready to supplant the colloidal tests on spinal fluids since the colloidal tests depend not wholly on the quantitative protein values but also on the *qualitative* one.

7. There is little, if any, correlation between the quantitative "protein pattern" of the spinal fluid and its content of reagin.

MID-WEST SURGICAL SUPPLY CO., INC.

Kaufman Building

Wichita 2, Kansas

FRED R. COZART

2437 N. W. 36th Terrace

Phone 8-2561   Oklahoma City, Okla.

CREDIT SERVICE

330 American National Building

Oklahoma City, Oklahoma

(Operators of Medical-Dental Credit Bureau)

★

We offer a dignified and effective collection service for doctors and hospitals located anywhere in the State. Write for information.

★

28 YEARS

Experience In Credit and Collection Work

Robt. R. Sesline, Owner and Manager

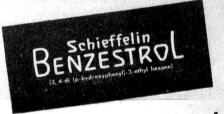

Uniform Satisfaction

Schieffelin BENZESTROL
(2, 4-di (p-hydroxyphenyl)-3-ethyl hexane)

Clinicians agree that Schieffelin BENZESTROL is a significant contribution to therapy in that it is both estrogenically effective and singularly well tolerated, whether administered orally or parenterally.

"In our hands it has proved to be an effective estrogen when administered either orally or parenterally and much less toxic than diethylstilbestrol at the therapeutic levels" (Talisman, M. R.—Am. Jour. Obstet. & Gynec. 46, 534, 1943)

"During the last two years I have used the new synthetic estrogen Benzestrol in patients in whom estrogenic therapy was indicated. The results have been uniformly satisfactory". (Jaeger, A. S. Journal Indiana State Med. Assn. 37, 117, 1944)

Schieffelin BENZESTROL is indicated in all conditions for which estrogen therapy is ordinarily recommended and is available in tablets of 0.5, 1.0, 2.0 and 5.0 mg.; in solution in 10 cc. vials, 5 mg. per cc.; and vaginal tablets of 0.5 mg. strength.

Literature and Sample on Request

Schieffelin & Co.

Pharmaceutical and Research Laboratories

20 COOPER SQUARE   •   NEW YORK 3, N.Y.

"Smoothage" IN THE CONSTIPATION OF PREGNANCY

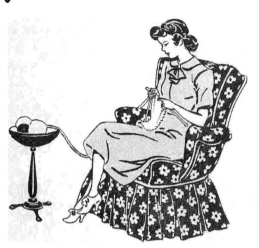

The constipation frequently encountered during pregnancy, due to pressure of the fetus on the pelvic bowel, lack of exercise, and restricted diet, is alleviated by Metamucil.

The Smoothage of Metamucil encourages easy, gentle evacuation. It does not interfere with the absorption of vitamins or other food factors:

METAMUCIL *is the registered trademark of G. D. Searle & Co., Chicago 80, Illinois*

"Smoothage" describes the gentle, nonirritating action of Metamucil—the highly refined mucilloid of a seed of the psyllium group, Plantago ovata (50%), combined with dextrose (50%).

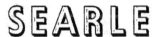

SEARLE

RESEARCH IN THE SERVICE OF MEDICINE

OFFICERS OF COUNTY SOCIETIES, 1945

★

COUNTY	PRESIDENT	SECRETARY	MEETING TIME
Alfalfa	W. G. Dunnington, Cherokee	L. T. Lancaster, Cherokee	Last Tues. each Second Month
Atoka-Coal	J. B. Clark, Coalgate	J. S. Fulton, Atoka	
Beckham			
Blaine			Second Tuesday
Bryan			Second Tuesday
Caddo	Preston E. Wright, Anadarko	Edward T. Cook, Anadarko	
Canadian			Subject to call
Carter	J. Hobson Veazey, Ardmore	H. A. Higgins, Ardmore	Second Tuesday
Cherokee			First Tuesday
Choctaw	Floyd L. Waters, Hugo	O. R. Gregg, Hugo	
Cleveland			Thursday nights
Comanche			
Cotton			Third Friday
Craig			
Creek			Second Tuesday
Custer	Ross Deputy, Clinton	A. W. Paulson, Clinton	Third Thursday
Garfield	Bruce Hinson, Enid	John R. Walker, Enid	Fourth Thursday
Garvin	M. E. Robberson, Jr., Wynnewood	John R. Callaway, Pauls Valley	Wednesday before Third Thursday
Grady			Third Thursday
Grant			
Greer	J. B. Lansden, Granite	J. B. Hollis, Mangum	
Harmon	W. G. Husband, Hollis	R. H. Lynch, Hollis	First Wednesday
Haskell			
Hughes			First Friday
Jackson	E. M. Mabry, Altus	J. P. Irby, Altus	Last Monday
Jefferson	F. M. Edwards, Ringling	J. A. Dillard, Waurika	Second Monday
Kay			Second Thursday
Kingfisher			
Kiowa			
LeFlore			
Lincoln	J. S. Rollins, Prague	Ned Burleson, Prague	First Wednesday
Logan	James Petty, Guthrie	J. E. Souter, Guthrie	Last Tuesday
Marshall			
Mayes			
McClain			
McCurtain			Fourth Tuesday
McIntosh	Dr. F. R. First, Checotah	W. A. Tolleson, Eufaula	First Thursday
Muskogee-Sequoyah			
Wagoner	R. N. Holcombe, Muskogee	William N. Weaver, Muskogee	First Tuesday
Noble			
Okfuskee			Second Monday
Oklahoma			Fourth Tuesday
Okmulgee	F. S. Watson, Okmulgee	C. E. Smith, Okmulge	Second Monday
Osage			Third Monday
Ottawa	C. F. Walker, Grove	W. Jackson Sayles, Miami	Second Thursday
Pawnee			
Payne			Third Thursday
Pittsburg			Third Friday
Pontotoc-Murray			First Wednesday
Pottawatomie	F. P. Newlin, Shawnee	Clinton Gallaher, Shawnee	First and Third Saturday
Pushmataha			
Rogers	W. A. Howard, Chelsea	P. S. Anderson, Claremore	Third Wednesday
Seminole			Third Wednesday
Stephens			
Texas	Daniel S. Lee, Guymon	E. L. Buford, Guymon	
Tillman			
Tulsa	John C. Perry, Tulsa	John E. McDonald, Tulsa	Second and Fourth Monday
Washington-Nowata	Ralph W. Rucker, Bartlesville	L. B. Word, Bartlesville	Second Wednesday
Washita	L. G. Livingston, Cordell	Roy W. Anderson, Clinton	
Woods			Last Tuesday Odd Months
Woodward	T. C. Leachman, Woodward	C. W. Tedrowe, Woodward	Second Thursday

*(Serving in Armed Forces)

THE JOURNAL
of the
OKLAHOMA STATE MEDICAL ASSOCIATION

| VOLUME XXXIX | OKLAHOMA CITY, OKLAHOMA, FEBRUARY, 1946 | NUMBER 2 |

Occupational Dermatitis

CARL BRUNDAGE, M.D.

OKLAHOMA CITY, OKLAHOMA

Most of the dermatoses considered in this paper are those encountered in the airplane industry as I have had more experience with the workers in this particular occupation.

In the January, 1937 issue of the Archives of Dermatology and Syphilology, Weber listed 588 occupations, with the various substances in each occupation which have been found responsible for producing a dermatitis.

An occupational dermatitis is a pathological condition of the skin, for which occupational exposure can be shown to be a major, causal or contributory factor. The distinguishing feature beween an industrial and an occupational disease is the fact that in the former the cause is sudden, whereas, the latter requires time. As far as therapy is concerned, the treatment for an occupational dermatitis is the same as for an industrial dermatitis, but from a medico-legal standpoint, it make a considerable difference, as occupational dermatoses are not compensatory in many states, including Oklahoma. Occupational dermatitis has increased a great deal in recent years. This increase has come about in the face of general improvements in safety measures and can only be explained by the increase in new materials, new processes of manufacture, new employees, and the shortage of protective wearing apparel.

C. Guy Lane states that 10 to 12 per cent of all dermatoses are of industrial origin. According to Louis Schwartz of the United States Public Health Service, occupational dermatoses comprise 70 per cent of the occupational diseases. The predisposing causes of occupational dermatoses are — race, type of skin, perspiration, diet, age, season of the year, allergy, lack of cleanliness and pre-existing skin diseases. Cleanliness is the most important preventive measure; a clean environment and personal cleanliness are important. It is important to remember that cleansing materials are often the cause of a dermatitis which had been attributed to the substances handled in the work. It is well known in industry that the negro is less susceptible to skin irritants and less likely to be hypersensitive to substances which he contacts in his work.

In normal times many factories will not employ persons with thin blonde skins in an occupation that would bring them in contact with potential irritants. Workers having thick oily skins can tolerate the action of fat solvents such as soaps, turpentine, naphtha and carbon tetrachloride better than the individuals with a dry skin. On the other hand, in occupations where oils, greases and waxes are apt to soil the clothing, the individual with hairy arms and legs and a seborrheic skin is more likely to develop acne-like lesions, folliculitis and furuncles. Occupational dermatitis is more prevalent in warm weather when light clothing is worn and contact with external irritants is more likely to occur.

Excessive perspiration combined with friction will macerate the skin and in this way make the skin less resistant to the action of external irritants, bacteria and fungi. Age is an important predisposing factor. In addition to the predisposition to acne at adolescence, age seems to have an influence on sensitivity to external irritants. Most of the workers with an acute dermatitis are young and new workers. This may be because they have not become immune or "hardened" to the chemicals or because they are less careful in handling them. On the other hand, the chronic eczematous types of occupational dermatitis, usually occurs in workers of middle age and beyond.

Workers may continue to work and their skin may become immune or "hardened" to substances handled if the dematitis is caused by irritation, but will get worse if it is due to hypersensitivity. The actual cause of occupational dermatitis is mechanical, physical, chemical and biological.

A large per cent of the cases of occupational dermatitis is caused by chemicals. Most of the employees, and many physicians, attribute the dermatoses of the aircraft workers to the aluminum that they handle.

Dural or duraluminum is an alloy consisting of 95 per cent aluminum, a small amount of copper, magnesium and manganese and a trace of silicon. According to Francis C. Prary, Director of the Aluminum Research Laboratory of the Aluminum Company of America, there could not be any reaction on the skin from dural but some workers are affected by the chromic acid coating or the protective oil which contains fish oil. Only four new workers at the Douglas Plant had a positive patch test to dural filings. However, either the protective oil or the chromic acid coating may have been the actual cause.

An analysis of 3,392 patients admitted to the Douglas skin clinic in a period of thirteen months are as follows: Approximately one per cent was industrial, 32 per cent non-industrial, 25 per cent occupational, and 42 per cent of the cases were either not seen by me or I was unable to determine whether or not the dermatoses was of occupational origin. Most all of the industrial dermatoses, usually generalized, followed the treatment of the minor burns and lacerations with the sulfonamides and butysin picrate ointment. It is my opinion that these dermatoses could be avoided.

Zinc chromate primer was found to account for a large majority of the occupational dermatoses. The next most common cause was Hi seal or lagging (trade name for secret formulas) which are used in the heat and vent department. These preparations contain a resin which is probably the sensitizer. We have had very few cases after employing negroes in this department and transferring the blondes to another department. Many of the cases of dermatitis in this department were caused by thinner, which was used to remove this glue-like substance from the skin. Approximately six per cent of the dermatoses was caused by petroleum products and a similar number from solvent and alkalis. About four per cent of the occupational dermatoses was caused by stone felt or spun glass. A small percentage of the dermatoses was caused by dyes, varnish and acids, particularly chromic acid. Several of the employees, such as salvage men and janitors, handled so many substances that are potential irritants to the skin that it is not practical to try to determine the offending agent.

There were three things that impressed me while examining these patients:

1. The incidence of skin eruptions which could be prevented;

2. The number of non-occupational dermatoses which workers would like to attribute to their occupation; and

3. The large number of employees who have been advised by physicians that they have aluminum or metal poisoning.

It was surprising to me to learn that the greatest number of unnecessary skin eruptions and the ones which caused the greatest number of days away from work, are those dermatoses which are secondary to the topical application of the sulfonamides, the skin of workers with lacerations, contusions and infections healed satisfactorily after washing the affected part with soap and water and the application of a sterile dressing. If the physician preferred, a dilute non-irritating watery or alcoholic solution of an antiseptic was applied before the sterile dressing. Such simple therapy gave satisfactory results in the majority of cases. Approximately 15 per cent of those using the sulfonamides locally became sensitized to them during the first course of treatment. Such sensitization usually precludes their use at a later date when the patient may urgently need them for the treatment of a serious infection, such as pneumonia. Other common and unnecessary skin eruptions are caused by ammoniated mercury, merthiolate and butysin picrate.

Harsh cleansing agents have frequently been found to be the actual cause of an occupational dermatitis which before investigation appeared to have been caused by the chemicals handled. Those workers who handle chemicals which are difficult to remove from the skin by ordinary toilet soap are the ones most commonly affected by dermatitis caused by the skin cleanser. Sulfonated oils, especially sulfonated vegetable oils, have been used in industry for a number of years. It is surprising how many workers can be kept at work despite the presence of a contact dermatitis if they use a sulfonated vegetable oil for cleansing their hands and forearms.

Approximately one-third of the cases with skin eruptions examined at the Douglas Plant were not connected in any manner with their work. Such common diseases as dermatomycosis, impetigo, psoriasis, seborrheic dermatitis, acne, pityriasis rosea, herpes zoster, nummular eczema, scabies and pediculosis, were some of the conditions frequently seen.

The most difficult cases to examine and treat were the workers who had been advised by a physician that they had aluminum or metal poisoning.

Diagnosis: There is no factor upon which a diagnosis of occupational dermatitis can be made. All of the following factors must be considered:

1. *History*.
   a. That the dermatitis was not present before the patient entered the occupation.
   b. It must be shown that the dermatitis developed during the period of industrial exposure.
   c. Knowledge of the substances handled will enable the physician to judge whether there is an exposure to known irritants.
   d. Finally, if the history shows that the dermatitis develops when he is at work, gets well or improves when he is away from work, and recurs upon his return to the job, then a definite causal relation is established between his work and the dermatitis.

2. *Site of eruption*: Occupational dermatitis usually begins on the exposed parts — the hands and forearms — if the irritant is a solid or a liquid, or on the face and neck if the irritant is a fine dust or vapor.

3. Patch tests of the patient's skin with substances handled in the occupation is a great deal of assistance in making a diagnosis of occupational dermatoses. The patch test is of the greatest value in cases of contact dermatitis in which substances contacted away from the work are suspected. Preemployment patch testing for the purpose of discovering those workers who are allergic is not advisable, because workers are not usually allergic to chemicals with which they have had no previous contact. Positive patch tests should be regarded as additional confirmation of the history and clinical findings and not considered as diagnostic.

Some of the important preventive measures in the treatment of occupational dermatoses are:

1. Personal and environmental cleanliness is essential.

2. Careful selection of employees with reference to the type of skin for occupations in which potential skin irritants are contacted.

3. New workers with skin eruptions caused by skin irritants should be given protective ointments to put over the exposed parts, proper protective clothing such as rubber gloves and aprons and kept on the job. In most of these cases the skin will develop immunity and the skin eruption will disappear.

The workers with dermatoses caused by hypersensitivity should be transferred to avoid the known or suspected skin sensitizer. The medical therapy of dermatitis must be undertaken with caution. The best results are usually obtained by the use of simple remedies.

In acute dermatitis consisting of erythema, vesiculation and edema, the application of cold wet compresses is advised. The following solutions have been found effective:

Two to four per cent boric acid solution, aluminum actetate solution — 1 to 20 and potassium permanganate solution — 1 to 10,000.

If the dermatitis is generalized, relief from itching may be secured by lukewarm baths containing starch, oatmeal or potassium permanganate. Calamine lotion with one-fourth to one-half of one per cent phenol is a valuable application for a mild dermatitis. A vanishing cream containing 3 per cent liquor carbonis detergens is a valuable preparation to apply following the use of wet compresses. Lassar's paste is an excellent soothing and protective application for sub acute dermatitis.

Complications such as infections and ulcerations must be treated with antiseptics. Infected follicles and furnucles should be opened daily and the lesions washed with soap and water, followed by the application of a five per cent solution of gentian violet.

If the infection is impetiginous, ammoniated mercury ointment — 3 to 5 per cent should be rubbed in thoroughly twice daily after washing with soap and water. Some skins are sensitive to ammoniated mercury and it must be stopped immediately if superimposed dermatitis appears.

Most occupational dermatoses are of acute nature and ointments are contraindicated as it prevents good drainage. If the skin is dry and scaly, oily substances are indicated. A mixture of equal parts of calamine lotion, olive oil and lime water is a satisfactory preparation.

In the chronic eczematous eruptions with marked thickening and lichenification of the skin, stimulating drugs such as crude coal tar, salicylic acid and fractional doses of X-Rays are indicated.

The sulfonamide ointments and powders should rarely, if ever, be used in the treatment of occupational dermatoses. With the exception of nickel, very few cases of dermatitis are caused by metals.

Physicians and nurses should not mention the words metal poisoning during the examination or while talking to industrial workers.

Pathologic Aspects of Certain Surgical Diseases of the Stomach and Duodenum

Charles Donovan Tool, M.D.

OKLAHOMA CITY, OKLAHOMA

This paper presents a brief review of some of the surgical lesions occurring in the stomach and duodenum. Of the 25 feet of hollow muscular tube constituting the gastro-intestinal tract, two feet or so is selected which exerts the major secretory function.

In any evaluation of gastro-intestinal complaints, it is well to remember that symptoms produced by surgical diseases in this area are carried over the same public address system and in the same tones as those produced by non-organic dysfunction or by purely reflex mechanisms initiated by dysfunction of other systems.

From any of these causes, the gastro-intestinal tract reacts through the mechanism of spasms and disturbed peristalsis from obstruction whether functional or organic. Above the site of obstruction is found dilatation and reverse peristalsis. But in our chosen area these symptoms are exaggerated because much of the secretory function is located in the stomach and duodenum, so that here these symptoms are intensified.

The common sites of obstruction are near the cardiac end of the stomach, with cardiospasm and a symptom complex suggesting a low esophageal obstruction; near the pyloric area with pylorospasm and vomiting of stomach contents without bile; above the papilla of Vater with the same symptoms; and below the papilla with symptoms of duodenal obstruction and bile in the vomitus. These mechanisms should be considered as the lesions are reviewed.

In infants, hypertrophic pyloric stenosis is fairly common,[1] and its recognition is vital. Too often medical treatment is continued until the patient is severely malnourished and the surgical risk is very poor, so that the resultant mortality rate is pitifully high.

The child, usually male and often the first born, does well for a week or two and then commences to vomit. He may improve spontaneously in a few weeks, or symptoms may continue until death supervenes. One physical examination, the pylorus may be felt as a round, firm, movable mass. At operation or necropsy, the pylorus is greatly thickened for a distance of a few centimeters along the pyloric canal, projecting into the duodenum. The lumen is obliterated by closely packed folds of mucosa, sometimes hardly admitting a probe. There is some dilatation and hypertrophy of the rest of the stomach wall. In the pylorus, the mass is caused by an enormous overgrowth of the circular layer of muscle. This condition has been reported in a seven-month fetus, so that it is apparently congenital, though a spastic element is evidently superadded.

Congenital stenosis of the duodenum is occasionally seen. While rare, it occurs often enough to be worth remembering. Almost always there is a membranous septum across the lumen. The symptoms depend on the site of the obstruction, and the degree. If above the papilla of Vater, the symptoms are those of pyloric obstruction. If below, bile is regurgitated.

These membranous obstructions of the duodenum fall into three groups. (1) In the first, the obstruction is complete, and death occurs soon after birth. In most of these cases, the obstruction is at or above the papilla of Vater. In the second group, the septum is incomplete, so that a small opening permits the passage of liquids. The child usually does well until changed from a liquid to a solid diet. In the third group, the obstruction is still less marked, and is often an incidental finding at necropsy. At times overindulgence in food or obstruction from solid food impacting at this point, precipitates an obstruction.

Diaphragmatic hernia[2] usually presents a difficult diagnostic problem. Occasionally there is a hemidiaphragmatic hiatus, which is usually incompatible with life, and the child dies in a few hours or days. The condition may arise from a congenitally short esophagus, giving a stomach with the cardia above and most of the fundus below the diaphragm. In the more frequent type a space between in the diaphragmatic crura allows the herniation, usually of the fundus, into the chest cavity. Symptoms of dyspnea and of partial high obstruction may both be present in these cases.

A condition which occurs in adult life is arterio-mesenteric occlusion of the duodenum, also known as duodenal ileus. Pressure from the superior mesenteric artery or its branches contained in a fold of the mesentery, caused by displacement of a loop of small bowel into the pelvis minor, may give rise to partial or complete obstruction of the duodenum. The same effect may come from an abnormally mobile ascending colon and cecum, giving rise to what may be termed an arteriomesocolic occlusion of the duodenum.[3] If obstruction is complete or if symptoms warrant, surgical measures may be necessary for relief. The condition may be precipitated spontaneously or by operation, trauma, or over-indulgence in food. Always there is great distention of both stomach and the proximal portion of duodenum, and there is nausea and profuse vomiting of bile-containing fluid.

A condition commonly seen is acute dilatation of the stomach. This usually follows abdominal operation, but may complicate surgery of other regions, occasionally severe injury or even spontaneous disease. It is characterized by sudden increase in size of the stomach, accompanied by vomiting, epigastric pain, abdominal distention and collapse. At times the dilatation ends at the pylorus, at others it extends as far as the point where the duodenum is crossed by the mesenteric folds and the superior mesenteric vessels, producing a secondary arterio-mesenteric occlusion. Early there is much gas, but later great quantities of fluid may be present. Apparently this is primarily a neuromuscular disturbance with both sympathetic and vagal fibers paralyzed, and there is a great thinning of the dilated vicus. Here the Wangensteen type of drainage is often life-saving.

Diverticula of the stomach are rare, but diverticula of the duodenum are more common. Spriggs and Marxer[4] found 134 cases in 1000 consecutive radiological examinations. Usually symptomless and discovered accidentally or at necropsy, the diverticulum, if large, may give rise to some obstructive symptoms. The usual site is in the neighborhood of the ampulla of Vater, and is along the line of entrance of the vessels. It is an extrusion of mucosa and muscularis mucosae through the muscular wall.

Acute and chronic gastritis are not surgical conditions, and acute ulcer is not of interest in this discussion. Chronic ulcer, on the other hand, is of interest to every clinician and surgeon. Peptic ulcer — for it is easier to consider chronic ulcer of the stomach and of the first portion of the duodenum together — is probably the most frequently encountered pathological condition of the stomach and duodenum. In a series of 4000 necropsies Stewart[5] encountered chronic gastric ulcer in 2.23 per cent of cases and chronic duodenal ulcer in 3.83 per cent — together more than 6 per cent of all cases. The etiology of peptic ulcer is beyond the scope of this paper. Whatever other factors are involved, most clinicians feel that probably a neurogenic factor is present[6], and certainly stress and overwork are important factors in any patient with a known ulcer.

The chronic ulcer of the stomach is curiously selective of its site. Over 80 per cent are located on the lesser curvature and are on the Magenstrasse — that pathway formed by the oblique muscle fibers. The ulcers are usually on the pyloric side of that v-shaped line which separates the acid-producing fundus region from the pyloric region. Less than 10 per cent of gastic ulcers are prepyloric, which is in direct contrast to carcinoma.

In the duodenum, chronic ulcer is almost always in the first portion, the duodenal bulb or pyloric cap, a region continually moistened by acid chyme. The X-ray evidence is distinctive.

The chronic ulcer is usually single, but in 5 to 10 per cent of cases it may be multiple. It has a punched-out appearance with abrupt, funnel-shaped, or terraced walls. The wall on the proximal side tends to be abrupt, that distally is usually terraced. The floor is hard and indurated. The duodenal ulcer has a similar appearance, but is often smaller.

Histologically, the usual ulcer presents a hyperplastic, piled-up mucosa at the edge, with the base composed of dense, cicatricial tissue. Endarteritis and periarteritis are common. Many inflammatory cells are seen. Granulation tissue lines the edges, and extends toward the base. If healing takes place, the granulation tissue thickens and fills in the depressed, indurated base. The mucosa gradually grows out from the edges. At first it is composed of a single layer of flat or cuboidal cells, which later become tall columnar. If too much tissue destruction has not taken place, a healed gastric ulcer may leave little scar at the former site. However, duodenal ulcers leave an easily recognizable and often deforming scar. Healing seems to depend upon the degree of protection from the gastric secretions.

The common complications of chronic ulcer are perforation, hemorrhage, and cicatricial contraction, resulting in disturbed peristalsis or obstruction. Perforation is the natural termination of the ulcer which continues to enlarge unchecked. It is more common in those ulcers presenting symptoms for only a few days. Those ulcers with continuous symptoms will perforate oftener than the remittent type. If the perforation is near one of the neighboring organs, adhesions form and generalized peritonitis may not result. As the usual ulcer is on the posterior wall of the stomach the liver or pancreas are the common organs involved. In the pancreas an indurated mass may be formed, but in the liver necrosis and abscess formation are more apt to form. The duodenal ulcer is more likely to perforate and to give rise to a generalized peritonitis.

Hemorrhage is the most frequent complication of chronic peptic ulcer. There are few ulcers in which occult blood cannot be found in the stool. Although usually a mere oozing, the hemorrhage may be severe or event fatal. In the stomach, severe hemorrhage is often from an ulcer astride the greater curvature. In the duodenum, on the other hand, hemorrhage is usually from an ulcer on the posterior wall, where the arteries lie.

Scarring is a late effect of all ulcers. Near the pylorus, a chronic ulcer may cause a pyloric stenosis. On the lesser curvature it causes the "hour-glass" stomach. Always there is a disturbance of motility at the level of the lesion, which may be seen on fluoroscopy.

Two conditions which may mimic peptic ulcer are chronic follicular gastritis and chronic duodenitis. In the first, there is a patchy thickening of areas of the wall of the pyloric region, covered by a shiny mucus. Clefts may but through the mucosa and reach the vessels of the submucosa, so that hemorrhage results. There is always thickening of the muscular coat. The etiology is unknown. It is best diagnosed by gastroscopy. In the chronic state the thickened areas develop polypoid processes — gastritis polyposis. In duodenitis, as Judd pointed out, there is congestion and often pinpoint mucosal ulcers stipple the duodenal mucosa. Histologically, the mucosa is usually intact but many inflammatory cells are seen in the tunica propria and submucosa. If the inflammation is extensive, scarring may result.

Carcinoma of the stomach is still probably the most common malignancy in the male. In the female it is less common than carcinoma of the cervix uteri and of the mammary gland. Most commonly the onset is in the sixth decade, but it may develop as early as the second or third. Sixty per cent of carcinomas and ten per cent of ulcers are in the prepyloric region. Any ulcer in the prepyloric region, therefore, should be regarded as a malignant lesion until proven benign..

Histologically, almost all carcinomas of the stomach are columnar cell carconomas. The more anaplastic types will usually contain fields where columnar cells forming acino-tubular structures may be seen.

A satisfactory classification is one based on gross morphology. We may divide the carcinomas into the fungating, the ulcerating, and the infiltrating types of carcinoma.

In the fungating, papillary or polypoid type the tumor forms a large, usually rather soft mass which projects into the lumen. Unfortunately it gives little distress until ulceration takes place, unless it obstructs the lumen. When ulcerated and infected the classical symptom complex of cachexia, hemorrhage and anemia appear. By this time metastases regionally and distally have usually made the prognosis very grave. In this variety the carcinoma is columnar cell, with well defined glandular structures. As would be expected from its histologic maturity, early surgical intervention is rather successful, because it does not metastasize as early as the more undifferentiated types.

One variety of the fungating carcinoma is the so-called gelatinous or mucinous carcinoma. The slimy gross appearance and the many signet-ring cells microscopically distinguish it from other well-differentiated carcinomas. Probably five per cent of all carcinomas of the stomach are of this kind, and the prognosis is that of the fungating type in general.

The type in which ulceration is an early and predominating characteristic is almost always prepyloric. This is the most usual kind of carcinoma. The edges of the crater are raised and rounded. Usually the crater of an ulcerating carcinoma is larger than that of a chronic peptic ulcer. McCarty's dictum that any ulcer over 2 cm. in diameter is probably a malignancy is still fairly safe in spite of exceptions. The histologic picture varies, but usually the cells are more anaplastic, with a tendency to form solid sheets or columns. The fibrous stroma varies and may be very dense, forming a "scirrhous" carcinoma. In the same preparation one may see areas of columnar cell carcinoma with well-formed or atypical acino-tubular structures, the signet-ring cells of mucinous carcinoma and the nests and cords of anaplastic, undifferentiated or "spheroidal-cell" carcinoma. The submucous and muscular coats are extensively infiltrated. Metastases are usually earlier and more extensive.

The infiltrating type presents no mass, and may not ulcerate. Instead, there is infiltration and induration of the stomach wall, local or diffuse. The local form is usually at the pylorus, where a dense ring of hard tissue forms and causes an intense stenosis with obstruction and dilation of the stomach. The diffuse form, the "leather-bottle stomach" or "linitis plastica" is of interest because while usually carcinomatous it is possibly not always so. In this condition varying amounts of epithelial cells or cell nests are seen in a very dense fibrous connective tissue stroma. Many sections from various parts may need examination before the neoplastic nature of the lesion can be ascertained. It is an interesting example of the desmoplastic power of a carcinoma. This type is of limited malignancy, for the carcinoma has been partly "smothered out" by the fibrous tissue reaction it has evoked. Metastases other than regional are rather rare, and death is usually from disturbed function.

It may be of interest to consider the manner of spread of gastric carcinoma. Local infiltration is such that tumor cells are usually found 1 to 2 cm. beyond the visible limits of growth. Usually the regional lymph nodes are next involved, then the liver, and pancreas, and frequently the omentum. The aortic and superior illiac lymph glands are involved, and those of the root of the mesentery. "Drop metastases" seed the peritoneal cavity, and account for the frequent peritoneal and ovarian metastases, the so-called Krukenberg tumor of the ovaries, and for Blumer's shelf. It is late when, by way of the thoracic duct, Virchow's node is involved. Blood spread is less frequent, but lungs, brain, and bone may be involved by this method.

Carcinoma of the duodenum is rare, and many of the reported cases have probably originated in the bile ducts or pancreatic ducts.

A few benign tumors of the stomach and duodenum should be mentioned. Leio-myomas, fibromas, fibroadenomas, lipomas and hemangiomas have been reported.[7] Symptoms vary with the amount of obstruction produced. Sarcomas constitute about one per cent of all gastric malignancies. Myosarcoma is most common, and often in young patients. The external forms are almost asymptomatic until late, when metastases draw attention to the condition. If inside the stomach wall, ulceration may occur and the symptoms resemble those of carcinoma.

The stomach and duodenum may be involved early in Hodgkin's disease, lymphosarcoma, or the leukemias. Symptoms may be very puzzling until other involvement is recognized.

This data briefly presented may serve to recall these conditions to mind, and to re-emphasize that the knowledge of the fundamental nature of disease is the only rational basis for diagnosis and treatment. Otherwise we descend to the level of the empirical or "cook-book" school of practice and lose most of the enjoyment of the practice of medicine.

BIBLIOGRAPHY

1   Cannon, Paul R. and Halpert, Bela: Congenital Stenosis of the Third Portion of the Duodenum with Acute Occlusion and Rupture of the Stomach. Arch. Path. 8, pp. 611-622, 1929.
2.   Weinberg, J.: Diaphragmatic Hernia, collective review Surg. Gynec. and Obst. Vol. 72, pp. 445-458, 1941.
3.   Halpert, Bela: Arteriomesenteric Occlusion of the Duodenum; An anatomical study. John Hopkins Hospital Bulletin, Vol. 38, pp. 400-422, 1926.
4   Spriggs, E. I. and Marxer, O.: Intestinal Diverticula, Quarterly Journal Medicine, Vol. 19, pp. 1-32, 1925.
5.   Hurst, A F. and Stewart, M J.: Gastric and Duodenal ulcers. Oxford University Press, London, 1929.
6.   Cushing, H.: Peptic ulcers and the Interbrain, Surg., Gynec. and Obst., Vol. 55, pp. 1-34, 1932.
7.   Eliason, E. L. and Wright, V. W. M.: Benign tumors of the stomach, Surg., Gynec. and Obst., Vol 41, pp. 461-472, 1925.

Surgical Treatment of Intestinal Obstruction *
Pre-Operative Preparation

J. H. ROBINSON, M.D.
OKLAHOMA CITY, OKLAHOMA

REPLACEMENT OF FLUIDS
After a diagnosis of intestinal obstruction has been made, preparation for operation is usually the next step. One of the first steps is to bring up the fluid balance. The patient is usually dehydrated from a reduced intake, sometimes over a period of several days, and a stepped-up output because of pain, nervousness, and often vomiting. Patients are invariably low in chlorides, therefore saline administration serves the dual purpose of water and chlorides.

Glucose in saline intravenously serves an additional purpose in furnishing nourishment. Where large quantities of fluid are required, 10 per cent glucose intravenously is recommended while at the same time normal saline is being given by hypodermoclysis.

*Read before the Oklahoma City Clinical Society at Oklahoma City, November 27, 1945.

If time permits, adequate preparation with 2,000 cc. each of saline and glucose in saline can easily be given within a 12 hour period. A nitrogen balance can also be improved by using amino-acids mixed with the saline and given intravenously. This can also be achieved through the use of plasma during the same 12 hour period.

Deflation is imperative and can be achieved by use of nasal suction while the fluids are running. By nasal suction the upper portion of the intestinal tract can be relieved of its contents and the existing pressure, thus adding to the comfort of the patient, and making the operation more acceptable to the patient.

The lower bowel must be emptied. This is done best by use of enemas and the colon tube. Enterostomy may be beneficial also in

a small per centage of the cases but this relieves only a small section of the intestinal
tract. Especially is it to be considered in a
small percentage of cases which have been
obstructed and distended a long period of
time.

Pain can best be relieved by use of opiates.
Preferably pantapon, or a mixture of morphine and scopalamine in the form of the
well-known H.M.C. If the patient is only un-
comfortable, sodium luminal is a good selection. If the patient's condition does not demand prompt operation, great improvement
may be expected within six to twelve hours,
even 24 hours of treatment is advantageous
in many a case.

The first step in the surgical management
of intestinal obstruction lies in the preparation. This is vitally important to the success of the second step which is the operation itself. At the time of operation we must
consider the anesthetic. Today I would select
a gas anesthetic of cyclopropane with the
added use of intocostrin intravenously at the
time of making the incision. Many would prefer a spinal anesthetic, which, of course,
would serve well in a large percentage of
cases. Given a patient in good general condition there are many anesthetic agents acceptable. Many of these obstructed patients are
in critical condition with shock, low blood
pressure, toxemia and exhaustion. A gas anesthetic by the endottachial method gives
adequate relaxation and has the advantage of
free use of oxygen and carbondioxide, as well
as the privilege of discontinuing the anesthetic agent at any time.

Fluids, such as were given during the preoperative period should be given the patient
intravenously while the operation is in progress. I believe it is generally agreed that a
patient expends about 1000 ccs. of fluid by
way of respiration, skin and kidneys during
a major operation lasting about an hour. This
amount can easily be given intravenously
during the operation. This is an excellent
way of preventing shock.

As the incision is made the surgeon has
for his aim a direct attack upon the obstructive mechanism. A one-stage operation
should be the aim. Here is where it is advantageous to have a well prepared patient.
When obstructing adhesions are found and
divided one should use ligatures freely to
make sure bleeding doesn't develop later. A
raw surface on the wall of a bowel many
times justifies the use of an autogenous fatty
patch to prevent this surface from re-attach-
ing elsewhere. This fat may be easily obtained from the omentum or subcutaneous fat.
When obstruction is due to involvement of
the bowel wall in an inflammatory process,

it is often advisable to anastomose around
the obstruction and leave the obstructed loop
rather than attempt removal with the danger of spreading the infection. When the pathology is exposed and a one-step operation
seems to be too much surgery for the patient
to tolerate or endure, some type of exteriza-
tion should be elected. In this event drainage
can be done and anastomosis done later. This
should be as close to the point of obstruction
as possible and leakage must not occur into
the operative fields.

ENTEROSTOMY

When obstruction of the small bowel has
prevailed a fairly long time and distention
exists, enterostomy is advisable in a fairly
large percentage of cases. This is done to relieve distention, drain off material which has
been held back, and relieve pressure upon
the damaged gut. The material which has
accumulated proximal to the point of obstruction is very septic and causes the patient to
become very toxic when it reaches the colon.
To drain this off makes for a much smoother
convalescence in the postoperative period.

A severe toxic psychosis may be avoided
by draining this material off. This should be
done proximal to the point of obstruction but
very close to it. A Witzel type of enterostomy
is an excellent method where it is not considered necessary to deviate the entire fecal
stream. This is done by fixing a catheter into
the bowel, pointing it downward and suturing it into a fold in the wall of the bowel
made lengthwise. Appendicostomy serves this
purpose well if the obstruction is in the first
half of the colon. Bringing a loop of ileum
through the abdominal wall may be necessary in a few severe cases.

The selection of the proper type of suture
material is important. Where suture material is used upon the intestinal tract I almost
invariably use chromic 00 with a swedged-on
needle. The swedged-on needle clips through
with the least possible damage, thereby safeguarding against leaking along the suture
line. In small children chromic five 0 should
be used.

The use of sulfa crystals about any operative field upon the intestinal tract below the
stomach seems helpful in preventing infection. It seems to do no harm. It should be
lightly sprinkled upon the suture line of an
anastomosis as well as upon any raw surface
left in the mesentery where a resection has
been done. The use of a drainage tube is
probably less necessary since sulfa crystals
have come into general use. In case of doubt
as to whether drainage is necessary I prefer
to drain. A soft collapsible rubber drain like
that of the Penrose drain can probably do
no harm, but is more likely to be beneficial.

POSTOPERATIVE CARE

Sedation is necessary. It can best be secured by use of opiates such as pantapon, H.M.C. or codeine. These preparations are far much less likely to cause nausea than morphine. Twenty-four to 48 hours after operation, sodium luminal in four grain doses aids in keeping the patient quiet. It does not relieve pain. When a patient returns from surgery saline and glucose should be started promptly. If the patient shows evidence of shock blood or plasma should be used. For the average sized adult about 3000 to 4000 ccs of fluid should be administered in the first 24 hours following operation. This can be gradually reduced as the patient begins taking liquids by mouth. Sufficient fluid should be given to keep the urinary output above 750 ccs. per each 24 hours period.

Nasal suction should be started promptly after operation. This relieves the stomach of the air accumulated during surgery. In a high per centage of patients there will be no distention if suction is started promptly after operation. This empties the stomach of both air and fluid and prevents it from passing into the duodenum. This, in turn, prevents distention.

AMERICAN COLLEGE
of
CHEST PHYSICIANS
500 North Dearborn Street

Chicago 10, Illinois

Announcement

A Postgraduate Course in Diseases of the Chest will be given under the auspices of the Illinois Chapter of the American College of Chest Physicians at Michael Reese Hospital, Chicago, Illinois, during the week April 1st to 6th, inclusive.

Doctors may elect to follow this week's formal course with practical instruction in the fields of thoracic surgery, bronchoscopy, pneumothorax, bronchography, and other methods and technics in the diagnosis and treatment of pulmonary disease.

Further information may be secured at the office of the American College of Chest Physicians, 500 North Dearborn Street, Chicago 10, Illinois.

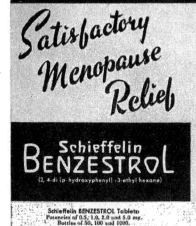

Satisfactory Menopause Relief

Schieffelin
BENZESTROL
(2, 4-di (p-hydroxyphenyl) -3-ethyl hexane)

● Clinical tests have demonstrated that this synthetic estrogen successfully relieves the distressing emotional and vasomotor symptoms comprising the so-called menopausal syndrome.

Its rapid and effective action, as well as the low incidence of untoward side effects, offer the physician a dependable means of administering estrogenic hormone therapy with a high degree of satisfaction.

Literature and Sample on Request.

Schieffelin BENZESTROL Tablets:
Potencies of 0.5, 1.0, 2.0 and 5.0 mg.
Bottles of 50, 100 and 1000.

Schieffelin BENZESTROL Solution:
Potency of 5.0 mg. per cc. In 10 cc.
Rubber Capped Multiple Dose Vials

Schieffelin BENZESTROL Vaginal Tablets:
Potency of 0.5 mg.   Bottles of 100.

Schieffelin & Co.
Pharmaceutical and Research Laboratories
20 COOPER SQUARE • NEW YORK 3, N. Y.

Clinical Pathological Conference

University of Oklahoma School of Medicine

Presented by the Departments of Pathology and Surgery

HARRY WILKINS, M.D.—BELA HALPERT, M.D.

DOCTOR HALPERT: The patient, whose story we are presenting this morning died of an inaccessible and thus an incurable neoplasm of the brain. A few decades ago such a patient would have presented an insoluble diagnostic problem. Today, as the result of tremendous advances in this field of study, it is possible, as a rule, to precisely localize the lesion and, more often than not, to correctly hypothecate as to the histologic characteristics of the neoplasm. In an ever increasing proportion of these cases, temporary alleviation of symptoms or complete cure is obtained. It is an education in itself to study the procedures and to analyze the processes by which a skilled neuro-surgeon elaborates a diagnosis and attacks a problem such as this. Dr. Wilkins will present the clinical aspects of this case.

PROCTOCOL

Patient: T. R. R., while male, age 5; terminal admission April 12, 1945; died April 21, 1945.

Chief Complaint: Vomiting for two months; general malaise for two months; staggering gait for five months; and visual disturbances for five months.

Present Illness: The patient was first admitted on April 12, 1944 with the above complaints. Five months prior to admission he was noticed to stagger, stumble and run into things. Shortly afterward he seemed to lose strength and energy. Three months later he developed high fever and vomiting and was diagnosed as having a urinary infection for which he was given sulfonamides. About the same time as the onset of this illness, it was noted that he had some difficulty in lateral deviation of the eyes.

Past History: Birth and development were normal until the present illness except for the usual childhood diseases and minor injuries.

Family History: Not obtained.

Physical Examination: On admission the patient was slightly depressed and the head was maintained in attitude of slight flexion, slightly deviated to the left. He deviated slightly to the left when walking and would sway to the left on Rhomberg test. Both hands were slightly clumsy, the right more

than the left. There was no apparent defect in the visual fields and no choking of the discs. He was unable to move his eyes laterally but vertical movement was relatively normal. Vertical nystagmus was present. There was a left facial weakness of nuclear or peripheral type. Tests of the remaining cranial nerves were negative. Superficial reflexes were absent. Deep reflexes were decreased in the upper extremities and increased in the lowed extremities. Pathologic reflexes were present in both extremities. No clonus was observed. There was no apparent impairment of cutaneous or deep sensations.

Laboratory Data: On April 13, 1944 the urine contained occasional squamous epithelial cells and rare white blood cells. The blood contained 12 Gm. Hb., 3,610,000 R.B.C. and 4,850 W.B.C./cu.mm. In the absence of pressure signs, lumbar puncture was deemed desirable. Spinal fluid examination on April 15, 1944 revealed no globulin, 15 mg. per cent total protein, 62 mg. per cent sugar; one lymphocyte. Spinal fluid Wassermann reaction and colloidal gold test were negative.

Clinical Course: On April 21, 1944 encephalograms revealed no evidence of block of the ventricular system, but did indicate slight posterior displacement of the floor of the 4th ventricle. These findings being compatible with a pontine tumor, deep x-ray therapy was started. The patient received a total of 1500 R to each of three fields. He improved moderately and was discharged on June 18, 1944 to be followed in the clinic. On October 23, 1944 he was readmitted because of recurrence of symptoms and received another 1500 R to each of three fields. From this he obtained a very satisfactory response and was discharged on November 11, 1944. He was again readmitted on February 16, 1945 because of recurrence of symptoms. Another course of deep x-ray therapy was given and the patient was discharged only moderately improved. He was admitted a fourth time on April 12, 1945 and x-ray therapy was again given. After three treatments his condition became much worse. X-ray therapy was discontinued and hypertonic solutions were given intravenously, as well as stimulants and other supportive measures. His condition became progressively worse; his temperature rose to 106 degrees F. and he expired on April 21, 1945.

DOCTOR WILKINS: It is a pleasure to present one of our cases before this group and I hope that it may be of practical value in illustrating some of the problems that will confront you. We hope to show you some things that you may need to arrive at a diagnosis in cases of this sort. It may seem odd to select a patient for our discussion about whom little can be done. I believe, however, that much can be gained by study of this case as to what can be done in other cases of a somewhat similar nature. Actually this case presents a better study from the students' standpoint than one in which good results were obtained, since we can examine the necropsy report and get precise information as to the type of neoplasm, its extent, etc.

On admission, we considered the possibility of a urinary tract infection as the major lesion. Certainly we can expect a febrile reaction and, when there is toxemia and fever, it is not unusual to experience headache and perhaps other symptoms which may be common also to primary disease of the central nervous system. The instability of posture and gait rather promptly asserted themselves as signs of major importance, however, and directed our attention to the central nervous system. The initial symptom in this case was stumbling. We had thought that the febrile reaction was probable due to cystitis and pyelitis. Now, immediately, with the history of instability dating back some five months, we must turn from this relatively simple initial diagnosis in order to determine the basis for the disturbance in equilibrium. A person in whom such a symptom is of sudden onset usually has a disturbance in the internal ear. The onset was not sudden in this case so that a more logical source of trouble seemed to be the cerebellum. It was considered that involvement need not be limited to the cerebellum, or perhaps the cerebellum proper might be involved at all, but rather the pathways leading to or from the cerebellar nuclei. If we had had no symptom or sign of the nature of unsteadiness to point to the cerebellum we would probably have considered a lesion in the immediate vicinity of the third ventricle. We did not have severe headache and vomiting in this case, however, which would be apt to result from obstruction of the third ventricle, only the unsteadiness. To consider again, for a moment, the obvious infection from which this child suffered, the fact that this infection responded well to sulfonamide therapy, but that, even during this improvement, symptoms relating to the central

nervous system continued to progress, is perhaps the strongest evidence of all that in addition to the infectious process, we were dealing with some more serious, entirely unrelated condition. The difficulty in ocular movements was very important; he often had double vision. Bilateral paralysis of the rectus muscles leads us to consider a lesion in the pons. The headaches of which this patient complained did not appear significant. Similarly, vomiting occured only during the period of sulfonamide therapy, and suggested central vagus irritation rather than increased intracranial pressure. Incidentally, you would be surprised how many people come from their family physician and outlying clinics with a diagnosis of anterior poliomyelitis when their symptoms are exactly these. There is one thing very noticeably missing from the "physical examination" and that is the visualization of the ocular fundi. That, as far as I am concerned is very important. In this patient, the fundi appeared quite normal. There was no indication of increased intracranial pressure. The child was unstable and exhibited various muscular paralyses. The defect in the left side of the face indicated a nuclear or peripheral paralysis which further narrowed the diagnosis to a pontine tumor. In such conditions the disturbances may appear in the motor pathways first. We also observed a loss of superficial reflexes which is a very important point in this case in that it indicates altered function of the corticospinal pathways. Particularly in children, one may observe a loss of muscular tone and hyporeflexia in cerebellar lesions. In such a case, however, superficial reflexes are retained and active. I believe that this pretty well covers the significant things as we saw them. Lesions of the pons do not affect the flow of cerebrospinal fluid as a rule. I am sure that when you encounter this multitude of abnormal neurologic findings, coming on over a period of time, and no increase in intracranial pressure, you have a very good reason to consider the primary lesion to be a tumor in the pons. Sensory changes are notable in their absence. In a five year old child it would be extremely difficult to detect such changes even though they were present.

CLINICAL DISCUSSION

QUESTION: Do you hesitate to do a spinal tap in a patient with a suspected brain tumor when there is absence of choked disc?

DOCTOR WILKINS: No; in the absence of choked discs, you would be justified in doing a spinal tap. This is an important part of a complete examination (unless contraindicated) and you will certainly gain much confidence from the patient and his family if you will explain to them that a thorough examination will often reveal more than an x-ray of the head. Often patients object to examinations other than of the head if it has been suggested that they have "head trouble". In this case we searched about for additional support of our diagnosis of pontine tumor and decided that if we could visualize the 4th ventricle we might find some evidence to support our belief. We did observe a slight posterior displacement of the fourth ventricle. At this time I might add that the only indication for surgical intervention in the case of a pontine tumor is if, due to enlargement of the pons, the subarachnoid pathways for cerebrospinal fluid become obstructed with a resultant increase in cerebrospinal fluid. In such a case we merely enlarge the tentorial notch, providing a new passageway for the fluid. This brings about only palliative relief, but may prolong life for several months.

QUESTION: Is it your opinion that this neoplasm was radio-sensitive?

DOCTOR WILKINS: I believe that in this case there was a definite response to irradiation. I do not know whether or not it was a reaction of the neoplasm itself or of the surrounding tissues. There may be some reduction in the edema of surrounding tissues which will produce a transient benefit. I believe that x-ray in this case prolonged life for about a year.

QUESTION: What was your opinion as to the type of neoplasm present?

DOCTOR WILKINS: Most often neoplasms, in this area, are spongioblastomas. I believe that this was a unipolar spongioblastoma.

ANATOMIC DIAGNOSIS

DOCTOR HALPERT: It was not a pathologist who gave us our present concept of neoplasms of the brain but a surgeon. The classification of primary brain tumors elaborated by Cushing and Bailey is now almost universally used. Going back in the embryologic evolution of the central nervous system, one finds primitive cells which have not as yet decided whether or not they will be nerve cells or glial cells. Neoplasms in which the cell type corresponds to these highly undifferentiated cells are called medulloblastomas. The next stage in differentiation of glial cells is represented by the spongioblasts. Tumors of this origin, spongioblastomas, show a great deal of variation in cellular size and shape. They infiltrate readily and fairly rapidly. Still further along in development are the astrocytes. They provide the supportive structure for the nerve tissue proper. Oligodendroglial cells are next in line. With this very brief and incomplete sketch of the various types of glial tumors and their precursor cells, let's proceed with this particular

case. The tumor which we found represents a type somewhat further differentiated than that which Dr. Wilkins postulated; it was a fibrillary astrocytoma. Its location was as Dr. Wilkins concluded. It lay mostly in the right side of the pons, but had invaded the left side also and had almost obliterated the normal pattern of the pons. There was no marked obstruction to the ventricular system although a cerebellar pressure cone was present and there was some flattening of convolutions. This was a manifestation, in large measure, of edema of the brain substance.

It would be a serious omission if we were to conclude this presentation without laying stress on one of the peculiarities of glial neoplasms, as a group, which is almost unique among malignant neoplasms. It is important to remember that, although such neoplasms invade, infiltrate and destroy nervous tissue *they do not metastasize to tissues outside of the central nervous system.* Although this fact is generally well appreciated, still we encounter, occasionally, a patient in whom visceral metastatic lesions are explained on the basis of primary brain tumor. Such cases do not occur. It must be remembered also that metastatic lesions in the brain from carcinomas make up a considerable proportion of "brain tumors". Those which are particularly apt to metastasize to the brain are: carcinoma of the mammary gland, lung, thyroid gland and kidney. Not infrequently a primary carcinoma of the lung will be of small size and give few or no symptoms pointing to the lung, and yet metastatic lesions in the brain or bone are outspoken.

DISCUSSION

QUESTION: What was the relationship between the last series of x-ray treatments and the rather sudden onset of cerebral edema?

DOCTOR WILKINS: Occasionally irradiation therapy will produce such a temporary change and this may be sufficient in some cases to cause death.

QUESTION: What was the immediate cause of death?

DOCTOR WILKINS: Respiratory failure.

QUESTION: What about the temperature of 106 degrees F. just before death?

DOCTOR WILKINS: Hyperthermia is not infrequent in lesions of the paraventricular area and brain stem proper. In fact any time one encounters hyperthermia of this degree it is most likely the direct effect of some alteration of the temperature regulating mechanism, either from mechanical injury of chemical injury, as in certain marked toxemias.

Special Article

The Tulsa County Medical Clinic

HOMER A. RUPRECHT, M.D.

Chairman, Clinic Committee
Tulsa County Medical Society

TULSA, OKLAHOMA

It is a frequent observation of the medical profession of the United States that most systems of indigent medical care are singularly devoid of system. This lack of system has in turn produced many abuses to the detriment of the doctor, the patient, and the community. Despite good intentioned efforts of government and medical leaders, many large cities and towns of the United States are completely lacking of a workable system whereby adequate medical and hospital care is made available to the indigent sick.

A problem of this character faced the physicians of Tulsa County in the years following the first world war. As the city grew, the burden of the indigent sick tended to increase. It became increasingly difficult for the employed medical personnel of the county health department to render the degree of medical care required by aged chronics and the indigent sick of the County. The Tulsa County Medical Society had long been aware of this problem, but it was not until the establishment of the Society's Executive Offices and the employment of an Executive Secretary in 1938 that facilities were created to adequately cope with the situation. At that time, the medical leaders of the Society succeeded in interesting government and community leaders in the idea of a free clinic staffed by a medical personnel consisting of specialists in all fields of medicine. From the Society's plan was evolved the Tulsa County Medical Clinic, believed to be representative of a modern and workable system of indigent medical care.

The members of the Tulsa County Medical Society had several objectives in creating the Tulsa County Medical Clinic. Foremost among these were:

1. Elimination of indigent medical care from political interference and the abuses of the political administration.
2. Creation of adequate facilities for an indigent medical care program and the concentration of such facilities into a single unit.
3. Reduction of the costs of operating the indigent care program.
4. Provision of facilities for clinical study and investigation by Tulsa physicians.

5. Maintenance of proper supervision of the medical personnel.

The idea of a Society-operated or supervised clinic was first broached during the depression years following 1929. It met with a consistently unfavorable reception and the idea was temporarily dropped. Later, in 1938, when the need was more apparent and acute, the proposals were revived. A special committee created by the Society did much investigative work and early in 1939 presented a workable plan of operation. Many Tulsa civic leaders and the local newspapers were interested in the project and their favorable reception of the idea created a strong support. After months of debate and ironing out operative details, the Board of County Commissioners approved the proposal on August 14, 1939.

The plan of operation of the Tulsa County Medical Clinic, which has remained unchanged in seven years of existence, consisted of several basic points:

1. The Society was to exert a general supervisory influence over the Clinic with details of operation entrusted to a county physician appointed by the Board of County Commissioners from physicians recommended by the Society.
2. The Society was to provide the services of its members without charge for regular clinics in each of the various medical specialties. Each member agreed to donate a certain amount of professional time to the Clinic each month.
3. All expenses of the Clinic were to be borne by the Board of County Commissioners with the exception of certain items to be paid by the Society.
4. Equipment, and the maintenance of equipment, was to be a responsibility of the Society.
5. Patients requiring hospitalization were to be sent to Tulsa hospitals with the cost borne by the Board of County Commissioners.

The Tulsa Welfare Building at 602 South Cheyenne, Tulsa, was selected as the site of the Clinic. The basement and first floor of the large rear addition of the Building were made available. Facilities were created to care for upwards of 2,500 patients monthly. Altogether, about 20 units were provided with diagnostic roms, administrative offices, specialized examination rooms, a dispensary, x-ray and pathological laboratories, and nursing quarters included.

Through the generosity of Mr. Waite Phillips, prominent Tulsa oil executive, the Society received the sum of $6,000.00, which was used in remodeling the quarters for use. Other groups contributed equipment and fixtures to complete the medical facilities.

A regular schedule of daily clinics was set up, enabling physicians to make a maximum use of their individual specialties. Facilities were then available without cost to the indigent sick which the average moderately situated family could not afford from private doctors.

The Tulsa County Medical Clinic opened its doors on Wednesday, November 14, 1939, at which time several hundred visitors inspected the premises. During the first month some 1,500 patients were seen. Costs of operating the county's charity program dropped sharply and it is conservatively estimated that the operation of the Clinic has saved taxpayers the sum of from $30,000.00 to $50,000.00 annually.

Since its opening, the Clinic has been under the capable supervision of Dr. J. J. Billington, county physician. An employed personnel consists of nurses, laboratory technicians, druggists, and clerical workers. Three physicians, including a full-time radiologist and two part-time assistant county physicians, complete the employed staff.

The Clinic has been fortunate in enjoying excellent relationships with the Board of County Commissioners. Such differences as have arisen have been amicably settled through mutual cooperation and understanding.

During the war years the number of patients at the Clinic has declined considerably, a condition due to the full employment program of the defense plants located in Tulsa, and in some measure to the requirements of the Selective Service Act. Since the end of hostilities, there has been a steady upswing in the number of patients handled and it appears that the number of indigents requiring medical attention is increasing. The Tulsa County Medical Society believes that a strong need for the Clinic will continue to exist. The success of the project is assured through the public's acceptance of the Clinic's community value.

So many Tulsa physicians have contributed to the creation and progress of the Clinic that it is not possible to give them credit here, but mention should be made in particu-

lar of the fine work of a few doctors instrumental in the Clinic's inception. These include Dr. A. W. Pigford, Dr. S. C. Shepard, Dr. Henry S. Browne, Dr. A. Ray Wiley, Dr. P. P. Nesbitt, Dr. J. C. Brogden, Dr. George R. Osborn, Dr. Charles H. Haralson, Dr. John F. Gorrell, and many others. To them, and others who have contributed so freely of their time, sincere thanks are due.

CREDIT SERVICE

330 American National Building

Oklahoma City, Oklahoma

(Operators of Medical-Dental Credit Bureau)

We offer a dignified and effective collection service for doctors and hospitals located anywhere in the State. Write for information.

28 YEARS

Experience In Credit and Collection Work

Robt. R. Sesline, Owner and Manager

NEUROLOGICAL HOSPITAL

Twenty-Seventh and The Paseo
Kansas City, Missouri

Modern Hospitalization of Nervous and Mental Illnesses. Alcoholism and Drug Addiction.

THE ROBINSON CLINIC

G. WILSE ROBINSON, M.D.
G. WILSE ROBINSON, Jr., M.D.

Cascara
Petrogalar

REG. U. S. PAT. OFF.

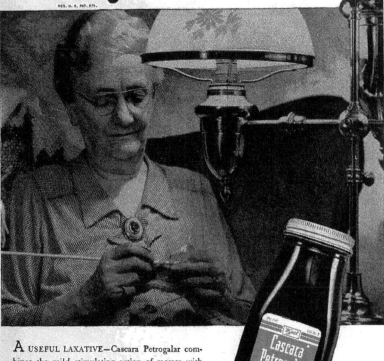

A USEFUL LAXATIVE—Cascara Petrogalar combines the mild stimulating action of cascara with the softening effect of homogenized mineral oil. Prompt, easy evacuation of soft, formed stools is assured without undue strain or discomfort. Especially useful in treating stubborn cases and in elderly persons, its pleasant, dependable action helps to restore "habit time" of bowel movement. CASCARA PETROGALAR—an aqueous suspension of Mineral Oil, 65%, with aqueous extract of Cascara Sagrada, 13.2%.

Supplied in 8 fl. oz. and pint bottles

WYETH INCORPORATED • PHILADELPHIA 3 • PA.

THE PRESIDENT'S PAGE

If we are to meet the demands of the people we serve, we must, as individuals, as well as an organizational unit, give information to the public as to what we expect to offer as a substitute for the program recommended by the National Government. This can only be accomplished by the doctors first acquainting themselves with what the Blue Cross and Physicians Service of our State has to offer and then, from mouth to ear, transmit that information and encourage and work with the administrative force of said organizations to get the service disseminated to every part of our State.

The Blue Cross and Physicians Service will, if properly explained, offset this demand and give us the needed help to forestall national legislation that is being proposed. If there are needed changes in the service to meet the demands of the rural districts, such changes should and must be made.

It is the general opinion of all those interested in this service that it must be offered to the public NOW and not wait for the economic need to exist. Therefore, an additional drive to acquaint the doctors with their responsibility is both just and demanding. The return of the men in service has and will relieve the personnel shortage for the administration of this service. The national health congress, as an aid to the state organizations, should also be encouraged and fostered in every way possible by each state organization and we should remember the old adage: "With complete unity there is strength; individually there can be little done. When there is inactivity of thought or interest there is failure."

President.

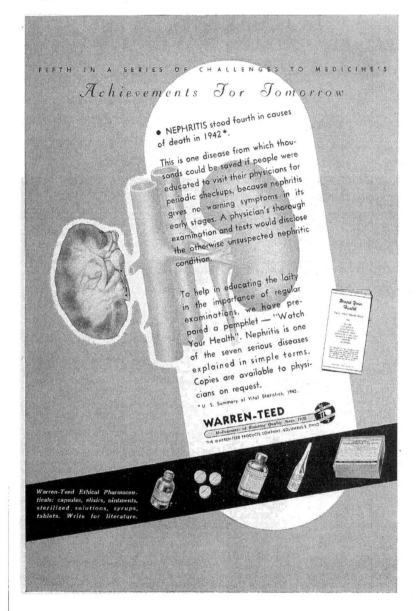

FIFTH IN A SERIES OF CHALLENGES TO MEDICINE'S

Achievements For Tomorrow

• NEPHRITIS stood fourth in causes of death in 1942*.

This is one disease from which thousands could be saved if people were educated to visit their physicians for periodic checkups, because nephritis gives no warning symptoms in its early stages. A physician's thorough examination and tests would disclose the otherwise unsuspected nephritic condition.

To help in educating the laity in the importance of regular examinations, we have prepared a pamphlet — "Watch Your Health". Nephritis is one of the seven serious diseases explained in simple terms. Copies are available to physicians on request.

* U. S. Summary of Vital Statistics, 1942.

WARREN-TEED
Medicaments of Enduring Quality Since 1920
THE WARREN-TEED PRODUCTS COMPANY, COLUMBUS 8, OHIO

Warren-Teed Ethical Pharmaceuticals: capsules, elixirs, ointments, sterilized solutions, syrups, tablets. Write for literature.

The JOURNAL Of The
OKLAHOMA STATE MEDICAL ASSOCIATION

EDITORIAL BOARD
L. J. MOORMAN, Oklahoma City, Editor-in-Chief

E. EUGENE RICE, Shawnee   BEN H. NICHOLSON, Oklahoma City

MR. DICK GRAHAM, Oklahoma City, Business Manager

JANE FIRRELL TUCKER, Editorial Assistant

CONTRIBUTIONS: Articles accepted by this Journal for publication including those read at the annual meetings of the State Association are the sole property of this Journal.

The Editorial Department is not responsible for the opinions expressed in the original articles of contributors.

Manuscripts may be withdrawn by authors for publication elsewhere only upon the approval of the Editorial Board.

MANUSCRIPTS: Manuscripts should be typewritten, double-spaced, on white paper 8½ x 11 inches. The original copy, not the carbon copy, should be submitted.

Footnotes, bibliographies and legends for cuts should be typed on separate sheets in double space. Bibliography listing should follow this order: Name of author, title of article, name of periodical with volume, page and date of publication.

Manuscripts are accepted subject to the usual editorial revisions and with the understanding that they have not been published elsewhere.

NEWS: Local news of interest to the medical profession, changes of address, births, deaths and weddings will be gratefully received.

ADVERTISING: Advertising of articles, drugs or compounds unapproved by the Council on Pharmacy of the A.M.A. will not be accepted. Advertising rates will be supplied on application.

It is suggested that members of the State Association patronize our advertisers in preference to others.

SUBSCRIPTIONS: Failure to receive The Journal should call for immediate notification.

REPRINTS: Reprints of original articles will be supplied at actual cost provided request for them is attached to manuscripts or made in sufficient time before publication. Checks for reprints should be made payable to Industrial Printing Company, Oklahoma City.

Address all communications to THE JOURNAL OF THE OKLAHOMA STATE MEDICAL ASSOCIATION, 210 Plaza Court, Oklahoma City 3

OFFICIAL PUBLICATION OF THE OKLAHOMA STATE MEDICAL ASSOCIATION

Copyrighted February, 1946

EDITORIALS

INQUIRE OF THE DEAD

If the medical great could be called from oblivion for an intimate chat over their coffee, no doubt they would discuss the art and science of medicine, without reference to the political strife and bickering they endured. If the sweepings from their hearts could be sifted they would reveal little of medical economics. Though doctors are now walking with peas in their shoes because of political pressure, they should accept the penance and undauntedly travel on.

When the time comes to check life's till the consciousness of work well done, the knowledge of unselfish response to the needs of life and the well-earned coin of gratitude will mean more than the world's heavy medium of exchange which has no value beyond the last horizon.

In the tradition of good medicine, dealing with the sick, day and night, develops tolerance and long suffering. Those who talk about the patience of Job should remember that Job never tried treating other peoples sores; never experienced the humility that comes through sharing other peoples suffer-

ing. But in medicine, where shadows are found, always there is light.

In the end it is more important to be diligent, efficient, generous, gentle and sympathetic than to gather in the golden quid.

MEDICINE'S SACRED DUTY REGARDING THE VETERANS ADMINISTRATION

In previous issues of the Journal the editorial comment on the reorganization of the Department of Medicine and Surgery in the Veterans Administration has emphasized a long delayed improvement of medical and surgical services to America's worthy veterans. The reorganization planned by General Bradley to be implemented by Major General Paul R. Hawley as Chief Medical Director will replace the previous setup under Civil Service and, of great importance, it will include a plan to associate medical personnel of the Veterans Administration with civilian medical associations and teaching centers.

Of even greater importance to the disabled veteran, the doctor and the people, is the plan to supplement the effort to give the best obtainable service by the appointment of outstanding authorities in specialized medical fields to assist General Hawley in the establishment of the highest possible standards. Also the appointment of medical and surgical specialists as consultants in the thirteen branch areas of the United States.

Through this long approach we have reached the crux of this editorial statement. For once it is agreed that United States civilian medicine is on trial. If the doctors of the thirteen branch areas do not respond to General Hawlay's call with promptness and with a will to give full cooperation in his proposed program for the area, whatever it may be, the case for civilian medicine will be lost and medicine will be open to the severest criticism from political circles and pressure groups because, after all the fuss about government medicine, we fail to measure up to our opportunities and our obligations.

Those who do not know General Hawley and who may wonder what all this is about may rest assured that all recommendations now coming out of the Veterans Administration are motivated by a sincere desire to give the disabled veteran medicine and surgery approximating the best available in civilian practice. This is the publicly avowed policy of General Hawley who bravely declares his medical policies in the face of political opinion whether favorable or unfavorable. It should be stated that civilian doctors will not be requested to work without pay. Those who accept service and conscientiously perform their duties can help carry the banner for civilian medicine.

INTRACARDIAC BLOOD TRANSFUSION

In the December American Review of Soviet Medicine, B. I. Iokhveds reports two cases brought back to life by intracardiac transfusions. The first case was that of a man 34 years of age suffering from infection requiring an operation on the knee joint. Five and a half hours after operation the patient was moribund. After subcutaneous and intravenous cardiovascular stimulants had failed and the cardiac and respiratory functions had ceased, the heart was punctured through the fourth interspace left of the sternum. The inserted needle remained immobile but after one cubic centimeter of one per cent epenephrine was injected there was a slight pulsation of the needle but no breathing or pulse could be detected and blood did not flow from an open vein.

With the needle in position, 250 cc. of citrated blood were injected, followed by 100 cc. of 40 per cent glucose and 250 cc. of physiologic sodium chloride. It is reported that

at the end of the transfusion the pulsation of the needle became stronger and the pulse could be felt in the radial artery. The patient regained color and manifested the normal responses to environment finally becoming conscious but after 21 hours he suddenly grew worse, failed to respond to ordinary stimulants and died.

The second case was that of a Red Army soldier 18 years of age who was dying from loss of blood following the blunt dissection of a large supraclavicular aneurysm due to trauma. When the heart sounds were inaudible and respiration ceased, a needle was introduced about 6 centimeters through the fourth interspace, 3 centimeters to the left of the sternal border, 500 cubic centimeters of normal salt solution were introduced and gradually signs of life returned, 300 cubic centimeters of whole blood were introduced followed by 250 cc. additional saline. During this procedure the subclavian artery was ligated and the hemorrhage did not recur. Later 300 cc. of blood were given intravenously and the patient made an uneventful recovery.

In the first case an autopsy revealed myocardial degeneration which, in all probability, accounted for the death of the patient. In the second case the clinical death was due to profuse hemorrhage, consequently restoration of the body functions led to complete recovery. In the course of the discussion the author states, "It cannot be demonstrated in this case that the injection of blood or saline solution into the right ventrical would have been preferable. It is important, however, that the injection into the left ventrical proved successful and as further observation showed caused no harm. In the available literature we could not find a report on the introduction of fluids into the left rather than the right ventricle."

HEAP BIG MEDICINE MAN

Under the Wagner-Murray-Dingle Bill the Social Security Administrator would carry the responsibility of giving medical, dental, laboratory, hospital and nursing service to 130 million people with the expenditure of approximately four billion dollars.

As though in response to an oracle from the Sibylline Books, the Social Security Administrator would stand forth as did Aesculapius of old. Behold the brave new god in a brave new world. How wonderful to get back to the cloying gods without the confusing clouds of Olympus!

Armed with man-made omnipotence, through powers delegated to otherwise impotent lesser gods including the Surgeon General of Public Health, who could not make an important decision without approval of the beneficent Administrator would prescribe for his people throughout the expanding peripheries of his domain, bringing health to his helpless suppliants shackled by the sheckles snatched from their thrift for the support of his throne. Every individual who learns through loss of freedom that there is no god but the Administrator, should face his mecca, bow down to earth and in sack cloth and ashes confess his bitter faith.

Before this happens every individual wi h a grain of common sense will pray to his own god for protection against such a violation of good government.

WHY WE ARE WHAT WE ARE

Man's life on earth is dependent upon two sets of factors, the hereditary and the environmental. The best he can do is to take what his progenitors provided and get on with his environment the best he can. If he makes three score and ten he is batting high. Regardless of his ability in this respect there is no alternative. At any time during life, what he is and what he does hinges upon these two sets of factors. He begins to die as soon as he is born because many of the environmental factors are unfriendly. He would not last long if it were not for resistant and restorative powers leading to incredible possibilities.

It would be interesting to see how many of the government officials in Washing on who prate about the need of better medical service could pass the induction center examinations. They have been in a position to have the best of medical care, at least they cou'd have the kind they wanted from doctors who certainly could not do better under government control. Obviously these advocates of socialized medicine could not qualify for war because of hereditary defects and the scars of an unfriendly environment, but there is comfort in the fact that the bulk of the world's work has been done by the physically handicapped. The politicians who advocate a change in medical practice may do well to remember the voters are among the important environmental factors which condition their lives.

OUR CREED

O Lord, we thank Thee for all blessings of the past. For the privilege of the present and the prospect of the future. Make us grateful for the bounty Thou has provided and help us share it with the harrassed and hungry throughout the world. Give us strength to meet our obligations with fitting fortitude and help us approach our opportunities with hope and industry. Make us worthy citizens of this great country and militant patrons of good government. Preserve within us the divine gift of personal freedom and the true spirit of democracy as planned by our fathers of old, giving us the right to choose our wives, our work, our church and our doctors — and to say so!

MEDICINE AND LABOR

In the atmosphere of the sacred pact of the present patient-doctor relationship characterized by intimate contact in the doctor's office and at the bedside, it is not uncommon for members of labor unions to admit their thralldom with the stolidity of a plantation mule under the coercion of the whip while enslaved by the halter.

These are the people who make up pressure groups in Washington and ostensibly vote enbloc built up by their unwanted leaders. Already they have lost their freedom to economic groups and against their wills or without their knowledge they vote collectively for national bureaucratic slavery.

Concerning the Fundamental Differences of Contagions

The fundamental differences of all contagions are seen to be three in number those infecting by contact alone, those only by contact and leaving fomites by which they are contagious such as scabies, phthisis, itch baldness, elephantitsia and others of this sort, I call fomites, clothing, screens and other things healthy themselves but apt to conserve the first seeds of infection and to infect through them and then several things which not only by contact, not only by fomites, but which transfer infection at a distance, such as pestilential fevers, and phthisis and certain ophthalmia and other exanthemata, which are called variola and the like. And these are seen to follow a certain rule, those which produce contagion from a distance are accustomed to infect both by fomites and by contact, those which are contagious through fomites are also contagious by contact. At a distance all are not contagious but all are by contact, thus it is most simple that we occupy ourselves with studying first that contagion, which infects solely by contact, and its cause inquiring in what manner it takes place and of what origin soon then studying other questions so that we may see whether there be any character common to all or differing in certain instances and what characteristic each one may have. *The Theory of Infection. Hieronymus Fracastorius Veronensis. Classic Descriptions of Disease. Ralph Major, M.D.*

As a rule, he fights well who has wrongs to redress; but vastly better fights he who, with wrongs as a spur, has also steadily before him a glorious result in prospect, —a result in which he can discern balm for wounds, compensation for valor, remembrance and gratitude in the event of death. *Lew Wallace; Ben Hur.*

In our country and in our times no man is worthy the honored name of statesman who does not include the highest practicable education of the people in all his plans of administration. He may have eloquence, he may have a knowledge of all history, diplomacy, jurisprudence; and by these he might claim, in other countries, the elevated rank of a statesman; but unless he speaks, plans, labors, at all times and in all places, for the culture and edification of the whole people, he is not, he cannot be, an American statesman. *Horace Mann. Lectures and Annual Report on Education.*

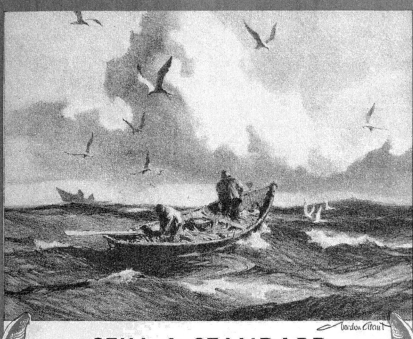

STILL A STANDARD

In appraising the potency and therapeutic value of antirachitic agents, the norm and standard still remains time-honored, time-proved cod liver oil.

Your patients obtain the wholly-natural vitamins A and D of cod liver oil itself when you prescribe any one of the three palatable, convenient dosage forms of

WHITE'S COD LIVER OIL CONCENTRATE

The economy factor of White's Cod Liver Oil Concentrate is important to many patients—*prophylactic antirachitic dosage for infants still costs less than a penny a day.*

3 Forms for your Prescription Convenience:

        LIQUID—for drop dosage to infants

        TABLETS—for youngsters and adults

        CAPSULES—for larger dosage

Ethically promoted—not advertised to the laity. White Laboratories, Inc., Pharmaceutical Manufacturers, Newark 7, N. J.

1946 A.M.A. MEETING IN SAN FRANCISCO JULY 1, 2, 3 AND 4

ASSOCIATION MAY SPONSOR SPECIAL TRAIN

The Board of Trustees of the American Medical Association has announced that the 1946 Session will be held in San Francisco, July 1, 2, 3 and 4. The Convention will revert to pre-war in all respects and it is anticipated that the attendance will rival that of pre-war years.

Dr. V. C. Tisdal, President of the Association has authorized the Executive Secretary to investigate the possibility of promoting a special train from Oklahoma to the Convention. This project is now under discussion with the railroads and every indication points to the possibility that it will be feasible to attempt such an undertaking. The railroads have tentatively committed themselves to being able to take care of a special train with their best rolling stock being made available. A preliminary discussion has indicated that a tour to include the Northwest, with specific stops being made at Crater Lake, Ranier National Park and Yellowstone, can be fitted into a fifteen day tour. Rates for such a tour have not yet been made available and further publicity concerning this activity will be carried in future issues of the Journal and communicated to the individual members of the Association.

ASSOCIATION TO STUDY HOME CARE FOR VETERANS

Dr. V. C. Tisdal, President, will shortly announce the appointment of a Veterans' Affairs Committee to work with the Veterans Administration in incorporating for the State of Oklahoma a plan whereby the individual ex-service man may receive treatment by the physician of his choice for service-connected disability.

Plans of this type are now in operation in the states of Michigan and Kansas and a preliminary discussion has been made by the Executive Office of the Association and Major P. B. Smith of the Veterans Administration.

The program will call for the complete cooperation of the medical profession and will give the profession an opportunity to prove conclusively to the public that it is in a position to meet the demands for medical care without government interference.

O. U. ALUMNI STARTS RESEARCH SURVEY

The O. U. Alumni is inaugurating its initial survey into the feasibility of conducting a campaign to raise approximately $5,000,000.00 for Research in Medicine in Oklahoma.

The survey is being conducted by Mr. Frank Woods of the Marts-Lundy Company, Inc. of New York City. He will be in the various counties of the state for the next eight weeks.

The Alumni Association, as announced in the December Journal, has completed its Councilor District organization with the following alumni acting as Councilor District Representatives: District 1—C. A. Traverse, M.D., Alva; District 2—J. E. Ensey, M.D., Altus; District 3—L. R. Wilhite, M.D., Perkins; District 4—Onis G. Hazel, M.D., Oklahoma City; District 5—Roy Emanuel, M.D., Chickasha; District 6—Ralph McGill, M.D., Tulsa; District 7—John Carson, M.D., Shawnee; District 8—Matt Connell. M.D., Picher; District 9—E. H. Shuller, M.D., McAlester; District 10—P. H. Lawson, M.D., Marietta.

Should any physician know of a person whom he believes would be interested in the Research Program of the Alumni Association, it is requested that he write to the Councilor District Chairman for his District.

HOTEL RESERVATIONS FOR ANNUAL MEETING MUST BE MADE EARLY

The Annual Meeting of the Association which has been announced for May 1, 2, and 3 in Oklahoma City at the Skirvin Hotel is presenting many problems for the committees in charge of the Meeting.

While the problem of food has improved over the previous months, there still remains an acute shortage of hotel reservations.

The Association is working with the Oklahoma City Chamber of Commerce to assure adequate hotel accomodations for the physicians in the leading hotels and it is suggested that those who know that they will be attending the Meeting, make their reservations at the earliest possible date. Reservations may be made direct with the hotel or can be addressed to the office of the Association, 210 Plaza Court, Oklahoma City 3, Oklahoma.

NATIONAL PHYSICIANS COMMITTEE HOLDS ST. LOUIS MEETING

Dr. V. C. Tisdal, President of the Association appointed Dr. James Stevenson, Tulsa; Dr. Floyd Keller, Oklahoma City and Mr. Dick Graham, Executive Secretary, to represent the Oklahoma State Medical Association at a meeting to discuss economic and political problems of the profession at a meeting held by the National Physicians Committee in St. Louis on January 18 and 19.

The National Physicians Committee which has taken a very aggressive attitude toward presenting to the public the problem of medical care is urging that each State Medical Association organize its County Societies and District Groups into well knit and cohesive organizations whereby they may disseminate information to allied groups and the public at large.

Dr. Stevenson and Dr. Keller will appear before the Council of the Oklahoma State Medical Association at its next meeting to make certain recommendations in this field for Oklahoma.

OKLAHOMA HOSPITALS APPROVED BY AMERICAN COLLEGE OF SURGEONS

The following hospitals in Oklahoma were approved by the American College of Surgeons for the year 1945. The approval was based on: modern physical plant; clearly defined organization; carefully selected governing board; competent, well-trained superintendent; adequate and efficient personnel; organized medical staff of ethical, competent physicians and surgeons; adequate diagnostic and therapeutic facilities under competent medical supervision; accurate, complete medical records, readily accessible for research and follow-up; regular group conferences of the administrative staff and medical staff to maintain a high plane of scientific efficiency, and a humanitarian spirit, the primary consideration being the best care of the patient:

Oklahoma City: Bone and Joint Hospital-McBride Clinic; Oklahoma Hospital for Crippled Children; Oklahoma City General Hospital; St. Anthony; University; Wesley.

Tulsa: Hillcrest Memorial; St. Johns.

Ada: Valley View.

Ardmore: Hardy Sanitarium.

Bartlesville: Washington County Memorial.

Claremore: Claremore Hospital.

Clinton: Indian Hospital; Western Oklahoma State Hospital; Western Oklahoma Tuberculosis Sanitarium.

Concho: Indian Hospital.

Cushing: Masonic Hospital.

El Reno: Federal Reformatory Hospital.

Enid: Enid General; St. Mary's; University Hospital Foundation.

Fort Supply: Western Oklahoma Hospital.

Lawton: Kiowa Indian.

McAlester: Albert Pike; St. Mary's.

Muskogee: Muskogee General; Oklahoma Baptist.

Normans Central Oklahoma State Hospital; Ellison Infirmary.
Pawnee: Pawnee-Ponca Hospital.
Ponca City: Ponca City Hospital.
Shawnee: A.C.H. Hospital; Shawnee Indian Sanatorium; Shawnee Municipal Hospital.
Stillwater: Stillwater Municipal Hospital.
Sulphur: Oklahoma State Veterans Hospital.
Tahlequah: William W. Hastings Indian Hospital.
Talihina: Eastern Oklahoma State Tuberculosis Sanatorium; Talihina Indian Hospital.

GUEST SPEAKERS FOR ANNUAL MEETING

Dr. J. H. Robinson, Chairman of the Scientific Work Committee has announced the following Distinguished Guest Speakers who will appear on the various Programs for the Annual Meeting which is to be held May 1, 2 and 3 in Oklahoma City. Other names will be published upon receipt of final acceptance.

Section on Obstetrics and Gynecology—M. Edward Davis, M.D., The University of Chicago, Department of Obstetrics and Gynecology, The Chicago Lying-In Hospital.

Section on Eye, Ear, Nose and Throat—H. Rommel Hildreth, M.D., St. Louis, Missouri.

Section on Neurology, Psychiatry and Endocrinology —George B. Fletcher, M.D., Hot Springs, Arkansas.

Section on Public Health—J. E. Moore, M.D., Baltimore, Md. H. E. Hilleboe, Medical Director, Chief Tuberculosis Control Division, U.S.P.H.S.

Section on Urology and Syphilology—A. I. Folsom, M.D., Dallas, Texas.

DR. WANN LANGSTON APPOINTED TEMPORARY DEAN OF MEDICAL SCHOOL

Dr. Wann Langston was appointed Temporary Dean of the University of Oklahoma School of Medicine December 11, 1945 by Dr. George L. Cross, President of the University.

Dr. Langston graduated from the University of Oklahoma School of Medicine in 1916, but even before his graduation was instructor in pathology and clinical microscopy. In 1917 he was made associate professor of pathology and clinical microscopy, and was officially appointed director of the laboratory, a position which he had filled without official recognition in the preceding year.

In the years 1918-19, Dr. Langston served with the Army, nine months of his service being overseas. After the Armistice, he was a member of the faculty and organizer of the Department of Bacteriology at the A.E.F. University at Beaune, France.

He again became associated with the School and Hospitals as Associate Professor of Clinical Pathology

and Medical Superintendent in 1920. In 1924 and 1925, Dr. Langston studied in Europe. In 1929 he was appointed Executive Assistant to the Dean and Superintendent of the Hospitals, and was Acting Dean in the absence of Dr. Long. Later his title was changed to Administrative Officer. He resigned this position in 1931 and was given the rank of Professor of Clinical Medicine and Director of the Outpatient Department. In 1944 he become Professor of Medicine and Chairman of the Department of Medicine.

Dr. Langston is a member of the American Medical Association and of the County and State Societies. He is a Fellow in the American College of Physicians and a Diplomate of the American Board of Internal Medicine.

POSTGRATUATE COURSE IN SURGICAL DIAGNOSIS TO START NEW CIRCUIT MARCH 18

The Committee on Postgraduate Medical Teaching wishes to report that the postgraduate course in Surgical Diagnosis is progressing satisfactorily. The course will begin in the 7th Circuit on March 18, 1946. This Circuit includes Enid, Fairview, Alva, Woodward and Guymon.

Physicians receiving the course in Surgical Diagnosis which is being given by Dr. Patrick Wu, are definitely enthusiastic. Doctor Wu is a very good speaker, is diplomatic, has the latest information in general surgery at his finger tips and attempts to make each lecture better that the preceding one and each circuit better than the preceding circuit.

Doctors in the 7th Circuit are urged to register for this course promptly.

BLOOD PLASMA TO BE MADE AVAILABLE TO HOSPITALS AND PHYSICIANS

Dr. Grady F. Mathews has announced that, through the cooperation of the American Red Cross, blood plasma will be placed in all approved hospitals and emergency centers such as the highway patrol stations, with a reserve supply being maintained at the Public Health Department at all times.

This blood plasma is being made available to the profession through the Plasma Program of the American Red Cross and physicians who utilize the plasma will be allowed to charge for its administration but not for the plasma itself. For the first quarter of 1946 there will be made available in Oklahoma approximately 5,000 units, running from 250 cc to 500 cc packages.

Physicians who are in need of plasma in treatment should contact the hospitals in which they practice. In rural areas where a physician finds it impractical to

WILLIAM E. EASTLAND, M.D.
F. A. C. R.

RADIUM AND X-RAY THERAPY
DERMATOLOGY

405 Medical Arts Bldg.

Oklahoma City, Oklahoma   Phone 3-1446

LIBRARY OF THE
COLLEGE OF PHYSICIANS

work through a hospital he may write direct to the Department of Health for information as to the best method of securing a supply.

All blood plasma packages will have plainly marked upon them that the contents of the package is gratis to the patient. Upon the issuance of the plasma, hospitals and physicians will be required to sign a receipt. The names of patients upon whom the plasma is used will be reported to the Department of Health.

Further details regarding the plan outlined above will be published at a later date.

REPORT OF THE MEDICAL ADVISORY COMMITTEE TO PUBLIC WELFARE DEPARTMENT

Meetings of the Medical Advisory Committee continue to be held quarterly. Review of new cases and those in which the county has some question as to incapacity continue to be the primary function of the Committee. At the present time consideration is being given to ways in which the Committee can assist the Department in securing treatment for patients as recommended. The personnel of the Committee at present is as follows: Dr. Mack I. Shanholtz, Chairman; Dr. Roy E. Emanuel, Dr. Hugh M. Galbraith, Dr. Joseph W. Kelso, and Dr. Walker Morledge.

The Committee continues to find the physicians co-operative in making examinations of aid to dependent children. The Committee recognizes that it would have been unable to function without the assistance of physicians over the State who were interested in making adequate reports of their examinations of persons who were applying for assistance.

At the time the Committee was organized the primary purpose was to assist in securing more adequate medical reports. This has been accomplished and at this time it seems we need to consider ways in which we can assist in developing plans which will make treatment available to individuals who are interested in following through on the physician's recommendations.

A statistical analysis of the work done in 1945 is submitted.

For the period January 1, 1945 to December 31, 1945.

1. Cases pending January 1, 1945   163
2. Cases referred to M.A.C.
   A. Applications   1152
   B. Cases receiving assistance   392
      1. Review examination requested
         by county department   81
      2. Reexamination requested by
         M.A.C. in previous review   311
   C. Hearings   5
3. Total cases under consideration   1712
4. Cases disposed of since last report   1547
   A. Review of M.A.C. completed   1513
      1. Disabled because of physical
         or mental incapacity   1396
      2. Able to engage in any normal
         physical activity   117
5. Cases pending, December 31, 1945   163

From this it is seen that 1152 new cases were submitted with 392 cases referred by the county as there was some question concerning whether or not the patient was incapacitated. A total of 1513 cases were reviewed by the Medical Advisory Committee during the year, of which 1396 were found to be incapacitated.

Following a physical reexamination the Medical Advisory Committee decided that one of the five cases studied for a hearing was incapacitated to the extent that his children were deprived of parental support and this case was reopened. Two of the cases were denied and two are still pending further medical information.

During the year 1945 a total of $4,497.50 for examinations and laboratory fees was paid 415 physicians. Transportation in connection with examinations to de-

termine eligibility amounted to approximately $273.60 for the calendar year.

A sample of 169 cases which had been reviewed by the Medical Advisory Committee were studied to determine the kind of treatment recommended and if the suggestion made had been followed. Treatment was suggested in 127 cases; examining physicians had made recommendations in 119 of the cases and in 8 the Medical Advisory Committee had recommended treatment. The following tables indicate the types of treatment, the way in which it was secured and the reasons treatment was not available.

Table No. 1—Type of treatment recommended for patient by whether or not treatment was provided

Type of Treatment Recommended	Total	Provided	Not Provided	Un-known
Total	127	49	73	5
Medicine	35	20	14	1
Physician's services	19	8	11	0
Surgery	16	4	11	1
Hospitalization	20	7	13	0
Rest	13	6	5	2
Diet	17	3	14	0
Appliances	1	1	0	0
Other	6	0	5	1

Table No. 2—Number of cases where treatment was provided by source of treatment.

Source of Treatment	Number
Total	49
Cost included in assistance plan	17
Hospitalization	10
Private Physician	10
Public health physicians	2
County commissioners	2
At home (rest)	6
Indian Agency	2

Table No. 3—Number of cases where treatment was not provided by reason treatment not provided

Reason treatment not provided	Number
Total	73
Facility not available	8
No funds available	22
Plans initiated but not completed	6
Patient refused	9
Agency made no plan	21
Unknown	7

Medical services and cost of hospitalization cannot be paid by the State agency; therefore, in those instances where individuals were able to secure physician's services or hospitalization in most instances this was free service or other interested individuals made arrangements to provide this care. The seventeen cases in which Public Assistance funds were used to provide treatment included only those in which special diet or medicine recommended by the physician were secured since these items may be included in the assistance plan. This fact is one of the difficulties in securing treatment as recommended and at the present time the assistance payments are not adequate to meet all of an individual's needs.

In a sample of the cases studied to determine whether or not treatment had been secured it was found that the average monthly unmet need per family was $48.08. According to the agency records, 61 per cent of the families receiving aid to dependent children on this basis of physical incapacity have no income other than assistance. The remaining 39 per cent have an average income of $14.60 per month. Thus the limited payment available to individuals with the limited hospital facilities in certain areas of the State may be a factor in less than one half of the patients receiving treatment for conditions which limit their activity to the extent they are unable to provide for their children.

Your 3 choices when treating diabetics...

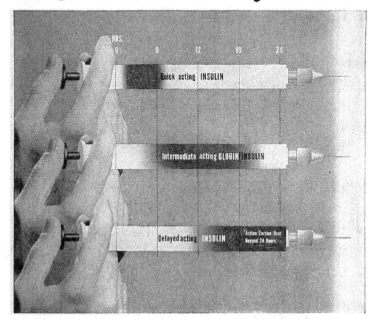

WHEN A PHYSICIAN decides that a patient needs more than diet to control diabetes, he can now choose from three types of insulin. One is quick-acting and short-lived. Another is slow-acting and prolonged. Intermediate between these, is the third—the new 'Wellcome' Globin Insulin with Zinc. Its action begins with moderate promptness yet is sustained for sixteen or more hours—adequate to cover the period of maximum carbohydrate ingestion. By night, activity is sufficiently diminished to decrease the likelihood of nocturnal reactions. Physicians who consider the many advantages of this new third type of insulin now have another effective method of treating diabetes.

'Wellcome' Globin Insulin with Zinc is a clear solution, comparable to regular insulin in its relative freedom from allergenic properties. Accepted by the Council on Pharmacy and Chemistry, American Medical Association. Developed in the Wellcome Research Laboratories, Tuckahoe, New York. U. S. Patent No. 2,161,198. Available in vials of 10 cc., 80 units in 1 cc., and vials of 10 cc., 40 units in 1 cc. Literature on request. 'Wellcome' trademark registered.

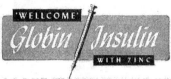

'WELLCOME'
Globin Insulin
WITH ZINC

BURROUGHS WELLCOME & CO. (U.S.A.) INC., 9 & 11 EAST 41ST STREET, NEW YORK 17, N.Y.

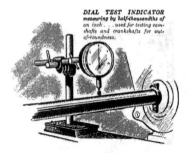

DIAL TEST INDICATOR measuring by half-thousandths of an inch . . . used for testing camshafts and crankshafts for out-of-roundness.

WHEN IT'S *Precision*

YOU REQUIRE . . .

FOR the treatment of pernicious anemia, medical science has found a specific in liver therapy.

But like the highly sensitive dial test indicator which measures within .0005 inch, liver extract—to give precise results—must be manufactured with the utmost care.

. . . And nothing less than precision will meet the requirements of the competent physician.

For these requirements, Purified Solution of Liver, Smith-Dorsey, deserves your confidence.

Its uniform purity and potency are traceable to the conditions under which it is produced—to the capably staffed laboratories, the modern facilities, the rigidly standardized testing procedure.

You may be assured of *precision* in liver therapy when you use

PURIFIED SOLUTION OF *Liver*

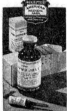

Supplied in the following dosage forms: 1 cc. ampoules and 10 cc. and 30 cc. ampoule vials, each containing 10 U.S.P. Injectable Units per cc.

THE SMITH-DORSEY COMPANY
Lincoln, Nebraska

Manufacturers of Pharmaceuticals to the Medical Profession Since 1908

Book Reviews

HYPERTENSION. A Manual for Patients With High Blood Pressure. Fourth Printing. Irvine H. Page, A. B., M. D., Charles C. Thomas, Springfield, Ill. $1.50. 80 pages. 1944.

A modest preface explains the origin of this helpful monograph prepared for patients suffering from high blood pressure. The next step is to state the purposes of the book. First, to explain the various examinations; second, to show what is meant by high blood pressure; and third, what can be done about it.

With these objectives in mind the author clearly presents the diagnostic methods usually employed in plain words and easy style so the patient may grasp the meaning of each procedure. The significance of the findings are discussed in such a way as to stay the fears which might otherwise arise or to allay fear and anxiety already present.

In the chapter dealing with the disease the author defines the words most commonly employed by the doctor when talking to patient and gives pictures and descriptions of blood vessels. Naturally the reviewer wonders if the patient can profitably make use of such knowledge. The description of malignant hypertension seems unwarranted for the average patient, also there is a discussion of surgical treatment and of kidney extract. While the book has its good qualities, the experienced doctor may find it easier to convey to the individual patient all needed knowledge rather than answer all the questions and allay the anxiety which the book may inspire.—Lewis J. Moorman, M.D.

CLASSIC DESCRIPTIONS OF DISEASE. Ralph M. Major, M.D., Professor of Medicine, University of Kansas School of Medicine. Beautifully printed, finely bound, 195 authors, 287 selections. 158 illustrations. Price $6.50. Charles C. Thomas, Publisher, Springfield, Ill. 1945.

The third edition of this treasure book of medical history should be in every doctor's library. The first and second editions are among our rare possessions and sell at a sizeable premium when made available. How can doctors hope to rise above the common level, unless they associate with those who have made the ascent?

Biographically Ralph Major brings the great men of medicine and their outstanding accomplishments to the bedside of every doctor who thinks enough of his own rating to purchase this valuable book.

When the candle burns low and the shadows baffle sleepy eyes, it is good to drop off, with the words of Hippocrates, Galen, Sylvius, Hunter, Sydenham, Louis, Laennec or Osler lingering in the subconscious minds. To those who know something of the past in medicine, the present is always brighter and better.

A sincere vote of thanks to Ralph Major for making this past so readily available to inquiring minds.—Lewis J. Moorman, M.D.

THE PHYSICIAN'S BUSINESS. Second Edition. George D. Wold, M.D., Assistant Clinical Professor of Otolaryngology, New York Medical College, Attending Laryngologist Sydeham Hospital, New York City; Fillon New York Academy of Medicine; Fellow American Medical Association. 384 pages, 57 illustrations. Price $5.00.

This book is valuable for either the general practitioner or the specialist. It is especially valuable for the physician starting practice, because it covers a subject not included in the regular medical curriculum of the usual medical school. This work begins with the completion of the medical course.

Chapter I gives some good information concerning hospital internship; choice of hospitals and the methods of appointment. Also discussions on the type of internships relative to the anticipated type of practice.

Chapters 2, 3 and 4 explain the various types of medical careers other than private practice giving the advantages, as well as the disadvantages. There is a discussion on specialization; reasons for specialization with comparative incomes and locations for specialists. A free discussion on the choice of location for the physician, giving advantages as well as the disadvantages with reference to the type of work he is interested in and the choice of a location for the physicians office giving advantages and disadvantages of various locations for various types of practice.

Chapter 5 contains a free discussion on ethics of professional contacts, explaining the physicians conduct with patrons, with colleagues and with the public. Explanation of affiliation with hospitals and dispensary is given and a choice of institutions and the attitude toward personnel.

Chapter 6 deals with the physician and his patient. Demonstrations of types of record forms for case histories; case records and financial accounts, how they should be used for the physicians convenience with the conservation of time for the physician. I am particularly impressed with the simplicity of the forms that are illustrated, also the discussion on fees with methods of collections are quite valuable.

Chapters 7 and 8 are on planning and equipping an office. Illustrations of plans for the greatest amount of convenience and conservation of time for both the physician and the specialist. Suggestions on equipment and how to acquire same; a good working equipment with suggestions as to the selecting of proper instruments with instructions in care and preservation.

This work also gives valuable information on forensic medicine; how to avoid law suits, physicians as witnesses in court, and definitions of expert testimony.

In a Chapter on Income tax there is a listing of exemptions and what is taxable and deductions are thoroughly discussed.

There is a good discussion on the present trends in medicine with the different forms of state medicine both local and foreign, with the various plans for Health Insurance. The merits and demerits of which are fully presented. The final chapter is an explanation of the present Workman's Compensation Laws and how they operate in various states.

The physicians business supplies a need for a manual in medical economics.—Morris Smith, M.D.

MY SECOND LIFE, AN AUTOBIOGRAPHY. Thomas Hall Shastid, M.D. George Wahr, publisher, Ann Arbor, Michigan. 1945. 1000 pages, Price $10.00.

Rarely is one privileged to review a book so formidable in appearance, that proves to be, throughout, so genuinely, entertainly and interestingly true. Having been born in Pike County, Illinois, which is the scene of this author's narrative, and with a grandfather and father both of whom began the practice of medicine in the same county, this book has a fascinating interest. Moreover, we were privileged to know, personally, most of the places described and many of the characters and anecdotes.

Stories of the early development of that part of Illinois and of the practice of medicine at that time, which my grandfather and father told me nearly half a century ago are brought back vividly in this narrative.

The life of a hardy frontier people, struggling against physical hardships, lack of educational facilities, lawlessness, law enforcement, superstition, ignorance, family devotion, tragedy and humor, history as it was being made in Western Illinois—all are woven into this autobiography. It depicts lives of men of medicine who, because of their inherent worth and indomitable courage, rose to high places over apparently unsurmountable obstacles. Examples of these are Dr. John T. Hodgen,

VON WEDEL CLINIC

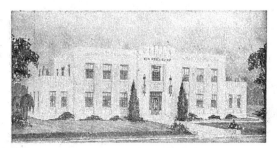

PLASTIC and GENERAL SURGERY
Dr. Curt von Wedel

TRAUMATIC and INDUSTRIAL
SURGERY
Dr. Clarence A. Gallagher

INTERNAL MEDICINE and DIAGNOSIS
Dr. Harry A. Daniels

Special attention to cardiac and gastro
intestinal diseases

Complete laboratory and X-ray facilities.
Electrocardiograph.

610 Northwest Ninth Street
Opposite St. Anthony's Hospital
Oklahoma City

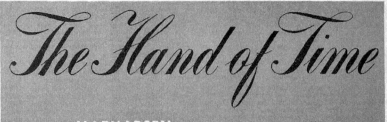

The Hand of Time

MAPHARSEN now entering its thirteenth year of active clinical use, has assumed a leading role among arsenical antisyphilitics. More than 150,000,000 doses of MAPHARSEN have been used clinically during the past five years with a minimum of reaction and maximum of therapeutic effect.

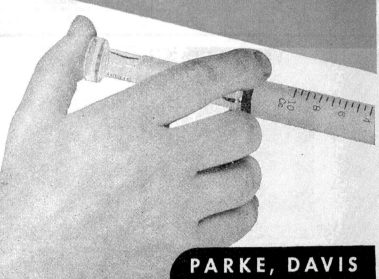

PARKE, DAVIS & COMPANY

and MAPHARSEN

United States Navy records[1] consistently show the relatively low toxicity of MAPHARSEN. Over the ten-year period, 1935-1944 inclusive, Navy reports indicate one fatality for every 167,826 injections of MAPHARSEN. Compare this to the Navy reports on neoarsphenamine for the same period which show one fatality in every 28,463 injections.

MAPHARSEN (meta-amino-para-hydroxyphenyl arsine oxide (arsenoxide) hydrochloride) offers another great advantage in that its solution does not become more toxic on standing, nor does agitation or exposure to air increase its toxicity. Stokes[2] states that no loss of efficacy or increase in toxicity result when the solution is allowed to stand for several hours exposed to the air. Therefore, haste need not be made in preparation of the solution for injection.

[1] U.S. Nav. M. Bull. 45:783, 1945, and previous annual Navy reports.
[2] Stokes, J.H., Beerman, H. and Ingraham, N.R.: Modern Clinical Syphilology, ed. 3, Philadelphia, W.B. Saunders Company, 1945, pp. 359, 300.

DETROIT 32, MICHIGAN

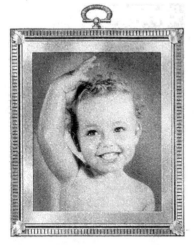

DOCTOR, MEET THE
DARICRAFT BABY

Perhaps you are "meeting" the Daricraft Baby every day in your own practice. If not, may we call to your attention the following significant points of interest about Vitamin D increased Daricraft:

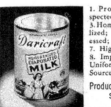

1. Produced from inspected herds; 2. Clarified; 3. Homogenized; 4. Sterilized; 5. Specially Processed; 6. Easily Digested; 7. High in Food Value; 8. Improved Flavor; 9. Uniform; 10. Dependable Source of Supply.

Producers Creamery Co.
Springfield, Mo.

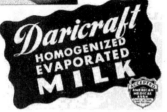

Daricraft
HOMOGENIZED
EVAPORATED
MILK

Dr. Henry Hodgen Mudd, and Dr. Joseph Nash McDowell.

Non-medical men who rose to a national level of importance also figure in this work. John Milton Hay, who later was Secretary of State of the United States and Ambassador to the Court of St. James; John G. Nicollet, private Secretary to President Lincoln and co-author with John Milton Hay on the "Life of Lincoln" —both attended school in Pittsfield, Illinois where Dr. Shastid practiced. The simple story of Nicollet's rise from a printer's helper to Editor-Publisher and Presidential Secretary is typical of many things that are depicted in this book. It shows too, with the keen appreciation, the development of medical education in those days, particularly with respect to those schools in the Middle West and describes, with great interest, practicing physicians "commuting" a hundred miles to teach classes.

These, in brief, are a few of the interesting sketches of Middle West life which make this a book of tremendous interest not only to the physician but to the historian and to the lay reader.—*George H. Garrison, M.D.*

STRUCTURE AND FUNCTION OF THE HUMAN BODY. Ralph N. Baillif, Ph.D., Assistant Professor of Anatomy, Louisiana State University School of Medicine, New Orleans and Donald L. Kimmel, Ph.D., Associate Professor of Anatomy, Temple University School of Medicine, Philadelphia. 328 pages, Price $3.00. J. B. Lippincott Co., Philadelphia, 1945.

This text book of anatomy and physiology gives the reader a brief review of anatomy and physiology. It is concise and carefully organized and the authors have used the simplest language and terminology.

The principle feature of this text is the correlation of the anatomy, both gross and microscopic, with the functions of the cellular and gross structures of the body. The subject matter is in four units. Unit One: discusses the structure and function of the cellular units as well as the primary tissues and membranes. Also the functions, structure and embryology of skeletal, muscular, circulatory, digestive, respiratory, urogenital and endocrine systems. Unit Two: devoted the skeletal and circulatory systems, gives the structure and function of bones and muscles, the muscular attachments and the muscular activities. Unit Three: digestive system and the respiratory system. Here the discussion is brief on structure of the systems with their functional relations. Unit Four: discussions on anatomy and physiology of both female and male reproductive organs and with explanations as to the manner of development.

The endocrine system is well presented, giving the principles of hormones and their regulation of tissue metabolism, control of muscular tone, digestive and sex and gland control.

This book, on account of its simplicity could be used for students of nursing and in other schools undertaking the task of teaching the fundamentals of anatomy and physiology.—*Morris Smith, M.D.*

The Lowdown From Franklin

Franklin on 19 March was skeptical about animal magnetism, but willing to think that the "delusion may, however, in some cases be of use while it lasts. here are in every great rich city a number of persons who are never in health because they are fond of medicines and always taking them, whereby they derange the natural functions and hurt their constitutions. If these people can be persuaded to forbear their drugs in expectation of being cured by only the physician's finger or an iron rod pointing at them, they may possibly find good effects though they mistake the cause." He was too ill to go to Paris and left it to the other commissioners to attend Deslon's clinic and study his modes of healing.—*Benjamin Franklin by Carl Van Doren, page 714. he Viking Press. New York. 1938.*

THE ANNUAL MEETING

of the

Oklahoma State Medical

Association

May 1, 2, & 3, 1946

Skirvin Tower Hotel

OKLAHOMA CITY, OKLAHOMA

. . . COMPLETE PROGRAM TO BE ANNOUNCED LATER . . .

MAKE YOUR HOTEL RESERVATIONS EARLY!

*For Circulatory and Respiratory Support
during and after operation
inject Metrazol intravenously*

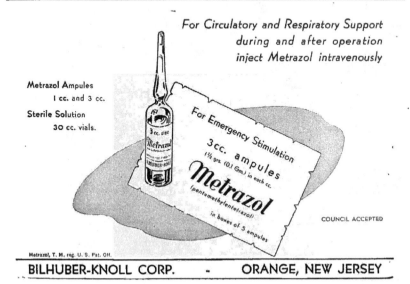

Metrazol Ampules
1 cc. and 3 cc.

Sterile Solution
30 cc. vials.

For Emergency Stimulation

3 cc. ampules
(1½ grs. (0.1 Gm.) in each cc.

Metrazol
(pentamethylentetrazol)

in boxes of 5 ampules

COUNCIL ACCEPTED

Metrazol, T. M. reg. U. S. Pat. Off.

BILHUBER-KNOLL CORP. - ORANGE, NEW JERSEY

Medical Abstracts

SURGERY OF THE MANDIBLE: THE AMELOBLAS-
TOMA. Louis T. Byars and Bernard G. Sarnat. Surgery, Gynecology and Obstetrics. Vol. 81, November,
1945. N. S. pp. 575-584.

This article although written concerning a rare condition, has some very valuable information for anyone
doing surgery or malignancies or surgery about the
mouth and face. First, in consideration of the diagnosis:
"The roentgenogram serves as a valuable adjunct in
the diagnosis of cystic lesions of the jaw, but the final
diagnosis depends on the gross and particularly the
microscopic examinations."

Second, the proper treatment: "Inasmuch as radiation
does not affect the ameloblastoma materially, the treatment of this tumor is primarily surgical. Both the
surgical approach and the procedure which is carried
out depend not only upon the diagnosis of the type of
the tumor but also upon its extent.

"An accurate microscopic diagnosis will give the
operator courage to do a radical operation, if necessary,
or will give him confidence in the less radical procedure.
The more accessible lesions are first removed locally. In
many instances this local excisions is adequate and not
deforming. In other instances (1) where a large portion
of the mandible is involved, (2) where the tumor has
definitely invaded beyond the confines of the bone, or
(3) where inaccessible areas of the mandible are involved so that local excision could not be adequate, resection of the mandible is the primary treatment of
choice.

"Wherever a resection is done some provision must
be made to maintain the remaining fragments of the
mandible in as near proper position as possible prior
to bone graft repair. If there has been disarticulation
in removal of the ramus, then only the anterior fragment
must be considered, and in this case the simplest and
best method of maintaining position is to wire the remaining teeth in occlusion until complete soft tissue
has taken place. However, if the resection has been
near the angle of the jaw so that the angle and ramus
remain as the posterior segment, some means must be
taken to maintain not only the space between fragments
but also the posterior fragment in its proper position.
Various methods have been used to control the posterior
fragment (reference to table of methods). It is essential that this space retention be maintained until
there is complete soft tissue healing.

"When healing is complete and only then do the
authors think that some form of restoration of the
mandible is to be considered. Several methods may
be used but in general a free bone graft is the most
desirable procedure.

"In order to carry out the procedure of a free bone
graft satisfactorily, certain things are necessary. The
fragments of the mandible which remain must be free
enough so that they can be not only placed but also
maintained in their proper position during the time that
the bone graft is healing in place. It is extremely important that the covering soft tissue be adequate in
quality and amount to give good covering and nourishment to a bone graft."—J.F.B., M.D.

CHRONIC POSTTRAUMATIC SYNDROMES LEADING
TO ENUCLEATION. Bertha A. Klien. American
Journal of Ophthalmology. Vol. 28, pp. 1193-1203. No-
vember, 1945.

There are several conditions developing after eye injuries which may lead to enucleation on suspicion of
sympathetic ophthalmia. The author's study includes
77 eyes which were selected from a total of 219 eyes
with penetrating injuries during the past 175 years.
The eyes selected had in common a chronic low-grade
painful state of irritation or inflammation which made
them suspicious of sympathetic ophthalmia. There were
eyes in which the terminal inflammation was continuous
with the immediate posttraumatic reaction; also eyes
in which a quiescent interval varying from several weeks
to years preceded the activated state of inflammation
which prompted their removal.

In chronic mild septic endophthalmitis the clinical
course was characterized by moderate photophobia and
pain, and moderate to marked ciliary injection of the
injured eyes; there was occasionally a moderate increase
in the number of free cells in the aqueous but without
corneal precipitates. In several cases there was an abscess somewhere along the intraocular path of the penetrating scar, in some instances with a foreign body in
the abscess. If such an eye would not be removed, an
atrophia bulbi with retinal detachment would be the
expected outcome.

Some of the eyes show extensive tissue necrosis. In
these the penetrating injury was accompanied by marked
contusion. The predominant clinical finding was a complete hyphema. Some of the eyes developed blood staining of the cornea, others showed secondary glaucoma.
Histologically, there was necrosis of large portions of
the uveal tract and the retina, and free hemorrhage
into the intraocular chambers. Extensive necrosis interferes with the mechanism for the absorption of hemorrhage; it also exerts a chemotactic stimulus for migration
of leukocytes, proliferation of various phagocytes, etc.

In cases with sympathetic ophthalmia there were some
which had no quiescent interval between injury and
enucleation; others had three weeks, even one year, and
the fellow eye was involved at the time of enucleation
in a small number of cases.

In another group of cases, there was considerable
time between the injury and the development of posttraumatic affection of the eye. The traumatic reaction
was occasional a chronic infiltrating iridocyclitis. This
type of reaction usually developed from 8 to 14 days
after the eye injury. The main characteristic of this
type of reaction is an iris densely packed with lymphocytes, or a mixture of lymphocytes and plasma cells and
a relative absence of inflammatory changes in the ciliary
body.

Other eyes showed endogenous iritis as a posttraumatic
reaction. In two cases the eye had suddenly become
painful and inflamed after 7 years and 40 years, respectively, in both patients during an attack of influenza.
In two other cases a tuberculous uveitis developed.

J. E. HANGER, Inc.

ARTIFICIAL LIMBS, BRACES, AND CRUTCHES

Phone: 2-8500   612 N. Hudson

L. T. Lewis, Mgr.   BRANCHES AND AGENCIES IN PRINCIPAL CITIES Oklahoma City 3, Okla.

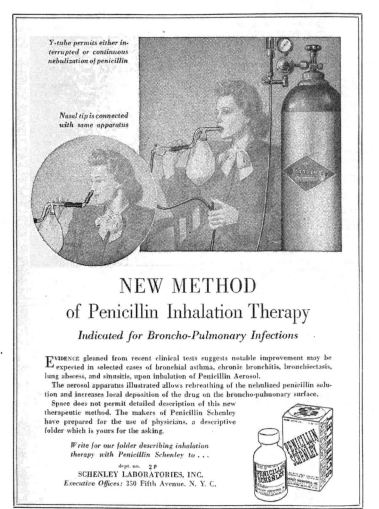

Y-tube permits either interrupted or continuous nebulization of penicillin

Nasal tip is connected with same apparatus

NEW METHOD
of Penicillin Inhalation Therapy

Indicated for Broncho-Pulmonary Infections

EVIDENCE gleaned from recent clinical tests suggests notable improvement may be expected in selected cases of bronchial asthma, chronic bronchitis, bronchiectasis, lung abscess, and sinusitis, upon inhalation of Penicillin Aerosol.

The aerosol apparatus illustrated allows rebreathing of the nebulized penicillin solution and increases local deposition of the drug on the broncho-pulmonary surface.

Space does not permit detailed description of this new therapeutic method. The makers of Penicillin Schenley have prepared for the use of physicians, a descriptive folder which is yours for the asking.

Write for our folder describing inhalation therapy with Penicillin Schenley to . . .

dept. no.   2 P
SCHENLEY LABORATORIES, INC.
Executive Offices: 350 Fifth Avenue, N. Y. C.

Your Local Distributor for **PENICILLIN** SCHENLEY is:

Caviness-Melton Surgical Company
OKLAHOMA CITY

Chronic hemophthalmos was occasionally seen. A typical case is that of a boy who, after an eye injury, was discharged with the right eye quiescent and with vision of only light perception. During the following four years there were several recurrent attacks of pain and redness in this eye. At the time of enucleation, four years after the injury, vision in the right eye was nil. There was marked photophobia and ciliary injection of the bulb. Through the upper clear two thirds of the cornea a mass of cholesterol crystals was visible in the anterior chamber; the lens was cataractous and partly absorbed. Formation of cholesterol tumors was characteristic for eyes with chronic hemophthalmos.

Nine enucleated eyes showed epithelial implants. In six, the implants sometimes extended through part of the anterior chamber and also parts of the more posterior structures. In three cases the epithelial implant was complicated with secondary glaucoma.

An old penetrating injury of the eye may also result in degeneration and rupture of the lens, or in extensive retinal disinsertion and detachment. In the author's series, six eyes exhibited this condition, in which mild late iritis necessitated enucleation. The iritis proved to be of an unspecific infiltrating type; it can be considered secondary to the long-standing retinal detachment.—M.D.H., M.D.

OSTEOPOROSIS CIRCUMSCRIPTA CRANII: ITS PATHOGENESIS AND OCCURENCE IN LEONTIASIS OSSEA AND IN HYPERPARATHYROIDISM. Frank Windholz. Radiology. XLIV, 14, Jan. 1945.

Osteoporosis circumscripta cranii was first described by Schuller as large, irregular, circumscribed areas of osteoporosis in the cranium. Sosman demonstrated a histological relationship between osteoporosis circumscripta and Paget's disease. For a time this evidence seemed to be corroborated, and the lesions were thought to be an atypical form of Paget's disease, ''probably

the absorptive or destructive phase with the productive phase held in abeyance''. Schmori first noted both gross and microscopic changes, which he considered to be the result of circulatory disturbance; they resembled hemorrhagic infarts, rather than the anatomical changes found in Paget's disease. A third histological picture was noted by Schellenberg, one which resembled osteitis fibrosa.

Of the published cases of osteoporosis circumscripta, 60 per cent have been associated with Paget's disease, and 20 per cent with leontiasis ossea, or bony tumors of the maxilla. In a case in which osteoporosis was associated with a condition believed to be leontiasis ossea, the latter was variously interpreted as leontiasis ossea, Paget's disease, osteitis fibrosa, osteofibroma, and osteoma. Recently the author observed a case of osteoporosis circumscripta with histologically verified leontiasis ossa (Virchow type).

Three cases are presented, two of leontiasis ossea, and one of hyperparathyroidism. One case was that of the Virchow type of leontiasis ossea. The histological picture was studied from a gum biopsy. This revealed: ''Complete transformation of the bone tissue with hyperplasia due to osteoblast activity and simple metaplasia; fibrous bone marrow containing inflammatory cells and capillary blood vessels; bone resorption by osteoclasts with formation of small cavities. No hyperplasia or hyperostoses were seen in the vault. It was felt that the vault changes (osteoporosis) were secondary to the leontiasis ossea, but not intimately and topically connected with it.

Pathologically, two types of osteoporosis are known: one represents circulatory disturbances, with hemorrhagic changes and decalcification, and the other, Paget's disease. The hemorrhagic form may be considered a primitive non-specific reaction common to many diseases of the cranium and one which may be followed by the

DIAGNOSTIC CLINIC OF INTERNAL MEDICINE AND ALLERGY

Philip M. McNeill, M. D., F. A. C. P.

General Diagnosis

CONSULTATION BY APPOINTMENT

Special Attention to Cardiac, Pulmonary and Allergic Diseases

Electrocardiograph, X-Ray, Laboratory
and Complete Allergic Surveys Available.

1107 Medical Arts Bldg.
Oklahoma City, Okla.　　　　　　　　　　　　Phone 2-0277

More pleasure to you, Doctor!

THREE nationally known research organizations recently reported the results of a nationwide survey to discover the cigarette preferences of physicians and surgeons.

Physicians all over the United States were asked the simple question: "What cigarette do you smoke, Doctor?" The question was put solely on the basis of *personal preference as a smoker.*

The thousands and thousands of answers from these physicians in every branch of medicine were checked and re-checked. The result:

More physicians named Camel as their favorite smoke than any other cigarette. And the margin for Camels was most convincing.

Certainly the average physician is busier today than ever before and is deserving of every bit of relaxation he can find in his day-by-day routine . . . a cigarette now and then if he likes. And the makers of Camels are glad to know that physicians find in Camels that extra margin of smoking pleasure that has made Camels such a favorite everywhere.

According to this recent nationwide survey:

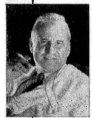

More Doctors
Smoke Camels
than any other cigarette

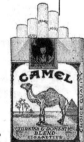

R. J. Reynolds Tobacco Company, Winston-Salem, N. C.

characteristis mosaic structure and fibrous bone marrow of Paget's disease.

The second case described was one of fibrous osteodystrophy which clinically resembled leotiasis ossea. There were extensive hyperostoses of the cranium, surrounded by wide areas of osteoporosis, giving the impression that the osteoprosis was a change largely involving the vault.

The third case was one of hyperparathyroidism, proved by the removal of a parathyroid adenoma, which weighed seven grams. The localization and outline of the osteoporotic areas closely followed those of Paget's disease. They developed five years after the first cranial changes, thus suggesting a circulatory disturbance.

The pathogenesis of these lesions lies in the circulatory disturbances caused by space-occupying lesions near the base of the skull or in the facial bones. Serial microscopy of biopsy specimens reveals obliterated blood vessels running into areas of quiescent bone tissue with no celluar reaction about the lamellae. Areas of primitive osteoporosis may undergo structural transformation corresponding to the demands of the statics of the vault.

Osteoporosis circumscripta cannot be regarded as a type or phase of Paget's disease or of any other disease entity. It occurs most often in Pagent's disease, however, and frequently may be transformed into it. The "primitive" form of osteoporosis circumscripta is a characteristic reaction of the bones of the cranium, and is probably caused by circulatory disturbances in the presence of bony hyperplasias or of bony tumors near the base of the skull.—E.D.M., M.D.

PENICILLIN IN OPHTHALMOLOGY: AN INTERIM REVIEW. Arnold Sorsby. The British Journal of Ophthalmology. Vol. 29. pp. 511-536. October, 1945.

Penicillin is still largely an impure product so that a final assessment of the ocular tolerance to this drug is not possible at present. Drops in a concentration of 5,000 units per ml are well tolerated by most patients, though some complain of a stinging sensation when drops are first instilled, while repeated instillation produces some reddening of the conjunctiva in most patients; drops in concentration of 2,500 units per ml are generally well tolerated. Subconjunctival injection of 1,250 units injected in 0.5 ml isotonic saline produces transitory stinging sensation; after 24 hours there is considerable conjunctivities or hyperemia and a second injection is distinctly painful; injections containing no more than 500 or 600 units are well tolerated.

Injection of penicillin was made also into the anterior chamber; 200 units of penicillin in 0.2 ml isotonic saline were well tolerated by experimental animals; within 24 hours there was some exudative reaction at the papillary margin, but it disappeared after 3 days. Intravitreal experimental injections resulted in vitreous opacities, and

development of a fibrous band, with final shrinkage of the eye globe. These observations of the author are substantially the same as reported by former investigators.

In man no penicillin has been detected in the tears when the drug is injected intravenously, intramuscularly or subcutaneously. Other observations show that the concentration of penicillin within the eyes does not reach a level which could be considered of any antibacterial value, neither in the equeous nor in the vitreous.

When the penicillin is locally applied, the drug penetrates readily through the cornea and the concentration of penicillin may reach a value of 40 Oxford units per ml in the iris half an hour after the application of 20,000 units of penicillin in one ml to the conjunctiva in form of drops. Subconjunctival injections may result in the same concentration of penicillin within the eye.

Penicillin has been used in various experimental infections of the eye with varying results. There is, as yet, no valid experimental evidence that local penicillin therapy is effective in infections of the outer eye. The evidence that penicillin, applied by corneal bath and by ionization, is effective against infection of the anterior chamber is more convincing. Intravitreal injection of penicillin into the experimentally infected vitreous appears to have given satisfactory results.

In contrast to this uncertainty there is adequate clinical experience as to the efficacy of penicillin in the external infections of the eye. This is most strikingly brought out in ophthalmio neonatorum, where concentrations of less than 2,500 units per ml were not found satisfactory, while the best results are obtained when drops of that concentration are put in at such frequent intervals as five minutes. In less severe infections, such as blepharitis, paints containing 1,000 units per ml, or even less, are adequate. Blepharitis is generally due, however, to staphylococcus aureus, an organism which is particularly susceptible to penicillin.

It appears that nothing is to be gained by using drops in a concentration of less than 2,500 per ml for the purulent or muco-purulent infections of the outer eye. It would seem, however, that the systemic administration of the drug has limited value. In this respect penicillin forms a striking contrast to the sulfonamides. The field of action for penicillin would, therefore, seem to be limited for the present to external infections and local applications.

For the present, penicillin has its widest application in those infections which have responded to general sulfonamide therapy, i.e., essentially the external infections of the eye. It is therefore recommended that on this field the sulfonamides should be replaced by penicillin.

The outstanding non-purulent infection of the outer eye is trachoma. Here local sulfonamide therapy has

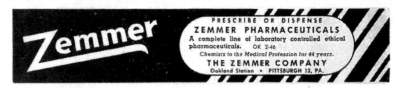

PRESCRIBE OR DISPENSE
ZEMMER PHARMACEUTICALS
A complete line of laboratory controlled ethical pharmaceuticals.   OK 2-46
Chemists to the Medical Profession for 44 years.
THE ZEMMER COMPANY
Oakland Station • PITTSBURGH 13, PA.

THE WILLIE CLINIC AND HOSPITAL

A private hospital for the diagnosis, study and treatment of all types of neurological and psychiatric cases. Equipped to give all forms of recognized therapy, including hyperpyrexia, insulin and metrazol treatments, when indicated. Consultation by appointment.

JAMES A. WILLIE, B.A., M.D.
Attending Neuro-psychiatrist

218 N. W. 7th St.—Okla. City, Okla.   Telephones: 2-6944 and 3-6071

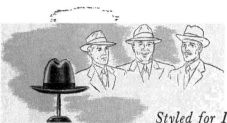

Styled for Individual Tastes

Neo-Synephrine for intranasal use is "styled" in three distinct forms too. All three provide the same real breathing comfort . . . prompt decongestion that endures for hours. Only the vehicles are different . . . isotonic saline, unflavored; Ringer's Solution, pleasantly aromatic; jelly in applicator tubes for convenience.

Neo-Synephrine
HYDROCHLORIDE
L-(HYD)-4 - HYDROXY-B - METHYLAMINO - 1 - PHENYL - ETHYL ALCOHOL HYDROCHLORIDE

For Nasal Decongestion

THERAPEUTIC APPRAISAL: Quick acting, long lasting . . . nasal decongestion without compensatory recongestion; relatively free from cardiac and central nervous system stimulation; consistently effective upon repeated use; no appreciable interference with ciliary activity; isotonic to avoid irritation.

INDICATED for symptomatic relief in common cold, sinusitis, and nasal manifestations of allergy.

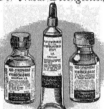

Samples Upon Request

ADMINISTRATION may be by dropper, spray or tampon, using the ¼ % in saline or in Ringer's solution in most cases— the 1 % in saline when a stronger solution is indicated. The ½ % jelly in tubes is convenient for patients to carry.

SUPPLIED as ¼ % and 1 % in isotonic salt solution, and as ¼ % in isotonic solution of three chlorides (Ringer's), bottles of 1 fl. oz.; ½ % jelly in ⅝ oz. collapsible tubes with applicator.

Frederick Stearns & Company
Division
DETROIT 31, MICHIGAN

NEW YORK   KANSAS CITY   SAN FRANCISCO   WINDSOR, ONTARIO   SYDNEY, AUSTRALIA   AUCKLAND, NEW ZEALAND.

Trade-Mark Neo-Synephrine—Reg. U. S. Pat. Off.

proved invaluable, while it is generally agreed that penicillin is ineffective against virus infections. Whether the drug should be experimented with in syphilitic affections of the eye remains a question. Most of the syphilitic affections of the eye (such as interstitial keratitis) are probably not spirochaetal in origin, but anaphylactoid, and penicillin cannot be of any help in allergic reactions.

The full exploitation of penicillin must await a fuller understanding of the mechanism of blood-aqueous carrier and the nature of intraocular inflammation.—M.D.H., M.D.

A METHOD OF TREATMENT OF CHRONIC INFECTIVE OSTEITIS. Ivor M. Robertson and John N. Barrow, St. Albans. England. The Journal of Bone and Joint Surgery. January, 1946. Vol. 28. No. 1, pp. 19-28.

"This complicated procedure requires the intimate co-operation of the orthopedic surgeon and the plastic surgeon."

The above is one of the sentences in the conclusion of a very interesting article. After reading the article one thoroughly agrees with the conclusion.

Chronic infective osteitis has certainly taxed the ingenuity and resourcefulness of anyone attempting to treat it. This article is a report on a method and is presented for further study and observation.

The following is the suggested treatment:

"The treatment is based on the principle of extensive excision of all diseased tissue, including skin, deep scar, and infected bone; and the replacement of soft tissue defects by muscle and skin flaps, and of bone defects by bone transplants. The aim is to remove the whole of the local disease and to establish normal conditions in the tissues. This requires either two or three operative stages as follows:

"Stage I. The excision of all diseased tissue and the application of a split skin graft to the wound surface.

"Stage II. The plastic repair of the soft tissues. The split-skin graft is removed and the area is covered by a skin and subcutaneous-tissue flap, muscle being included where necessary.

"Stage III. The repair of the bone defect."—J.F.B., M.D.

ESOPHAGEAL FOREIGN BODIES AND THEIR COMPLICATIONS. R. L. Flett. The Journal of Laryngology and Otology, London. Vol. 60, pp. 1-15. January, 1945.

The author reports on his experiences with endoscopy. He removed about one hundred foreign bodies by means of esophagoscopy. When a patient reports after swallowing a foreign body, it is very difficult in some cases to assess the symptoms so as to find out whether the condition is worth further investigation. Before esophagoscopy, the patient should be examined by negative screening, x-ray plates, and a barium swallow. With a positive result from x-ray investigation, esophagoscopy is essential. Nervous patients with indefinite symptoms should get no treatment. Patients with some complaints, who feel that esophagoscopy is necessary, should be given carbolic lozenges.

After removal of a foreign body the patient should be kept in the hospital for 24 hours. If there is slight injury to the esophageal wall, he should be given nothing by mouth except sterile water for 12 hours.

The large majority of the author's cases included the swallowing of coins. The next most numerous type of foreign body is described as a "meat bone". One dish which causes this trouble very frequently is the Irish stew, and the other, the chicken stew (the American chicken ala king). The post-cricoid stricture of the esophague due to hypochromic anemia is very often obstructed by a small bolus of meat.

Among the complications of foreign bodies of the esophagus is the edema of the esophageal wall. If there is no perforation of the wall, this edema may disappear in two or three days. Other patients may show cellulitis or abscess formation, and sometimes a prophylactic mediastinotomy may be required. Mediastinal infection is often suspected but it does not always occur, even when an open safety pin perforates the esophageal wall. In one case an old man swallowed a complete upper dental plate which stuck in the cervical esophagus; though there were severe lacerations of the esophageal mucosa, no mediastinitis developed.

Difficulty in swallowing may be due not to a foreign body but (in elderly women) to an anemic web or post-cricoid stricture, which is most often associated with a carcinoma in the lower third of the esophagus.

The mortality in esophageal foreign body injuries was formerly rather high, especially on account of the complicating mediastinitis. If there is a perforation, the author recommends internal dilatation of the perforation by means of forceps, punch forceps or scissors. This may be followed by nursing in the head-down position. A feeding tube may be inserted into the stomach; gastrostomy may be also performed. If, however, the patient is still very ill, or the cavity seen through the perforation is large, then external operation should be performed.

Sometimes the swelling of the esophageal wall will not permit the passage of an esophagoscope. In this case an external opening should be made, with an attempt to find the perforation, to dilate this by scissors until the esophagoscope can be passed, or a feeding tube inserted. If an incision is to be made in the esophagus, it is made

Anal Dilatation often Helpful in Pediatrics   Young's **RECTAL DILATORS**

Many pediatricians secure remarkable results through anal dilatation in constipation, especially in children with an atonic colon in association with a tight or spastic anal sphincter.

YOUNG'S RECTAL DILATORS are sold on physician prescription only, not advertised to the laity. Obtainable from your surgical supply house or ethical drug store. Bakelite, 4 graduated sizes. Children's set $4.50, adult $4.75. Write for brochure.

F. E. YOUNG & COMPANY   -:-   424 E. 75th St., Chicago 19, Ill.

In *Cheilitis* from LIPSTICK

Intractable exfoliative lip dermatoses may often be traced to eosin lipstick dyes. Remove the offending irritants, and the symptoms often disappear. In lipstick hypersensitivity, prescribe AR-EX NON-PERMANENT LIPSTICK—so cosmetically desirable, yet free from all known irritants. *Send for Free Formulary.*

PRESCRIBE

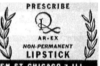

AR-EX NON-PERMANENT LIPSTICK

AR-EX COSMETICS, INC.   1036 W. VAN BUREN ST. CHICAGO 7, ILL.

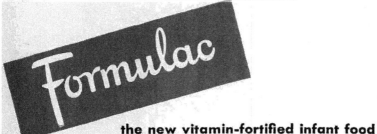

the new vitamin-fortified infant food

FORMULAC was developed by E. V. McCollum.
It is a reduced milk, in liquid form, fortified by
vitamins and minerals to meet the nutritional
needs of infants *without supplementary
administration.* Incorporation of vitamins
into the milk itself eliminates
the risk of human oversight or error.

FORMULAC has been tested clinically,
and proved satisfactory in
promoting infant growth and development.

FORMULAC presents a flexible basis for
formula preparation. Supplemented
by carbohydrates at your discretion,
it may readily be adjusted to meet each
child's individual nutritional needs.

FORMULAC is inexpensive. Priced
within the range of even low income
groups, it is on sale at
most drug and grocery stores.

FORMULAC IS PROMOTED ETHICALLY

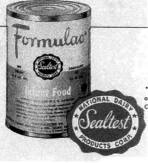

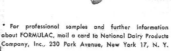

* For professional samples and further information
about FORMULAC, mail a card to National Dairy Products
Company, Inc., 230 Park Avenue, New York 17, N. Y.

Distributed by KRAFT FOODS COMPANY
NATIONAL DAIRY PRODUCTS COMPANY, INC.
New York, N. Y.

best in the posterior wall as in Seiffert's splitting operation. These methods are to be advocated in every case of mediastinitis associated with a sharp pointed foreign body.

When a smooth or rounded foreign body is present and had been in situ for such a time as to cause mediastinitis, the mediastinal condition may be dealt with and time may be allowed for the esophageal swelling to subside and allow esophagoscopy.

Prophylactic mediastinotomy is rather of questionable value. Often it may quicken the spread of infection. In the case of a much injured esophagus, the insertion of drainage tubes through an external wound has a very good hypnotic action on the surgeon.

Sulfonamides have reduced the necessity of external operation. Also penicillin by intramuscular injection, and local use in an external wound, should render the very severe complications of esophageal foreign bodies much less dangerous to life.—M.D.H., M.D.

REACTION OF THE HUMAN CONDUCTION MECHANISM TO BLAST. H. B. Perlman. The Laryngoscope, Vol. 55, pp. 427-443. August, 1945.

When T.N.T. explodes, a small volume of solid changes into a large volume of gas in ca. 10 microseconds; this causes high pressure in the air, which lasts about 1/1000 second, followed by a negative pressure lasting over 1/100 second, to give way to normal pressure again. The positive pressure wave is the shock pulse. The pressure wave is a sound wave of great condensation and great initial velocity; the peripheral ear will respond to these pressure changes in the atmosphere. If the pressure of the shock pulse is great enough, gross damage to the conducting mechanism may result; sustained pressure of 200 to 400 mm Hg is sufficient to rupture the ear drum. The malleus goes into oscillation. The movement of the stapes foot-plate is already under the influence of a much reduced shock pulse. The principal

oscillation delivered to the end-organ by the stapes foot-plate is largely negative in phase.

Rupture of the drum appears to have a protective effect on the end-organ. A perforated drum results in a reduction in the amplitude of an induced movement of the ossicles to large stimuli. Contraction of the stapedius and tensor tympani muscles also reduce the amplitude of oscillation of the ossicular chain, but the chronazia of reflex muscle contraction is slower than the propagation of the shock pulse. Shielding the ear from the pulse can be effected by covering the external meatus, opening the Eustachian tube, use of ear flaps, obturators (beeswax or wet cotton).—M.D.H., M.D.

KEY TO ABSTRACTORS

J.F.B., M.D. ....John F. Burton, M.D.
　　　　Oklahoma City, Okla.

M.D H., M.D. ....Marvin D. Henley, M.D.
　　　　Tulsa, Okla.

E.D.M., M.D. ....Earl D. McBride, M.D.
　　　　Oklahoma City, Okla.

MAKE YOUR HOTEL
RESERVATIONS
EARLY
ANNUAL MEETING — MAY 1, 2, 3
OKLAHOMA CITY

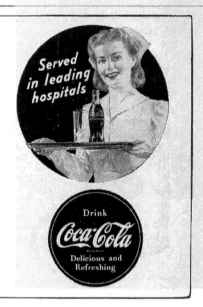

Pure..
Wholesome..
Refreshing

Safeguarded constantly by scientific tests, Coca-Cola is famous for its purity and wholesomeness. It's famous, too, for the thrill of its taste and for the happy after-sense of complete refreshment it always brings. Get a Coca-Cola, and get the feel of refreshment.

Served in leading hospitals

Drink
Coca-Cola
Delicious and Refreshing

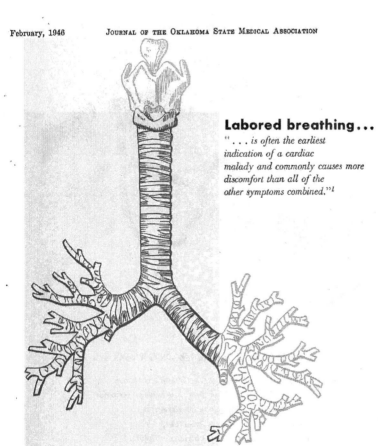

Labored breathing...

" . . . is often the earliest
indication of a cardiac
malady and commonly causes more
discomfort than all of the
other symptoms combined."[1]

AMINOPHYLLIN-SEARLE, by relaxing the bronchial musculature, encouraging resumption of a more normal type of respiration, reduces the load placed on the heart and helps prevent further damage.

Aminophyllin-Searle is indicated in paroxysmal dyspnea, Cheyne-Stokes respiration, bronchial asthma (particularly in epinephrine-fast cases) and in selected cardiac cases.

Aminophyllin-Searle contains at least 80% anhydrous theophyllin. G. D. Searle & Co., Chicago 80, Illinois.

1. *Harrison, T. R.: Cardiac Dyspnea,*
Western J. Surg., 52:407 *(Oct.) 1944.*

SEARLE *Research in the Service of Medicine*

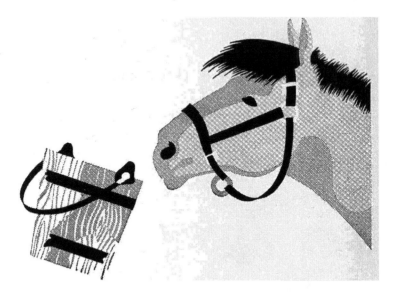

You can lead a horse...

and the same is unfortunately true of too many human
beings for whom well rounded diets have been prescribed.
When long-standing eating habits interfere with
conversion, the use of potent, easy to take,
and low cost supplementation with reliable Upjohn
vitamins can help assure vitamin adequacy.

UPJOHN VITAMINS

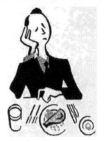

FINE PHARMACEUTICALS
SINCE 1886

The Preference
is Overwhelming

A comprehensive report published in *Human Fertility*[1] shows an overwhelming preference by experienced clinicians for the "Diaphragm and Jelly" method of conception control.

The report covering 36,955 new cases shows that the diaphragm and jelly method was prescribed for 34,314, or 93%.

On the evidence supplied by competent clinicians we continue to suggest that for the optimum in protection the physician should prescribe the combined use of a vaginal diaphragm and spermatocidal jelly.

When you specify "RAMSES"* a product of highest quality is assured.

Gynecological Division
JULIUS SCHMID, INC.
Established 1883
423 West 55th Street   New York 19, N. Y.

1. Human Fertility. 10:25, March, 1945.

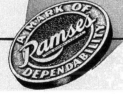

*The word "RAMSES" is a registered trademark of Julius Schmid, Inc.

Eye-witness
Reports...

IT is one thing to *read* results in a published research. Quite another to see them with your own eyes.

PUBLISHED STUDIES* SHOWED WHEN SMOKERS CHANGED TO PHILIP MORRIS SUBSTANTIALLY EVERY CASE OF THROAT IRRITATION DUE TO SMOKING CLEARED COMPLETELY, OR DEFINITELY IMPROVED.

But may we suggest that you make your own tests?

PHILIP MORRIS

PHILIP MORRIS & CO., LTD., INC.
119 FIFTH AVENUE, NEW YORK, N. Y.

*N. Y. State Journ. Med. 35 No. 11,590
Laryngoscope 1935, XLV, No. 2, 149-154

TO THE DOCTOR WHO SMOKES A PIPE: We suggest an unusually fine new blend—COUNTRY DOCTOR PIPE MIXTURE. Made by the same process as used in the manufacture of Philip Morris Cigarettes.

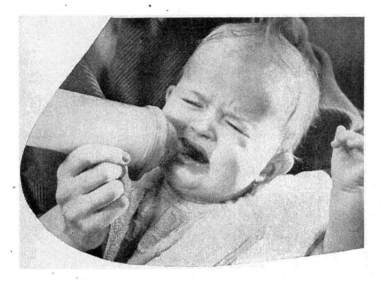

Battle dress

Too often it's on with the bib, on with the battle! The fruitless struggle between mother and baby goes on at every feeding. Mealtime can again be "peace time" when 'Dexin' brand High Dextrin Carbohydrate helps form good feeding habits without the commando tactics that leave both mother and baby exhausted, upset.

'Dexin' helps assure uncomplicated feeding because its high dextrin content (1) diminishes intestinal fermentation and the tendency to colic and diarrhea, and (2) promotes the formation of soft, flocculent, easily digested curds. Palatable and not over-sweet, 'Dexin' encourages a healthy appetite. Readily soluble in hot or cold milk, it supplements other bland foods. 'Dexin' does make a difference.

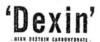
- HIGH DEXTRIN CARBOHYDRATE -

Composition—Dextrins 75% • Maltose 24% • Mineral Ash 0.25% • Moisture 0.75% • Available Carbohydrate 99% • 115 calories per ounce • 6 level packed tablespoonfuls equal 1 ounce • Containers of twelve ounces and three pounds • Accepted by the Council on Foods and Nutrition, American Medical Association.
'Dexin' Reg Trademark

Literature on request

BURROUGHS WELLCOME & CO. (U.S.A.) INC., 9 & 11 East 41st St., New York 17, N. Y.

OFFICERS OF COUNTY SOCIETIES, 1946

★

COUNTY	PRESIDENT	SECRETARY	MEETING TIME
Alfalfa	W. G. Dunnington, Cherokee	L. T. Lancaster, Cherokee	Last Tues. each Second Month
Atoka-Coal	J. B. Clark, Coalgate	J. S. Fulton, Atoka	
Beckham			Second Tuesday
Blaine			
Bryan	W. K. Haynie, Durant	Jonah Nichols, Durant	Second Tuesday
Caddo	Preston E. Wright, Anadarko	Edward T. Cook, Jr., Anadarko	
Canadian	G. L. Goodman, Yukon	W. P. Lawton, El Reno	Subject to call
Carter	J. Hobson Veazey, Ardmore	H. A. Higgins, Ardmore	Second Tuesday
Cherokee			First Tuesday
Choctaw	Floyd L. Waters, Hugo	O. R. Gregg, Hugo	
Cleveland	James O. Hood, Norman	Phil Haddock, Norman	Thursday nights
Comanche			
Cotton	G. W. Baker, Walters	Mollie Scism, Walters	Third Friday
Craig			
Creek			Second Tuesday
Custer	Ross Deputy, Clinton	A. W. Paulson, Clinton	Third Thursday
Garfield	Bruce Hinson, Enid	John R. Walker, Enid	Fourth Thursday
Garvin	M. E. Robberson, Jr., Wynnewood	John R. Callaway, Pauls Valley	Wednesday before Third Thursday
Grady	Roy Emanuel, Chickasha	Rebecca H. Mason, Chickasha	Third Thursday
Grant	I. V. Hardy, Medford	F. P. Robinson, Pond Creek	
Greer	J. B. Lansden, Granite	J. B. Hollis, Mangum	
Harmon	W. G. Husband, Hollis	R. H. Lynch, Hollis	First Wednesday
Haskell			
Hughes			First Friday
Jackson	E. W. Mabry, Altus	J. P. Irby, Altus	Last Monday
Jefferson	F. M. Edwards, Ringling	J. A. Dillard, Waurika	Second Monday
Kay	L. G. Neal, Ponca City	J. C. Wagner, Ponca City	Second Thursday
Kingfisher	John W. Pendleton, Kingfisher	H. Violet Sturgeon, Hennessey	
Kiowa			
LeFlore			
Lincoln	J. S. Rollins, Prague	Ned Burleson, Prague	First Wednesday
Logan	James Petty, Guthrie	J. E. Souter, Guthrie	Last Tuesday
Marshall			
Mayes			
McClain			
McCurtain			Fourth Tuesday
McIntosh	F. R. First, Checotah	W. A. Tolleson, Eufaula	First Thursday
Muskogee-Sequoyah			
Wagoner	R. N. Holcombe, Muskogee	William N. Weaver, Muskogee	First Tuesday
Noble			
Okfuskee			Second Monday
Oklahoma			Fourth Tuesday
Okmulgee	F. S. Watson, Okmulgee	C. E. Smith, Okmulgee	Second Monday
Osage			Third Monday
Ottawa	C. F. Walker, Grove	W. Jackson Sayles, Miami	Second Thursday
Pawnee			
Payne			Third Thursday
Pittsburg	Millard L. Henry, McAlester	Edward D. Greenberger, McAlester	Third Friday
Pontotoc-Murray	John Morey, Ada	R. H. Mayes, Ada	First Wednesday
Pottawatomie	F. P. Newlin, Shawnee	Clinton Gallaher, Shawnee	First and Third Saturday
Pushmataha			
Rogers	W. A. Howard, Chelsea	P. S. Anderson, Claremore	Third Wednesday
Seminole	Clifton Felts, Seminole	Mack L. Shanholz, Seminole	Third Wednesday
Stephens	Evert King, Duncan	Fred L. Patterson, Duncan	
Texas	Daniel S. Lee, Guymon	E. L. Buford, Guymon	
Tillman	H. A. Calvert, Frederick	O. G. Bacon, Frederick	
Tulsa	John C. Perry, Tulsa	John E. McDonald, Tulsa	Second and Fourth Monday
Washington-Nowata	Ralph W. Rucker, Bartlesville	L. B. Word, Bartlesville	Second Wednesday
Washita	L. G. Livingston, Cordell	Roy W. Anderson, Clinton	
Woods	John F. Simon, Alva	O. E. Templin, Alva	Last Tuesday Odd Months
Woodward	T. C. Leachman, Woodward	C. W. Tedrowe, Woodward	Second Thursday

*(Serving in Armed Forces)

THE JOURNAL
of the
OKLAHOMA STATE MEDICAL ASSOCIATION

| VOLUME XXXIX | OKLAHOMA CITY, OKLAHOMA, MARCH, 1946 | NUMBER 3 |

Remarks on the Treatment of Essential Hypertension*

S. Marx White, M.D.
MINNEAPOLIS, MINNESOTA

In a small percentage of cases of arterial hypertension an easily discoverable cause may be found. In one group we may find nephritis or polycystic kidneys, or urinary obstruction. Congenital coarctation of the aorta may be present. A tumor of the adrenal cortex may give paroxysmal hypertension. It is noted at times in congestive heart failure, as an accompaniment of pain, or after exertion or excitement, and it may attend a thyrotoxicosis. It may develop as a result of increased intracranial pressure.

The great majority of cases, some statistics give as high as 95 per cent, however, have no such demonstrable cause. This is the group, to the treatment of which attention is here directed. It has been called also "vascular" and "primary" hypertension, and the term "hyperpiesia" has been applied but has had very little use in this country.

There is general agreement now as to the mechanism and background for the development of essential hypertension. Certain brief statements may be made:

1. The claim that the structural changes in the arterioles are the causative factor in the increased intra-arterial pressure, has been generally abandoned.

2. That hereditary factors predispose in certain families with a high incidence of hypertension has been repeatedly shown, but that such factors play an important part in the heterogenous heredity background has not had a well controlled and analytical demonstration.

3. The group might be also designated as "neurogenic" hypertension as it is supposed that there is an increased number of nervous impulses carried by vasomotor nerves, result-

ing in increased peripheral resistance through widespread arteriolar contraction.

Psychiatric participation in the treatment of this group may be indicated by the manifestations of neurosis, a not uncommon accompaniment of hypertension.

This point is stressed because if this viewpoint is correct, practical, pragmatic, then the proper fundamental approach to the problem is through this segment of medicine, rather than by means of unilateral nephrectomy, ablation of the sympathetic nervous system or even by drugs.

An experience covering forty years of specific interest in this field leads the author to desire to encourage and develop this approach.

4. The so-called "Diencephalic Syndrome" is mentioned principally to warn against subtotal thyroidectomy in the case with this syndrome simply because of the marginal elevation of the basal rate (plus 10 to plus 30) along with slight diffuse enlargement of the thyroid gland, tachycardia and hyperperistalsis, and irregular flushing over the upper parasympathetic area—the face, neck and upper chest. The characterization as the "Diencephalic Syndrome" is due to the similarity of the above phenomena along with a labile hypertension with the signs which can be brought on by diffuse stimulation of the diensephalon in human beings.

Much is heard today about psychosomatic medicine. The term is misleading if we mean only the effect of the psyche, the mind, soul, or spirit, on the soma. If, however, we mean to include emotion, any agitated or intense state of mind, or more specifically any affective state in which joy, sorrow, fear, hate or the like is experienced as distinguished from cognitive and vo'itional states of consciousness, then we are on ground familiar to all of us.

*Presented at the Oklahoma City Clinical Society, November 28, 1945.

Arterial hypertension provides an illustration of some of the ultimate effects of emotional states (using the term in its broad sense as used in psychology) upon the whole body, acting through the cardiovascular system.

Whether or not we agree as to the usefulness of Hines' cold pressor test as a routine in clinical practice, we must admit that his studies have brought to the fore the importance of arterial pressor hyperreaction as a forerunner and probably a causative factor in the essential form of arterial hypertension. The clinical picture is one of the most familiar in the practice of medicine. Under this concept, repeated elevations of blood pressure stimulated by emotional responses to enviromental factors result eventually in presistent elevation, cardiac hypertrophy, arteriolar and arterial sclerosis, and eventual organ damage of vascular origin.

The influences that determine whether one case will remain benign in its manifestations and another become "malignant" remain obscure. We do know however that time, frequent repetition of pressor states, and higher pressure values tend to turn the balance toward "malignant" manifestations, and hence we often speak of the "malignant phase" of hypertension.

In attempting to explain the occurrence of cases in which the process seems malignant early and without the prolonged benign phase, an undue vulnerability of the cardiovascular system may be adduced as an explanation. Hereditary factors can play a part here as well as in providing a hyper-reactive pressor mechanism.

Whether slow or rapid in onset, benign or malignant when first seen, it is of extreme importance to recognize at the earliest possible moment, the earliest and more labile phases of the malady,

All of this preliminary is sketched in order to emphasize the unescapable need for attention to the part which environment and emotional responses thereto play in the evolution of hypertension in each individual case. It is here the physician needs to take stock. Is he trained and capable in the procedures and considerations needed to influence the daily life of his patient? I do not mean he must become a psychiatrist, a mental hygienist, or an occupational advisor. It should be stated at once that there are cases of maladjustment, or of psychiatric states, in which special training only can provide an adequate answer to the need. This should be recognized early.

The great majority of cases, however, need only the guidance of the wise physician, trained by experience in personality problems and willing to devote some time to the elucidation of the character of the problem so that the physician can give the patient himself some understanding of it. This takes time, patience in instruction, and tact.

The doctor is not in control of the environment. He can only indicate how favorable changes may be brought about. He cannot relax for the patient but he can provide instruction as to how to relax, and give guidance so that at least periods are secured during each day in which relaxation may be practiced and the ability to secure prompt relaxation developed.

The view about to be expressed may be iconoclastic, but I have never been impressed with the value of much reading by patients about medical matters which concern themselves. With an inadequate background the patient usually gets only a segment of the important and needed knowledge and persistently manipulates this to his detriment rather than to his advantage. There is, however, one little book for popular use which I have found to be helpful to many people. There is a well developed scientific basis for what the author has to say, and it is brief. Jacobson's "You Must Relax" has no fads or fancies to promote and it really teaches people to relax.

One of the greatest needs of the hypertensive patient is to protect him against the well-meant discussions of his malady by neighbors, friends, and members of his family. To do this requires adequate instruction by the physician at the earliest opportunity in the management. Groundless fears, as of complications, need to be removed. I usually try to impress the patient with a fact they will recognize, and that is that anything a layman tries to tell them about themselves is certain to be wrong, and further, that more well-conceived and well-directed programs for medical care are wrecked by neighborhood medicine than by any other influence.

Many among us are too busy delivering babies, removing tonsils, appendices or ovaries, to care to spend time in the instruction and guidance necessary. in the fundamental approach to the problems of the hypertensive. In this case it should not be attempted, but the problem should be entrusted to a colleague, or if necessary, even a rival.

While the barbiturates have an important place in the practice of medicine, that place is not in the routine treatment of arterial hypertension as such. A very common practice of doling out preparations touted by detail salesmen as effective for hypertension and containing phenobarbital is slovenly, inadequate and dangerous, and must not be indulged.

After attention has been given to the considerations above outlined, there remain certain procedures aimed at the amelioration of the hypertensive situation.

Most important for consideration are: reduction of weight in the obese; biological and chemical substances lowering blood pressure; surgical procedures.

Treatment of the obesity and overweight often associated with hypertension requires no comment except to say that it is only a part, but sometimes a very valuable part of the environmental management. The chief barrier to an effective weight-reduction campaign is the fear of weakness and fatiguability as a consequence of the dietary regime, and in women the development of wrinkles.

Many a woman has quit a favorable beginning when accosted by a so-called friend with the remark, "What's the matter; you look terrible." or words to that effect. It seems to be as difficult for the obese man or woman to reduce as for the rich man to enter the kingdom of heaven or the camel to pass through the proverbial needle's eye.

It has been possible to induce more women to adhere faithfully to a weight reduction program since I have begun quoting Edna Ferber than it was before. Edna coined the phrase, "A vast waddle of womanhood." To dangle that picture before the eyes of a fat woman is a stimulus of untold value.

The use of a kidney extract such as that of Page and his co-workers is still an experimental procedure. These extracts must be given parenterally, the results are complicated by anaphylactoid reactions which tend to obscure the effects of the extracts, and there is as yet no chemical knowledge of the active principle to guide in the separation of the desired agent. They must remain as yet experimental, although of great value in the effort to elucidate the mechanism of their activity and indeed of the chemical mechanisms of hypertension.

As of today, thiocyanate is the most effective drug generally available. The exact mechanism of action is not known, but there are three ways in which some effects are believed to occur: slight depressant action on the central nervous system; relaxation of smooth muscle fiber; reduction of basal metabolic rate.

Furthermore in experimental cholesterol atherosclerosis, thiocyanate has been shown to retard lipid deposition. If effective in any degree in man this effect should be to lessen the atherosclerotic component of the vascular changes induced or accelerated by arterial hypertension.

Since Barker in 1936 showed how to determine the level of thiocyanate in the blood, this drug has regained a wide use after having previously acquired a reputation as being dangerous and having been abandoned generally on that account.

A serious danger at this time is the resumption of its use without frequent control of blood levels, and observation for symptoms and signs of toxicity including the examination of the blood for effects on the bloodmaking organs: these will not be detailed here. They are mentioned only to urge that no one should be guilty of administering thiocyanate unless prepared to study serum levels and all forms of toxic manifestation including those to be found in the blood. The procedures are within reach of any laboratory.

The principal object of this discussion of the treatment of hypertension is to bring out the wide variations in dosage and effects of thiocyanate as observed over the years since Barker's method came to our aid.

Administration is begun with three one-grain (65 mg.) tablets potassium thiocyanate per day. At the end of two weeks, the blood level is determined and morphologic blood study made. I now have records of three patients in whom a very satisfactory reduction in both systolic and diastolic pressures developed with this dosage although the blood level did not rise above 4 mg. per cent. This is exceptional, and large doses are usually needed.

With many patients, weekly studies are too great a burden and the two-week period of study is the rule. Blood thiocyanate level is determined and blood morphology is studied. Doses are increased after each determination by adding one grain to the total daily dose until either a satisfactory level is reached, or as in some instances this increment appears to raise the level too slowly to be practical. In one case for example, 9 grains a day resulted in only a four to six mg. per cent level without demonstrable effect on pressure readings. It was only after 18 grains a day were given and a serum level of approximately 12 mg. secured that a considerable reduction in pressure developed.

When doses larger than 9 to 10 grains a day are necessary, 3 grain instead of 1 grain tablets are used. In some cases where a rather fine adjustment is necessary, as when 9 grains are not enough but 12 too much, combinations of three and one grain tablets are used. The patients readily recognize the difference in size and can regulate the total daily dosage accordingly.

The variation in dosage necessary to produce a given level, the variations in effective level, and the variations in susceptibility to toxic manifestations make it necessary to watch this drug unremittingly. To this is to be added the fact that a dosage tolerated over a long time without toxic effects may suddenly and for no known reason be productive of severe toxic effects.

It is interesting to note the considerable number of patients in whom the lower levels of serum thiocyanate are accompanied by satisfactory lowering of blood pressure. While most discussions of the subject give about 8 mg. as the level to be attained or exceeded, I have numerous instances of good results at levels between 4 and 7 mg. per cent. The dosage necessary to attain this has varied from 3 to 12 and even 15 grains a day.

It appears to be generally believed that a level of 15 mg. should not be exceeded. In one case after a year and a half of an 18 grain daily dosage with serum levels ranging closely around 12 mg., a routine examination revealed a serum level at 19 mg. without toxic manifestations but the dosage was promptly reduced nevertheless. In such an instance toxic manifestations would be likely to develop rapidly and might be fatal. Experience teaches that if results are to be secured they commonly appear at levels of 8 to 12 mg., even lower as already indicated. It seems desirable to consider 15 mg. the upper limit to be permitted.

If after about two months of thiocyanate therapy, and the attainment of adequate level in the serum, a fall of pressure or other evidence of benefit does not occur, the drug should be discontinued. Such other benefits, which may or may not be accompanied by a considerable fall of blood pressure, are relief of headache, dizziness, or tinnitus.

Contraindications to the use of thiocyanate are: cardiac decompensation; depression of renal function such as revealed by phenol-sulfonephthalein; severe arteriosclerosis especially cerebral; in general, patients over 60 years of age. Although symptomatic relief and moderate lowering of blood pressure has occurred in some patients in the 7th decade, thiocyanate has not been used in my clinic in any patient over 68 years of age.

With the development of papilledema and other indications of the malignant phase, the drug loses its efficacy. It is not beneficial in the hypertension of the toxemia of pregnancy. It is rare to secure relief of the anginal syndrome or of dyspnea on exertion. The anginal syndrome is often exaggerated by its use.

Not all hypertensives require thiocyanate. In fact, nearly half of the moderate labile hypertensives seen in our clinic are carried on without the drug since we attempt to rely upon environmental adaptation, instruction in relaxation, and the general measures believed to more fully recognize the causative factors.

Also when the drug is administered these considerations are not neglected, and, there is reason to believe, with benefit,

Treatment by unilateral nephrectomy may conceivably be justified in a very small number of cases studied in a free clinic by a highly expert group, including urologists and internists. Personal experience has been limited to cases of arterial hypertension in which a nephrectomy has been performed for the condition of the kidney and not for the hypertension. I have been called upon to study too many patients on whom a nephrectomy has been done under what has seemed to be to be inadequate indications, in whom hypertension has recurred or not even been relieved.

The story with regard to surgical treatment of hypertension is a similar one. For fifteen years I have been conscientiously trying to find a case in which the circumstances seemed suitable. I have so far failed. I have seen a number of patients in which it has been done. When successful, postural hypotension replaces the hypertension for a few months at least. The really commendable and satisfactory results I have seen are in some of the cases of malignant hypertension in which a temporary reprieve from very annoying and intractable conditions has been achieved.

ANNUAL MEETING

OKLAHOMA STATE

MEDICAL ASSOCIATION

MAY 1, 2, 3

SKIRVIN TOWER HOTEL

Oklahoma City

Make Your Reservations Now!

Weil's Disease

CLARENCE E. BATES, LT. COL., M.C., AUS
WILLIAM GORDON HARTNETT,
MAJOR, M.C., AUS
VETERANS HOSPITAL, MUSKOGEE, OKLA.

The returning soldiers are bringing back many medical souveniers from foreign countries in which they have served. Malaria, trench foot, jungle rot, and fungus infection, are common. There are many uncommon tropical diseases, such as schistosomiasis, trypanosomiasis, filariasis, and Weil's disease, now being encountered in localities wherein these afflictions have never been seen before.

Weil's disease, or infectious jaundice, is quite rare in the United States. Most of the literature on the disease, is gleaned from foreign journals. Kromer states that from 1922 to 1940 there were only 23 authentic cases reported in the American Literature.

Writing on the diagnosis of the disease, d'Silva, after treating 250 cases, from 1937 to 1939, in the Andaman Islands, says fever, prostration, albuminuria, and jaundice, are the most prominent symptoms. Jaundice appears on the fifth to seventh day. He states that serological diagnosis is helpful after the tenth day of the disease.

Of the signs and symptoms, prostration is found to be out of proportion to the fever which runs between 100 and 102:

Pain. The pain is excruciating in the muscles of the lower limbs, neck, and to a lesser extent in the arms, and body, at the onset. Conjunctival injection is one of the earliest signs, and associated with patchy hemorrhages.

Fever. The temperature runs from 100 to 102 persisting for 3 or 4 days to as long as from 7 to 10 days. A small secondary rash occurs usually after about a week.

Jaundice. The icterus appears about the third day in about 50 per cent of the cases. An unusual feature of the jaundice is the absence of pruritis.

Renal. Albuminuria is present in 95 per cent of the cases on the second to third day and lasts two days to a week. Furthermore, retention of the urine may appear. The respirations are shallow and slow and bronchopneumonia may co-exist. Pulse rate usually is in the neighborhood of 100. Liver and gall bladder enlargements are noted in 50 per cent of the cases and the spleen is rarely enlarged.

Hemorrhage. Bleeding is usually manifest about the fourth or fifth day of the disease and occurs as either epistaxis, or hemoptysis. Hematuria is rare. Gastrointestinal symptoms are absent.

Laboratory. There is usually a leukocytosis from 10,000 to 15,000, with 70 per cent to 85 per cent polys. Blood cultures are usually positive the first week. Guinea pigs will show the leptospirilla if inoculated after the seventh day of the disease.

Urine. Spirochetes are found after the tenth day, in some cases they cannot be found until as long as the 35th day.

TREATMENT

Bulmer describes treatment with penicillin and states that the disease is spread by infected rats who pass the leptospirilla in their urine and the source of infection is water used for washing. He reports on 39 cases in Normandy during World War II. Mortality rate was four cases in this 39. One case showed meningeal involvement as shown by spinal fluid examination. Penicillin was used on 16 cases, an average of 1,125,000 units being given in doses of 40,000 every three hours. Of the fatal cases, two cases died with anuria, one died with auricular fibrillation and one died of mycarditis. Of the 16 cases treated with penicillin the conclusions drawn were: 1. there was shortening of the general effects of the disease. 2. the penicillin did not influence the degree nor the duration of the cholemia. 3. penicillin did not affect the degree of nitrogen retention. 4. penicillin-treated cases showed marked improvement in 36 hours.

Cross reports one case which had typical symptom complex of Weil's disease, and was of the severe form, with delirium and incontinence. He was treated with 60 cc of serum. Urine was negative for spirochetes until the fourteenth day, and a guinea pig inoculated died ten days after inoculation and showed typical lesions. When the diagnosis was thus established, penicillin was started on the fourteenth day. One hundred twenty thousand units were given and the leptospirilla promptly disappeared from the urine. In all, 800,000 units were given in seven days, with uneventful recovery.

Hart reports one case treated with penicillin. His case began with symptoms of pneumonia, and the x-ray of the chest was reported as suggestive of atypical pneumonia. On the sixth day, jaundice developed. There was no hemorrhagic tendency. He concluded, that the diagnosis must be established before penicillin was given, as it may obscure the picture, and also that penicillin did not hasten recovery.

Strausburger and Thill state that only half of their cases showed splenic enlargement, and jaundice is frequently absent. Nephritis and uremia appear early but no edema. They state that in Japan, the mortality rate may be 30 per cent. In their two cases, they report that infection seemed to take place from swimming.

Clopper, Muir, and Myers, reporting on 13 cases, re-emphasize the frequency of meningeal involvement. Meningismus was present in three cases, with stiffness in the neck, a positive Kernig's and Brudzinski's sign, headache and vomiting. One case developed convulsions, and had a spinal cell count of 990. The other cases had normal cell counts, with elevated spinal pressure.

Heilman, in an experimental study on Weil's disease, concludes that penicillin was more effective than streptomycin, and it was suggested that the streptomycin may be useful as an adjunct to penicillin therapy in the treatment of spirochetal infections in man.

CASE REPORT

Mr. E. C. E., 24 years of age, entered the hospital on December 1, 1945, with admitting diagnosis of malaria and tonsillitis. He was seen by the O. D., who noted that the patient's temperature was 105 on admission. The patient was put on penicillin 2 cc q 5 hours. The following day, one of us saw the patient and made a note that the patient showed icterus, conjunctivitis, sore throat, rigidity of the neck, enlarged spleen. The patient stated that he had been sick for one week and he began to be ill with a sore throat. He had been taking atabrine and sulfathiazole together with penicillin at home and the note continues to say that a diagnosis of Weil's disease is in order. The history shows that the patient complained of chills and fever, headache and sore throat. His temperature continued high and he had intermittent chills, headaches, stiffness of his back muscles, discoloration of his skin and rigidity of his neck. The patient had recently been discharged from service, and on the way home had stopped over in Hawaii for a week. On the second day at home the patient had taken ill.

The examination showed the temperature to be 104, the pulse 120, respiration 24,

weight 144 pounds. Patient a 24 year old white male lying in bed apparently acutely ill. The eyes reacted to light and accommodation. There was marked injection of the conjunctivae and sclera. The ocular motions were normal. The nose showed the mucous membrane to be highly injected and swollen. The ears showed no abnormality. The tongue was furred, the teeth in fair condition, the tonsil on the right side was swollen and had a false membrane. The left tonsil was swollen and cryptic.

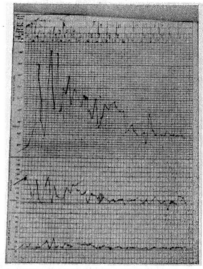

1. Temperature; 2. Pulse; 3. Respiration
Temperature Chart of Case Report of Weil's Disease

The neck showed enlarged cervical glands bilaterally, and was tender to touch. The thyroid was not enlarged, there was no unusual pulsation and the cervical veins were not dilated. There was considerable resistance in trying to bend the neck on the chest. The patient seemed very sensitive to any movement of his head. Expansion of the chest was limited, the respirations were rapid and the chest was resonant throughout. There were some moist rales heard in the right base. The PMI was in the 5th interspace within the MCL. There was no thrill or shock. The cardiac borders were within normal limits. The heart tones were normal in quality, and intensity and short in duration, regular sinus rhythm with a tachycardia.

The abdomen was soft and there was tenderness over the spleen. The spleen was felt two fingers breadth below the left costal margin. The liver was not enlarged, there were no masses, no rigidity, no tenderness. The extremities proved negative and there was no hernia present. Rectal examination was negative. The diagnosis was made of Weil's disease, bronchopneumonia and streptococcic sore throat.

The laboratory work showed an icterus index of 33; the Wassermann and Kahn were negative. The blood count was 5,640,000 red cells, 12,900 white blood count, 87 per cent polys, and 18 per cent lymphocytes. The hemoglobin was 85 per cent. The urine was yellowish in color, acid in reaction, specific gravity 1020, there was one plus albumin, no sugar, otherwise negative. A throat smear showed many gram positive cocci. Spinal fluid on the third day after admission showed a spinal fluid pressure of 11 mm. of mercury, which on pressure over the jugulars rose to 22 and returned to 11. There was no bacteria seen, globulin was not increased, cell count was 3, the Wassermann was negative and the gold curve was normal. Repeat blood count on the 6th of December showed a red count of 3,350,000 with a white count of 11,400. The differential was polys 81 per cent, the lymphocytes 13, the monocytes 6. The hemoglobin was 65 per cent. On December 6 the icterus index was 21.4, agglutination for bacillus abortus, tularemia, typhoid, paratyphoid, proteus OX 19, were all negative. On December 8 the urine was examined for leptospirilla and daily specimens were examined from that time until January 11, 1946, and in no specimen was the leptospirilla seen. On December 17, 1945, the icterus index had fallen to 12.7. On December 26, blood count had reached 4,900,000, with a total leukocyte count of 7,200, with a differential showing 64 per cent polys, 28 per cent lumphocytes. The icterus index the same date was 6.9. The galactose tolerance test gave normal results. The total protein on January 7, 1946, was 6.49; January 9, the NPN was reported as 38, the creatinin 1.3, the total protein 7.32. A serum was sent to Chicago, for agglutination test for Weil's disease. Bromsulfalein test on January 10, 1946, showed .4 per cent retention in one hour. X-ray examination on the second hospital day showed the heart and aorta normal. There is a poorly demarcated area of bronchopneumonic infiltration at the level of the 4th right interspace anteriorly.

Penicillin was given in 20,000 unit doses every three hours from the first of December, 1945, to the 21st of December, 1945. His temperature came down by reaching normal on the twelfth day. On the fifteenth day there was a slight rise in temperature to 100, promptly came down to normal and stayed

until the date of his discharge which was the 13th of January, 1946.

Serum agglutination was positive in dilutions of 1 to 1000 on December 18 and again on December 28 for leptospirilla icterhaemorrhagia.

The conclusions drawn from the treatment of a case of Weil's disease treated with penicillin are that the penicillin evidently destroys the spirochetes in both the urine and the blood stream, however, the disease ran its regular clinical course without any demonstrable effects from the penicillin.

BIBLIOGRAPHY

1. Kramer, David W.: Weil's Disease: Incidence, Diagnosis, and Treatment; Report of Two Cases, Pennsylvania Medical Journal, Vol. 45, page 1298. September, 1942.
2. D'Silva, H. A. H.: Weil's Disease with Special Reference to Its Diagnosis and Treatment, Indian Medical Gazette, Vol. 77, page 200. April, 1942.
3. Bulmer, Ernest: Weil's Disease in Normandy: Its Treatment with Penicillin. British Medical Journal, Vol. 1, page 113. January 27, 1945.
4. Cross, R. M.: Penicillin in Weil's Disease, Lancet, Vol 248, page 211. February 17, 1945.
5. Hart, V. Lloyd: A Case of Weil's Disease Treated with Penicillin, British Medical Journal, Vol. 2, page 720. December 2, 1944.
6. Strasburger, J. and Thill, O.: Clinic of Weil's Disease, with a Report on Two New Cases, Klinische Wochenschrift. Vol. 8, page 1391 July 23, 1929.
7. Clapper, Muir and Myers, Gordon V.: Clinical Manifestations of Weil's Disease with Particular Reference to Meningitis. Archives of Internal Medicine, Vol. 72, page 18. July, 1943.
8. Havens, W. Paul, Bucher, Carl J. and Heimann, Hobart A.: Leptospirosis: A Public Health Hazard. Report of a Small Outbreak of Weil's Disease in Bathers, Journal of the American Medical Association, Vol. 116, page 289. January 25, 1941.
9. Heilman, F. R.: Streptomycin in the Treatment of Experimental Relapsing Fever and Leptospirosis Icterohaemorrhagica (Weil's Disease), Proceedings of the Staff Meetings of the Mayo Clinic, Vol. 20, page 169. May 30, 1945.

Annual Prize Contest Announced

The American Association of Obstetricians, Gynecologists and Abdominal Surgeons Foundation announces that the annual prize contest will be conducted again this year. For information address Dr. Jas. R. Bloss, Secretary, 418-11th Street, Huntington 1, W. Va.

Manuscripts Invited for Norton Medical Award

The book publishing firm of W. W. Norton & Company announce that they are again inviting manuscripts for submission to be considered for the Norton Medical Award of $3,500.00 offered to encourage the writing of books on medicine and the medical profession for the layman. The first such award was made to "The Doctor's Job" Dr. Carl Binger's book, published last spring, which gave the doctor's point of view on his work. Announcement will be made shortly of the winning book for 1946. Closing date for submission of manuscripts this year is November 1, 1946. All particulars relating to requirements and terms may be had by addressing W. W. Norton & Company, Inc., 70 Fifth Ave., New York 11, N. Y.

The best books for a man are not always those which the wise recommend, but oftener those which meet the peculiar wants, the natural? thirst of his mind, and, therefore, waken interest and rivet thought. *William Ellery Channing: Self-Culture. Address Introductory to the Franklin Lectures.*

Books are the best things, well used; abused, among the worst. *Emerson: Miscellanies.*

It is just those books which a man possesses, but does not read, which constitute the most suspicious evidence against him. *Victor Hugo: The Toilers of the Sea.*

Clinical Pathological Conference

University of Oklahoma School of Medicine

Presented by the Departments of Pathology and Medicine

WANN LANGSTON, M.D.—HOWARD C. HOPPS, M D.

OKLAHOMA CITY, OKLAHOMA

DOCTOR HOPPS: The major diagnosis of the case to be presented this morning is probably obvious to you from having studied the protocol. It is not common these days to have an opportunity to study at necropsy a patient dying of pernicious anemia. In this sense pernicious anemia is, today, analogous to diabetes mellitus. Before the advent of insulin, diabetes was a disease which eventually terminated in starvation and death. Similarly with pernicious anemia in the days before liver therapy this disease was truly pernicious in that it was relentlessly progressive leading to a degree of anemia incompatible with life.

The historical aspects of this disease are of special interest because they tell the story of an important conquest of disease by medicine. You are familiar with the fact that Addisonian is a name frequently applied to this condition because of Addison's classic studies and description in 1855. Biermer also deserves credit since he wrote an even more comprehensive account of this disease (1872), apparently without knowledge of Addison's previous studies. It was at about this time that Pepper and Cohnheim first observed and correlated the changes which occur in the bone marrow. Shortly thereafter, Ehrlich described in detail the changes in the peripheral blood. To my mind, Ehrlich is one of the outstanding figures in medicine. You are all familiar with the fact that he introduced chemotherapy to medicine by his discovery of "606" or arsphenamine. Few of you probably recall, however, that his studies in staining characteristics of tissue and bacteria provided us, among other things, with the acid-fast stain for tubercle bacilli, or that he did pioneer work in the field of nutrition, and first isolated one of the amino acids. George Whipple who, as you know, has been awarded a Nobel prize for his studies on the formation of blood and hemoglobin, demonstrated experimentally the value of liver and other foods in restoring erythrocytes in anemia from blood loss, and suggested in 1922 that pernicious anemia might be the result of a deficiency in certain materials necessary for the formation of red

cell stroma. It was not until 1926, however, that Minot and Murphy proved the value of liver therapy in pernicious anemia. From this time on the term "pernicious" no longer carried the same implication as formerly. Pernicious anemia is now a deficiency disease for which adequate substitution therapy is available.

Dr. Langston will present and analyze the clinical data on our case for today.

PROTOCOL

Patient: G. C. F., Mexican male "preacher", age 66, admitted July 23, 1945; died July 23, 1945.

Chief Complaints: (Terminal Admission) Weakness, epigastric distress following meals, sore tongue, abdominal distention, dyspnea, nocturia, precordial pain, edema of the feet and ankles and stiffness and numbness of the legs.

Present Illness: Dates to January 1929 when the patient (at that time 50 years old) complained of weakness, shortness of breath, "gas on the stomach", sore mouth and constipation. This grew worse and on June 18, 1929 he came to the O.P.D. of the University Hospital. The impression was "generalized toxemia". On June 25 he was again seen and fluoroscopy revealed marked irregularity of the pyloric end of the stomach. On July 8, 1929 he was admitted to this hospital. Physical examination revealed a roughened mitral 1st sound, abdominal distention and a palpable spleen. There was slight jaundice. Fluoroscopy and x-ray plates disclosed a nonfilling gallbladder and a pyloric irregularity "apparently on the outer curvature". RBCs numbered 1.55/cmm. and Hb was 55 per cent of normal; no nucleated red cells seen. WBCs numbered 4,400/cmm. He was given a "high liver pernicious anemia diet" and on July 30, 1929 Hb was 90 per cent and RBCs numbered 2.60/cm. A laparotomy was performed on August 19, 1929 with preoperative diagnosis, possibly carcinoma of stomach. No neoplasm was discovered at operation and the postoperative diagnosis was chronic pancreatitis. Recovery was uneventful and he was discharged from the hospital on a regular diet.

Although he was not well, he felt better and worked during most of 1930. On April 28,. 1931 returned to the O.P.D. with his former complaints plus tingling of the fingers and toes and some swelling of the feet and of the face. There was marked pallor. Impression was pyloric spasm due to duodenal ulcer and he was treated with alkaline powders and belladonna. Fluoroscopy showed a marked pylorospasm and poor filling of the duodenal cap, "apparently due to ulcer of duodenum" (July 16, 1931). On July 21, 1931, fluoroscopic examination revealed a pyloric irregularity "characteristic and suggestive of syphilis". The Wassermann reaction was negative. On September 4, 1931 Hb was 38 per cent, RBCs numbered 1.55 and WBCs 3,600,' cmm. He was given iron ("Blaud's Mass") until September 15, 1931 when he was readmitted to the hospital because of severe upper respiratory infection. He was given ventriculin and later ½ lb. of raw liver b.i.d. HCl was given by mouth. He improved rapidly, returned home and continued to eat large amounts of liver. He was seen at frequent intervals in O.P.D. and repeated blood studies were made. Later he was given concentrated liver extract orally. During this time his red count average about 3.5/cmm. with 75-80 per cent hemoglobin. He remained well except during the winter and fall months when he had many upper respiratory infections. On September 11, 1935 intramuscular injections of liver extract (10 cc.) were begun. He was able to work regularly until May 19, 1937 when he "began to feel tired" and developed headaches and frequent colds. At this time RBCs numbered 4.74/cmm. and Hb 95.2 per cent. He was unable to secure liver extract and was placed on a regime of Lextron and liver by mouth. He did well until the spring of 1945. Liver therapy had been given by two local physicians until March 17, 1945 when he contracted a severe respiratory infection and returned to O.P.D. Gastric analysis revealed 23° combined acid and 0 free acid. Admission was advised because of generalized edema. Because of crowded conditions admission was delayed for a month. At this time Hb measured 11 Gm, RBCs numbered 2.90 and WBCs 6,200/cmm. Reticulocytes varied from 1.8 per cent to 7.8 per cent. Total plasma protein was 4.5 Gm. per cent and icteric index 8. He was treated with liver extract and placed on a high protein diet with slight improvement. He was discharged on June 16, 1945 and readmitted on July 21, 1945.

Past and Family History: Noncontributory.

Physical Examination: (July 20, 1945). On admission the patient appeared well developed and well nourished. He was lying quietly in bed but breathing with some difficulty. He appeared about 15 years younger than the stated age of 66. There were bilateral pterygia. Conjunctiva and other mucous membranes were pale and the tongue appeared smooth over the edges and tip. The chest was essentially negative except for moist rales bilaterally. The heart was essentially normal on physical examination. The blood pressure was 152/100 and the pulse rate was 105/minute. The abdomen was moderately distended and there was dullness extending from the right flank to the mid-clavicular line. No abnormal masses were palpated. Genitalia and lower extremities exhibited marked pitting edema.

Laboratory Findings: The urine contained 4 plus protein, occasional WBCs and occasional RBCs. Hb measured 4 Gm. and there were 1.57 RBCs and 11,950 WBCs/cmm.

Clinical Course: On July 21, 1945 the patient was "found in uremic coma". Emergency measures were of no avail and he died July 23, 1945.

CLINICAL DIAGNOSIS

DOCTOR LANGSTON: I have known G. C. Flowers rather intimately and have followed his course with great interest for a number of years so that my presentation cannot be of the type that has been so popular at the Massachusetts General Hospital in which the clinician handles the case as an unknown with only that information present on the chart as a guide.

· Because pernicious anemia is so uncommon in negroes, there was great interest in the race to which this patient belonged. Many considered him to be a negro, but this I know was not so. Flowers, although married to a negress and although he was hospitalized in the negro ward (by his own choice) was actually a Mexican.

We note that under the Chief Complaints there is listed weakness. Although this directs our attention along certain channels, this complaint characterizes so many diseases that we can draw no definite conclusions. Epigastric distress suggests the possibility of peptic ulcer, but the story of distress *following* meals is quite atypical for peptic ulcer. Symptoms of this type often characterize gastritis, carcinoma of the stomach and, occasionally, achlorhydria. Abdominal distention is another symptom which may be associated with almost any disease. Often it acts to divert attention away from the primary disease. This is especially true with cardiac patients; they often complain more of their abdomen than of their chest. Dyspnea is an important diagnostic symptom, because it is not common to so many diseases. As a rule, dyspnea, especially exertional dyspnea, immediately directs the doctor's thoughts to cardiac insufficiency. This is a logical thought but should not, in itself, lead to a definite conclusion. Severe anemia readily produces such a symptom and was the basis for this complaint here. Occasionally severe anemia may produce practically all the symptoms of heart failure, but you must not confuse these two conditions. We could take the full period on this symptom alone but we must hurry along. This patient complained also of nocturia. I believe we may dismiss prostatic hyperplasia as a cause here. In a normal individual, the urinary output for the waking hours exceeds several times the urinary output for the sleeping hours. In cardiac disease, just the opposite may be true. Often an investigaton of nocturia may give the first clue of cardiac insufficiency. Renal disease, diabetes and certain physiologic states must also be considered. Glossitis was a prominent symptom from the first in this case. Sore mouth and tongue are frequently important symptoms in pernicious anemia, but are often perminent in other conditions, e.g., pellagra and certain other vitamin deficiency states, chronic inflammatory glossitis and, occasionally, achlorhydria. Another symptom was numbness of the legs. This often characterized pernicious anemia, but one must remember that any severe anemia, regardless of its cause or type, may be associated with numbness and tingling in the fingers and toes. Similarly, any severe anemia may produce dependent edema, another symptom which may be incorrectly interpreted and attributed to heart failure. There are a great many cases of edema, particularly in hot weath and especially if the patient stands on his feet a good deal of the time. In addition to such obvious things as cardiac failure and nephritis, one must consider local circulatory phenomena e.g., thrombophlebitis, varicose veins etc. When you observe an individual with edema, next determine whether or not he has exertional dyspnea and orthopnea. If the patient is more comfortable lying flat in bed than with his head elevated, the edema is not on the basis of cardiac insufficiency.

Laboratory data reveals that the patient had no free HCl which is an important finding in this case in that it correlates with our tentative diagnosis. It in itself means very little. Approximately 10 per cent of adults will fail to show free HCl in response to the ordinary test meal, or upon a random analysis. In the older age groups the percentage is much greater. If Flowers had had free gastric HCl it would have immediately presented a very serious obstacle to the diagnosis of pernicious anemia. Another physical finding of importance here is the decreased vibratory sensation. All in all, then, the evidence strongly suggests pernicious anemia. I was never convinced that this was a true case of penicious anemia, however, since on the several occasions which I examined smears from this patient, marcrocytosis and/ or hyperchromatism were not particularly evident. In pernicious anemia, even a cursory examination of a good blood smear should reveal many erythrocytes definitely larger than normal—and the color of these cells will be good. The last criterion for diagnosis is the response to specific therapy. This poor fellow was fed for three weeks an emulsion of raw liver. He gained weight, his blood count rose and throughout the years, as long as he took adequate amounts of liver, he got along fairly well. Although the most dramatic responses to liver therapy are met with in cases of pernicious anemia, it may improve many macrocytic anemias. It was my impression that this man's anemia was probably not a true pernicious anemia, but on the basis of some other deficiency.

The terminal uremic state and things of this sort I will not have time to discuss. The anasarca was probably on the basis of protein deficiency with perhaps the added factor of some acute nephritic process. A very interesting thing about this patient was certain of the gastric signs and symptoms which were never explained. At one time he was suspected of having a gastric cancer and operated on. No evidence of cancer was found.

ANATOMIC DIAGNOSIS

DOCTOR HOPPS: I think that Dr. Langston gave an excellent discussion of this patient and many aspects were so well covered that I will not again discuss them in detail. This case illustrates well that one of the very important reasons for doing autopsies is not merely to learn why the patient dies, but to learn the whys and wherefores. I believe that from our necropsy findings we can satisfactorily explain every sign and symptom which this patient presented. Dr. Langston had an advantage which I did not have in evaluating this case, but from my studies and a review of the clinical data available in the case history, I cannot understand his hesitancy in accepting this as a typical case of pernicious anemia. I did not study blood smears from this patient but upon repeated occasions (when the patient was not taking liver) his color index was well above 1.0— at one tme it was 1.8. From this degree of hyperchromaticity we can assume a comparable macrocytosis. The two together, without any other information make pernicious anemia a probability. Then when we consider the glossitis, decreased vibratory sensation, absence of free HCl, response to liver therapy etc., pernicious anemia, in my mind, becomes a certainty. Furthermore, our studies of the bone marrow and spleen reveal the typical changes of pernicious anemia i.e., marked hyperplasia of erythropoietic elements. There were no abnormalities of the liver, spleen or other organs which would not fit the picture of pernicious anemia and which might have been the primary basis for such an anemia. The stomach also presented changes characteristic of the disease and changes which explain the lack of free HCl, chronic atrophic gastritis. We found evidence there also to explain the gastric signs and symptoms which, as Dr. Langston said, were never explained clinically. You will recall that various roentgenologic examinations suggested on different occasions, gastric syphillis, carcinoma of the stomach and duodenal ulcer with scarring. Actually, the patient had gastric polyposis. Of the three polyps present, the one on the greater curvature was largest. It lay at approximately the juncture of the pyloric and fundal portions and measured 2½ cm. in diameter. Only in the last few years have we become aware of the fact that gastric polyposis is relatively common in pernicious anemia and, furthermore, that the incidence of carcinoma of the stomach in patients with pernicious anemia is several times the normal. In this patients this largest polyp showed very clear-cut evidence of beginning malignant change; it was still quite localized however. You are all aware of the fact that gastric polyps represent a definite precancerous lesion. Some figures indicate that as many as 40 per cent of these will undergo malignant change if they are not removed. Several clinics throughout the country are examining all patients with pernicious anemia at 6 month intervals in order to detect gastric polyps and remove them before they become cancers. Our case of this morning is an illustration of why such a procedure is warranted.

So far then we have explained the cause of the anemia and have related the glossitis, weakness and dyspnea to the pernicious anemia. We were not permitted to examine the spinal cord, but had we done so I am sure that we could present a morphologic basis for the numbness and decreased vibratory sensation in the legs, changes also related to pernicious anemia. We have explained the epigastric distress following meals as on a basis of chronic atrophic gastritis and have demonstrated gastric polyps to explain the various roentgenologic abnormalities in the stomach.

There are several terminal conditions in this patient which, acting together, formed the precipitating cause of death. The most important of these was an active subacute glomerulonephritis which, microscopically,

was seen to be in the proliferative phase. The kidneys were each enlarged about 2 x (240 and 260 grams); they were pale and tense—cut surfaces bulged markedly. This is the obvious explanation of the proteinuria, hematuria and terminal uremic coma. It also explains in large measure the marked pitting edema and the mild hypertension (152/100) which had not previously been present. Hypoproteinemia was probably an additional cause of anasarca. Sixty-six years is certainly not the usual age period in which acute or subacute glomerulonephritis is found so that when it does occur in this older age group it is frequently missed clinically. In addition to this the patient had marked pulmonary edema, hyperemia and bronchopneumonia. This was sufficiently extensive in itself to be a major cause of death. The left lung weighed three times the normal (925 grams) and the right almost five times the normal (1500 grams). Also, adding insult to injury, there were approximately 2 liters of serous fluid in the left pleural cavity and 2 liters in the peritoneal cavity. Then as the final precipitating cause of death, we found an 8 cm. thrombotic embolus in the right atrium of the heart. Changes of secondary importance included marked fatty change, dilation and moderate hypertrophy of the heart and marked fatty change in the liver —both related to the severe anemia which this man had had off and on for many years. We found also an obliterative fibrous pleuritis of the right lung with adhesions to and fibrous obliteration of the pericardial sac. This, I believe, was the effect of an old tuberculous process on this side which, at the time of death, was manifested by a "healed" tuberculous primary complex. It is this lesion that probably accounted for an episode of chest pain some ten or twelve years previously.

DISCUSSION

QUESTION: How often does pernicious anemia occur in negroes?

DOCTOR HOPPS: At Johns Hopkins Hospital, 3.3 per cent of pernicious anemia occure in negroes.

QUESTION: Was there evidence of chronic pancreatitis?

DOCTOR HOPPS: No.

QUESTION: What was the basis of the peculiar yellowish color which this patient presented?

DOCTOR HOPPS: That is characteristic of pernicious anemia and occurs because of an increased destruction of erythrocytes,—in other words it represents a mild hemolytic icterus. The defect in maturation renders the erythrocytes unduly fragile and provides for increased destruction. Many of these improperly formed red cells are destroyed in the bone marrow before they ever get out into the peripheral circulation.

QUESTION: Is there any explanation for this increased tendency for patients with pernicious anemia to develop gastric neoplasms?

DOCTOR HOPPS: The most likely explanation relates to the fact that chronic irritation is one of the most important known causes of cancer. Patients with pernicious anemia have, almost invariably, a chronic atrophic gastritis characterized by a persistent low grade inflammatory reaction and an often dramatic metaplasia of the gastric mucosa so that it comes to closely resemble the epithelium of the colon.

QUESTION: Do you believe that the terminal marked anemia represented a "relapse" of the patient's pernicious anemia?

DOCTOR HOPPS: There was no macrocytosis or hyperchromia during this terminal episode and I believe that this anemia was a manifestation of toxic depression of the bone marrow by the subacute glomerulonephritis rather than pernicious anemia in relapse.

MID-WEST SURGICAL SUPPLY
CO., INC.

Kaufman Building
Wichita 2, Kansas

FRED R. COZART

2437 N. W. 36th Terrace
Phone 8-2561   Oklahoma City, Okla.

RADIUM

(Including Radium Applicators)

FOR ALL MEDICAL PURPOSES

Est. 1919

Quincy X-Ray and Radium Laboratories
(Owned and directed by a Physician-
Radiologist)

HAROLD SWANBERG, B.S., M.D., Director

W.C.U. Bldg.   Quincy, Illinois

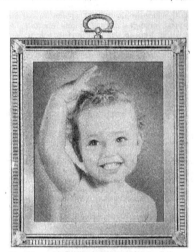

DOCTOR, MEET THE DARICRAFT BABY

Perhaps you are "meeting" the Daricraft Baby every day in your own practice. If not, may we call to your attention the following significant points of interest about Vitamin D increased Daricraft:

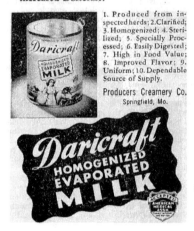

1. Produced from inspected herds; 2. Clarified; 3. Homogenized; 4. Sterilized; 5. Specially Processed; 6. Easily Digested; 7. High in Food Value; 8. Improved Flavor; 9. Uniform; 10. Dependable Source of Supply.

Producers Creamery Co.
Springfield, Mo.

Daricraft
HOMOGENIZED
EVAPORATED
MILK

Special Article

The Variety Club Health Center

OKLAHOMA CITY, OKLAHOMA

Georgia M. Bowen, Public Relations Director
Oklahoma County Health Association

On the cover of this month's Journal is pictured Variety Club Health Center, the 32 room Colonial building located at 600 S. Hudson, which houses the dozen or more clinics and health services operated by the Oklahoma County Health Association, a voluntary or non-official (as distinguished from official, tax-supported agencies) aggregation of health projects. Or as the swinging sign hanging below the gilt lettered name: "Variety Club Health Center", reads: "Home of Oklahoma County Health Association, a Community Fund Agency".

To the well informed medical man and layman, this seems a primer statement. Yet it is amazing how much confusion appears in the public mind regarding these rather cumbersome titles which are so often seen as two overlapping services, rather than the name of a building which is the home, or workshop of a collection of health agencies, theoretically all non-tax supported health services in Oklahoma County and all having specific national affiliations. It was to lessen this confusion that the swinging sign was hung from the portico not long ago. The institution is unique and without duplication anywhere in America.

Variety Club of Oklahoma, Tent 22, built and owns Variety Club Health Center. It pays physical or maintenance costs—heat, light, gas, water, janitor service. The story of the erection of the $60,000.00 building, formally opened June 26, 1941, as a project of the genial motion picture men of the State, has romance and history behind it, but space prevents its repetition here, as likewise does it prevent the repetition of how service upon service was added to the original half dozen, how they were extended until today they are bulging the seams of the pretentious building, and obviously, an annex or additional property is indicated before other services can be taken under the protective wing of Oklahoma County Health Association.

Yet the dedicatory plaque on the building stipulates the purpose :"For the preservation of the health of the community", and to meet this objective, services must be added as community needs arise. At present, there is recognized need for a mental hygiene department, diagnostic clinics for heart and cancer, a children's eye clinic, an ear, nose and throat clinic to aid and abet the work of the speech and hearing department. Enlargement of the mother's milk bank is imperative if this baby-saving service is to carry out its purpose and provide human breast milk for sick and premature infants beyond the County boundary lines, for it must be borne in mind, Oklahoma County mother's milk bank is the only human milk dispensary in the Southwest, and one of only 19 in the entire country.

Established services today include: maternity department, with pre and postnatal clinics, and child health clinic; mother's milk bank; children's dental clinics; tuberculosis clinics; speech and hearing clinics; social hygiene, nutrition, health information and education, public relations departments. There is one of the finest X-ray and laboratory departments to be found anywhere; an up-to-the-minute health library, open to the health-concerned public, an auditorium equipped with motion-picture apparatus and a wide array of health films ready to serve at the call of schools, clubs, or any group in the County.

All services and clinics are supported by the United Community and War Fund with the exception of two, i. e., the tuberculosis clinics and year-round program, financed by the annual sale of Christmas Seals, and the mother's milk bank, a private philanthropy established and financed by C. A. Vose, President of the First National Bank.

So much for the basic information which should be on the tip of the tongue to everyone concerned with "the preservation of the health of the community."

How assiduously is OCHA moving toward this objective? Obviously, from figures coming out of induction centers, OCHA along with other voluntary and official health agencies, parents, schools, and welfare institutions throughout the country, has fallen short of the mark, as is evinced in the thousands

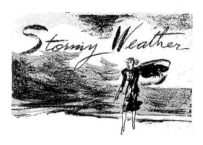

WHEN the menopausal storms set in—vasomotor disturbances, mental depression, unaccountable pain and tension—physicians today can take prompt, positive action to alleviate symptoms.

By the administration of a reliable solution of estrogenic substances, you may exert a gratifying measure of control.

For control of menopausal symptoms, you may turn with confidence to Solution of Estrogenic Substances, Smith-Dorsey . . . manufactured in the fully equipped, capably staffed Smith-Dorsey Laboratories . . . meeting rigid standards of purity and potency.

With such a medicinal, you can indeed *do something* about "stormy weather."

SOLUTION OF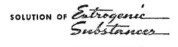

SMITH-DORSEY

Supplied in 1 cc. ampuls and 10 cc. ampul vials representing potencies of 5,000, 10,000 and 20,000 international units per cc.

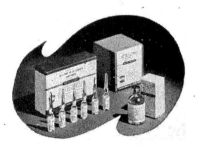

THE SMITH-DORSEY COMPANY
LINCOLN • NEBRASKA
Manufacturers of Pharmaceuticals to the Medical Profession Since 1908

of young men—and women—found "unfit" physically, mentally, emotionally to serve their country.

We have purposely excluded the medical profession from this indictment uncovered by war. Sir William Osler, that forthright physician and teacher of medicine declared: "The battle against tuberculosis is not a doctor's affair; it belongs to the entire public". The same may be said of any infectious and contagious disease. A doctor cannot pick his patients off the curb and drag them to his office for examination and treatment, even though he may recognize the need. In America, people go to doctors to be healed when they are sick—often too late for effective medical aid. The "heathen Chinee" paid doctors to *keep* them in health.

America must revert to this policy, according to Dr. Walker Morledge, associate professor of medicine in Oklahoma University's School of Medicine, who was the luncheon speaker at Oklahoma County Health Association's annual meeting in the Chamber of Commerce, February 6, which was keyed significantly to "Reconversion to Peacetime Health". Dr. Morledge spearheaded his remarks toward a larger degree of prevention —not only through a wider use of vaccines, antitoxins, and known immunization procedure and preventive techniques, but through an ever widening and unceasing barrage of health education. "Eternal vigilance is the price of health," Dr. Morledge warned.

While purely service departments, such as social hygiene, nutrition, health education, have always been open to, and directed toward all who wished to avail themselves, OCHA's clinical services, including tuberculosis, have been limited in scope to the indigent and the low income groups, both negro and white.

In the near future a mobile X-ray unit will be purchased, and a program of mass radiography launched. The contemplated Variety Health Wagon will roll health service and health education to remote corners of city and county, not only with portable X-ray equipment, but with health films, literature, talks—the oldtime "medicine show" shorn of snake-oils, "scare" techniques and quackery, and geared to the highest ideas and ideals of public health practice.

Reconversion will take time. It will mean revision of certain policies and a definition thereof, but with representatives of both county medical and dental societies on the 41-man board of directors, kinks should be easily smoothed out, and the entire health coalition set determinedly on the road to preservation of community health through education, prevention, early diagnosis and effective treatment.

FITTING ESTROGENIC THERAPY TO THE CASE

"Premarin" Liquid, No. 869 . . . for greater flexibility of dosage, and to provide a graduated estrogenic intake where required. Each teaspoonful is the equivalent, in potency, of one "Premarin" Half-Strength Tablet, No. 867.

"Premarin" Tablet, No. 866 . . . for severe estrogenic deficiencies requiring a highly potent yet essentially safe and well-tolerated preparation. Full therapeutic doses of "Premarin" induce a prompt response as judged by vaginal smears and by relief of subjective symptoms.

"Premarin" Tablet, Half-Strength, No. 867 . . . for "average" cases which can be controlled with less than full therapeutic doses. It is recognized that, in the menopause, the smallest effective dose of an estrogen is the *optimal* dose.

Highly Potent • Orally Active • Water Soluble • Naturally Occurring • Essentially Safe • Well Tolerated • Imparts a Feeling of Well-Being.

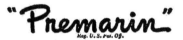

"Premarin"
Reg. U. S. Pat. Off.

AYERST, McKENNA & HARRISON LIMITED • 22 East 40th Street, New York 16, N. Y.

THE PRESIDENT'S PAGE

The House of Delegates of the American Medical Association heartily endorse the Councilor District Meetings attended by the officers of the State Association or their representatives and will insist on the following subjects discussed to acquaint the County Medical Societies with the national problem that is confronting the medical profession.

The suggested program is in line with our four point program of education that was endorsed by the House of Delegates at our last Annual Meeting with:

1. A suggested re-organization of the County Medical Societies wherein there are so few in number in the sparsely settled counties that it makes meeting uninteresting.

2. State wide publicity and educational program on medical care and public health

    A. Through public relations and advertising agencies.

    B. Financing of program.

3. Explanation of the Wagner-Murray-Dingell Bill brought to them in a way of hearing before the senate committee. In this manner bringing out points of the Bill and discussing it in a more enlightening way than has been practiced in the past.

4. They also advocate an allied professional committee which is advocated in the national health congress working with the state dental, hospital, nurses and drug organizations. Thus creating a unified front that will make it possible to contact every individual in a given community.

President.

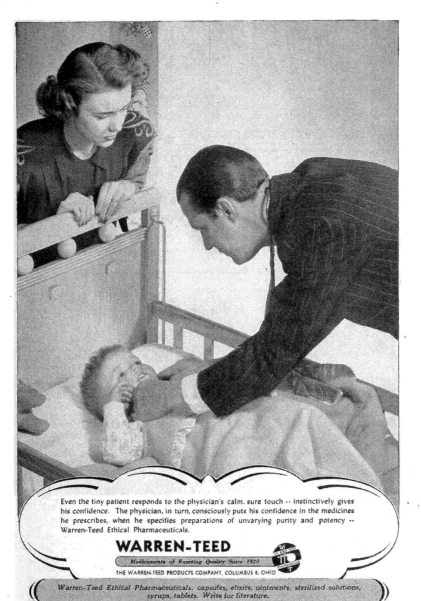

Even the tiny patient responds to the physician's calm, sure touch -- instinctively gives his confidence. The physician, in turn, consciously puts his confidence in the medicines he prescribes, when he specifies preparations of unvarying purity and potency -- Warren-Teed Ethical Pharmaceuticals.

WARREN-TEED

Medicaments of Exacting Quality Since 1920

THE WARREN-TEED PRODUCTS COMPANY, COLUMBUS 8, OHIO

Warren-Teed Ethical Pharmaceuticals: capsules, elixirs, ointments, sterilized solutions, syrups, tablets. Write for literature.

The JOURNAL Of The
OKLAHOMA STATE MEDICAL ASSOCIATION

EDITORIAL BOARD
L. J. MOORMAN, Oklahoma City, Editor-in-Chief

E. EUGENE RICE, Shawnee   BEN H. NICHOLSON, Oklahoma City

MR. DICK GRAHAM, Oklahoma City, Business Manager

JANE FIRRELL TUCKER, Editorial Assistant

CONTRIBUTIONS: Articles accepted by this Journal for publication including those read at the annual meetings of the State Association are the sole property of this Journal.

The Editorial Department is not responsible for the opinions expressed in the original articles of contributors.

Manuscripts may be withdrawn by authors for publication elsewhere only upon the approval of the Editorial Board.

MANUSCRIPTS: Manuscripts should be typewritten, double-spaced, on white paper 8½ x 11 inches. The original copy, not the carbon copy, should be submitted.

Footnotes, bibliographies and legends for cuts should be typed on separate sheets in double space. Bibliography listing should follow this order: Name of author, title of article, name of periodical with volume, page and date of publication.

Manuscripts are accepted subject to the usual editorial revisions and with the understanding that they have not been published elsewhere.

NEWS: Local news of interest to the medical profession, changes of address, births, deaths and weddings will be gratefully received.

ADVERTISING: Advertising of articles, drugs or compounds unapproved by the Council on Pharmacy of the A.M.A. will not be accepted. Advertising rates will be supplied on application.

It is suggested that members of the State Association patronize our advertisers, in preference to others.

SUBSCRIPTIONS: Failure to receive The Journal should call for immediate notification.

REPRINTS: Reprints of original articles will be supplied at actual cost provided request for them is attached to manuscripts or made in sufficient time before publication. Checks for reprints should be made payable to Industrial Printing Company, Oklahoma City.

Address all communications to THE JOURNAL OF THE OKLAHOMA STATE MEDICAL ASSOCIATION, 210 Plaza Court, Oklahoma City 3

OFFICIAL PUBLICATION OF THE OKLAHOMA STATE MEDICAL ASSOCIATION
Copyrighted March, 1946

EDITORIALS

VOLUNTARY MEDICAL AID AND CRIME DETECTION

The medical profession continued interest in public service is well illustrated by the proffered free services of doctors from a University of Oklahoma Medical group. Doctors W. F. Keller and H. C. Hopps, representing this group met with city, county and state criminal investigators and worked out a plan whereby from the designated group a doctor will accompany homicide or murder squads for the investigations of the causes of death and for the discovery of clues in criminal acts, etc.

Under this plan the scientific methods of crime detection worked out by members of the medical profession will be applied. It is anticipated that the plan will lead to suitable legislation for the purpose of establishing a tax supported criminology laboratory whereby approved standards and methods of investigation will be made available. Such a laboratory would serve as a clearing house for all unexplained deaths where crime is suspected and provide facilities for examination of specimens and the discovery and pursuit of clues. Naturally such a laboratory would become more proficient in the speedy discovery of clues and the detection of crime than the private laboratory occasionally engaged by criminal investigators. The state wide movement anticipates a doctor in each county specially trained to take up this work in cooperation with the coroner in handling the medical phase of each case.

Drs. Keller and Hopps have devoted much time and thought to this subject, gleaning the best points from long established services in Boston and New York for the purpose of adapting them to local needs. Certainly they are to be congratulated for sponsoring such a movement and giving so freely of their time and talent. Every doctor in the state should use his influence in behalf of the proposed legislation.

A CHANCE TO CHALK UP YOUR CHARITIES

In the A.M.A. Journal of February 9 there is an editorial entitled "Income Tax Credit for Charity Practice of Physicians". The Journal points out the fact that Representative Clare Booth Luce of Connecticut, recognizing the tremendous contribution made by physicians for public weal, has introduced a bill known as H. R. 5296. Commencing with the year 1946 the Bill provides that physicians, surgeons and dentists shall be allowed a credit for time devoted to charity, to free clinic work and public research.

Concerning the current proposals for various kinds of governmental control of medicine, Representative Luce said, "None of these proposals is a logical development of the American system of recognizing, promoting and rewarding individual choice and achievement. In our earlier history pioneer medicos were rewarded for their frequently ill paid devotion by a very special place in the community, high respect from their fellow citizens and patients, and payment in lovingly prepared delicacies where cash was scarce. Those times have largely vanished. To become a doctor, a surgeon, a dentist now requires some eight or nine years of unremunerative and expensive schooling. Until he has completed all this, usually by the time he is 29 or 30, the doctor cannot even begin to earn his own bread and salt, much less begin to repay himself for the costs of learning his profession."

In connection with the unpaid services which practically every physician renders, she goes on to say, "Surveys as to the amount of these unpaid services indicate that the percentages range from around 30 to 45 per cent of all treatments given. This is a direct contribution on the part of the physician, surgeon or dentist to the public welfare. In addition are the hours spent without pay in public research work, on hospital boards and on boards of charitable organizations. All this must be chalked up to professional devotion, since it results in no return and often requires the practitioner to lengthen his working day to fifteen or sixteen hours or more in times of epidemic. There are no limits possible on a doctor's working day."

The editorial states that this measure is now before the House Committee on Ways and Means and that it may be given consideration before the Committee in connection with its program to revise the income tax law.

Regardless of the ultimate outcome of this proposed legislation, the people and medical profession of the United States are indebted to Representative Luce for calling attention to this voluntary service. If the proposed legislation should be approved by Congress, in fairness to all tax payers, doctors should lean backward in order to make their deductions conform to reasonable estimates of services actually rendered.

THE VIRTUE OF VOLUNTARY MEDICINE

Since the days of Hippocrates when the level gaze of Greek medical minds initiated the age of enlightenment, voluntary, independent medical practice and research have marched hand in hand throughout history, with continuity seldom broken by selfishness and greed.

The progress of medical science and age-old drama which must find new players when we are dead and gone. Life is temporary and relatively unimportant in the course of history. If socialized medicine should come to this country it will pass and be recorded as a political blunder while the thread of continuity pierces the unfortunate period.

Orthodox medicine is too fundamental, too sacred to escape survival. It comes natural to people and they will not long live without it. It is an essential part of humanity, weighed with friendship, goodwill and personal service.

THE HEARING CLINIC AT BORDEN HOSPITAL

During a recent visit to Chickasha for an inpection of Borden Hospital, immediate duties were constantly assailed by insistant memories. More than 40 years ago when the writer left his muddy ponies at the hitching rack and climbed the dingy stairway to his dreary office where days and weeks were spent waiting for calls that never came, he would have welcomed a still, small voice but there were no hearing aids. He would have given his kingdom to know what was on the lips of Fate but there was no lip reading service. Today the most effective hearing and lip reading clinic in the world is connected with Borden Hospital in Chickasha, Oklahoma.

Col. E. R. Gentry, in charge of the hospital, deserves great credit for his unfailing support of this service. The young men in charge deserve the highest commendation, not only for daily duties well permored but for original work done at this hearing center. During the war, the Army had three such centers, today, Chickasha is the only one left. With a meticulously planned plant costing more than $90,000.00 over and above the highly specialized equipment, manned by fifty trained personnel, the work has progressed with enthusiasm and ever widening horizons. Special methods and newly devised techniques have given rise to much original work. The maximum patient capacity is 600. Since late 1943, 4,000 patients have passed through the clinic, all of whom have been helped.

Capt. W. P. Work expressed belief that the load will increase during the next 20 years. He explained that the fenestration operation is not done at this Clinic, chiefly because otosclerosis is not of Army origin. It was indicated that all patients need counseling service and than ten to fifteen per cent have

been referred for neuropsychiatric consultation. Of special interest is a small building
unit representing the initiative and ingenuity of the young doctors on the grounds. It
consist of a small room, isolated, insulated,
floated on cork, thickly padded within and
safeguarded by every known device to shut
out the noise and vibration which may come
from the realm of inaudibility. Standing
in this domicile of silence recalled the fact
that George Elliott once said that if we could
hear what goes on in the land of silence we
would be deafened by the noise.

In the medical mind a serious question a-
rises. Now that the war is over and Borden
Hospital may soon be closed, what will be
the fate of this hearing clinic? Being familiar with the mental operations of young
scientists the seasoned medical observer anticipates that having lost the stimulus of
war, these young men will not be content to
carry on in an isolated spot without the stimulating influences of a University atmosphere
where research in other fields may supply
its interlocking interests and thus stimulate
further research in this particular realm|
While we would like to hold this significant
scientific project in the State of Oklahoma
we must remember that manifest destiny
may decide the issue. It might be well for
the University of Oklahoma to take the cue.

ACROSS THE BORDER

On February 12 Dr. J. D. Osborn of Frederick, Oklahoma, already a member of the
National Board of Medical Examiners, was
made President-Elect of the Federation of
Medical Boards. Since he held down that
160 acres west of Lawton, he has proved up
many other calims and turned much new soil.

At the Conference of State Presidents and
Officers of State Medical Associtions, meeting
in Chicago during the A.M.A. Session of the
House of Delegates, Dick Graham was elected
to the Executive Committee for a period of
three years.

While Jim is busy helping all State Boards
pass upon the merits of those who are to
render medical service to our people, and
Dick is engaged in the task of bringing adequate health service to all the people according to the plans of the Conference of State
Presidents, we can count on high standards
and sound health services being promulgated
for the benefit of the people.

A TOAST TO THE TULSA WORLD

On February 6, editorially, the Tulsa World
voices a vigorous protest against the trend
toward further socialization of American
medicine through exaggerated sob stories
with false implications. Referring to a pa'd
advertisement under the title "More Import-

ant . Than Reaching the Moon — Child
Health", the World says this is not the first
time pious purposes and rank propaganda
have been associated. '

After uncovering the camouflaged design
of this advertisement and making clear its
false connotations, the World goes on to say,
"The advertisement tells a touching story of
infant deaths and maternal unpreparedness
—as if nothing had ever been done by doctors
and agencies to better family conditions. Apparently, under the new scheme, whatever
it may be, the families themselves and the
communities and the doctors and agencies
are to be relieved of all responsibility and are
expected to admit inefficiency and calousness.
There is lofty ignoring of what has been done
in millions of instances to help mothers and
babies. There is, as a matter of fact, a widespread organization for this specific field.

"What we see in this advertisement is a
big and raw socialistic scheme. It bears the
brand of politics rather than humanity. It
is a reach into the cradle to bring people up
in the true socialistic faith and to commit
all and sundry to non-effort, dependence, sub-
servience, to unidentified authority and ab-
ject surrender of personal responsibility and
volition. All such pious-looking approaches
should be examined with a microscope and
a meat-axe."

The advertisement which appears in the
Tulsa Tribune of Tuesday, February 5, closes
with these words in bold type, "Presented As
a Public Service by International Latex Corporation, Playtex Park, Dover, Delaware,
Paid Advertisement . . . Buy Victory Bonds."
The last three words make of this a sad paradox . . . Buy Victory Bonds . . . and Socialized
Free Enterprise.

TULSA COUNTY'S COMMENDABLE PROGRAM

In the February Bulletin of the Tulsa
County Medical Society, the 1946 Scientific
Program is announced. The Tulsa County
Medical Society is to be congratulated for
securing such outstanding speakers and planning this fine educational program for the
period of reconversion.

The first meeting under this plan was addressed by Colonel Howard E. Snyder, former consulting surgeon to the Fifth Army.
His subject was "War Wounds of the Abdomen". Other scheduled speakers are listed
as follows: Evarts A. Graham, M.D., Professor of Surgery, Washington University
School of Medicine, St. Louis, Missouri, Chicago, Ill.; T. E. Jones, M.D., Chief Procto-
logical Surgeon, Cleveland Clinic, Cleveland,
Ohio; Raymond W. McNearly, M.D., Associate Professor of Surgery, Northwestern Uni-

versity School of Medicine, Chicago, Ill.; W. Alton Schsner, M.D., Professor of Surgery, Tulane University School of Medicine, New Orleans, La.; Urban H. Eversole, M.D., Chief of Anesthesia Department; John A. Billingsley, M.D., Professor of Ophthalmolomy, University of Kansas School of Medicine, Kansas City, Kansas.

If the above speakers appear as scheduled it is easy to be seen that Tulsa County will have presented an outstanding postgraduate course staggered throughout the year.

VOLUNTARY PREPAYMENT SICKNESS PLANS

In another section of the Journal is printed a very significant and far-reaching article. It is a report from the American Medical Association in regard to the action taken by the Board of Trustees in definitely establishing a policy of endorsement of voluntary prepayment sickness plans.

This action is one of the most important that the Board has made in the past 25 years, not only from its content of statement, but also because of its broad social and economic implication. Here, in definite and concise language is offered the American people a plan to meet catastrophic illness expenses. A plan originated by the medical profession, with dignity of purpose, carrying out the

age-old relationship of patient and physician, yet at a financial level that is in keeping with the individual's income.

Such constructive action goes further to meet the question of government medicine than anything the doctors have propsed before.—J.F.B., M.D.

Wondrous, indeed, is the virtue of a true book. Not like a dead city of stones, yearly crumbling, yearly needing repair; more like a tilled field, but than a spiritual field; like a spiritual tree, let me rather say, it stands from year to year, and from age to age (we have books that already number some hundred and fifty human ages); and yearly comes its new produce of leaves (commentaries, deductions, philosophical, polietal systems, or were it only sermons, pamphlets, journalistic essays), every one of which is talismanic and thaumaturgic, for is can persuade men. *Carlyle: Sartor Resartus.*

The freedom of the press has never been denied to us, and that in all our history those who have sought the companionship which is found in good books, whether for the light which they shed upon the mind, or the consolation which they bestow upon smitten hearts, have not sought it in vain. *Joseph Anderson: Address. The Growth of a Christian Literature.*

We do not die wholly at our deaths: we have mouldered away gradually long before. Faculty after faculty, interest after interest, attachment after attachment disappear; we are torn from ourselves while living, year after year sees us no longer the same, and death only consigns the last fragment of what we were to the grave.—*Hazlitt: Table Talk.*

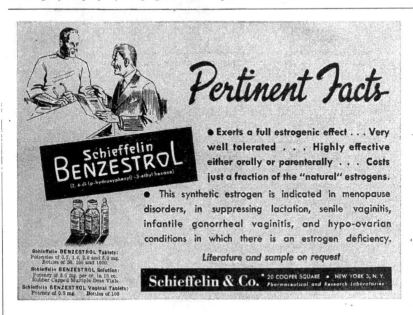

Pertinent Facts

Schieffelin BENZESTROL
(2, 4-di (p-hydroxyphenyl) -3-ethyl hexane)

● Exerts a full estrogenic effect . . . Very well tolerated . . . Highly effective either orally or parenterally . . . Costs just a fraction of the "natural" estrogens.

● This synthetic estrogen is indicated in menopause disorders, in suppressing lactation, senile vaginitis, infantile gonorrheal vaginitis, and hypo-ovarian conditions in which there is an estrogen deficiency.

Literature and sample on request

Schieffelin BENZESTROL Tablets:
Potencies of 0.5, 1.0, 2.0 and 5.0 mg.
Bottles of 50, 100 and 1000.
Schieffelin BENZESTROL Solution:
Potency of 3.0 mg. per cc. in 10 cc.
Rubber Capped Multiple Dose Vials.
Schieffelin BENZESTROL Vaginal Tablets:
Potency of 0.5 mg.   Bottles of 100

Schieffelin & Co.   20 COOPER SQUARE · NEW YORK 3, N. Y.
Pharmaceutical and Research Laboratories

ATTENTION VETERANS INCOME TAX QUESTIONS AND ANSWERS FOR THE RETURNED SERVICEMAN

Q. Are members of the armed forces exempt from tax? A. They are not themselves exempt, but most of their military pay is exempt. All pay of enlisted men and women is exempt; the first $1,500 of officers' pay is exempt. In both cases, any outside income is taxable.

Q. Suppose a serviceman does owe some tax but is overseas. When must he file his return and pay his tax? A. He must file his return within 5½ months after the month in which he returns. He may, however, apply for a postponement of the payments.

Q. What arrangements can be made for postponing the payments? A. Usually, the law allows payment, without interest, in 12 quarterly installments over a three year period. Application for such installment payments must be made before the first installment date to the collector to whom the tax is due.

Q. When is the first installment date under this plan? A. For men or women discharged prior to December 1, 1945, the first installment date is May 15, 1946; for those discharged during succeeding months the dates are—December, June 15, 1946; January, July 15, 1946; February, August 15, 1946; March, September 15, 1946; April, October 15, 1946; May, November 15, 1946. For all persons in service after November 30, 1946, the date is June 15, 1947. These dates apply to taxes owed for the years 1940-1945, inclusive.

Q. What other exemptions are granted discharged veterans? A. In addition to the usual exemptions allowed civilians, they are exempt on mustering-out pay, disability pensions, and educations benefits.

J. D. OSBORN PRESIDENT-ELECT OF FEDERATION OF MEDICAL BOARDS OF UNITED STATES

Word was received on Wednesday, February 13, that J. D. Osborn, M.D., Frederick, Secretary of the Oklahoma State Board of Medical Examiners, is the newly elected president-elect of the Federation of Medical Boards of the United States. Dr. Osborn was elected to serve in 1947. The election was held on February 12 in Chicago in connection with the annual convention of the Federation. Dr. Osborn was elected a member of the National Board of Medical Examiners at a convent of the American Medical Association in Chicago in June of 1943.

VETERANS ADMINISTRATION APPOINTMENTS AVAILABLE FOR DOCTORS

Managers of Veterans Administration Regional Offices and hospitals have been authorized by the Central Office at Washington to make temporary appointments of doctors and dentists to full grade, B. C. Moore, deputy administrator of the St. Louis Branch Office announced.

This grade will enable both physicians and dentists to go to work immediately in Veterans Administration hospitals, clinics and offices at a salary of $5,180.00 to $6,020.00 a year. The grade would permit a physician to become assistant to the chief of service or section; for the dentists the grade would permit the doctor to become assistant chief or chief of the dental service at a Veterans Administration hospital of the assistant chief of dental service in a regional office.

"The Veterans Administration will put to work all dentists and physicians it can secure under this program," Moore said. "They will be given a preference as to location insofar as possible in the area administered by the St, Louis Branch Office."

The doctors and dentists may be interviewed in the Branch Office in St. Louis or any Veterans Administration Regional Office or hospital in Missouri, Kansas, Oklahoma or Arkansas.

A doctor, to qualify for these full grade jobs, must be a citizen of the United States, be a graduate of a school of medicine approved by the Administrator of Veterans Affairs, be licensed to practice as a physician in a state or territory of the United States, meet the physical requirements of the department, and have the required professional experience.

The qualifications for a dentist are the same as those for a physician except that he must have been graduated from a dental school approved by the Administrator of Veterans Affairs and be licensed to practice dentistry in any state or territory of the United States.

INSURANCE PROGRAM MAKING GOOD PROGRESS

Dr. V. K. Allen, Chairman Insurance Committee of the Oklahoma State Medical Association, reports fine progress being made by Mr. Joe H. Jones, Manager, North American Accident Insurance Company, Tulsa, Oklahoma, in connection with the Accident and Health Program.

To date Mr. Jones has contacted the members of 14 County Societies with approximately 95 per cent participation.

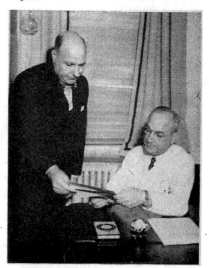

Mr. Joe H. Jones, Tulsa; Dr. V. K. Allen, Tulsa

Each County Society in the state will be contacted at the earliest date possible. Dr. Allen urges that the officers and members of each County Society make a special effort to learn full and complete details with reference to the Accident and Health Insurance Program at the time Mr. Jones visits their County Society. Dr. Allen points out that if application is made at that time, each doctor under age seventy will have an opportunity to participate, regardless of age or physical condition at the same low rate.

It is not necessary to discontinue any present accident and health insurance in order to participate in this program. These policies very nicely dove-tail with any insurance now in force. The individual policy is non-cancellable and covers all diseases and all injuries. Benefits are very liberal and the cost is very reasonable.

Dr. Allen, Dr. LeRoy Long and Dr. J. T. Phelps, members of the Insurance Committee, worked about two years, arranging for this broad coverage, low cost Accident and Health Insurance. The matter was then submitted to the Council through Dr. Tisdal on October 7, 1945, and received approval.

Dr. Allen is very enthusiastic and purchased Policy No. 1.

CONDITIONS GOVERNING POSTGRADUATE FELLOWSHIPS OFFERED BY COMMONWEALTH FUND

Fellowship aid shall be limited to honorably discharged physicians who have seen service for six months or longer, since 1940, in the armed forces of the United States, and who plan to take up residence and to practice in a community having a population of 25,000 or less, situated in Mississippi, Oklahoma, or Tennessee.

Physicians who qualify may be considered for a fellowship which provides postgraduate study for one to four months at an approved institution. The course or courses of study shall be subject to approval by the Fund and may include general medicine and diagnosis, pediatrics, obstetrics, medical gynecology, or minor surgery, or combinations of two or more of these subjects.

The Fund shall assume no responsibility for the registration of a fellow in a particular course; this arrangement must be made by the individual with the institution where the work is offered. Courses shall be taken in continuous term and shall not depart from the approved schedule without special authorization.

The applicant shall be a graduate of a reputable medical school and have completed a satisfactory internship. He shall furnish a record of a recent physical examination, and a personal interview with a member of the Fund staff may be required.

The rate of the fellowship shall be uniform at $100.00 a month for the duration of the award, one to four months. Application for fellowship shall be made on forms furnished by the Commonwealth Fund, Division of Public Health, 41 East 57th Street, New York 22, N. Y.

A.M.A. ESTABLISHES STANDARDS OF ACCEPTANCE FOR MEDICAL CARE PLANS

The Board of Trustees of the American Medical Association and the Council on Medical Service of the American Medical Association at a meeting just completed in Chicago have taken a long step toward protection of the American people against the costs of sickness through participation in a voluntary prepayment sickness plan now developed under the authority of the American Medical Association.

The fundamental step in the development of this plan was the establishment of standards of acceptance for medical care plans which have the approval of the Council on Medical Services of the American Medical Association. Any plan which meets the standards of the Council will be entitled to display the seal of acceptance of the American Medical Association on its policies and on all of its announcements and promotional material. In order to qualify for acceptance, the prepayment plan must have the approval of the state or county medical society in the area in which it operates. The medical profession in the area must assume responsibility for the medical services included in the benefits. Plans must provide free choice of a qualified doctor of medicine and maintain the personal, confidential relationship between patient and physician. The plans must be organized and operated to provide the greatest possible benefits in medical care to the subscriber.

Medical care plans may be in terms of either cash indemnity or service units, with the understanding that benefits paid in cash are to be used to assist in paying the costs incurred for medical service. The standards also include provisions relative to the actuarial data that are required, systems of accounting, supervision by appropriate state authorities and periodic checking and reporting of the progress of the plan to the Council.

Coincidentally with the announcement of these standards of acceptance, there was organized, as a voluntary federation, an organization known as Associated Medical Care Plans, Inc. This independent association will include as members all plans that meet the minimum standard of the Council on Medical Service of the American Medical Association. The Associated Medical Care Plans will undertake to establish coordination and reciprocity among all of these plans so as to permit transference of subscribers from one plan to another and use of the benefits in any state in which a subscriber happens to be located. Under this method great industrial organizations with plants in various portions of the United States will be able to secure coverage for all of their employees. Moreover, it will be possible for the Veterans Administration, welfare and industrial groups as well as government agencies, to provide coverage for the people in any given area through a system of national enrollment. In addition, the Associated Medical Care Plans, Inc., will undertake research and the compilation of statistics on medical care, provide consultation and information services based on the records of existing plans and engage in a great campaign of public education as to the medical service plan movement under the auspices of state and county medical societies.

Sparks

We are like giddy, wild sparks rising from a glowing camp fire. We have our impetous whirl, our ultimate upward flight, and, with little time for accomplishment, we vanish in the darkness. If our ascent is sustained by worthy aspirations and brave deeds, we may pass into poetry and dwell among the stars.

WILLIAM E. EASTLAND, M.D.
F. A. C. R.

RADIUM AND X-RAY THERAPY
DERMATOLOGY

405 Medical Arts Bldg.

Oklahoma City, Oklahoma   Phone 3-1446

LEWIS J. MOORMAN APPOINTED CONSULTANT TO VETERANS ADMINISTRATION

On February 8 Dr. Lewis J. Moorman, Oklahoma City was appointed Consultant by the Veterans Administration in line with their policy to bring civilian medical consultant service into the Veterans Medical Program.

Dr. H. L. Mantz and Dr. John Barnwell were in Oklahoma City on February 12 for the purpose of inspecting Borden General Hospital at Chickasha and the University of Oklahoma School of Medicine and University Hospital.

TRI COUNTY MEDICAL MEETING IN MIAMI

On February 28 a war casualty was again restored to activeness through the first postwar meeting of the Tri County Medical Association consisting of Ottawa County in Oklahoma, Cherokee County in Kansas and Newton County in Missouri.

The meeting was held at the County Club in Miami and representatives were present from the local Society, Baxter Springs, Columbus, Joplin and Carthage. Dr. James Stevenson of Tulsa and Mr. Dick Graham of Oklahoma City presented a program consisting of a mock Senate hearing on the Wagner-Murray-Dingell Bill.

Forty-seven members and guests were present. Among the guests was Dr. W. A. Howard of Chelsea and Dr. Ralph McGill of Tulsa. Dr. W. Jackson Sayles, Secretary of the Ottawa County Medical Society presided in the absence of Dr. C. F. Walker of Grove, President, who was unavoidably detained.

PLANS PROGRESSING FOR SPECIAL TRAIN TO A.M.A. CONVENTION

Plans are in the making for a Special Train, All-Expense Tour for the members of the Oklahoma State Medical Association and other interested Medical Associations for a Special Train Tour to San Francisco for the A.M.A. Convention in July.

Details have not as yet been worked out, however, tentative plans include a three week tour, going from San Francisco to the northwest section and returning by way of Yellowstone Park. Members of the Association will be contacted by letter as soon as final plans are completed.

MEDICAL MEN NEEDED BY CHINA

The United Nations Relief and Rehabilitation Administration has announced openings in the medical field for the China program. The existing needs include specialists in such things as general surgery, orthopedic surgery, genito-urinary surgery, ophthalmology, ear, nose and throat, pediatrics, etc. There is also a need for public health officers and administrators in the higher brackets. Compensation for the openings excellent.

For further information write to Goodrich C. Schauffler M.D., Field Operations Officer, Health Division, United National Relief and Rehabilitation Administration, 1344 Connecticut Avenue, Washington 25, D. C.

STATE NATIONAL LEGISLATIVE COMMITTEE APPOINTED BY PRESIDENT

The following have been appointed by V. C. Tisdal, President of the Association to act as a National Legislative Committee to study national legislation affecting the medical profession: McLain Rogers, M.D., Clinton, Chairman; Finis W. Ewing, M.D., Muskogee; J. D. Osborn, M.D., Frederick; Louis H Ritzhaupt, M.D., Guthrie; O. W. Starr, M.D., Drumright.

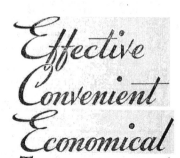

THE effectiveness of Mercurochrome has been demonstrated by more than twenty years of extensive clinical use. For professional convenience Mercurochrome is supplied in four forms—Aqueous Solution in Applicator Bottles for the treatment of minor wounds, Surgical Solution for preoperative skin disinfection, Tablets and Powder from which solutions of any desired concentration may readily be prepared.

Mercurochrome

(H. W. & D. brand of merbromin, dibromoxymercurifluorescein-sodium)

is economical because stock solutions may be dispensed quickly and at low cost. Stock solutions keep indefinitely.

Mercurochrome is antiseptic and relatively non-irritating and non-toxic in wounds.

Complete literature will be furnished on request.

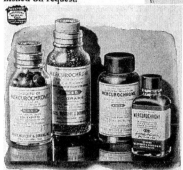

HYNSON, WESTCOTT & DUNNING, INC.
BALTIMORE, MARYLAND

A REAL VALUE!

┌─ **Broad Coverage** ─┐

Low Cost

ACCIDENT

and

HEALTH

└─ **INSURANCE** ─┘

for

Oklahoma Doctors

Approved by the Council Oklahoma State Medical Association

Write or Call for Complete Information

NORTH AMERICAN ACCIDENT INSURANCE CO.

OF CHICAGO, ILLINOIS

Old Line Stock Company   Established 1886

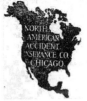

C. W. CAMERON
Southwestern Div. Mgr.
2305 Apco Tower
Oklahoma City, Okla.

JOE H. JONES
Tulsa District Mgr.
312 National Mutual Bldg.
Tulsa, Okla.

The symbol of safety and service

HENRY H. TURNER SPEAKS IN CHICAGO

The Annual Clinical Conference of the Chicago Medical Society was held at the Palmer House in Chicago on March 5, 6, 7 and 8. Dr. Henry H. Turner of Oklahoma City was one of the guest speakers and gave a discussion of ''Endocrine Problems of Childhood''.

SURPLUS BLOOD PLASMA MADE AVAILABLE

The following is a list of the hospitals throughout the state where the Blood Plasma offered by the Red Cross is available. Since the appearance of the article in last month's Journal, it has been decided not to require the report of the names of patients upon whom the plasma is used since it is available to all without charge regardless of financial ability. It is not necessary that the form enclosed with each unit of plasma be filled out and sent either to the Army or Navy or State Health Department.

Place	Hospital or Health Unit
Ada	Breco Memorial Hospital
Ada	Cottage Hospital
Ada	Valley View Hospital
Allen	Morris Clinic and Hospital
Altus	Altus Hospital
Alva	Alva Osteopathic Hospital
Anadarko	Caddo County Health Department
Ardmore	Carter County Health Department
Ardmore	Hardy Sanitarium
Bartlesville	Washington County Memorial
Blackwell	Riverside Osteopathic Hospital
Boley	Sanders Hospital
Bristow	Cowart-Sisler
Broken Arrow	Franklin Hospital
Carnegie	Hinton Clinic and Hospital
Checotah	Osteopathic Hospital
Chelsa	Jennings Hospital
Cherokee	Osteopathic Hospital
Chickasha	Cottage Hospital
Chickasha	General Hospital
Chickasha	Oklahoma Hospital
Claremore	Claremore General Hospital
Clinton	District IV Health Department
Clinton	Western Oklahoma Hospital
Comanche	Comanche Hospital
Commerce	Dr. Week's Hospital
Concho	Cheyenne Arapaho Indian Hospital
Cordel	Florence Hospital
Cushing	Masonic Hospital
Duncan	Lindley Hospital
Duncan	Patterson Hospital
Duncan	Stephens County Health Department
Duncan	Weedn Hospital
Durant	Bryan County Health Department
Durant	Durant Hospital
Durant	Haynie Hospital
Elk City	Community Hospital
Elk City	Tisdal Hospital
Enid	Enid General Hospital
Enid	Enid Osteopathic
Enid	University Hospital
Fairview	Fairview Hospital
Frederick	Frederick Hospital
Frederick	S. A. & A. Hospital
Freedom	Freedom Clinic and Hospital
Grandfield	Grandfield Hospital
Granite	Lewis Hospital
Guthrie	Cimarron Valley Wesley
Guthrie	Logan County Health Department
Guymon	District III Health Department

CREDIT SERVICE

330 American National Building

Oklahoma City, Oklahoma

(Operators of Medical-Dental Credit Bureau)

We offer a dignified and effective collection service for doctors and hospitals located anywhere in the State. Write for information.

28 YEARS

Experience In Credit and Collection Work

Robt. R. Sesline, Owner and Manager

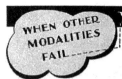

YOUNG'S Rectal Dilators

WHEN OTHER MODALITIES FAIL

Treatment of CONSTIPATION by dilation usually proves effective when habit forming laxatives and cathartics have proved inadequate or not tolerated. Set of 4 graduated bakelite dilators, adult $4.75, childrens size $4.50. Obtain at your pharmacy or surgical supply dealer. Write for brochure. Sold on prescription only.

F. E. YOUNG & CO.   424 E. 75th Street, Chicago 19, Ill.

J. E. HANGER, Inc.

ARTIFICIAL LIMBS, BRACES, AND CRUTCHES

Phone: 2-8500   612 N. Hudson

L. T. Lewis, Mgr.   BRANCHES AND AGENCIES IN PRINCIPAL CITIES   Oklahoma City 3, Okla.

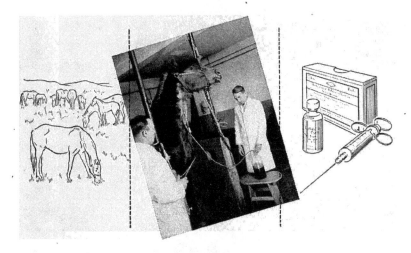

"NOT HOW MUCH... BUT HOW WELL"

U. S. STANDARD PRODUCTS CO.

BIOLOGICALS

AMPULS AND STERILE SOLUTIONS
FOR PARENTERAL ADMINISTRATION

An ideal location in a small rural community favors concentration on the important work in which we specialize—

Patented processes confer distinct therapeutic advantages—

Methods and thinking based upon the advanced frontiers of progress—

—These are factors contributing to the established acceptance of U. S. Standard Products by those of the medical profession who have come to regard them as essential.

U. S. Standard Products are now available at leading pharmacies throughout most of the United States. May we send you detailed information?

OUTSTANDING U. S. STANDARD BIOLOGICALS:

DIPHTHERIA TOXOID
SMALLPOX VACCINE
TETANUS ANTITOXIN
TYPHOID VACCINE

Also a representative list of glandular products and pharmaceuticals.

U. S. STANDARD PRODUCTS CO.
WOODWORTH, WISCONSIN, U. S. A.

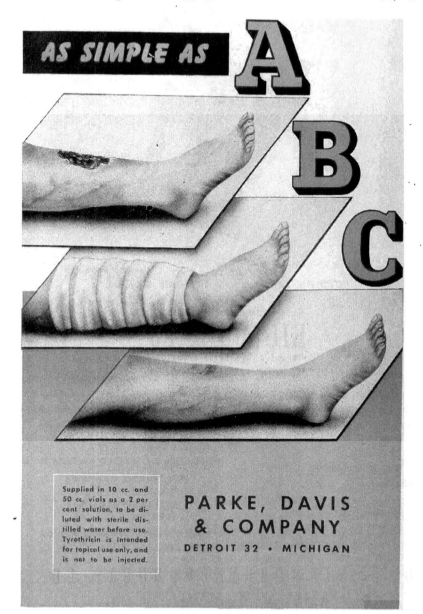

AS SIMPLE AS A B C

Supplied in 10 cc. and 50 cc. vials as a 2 per cent solution, to be diluted with sterile distilled water before use. Tyrothricin is intended for topical use only, and is not to be injected.

PARKE, DAVIS
& COMPANY
DETROIT 32 • MICHIGAN

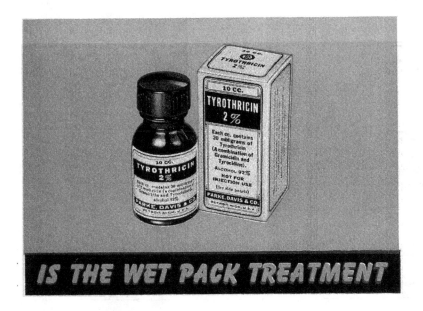

IS THE WET PACK TREATMENT

of superficial indolent ulcers and other skin lesions with
TYROTHRICIN . . . a most important antibiotic agent.

TYROTHRICIN

used in wet packs or by irrigation, is effective against
streptococcic, staphylococcic and pneumococcic infections of superficial tissues, deeper tissues made accessible by surgical procedures, and body cavities in which
there is no direct communication with the blood stream.

O

Harrah ....Devine's Clinic
Hinton ....Hinton Clinic and Hospital
Hobart ....General Hospital
Holdenville ....Holdenville General
Hugo ....Choctaw Health Department
Hugo ....Hugo Hospital
Hugo ....Johnson Hospital
Hugo ....Medical Arts Hospital
Kingfisher ....Kingfisher County Health Department
Lawton ....Angus Hospital
Lawton ....Comanche County Health Department
Lawton ....Southwestern Clinic
Lindsay ....Lindsay Hospital
Madill ....Madill Hospital
Madill ....Marshall County Health Department
Marlow ....Talley Hospital
McAlester ....Pittsburg County Health Department
McAlester ....St. Mary's Hospital
Medford ....Dr. T. V. Hardy, Supt. of Health
Meeker ....Bell Hospital and Clinic
Miami ....Miami Baptist Hospital
Miami ....Ottowa County Health Department
Moorland ....Northwest Community Hospital
Muskogee ....Muskogee County Health Department
Muskogee ....Oklahoma Baptist Hospital
Norman ....Cleveland County Health Department
Norman ....Norman City Hospital
Nowata ....Clinic Hospital
Okemah ....Clinic Hospital
Okemah ....Okemah Hospital and Clinic
Oklahoma City ....Capitol Hill General
Oklahoma City ....McBride's Hospital
Oklahoma City ....Oklahoma General
Oklahoma City ....Polyclinic Hospital
Oklahoma City ....St. Anthony's Hospital
Oklahoma City ....University Hospital
Oklahoma City ....Wesley Hospital

Okmulgee ....City Hospital
Okmulgee ....Oklahoma County Health Department
Pauls Valley ....Johnson and Lindsey Hospital
Pauls Valley ....Holman Hospital and Clinic
Pawhuska ....Osage County Infirmary
Pawhuska ....Pawhuska Municipal
Pawnee ....Pawnee Municipal
Pawnee ....Pawnee Ponca Indian Hospital
Picher ....Picher Hospital
Ponca City ....Ponca City Hospital
Poteau ....Beville-Rolls Hospital
Pryor ....Herrington Hospital
Pryor ....Whitaker Hospital
Purcell ....McCurdy Hospital
Sayre ....Sayre Hospital
Seminole ....Harber Hospital
Sentinel ....McMurry and Stowers Hospital
Shattuck ....Shattuck Hospital
Shawnee ....A. C. & H. Hospital
Shawnee ....Pottewatomie County Health Department
Shidler ....Wells-Lee Hospital
Stillwater ....Stillwater Municipal Hospital
Stroud ....Glendale Hospital
Sulphur ....Oklahoma Veterans Hospital
Tahlequah ....Tahlequah Hospital
Talihina ....Talihina Indian Hospital
Thomas ....Thomas Hospital
Tonkawa ....Tonkawa Hospital
Tulsa ....Byrne Hospital
Tulsa ....City Health Department
Tulsa ....Flower Hospital
Tulsa ....Hillcrest Hospital
Tulsa ....Medical and Surgical Hospital
Tulsa ....Mercy Hospital
Tulsa ....Moten Memorial (Negro)
Tulsa ....Oklahoma Osteopathic Hospital
Tulsa ....Salvation Army Hospital
Tulsa ....St. John's Hospital
Tulsa ....Tulsa County Hospital
Vinita ....Vinita Hospital

DIAGNOSTIC CLINIC OF INTERNAL MEDICINE AND ALLERGY

Philip M. McNeill, M. D., F. A. C. P.

General Diagnosis

CONSULTATION BY APPOINTMENT

Special Attention to Cardiac, Pulmonary and Allergic Diseases

Electrocardiograph, X-Ray, Laboratory
and Complete Allergic Surveys Available.

1107 Medical Arts Bldg.
Oklahoma City, Okla.   Phone 2-0277

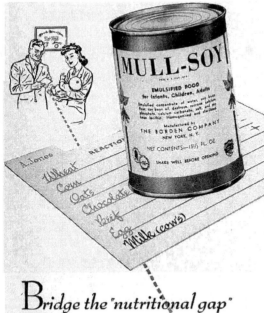

Bridge the "nutritional gap"

The nutritional benefits of milk need not be deprived the "milk-sensitive" patient, even though successful treatment demands complete elimination of the offending food from the diet.

Clinical evidence has established MULL-SOY as an effective hypoallergenic substitute for cow's milk. This concentrated, emulsified soy bean food—homogenized and sterilized—closely approximates cow's milk in protein, fat, carbohydrate and mineral content. It is palatable, well tolerated, easy to digest and easy to prepare. Infants (particularly) thrive on MULL-SOY, and take it readily.

Write for copies of "TASTY RECIPES FOR MULL-SOY IN MILK-FREE DIETS", for your milk-allergic patients.

BORDEN'S PRESCRIPTION PRODUCTS DIV., 350 MADISON AVE., NEW YORK 17, N. Y.

MULL-SOY

HYPOALLERGENIC SOY BEAN FOOD

MULL-SOY is a liquid emulsified food prepared from water, soy bean flour, soy bean oil, dextrose, sucrose, calcium phosphate, calcium carbonate, salt and soy bean lecithin; homogenized and sterilized. Available in 15½ fl. oz. cans at all drug stores.

Walters ....Walters Memorial Hospital
Waurika ....Waurika Hospital
Weatherford ....Weatherford Emergency
Wewoka ....Medical Arts Hospital
Wewoka ....Seminole County Health Department
Wewoka ....Wewoka Hospital
Woodward ....Woodward Memorial Hospital
Wynnewood ....Wynnewood Hospital

James Worrall Henry, M.D.
1888-1946

Dr. James Worrall Henry, former Oklahoma City physician died January 14 at the home of friends in Anadarko.

Dr. Henry came to Oklahoma in 1893 from Michigan. He entered medical school at the University of Oklahoma but received his medical degree from Columbia University in 1912. After serving internship at Polyclinic Hospital in New York City, he came to Oklahoma City where he practiced for a number of years. From Oklahoma City, Dr. Henry went to Chyenne where he practiced until his death. He was a member of the Beckman County Medical Society, the Oklahoma State Medical Association and the American Medical Association.

Surviving Dr. Henry are his wife and a cousin, Mrs. Dave Harriman.

J. R. Preston, M.D.
1876-1945

Dr. J. R. Preston, Weleetka, passed away on December 10, 1945 in a Kansas City Hospital.

Dr. Preston was born in 1876 in Johnson County, Kentucky. In 1907 he received his medical degree from the Lincoln Memorial Medical School in Knoxville, Tennessee, after which he came to Oklahoma and settled at Adair where he remained until 1917. At this time he moved to Weleetka where he remained until his death.

Dr. Preston was interested both in his profession and public welfare. He served for sometime as City Physician, Associate County Physician and President of the Okfuskee County Medical Association. He was Mayor of Weleetka for eight years. He was a member of the Oklahoma State Medical Association and the American Medical Association; the Masonic lodge in Weleetka and the Weleetka Christian Church.

Surviving Dr. Preston are his wife, Mrs. Madge Preston, three brothers, two sons and three stepsons.

Supplementary list of Medical Corp Officers released from service

Adams, J. W., Jr. ....Chandler
Aldredge, W. M. ....University Hosp., Okla. City
Anderson, W. D. ....Walker Bldg., Claremore
Atkins, Paul N., Jr. ....Braniff Bldg., Tulsa
Beaty, C. Sam ....Veterans Hosp., Muskogee
Best, Ralph L. ....Tulsa
Bishop, Calmes P. ......1944 Pennington Rd., Trenton, N.J.
Bohlman, W. F. ....Watonga
Borecky, George L. ....Okla. City
Bradshaw, John O. ....Welch
Branham, Donald W. ....Med. Arts Bldg., Okla. City
Buel, A. L. ....225 E. Boyd, Norman
Buffington, F. C. ....640 Okmulgee, Norman

Bush, Jordan M. ....827 N. E. 20, Okla. City
Cantrell, Wm. ....Med. Arts Bldg., Okla. City
Conover, George W. ....602 W. Virginia, Anadarko
Cordonnier, Byron, Jr. ....Broadway Tower, Enid
Cotteral, John ....Henryetta
Darrough, James B. ....Vinita
Deaton, A. N. ....Wewoka
Denyer, Hillard ....Wesley Hosp., Okla. City
Duer, Joe L. ....Woodward
Duff, Kenneth R. ....712 B Ave., Lawton
England, Myron ....Woodward
Ewell, Wm. C. ....1307 S. Main, Tulsa
Felts, Clifton ....Seminole
Ford, Richard B. ....Braniff Bldg., Tulsa
Fox, Raymond H. ....Altus
Freeman, Charles ....Rocky
Fry, Powell E. ....Stillwater
Fryer, Sam ....1912 N. W. 18, Okla. City
Fulton, C. C. ....Okla. City
Gallaher, Paul ....Shawnee
Gayman, Byron R. ....Veterans Hosp., Muskogee
Goggin, Chester ....525 S. Serrano, Los Angeles, Calif.
Graening, P. K. ....Med. Arts Bldg., Tulsa
Haddock, Phil ....231 E. Gray, Norman
Hardman, Thomas J. ....502 Med. Arts Bldg., Tulsa
Harrison, S. P. ....1701 N. W. 31, Okla. City
Hays, Luvern ....Tulsa
Hendren, Walter S. ....501 N. W. 12, Okla. City
Henry, Gifford ....Tulsa
Hinson, Bruce R. ....1017 W. Wabash, Enid
Howard, Robert B. ....Osler Bldg., Okla. City
Huston, Evans G. ....Okla. City
Karlick, Joseph R. ....204 Gilbert Bldg., Ardmore
Kreger, Glenn S. ....Tonkawa

(Continued on Page 140)

As friends and companions, as teachers and consolers, as recreators and amusers, books are always with us, and always ready to respond to our wants. We can take them with us in our wanderings, or gather them round us at our firesides. In the lonely wilderness and the crowded city, their spirit will be with us, giving a meaning to the seemingly confused movements of humanity, and peopling the desert with their own bright creations. *John Alfred Langford: The Praise of Books. Preliminary Essay.*

NEUROLOGICAL HOSPITAL

Twenty-Seventh and The Paseo
Kansas City, Missouri

Modern Hospitalization of Nervous and Mental Illnesses, Alcoholism and Drug Addiction.

THE ROBINSON CLINIC

G. WILSE ROBINSON, M.D.
G. WILSE ROBINSON, Jr., M.D.

PRESCRIBE OR DISPENSE
ZEMMER PHARMACEUTICALS
A complete line of laboratory controlled ethical pharmaceuticals.   OK 3-46
Chemists to the Medical Profession for 44 years.
THE ZEMMER COMPANY • Oakland Station • Pittsburgh 13, Pa.

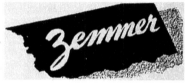

Your 3 choices when treating diabetics...

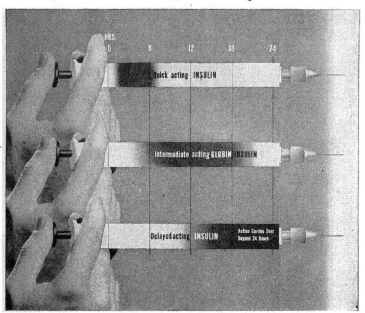

WHEN A PHYSICIAN decides that a patient needs more than diet to control diabetes, he can now choose from three types of insulin. One is quick-acting and short-lived. Another is slow-acting and prolonged. Intermediate between these, is the third—the new 'Wellcome' Globin Insulin with Zinc. Its action begins with moderate promptness yet is sustained for sixteen or more hours—adequate to cover the period of maximum carbohydrate ingestion. By night, activity is sufficiently diminished to decrease the likelihood of nocturnal reactions. Physicians who consider the many advantages of this new third type of insulin now have another effective method of treating diabetes.

'Wellcome' Globin Insulin with Zinc is a clear solution, comparable to regular insulin in its relative freedom from allergenic properties. Accepted by the Council on Pharmacy and Chemistry, American Medical Association. Developed in the Wellcome Research Laboratories, Tuckahoe, New York. U. S. Patent No. 2,161,198. Available in vials of 10 cc., 80 units in 1 cc., and vials of 10 cc., 40 units in 1 cc. Literature on request. 'Wellcome' trademark registered.

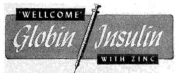

'WELLCOME'
Globin Insulin
WITH ZINC

BURROUGHS WELLCOME & CO. (U.S.A.) INC., 9 & 11 EAST 41ST STREET, NEW YORK 17, N. Y.

FUND FOR ADVANCEMENT OF
MEDICAL SCIENCE CREATED

O. U. ALUMNI PLAN $3,100,000.00

RESEARCH PROGRAM

At a meeting of the Council of the Alumni Association of the University of Oklahoma School of Medicine in Oklahoma City on February 3, there was created the Board of the Fund for the Advancement of Medical Science in Oklahoma. The creation of this Board to sponsor a $3,100,000.00 Endowment Fund for the establishing of a Research Institute is probably the greatest forward step medicine has taken in Oklahoma in the history of the state. The medical profession, by and large, must give this newly created organization its complete support both through its time and effort in the behalf of the Fund and by liberal financial contributions.

JOHN H. LAMB, M.D., CHAIRMAN OF TEMPORARY BOARD

The Council of the Alumni Association, which is serving as the temporary Board for the Fund, has selected Dr. John H. Lamb of Oklahoma City as the Chairman and Dr. Mark R. Everett, Secretary-Treasure. Dr. Lee K. Emenhiser, President of the Alumni Association and the following Councilors will continue to serve on the temporary Board until such time as the organization is made permanent Dr. C. A. Traverse, Alva; Dr. J. E. Ensey, Altus; Dr. L. R. Wilhite, Perkins; Dr. Onis G. Hazel, Oklahoma City; Dr. Roy Emanuel, Chickasha; Dr. Ralph McGill, Tulsa; Dr. John Carson, Shawnee; Dr. Matt Connell, Picher; Dr. E. H. Shuller, McAlester; Dr. P. H. Lawson, Marietta.

PROPOSED PROGRAM FOR RESEARCH INSTITUTE

The temporary Board at its organizational meeting adopted, in principle, the following program for the Research Institute:

Estimate of Costs for:

(A) Construction and Continued Maintenance of Research Institute Building.

(B) Operation of the Institute at capacity of a 10 year period.

(A) Construction of building (40,-000 sq. ft. floor space and permanent built-in equipment) $450,000
Installation of permanent movable experimental equipment (larger apparatus, furniture, etc.) 150,000
Endowment for c o n t i n u e d maintenance of building (utilities, insurance, janitor service, repairs, remodeling, salary of business manager and assistant, at yearly cost of $22,-500) 750,000
TOTAL $1,350,000

(B) Operation of the Research Institute for a 10-year period. The operation to consist of specific projects financed from ear-marked funds and from general fund allocations by the board.

I. Funds for Research Grants (specified and general, to include contributions made from time to time by individuals, federal grants, corporations, clinical institutes associated with the Medical School, etc.

(1) Allocations for salaries of research personnel (Estimate based on number of workers that can be conveniently accommodated in the Institute, tentatively itemized as:

3 Research Investigators, $10,000 each annually
3 Research Investigators, $6,000 each annually
6 Research Fellows, $3,500 each annually
12 Technical assistants $2 000 each annually   940,000

(2) Allocation for purchase of expendable equipment, publications, and special temporary services such as, special nursing, construction of special equipment etc., $50,000 annually 500,000

(3) Allocation for necessary care of selected patients beyond that which the University Hospitals can afford by law, $15,000 annually 130,000

II. Fund for salaries of Director of the Institute and of 3 permanent employees (secretaries, machinist) $16,000 annually 160,000

TOTAL   1,750,000

GRAND TOTAL $3,100,000

(Note: To start operation of the Institute approximately $2,000,000 must be obtained initially; the remainder could be pledged for contribution during a period of 3 to 5 years following the opening of the Institute)

SURVEY PROGRESSING SATISFACTORILY

The Board has been actively assisting Mr. Frank Wood, the Alumni Association's representative, in starting the survey of the project. The Councilors of the Association have been engaged in supporting this work. Dr. Lee Emenhiser, Dr. Onis Hazel and Dr. John Lamb comprise the Executive Committee for the first part of the survey in the Oklahoma City area, which has been completed. Fifty-two prominent citizens, including attorneys, bankers, merchants, petroleum executives, and other civic leaders have been consulted with most encouraging results. Only two of these citizens were not interested in the Alumni project. Many offered their services, financial and other assistance, in support of a campaign for funds. A number of these influential citizens stated that the project to create a Medical Research Institute was a very desirable and necessary philanthropy, and that Oklahoma has developed to a stage where it should naturally be expected to support the endeavor. Some indicated that an even larger project should be undertaken, while others believed that it was sufficient as planned. Several citizens thought that Oklahoma should attempt to build a medical center pre-eminent in the entire Southwest.

The Oklahoma City phase of the survey has been encouraging to the officials of the Alumni Association and the Board, and has given them the stimulus required for the considerable time and energy needed for their work. The next phase of the survey is to start in Tulsa. At the meetings of Alumni held in Tulsa, Dr. Ralph A. McGill, Alumni Councilor for the area, accepted the task of organizing an Executive Committee to assist Mr. Wood. Other Alumni who have offered to assist Dr. McGill include Dr. Fred Woodson, Dr. John Perry and Dr. E. O. Johnson. Councilors in other Oklahoma cities

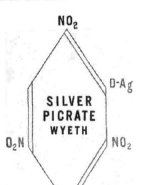

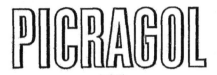

PICRAGOL is an effective agent in the treatment of urethritis and vaginitis. Its specific action is especially valuable for the control of trichomoniasis or moniliasis of the vagina and for trichomonas infections of Bartholin's or Skene's glands.

PICRAGOL CRYSTALS, Bottles of 2 grams. • COMPOUND PICRAGOL POWDER, Silver Picrate Wyeth, 1 per cent, in a kaolin base. Packages of six 5 gram vials. • VAGINAL SUPPOSITORIES PICRAGOL, Silver Picrate Wyeth, 0.13 grams, in a boroglyceride-gelatin base. Packages of 12 • VAGINAL SUPPOSITORIES PICRAGOL, *for infants*, Silver Picrate Wyeth, 65 mg., in a boroglyceride-gelatin base. Packages of 12.

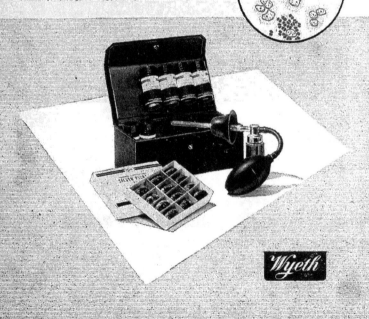

WYETH INCORPORATED • PHILADELPHIA 3 • PA.

are also doing their share in organizing the state-wide survey which is to follow the Tulsa study.

While a campaign for funds is not to be started until the survey has been completed, several contributions have already been made to the Fund for the Advancement of Medical Science. The available list includes the following: Dr. Daisy G. Cotton, Oklahoma City; Dr. J. Wm. Finch, Hobart; Dr. John A. Haynie, Durant; Dr. John H. Lamb, Oklahoma City; Dr. Lewis J. Moorman, Oklahoma City; Dr. Harry Nesh, Brooklyn, N. Y.

The first donation was received from Dr. John A. Haynie. Dr. John Lamb has allocated his contribution

to the creation of a research fellowship in pharmacology, in memory of the late Dr. A. B. Chase, formerly Professor of Medicine at the School of Medicine. Details of this fellowship will be announced elsewhere. It should also be mentioned that Dr. Coyne Campbell of Oklahoma City established the John Archer Hatchett Memorial Research Fund to support research fellowships at the medical school before the Alumni project was begun. Several Oklahoma City physicians, and Mr. and Mrs. John C. De Lana of El Reno, have contributed to this fund, which amounts to $3,900.00 at present.

Medical Abstracts

NEUROSURGICAL ASPECTS OF LUMBAR AND SCIATIC PAIN. Edgar F. Fincher. Journal of Medical Association of Georgia: 34: 149-154. 1945.

Fincher deals chiefly with cartilage damage, spinal cord tumors, and neuroses. A careful chronological history is of first importance. All cartilage ruptures are due to trauma, even if the frank displacement was precipitated by violent sneezing. One may get a history of trauma in tumors of the spinal cord, but this is merely coincidental. The patients with compensation neuroses all give a history of trauma.

The character of the back pain in patients with cartilage damage is important. The pain is exaggerated on motion and intensified by coughing or sneezing, and is alleviated by complete rest. In intradural tumors the onset of pain is insidious and slow in development; it is primarily radiating, and back pain may be absent. The pain is consistently exaggerated by rest. Patients get out of bed and walk for relief. In the psychological cases the patient strives to impress the doctor with the intensity of his suffering. The back pain is diffuse in location; the extremity pain is likely to involve the entire limb, and does not follow a nerve distribution. It is always exaggerated by work and not helped by rest.

Pain due to other causes is discussed. Important signs in cartilage cases are a flattening of the lumbar curve, and a sciatic list away from the painful extremity. There is muscle splinting on the painful side. The pelvis may tilt, and patients often limp. Calf atrophy can often be determined by measuring. In cord tumors, nothing is noted on inspection in most cases. In compensation cases bizarre positions may be assumed.

The differential diagnosis is discussed. Roentgenograms are necessary; stereoscopic anteroposterior films and lateral films are made. In disc cases the films show (1) straightening of the lumbar curve; (2) narrow-

ing of the intervertebral space, and (3) "sciatic list". Opaque injections to visualize the spinal canal are not necessary in cartilage cases, but are of value in tumor cases. They are severely condemned in psychological cases, and surgery is to be avoided in these cases.

There is much good common sense in this article, and many practical points in differential diagnosis.—E.D.M., M.D.

REPAIR OF LARGE ABDOMINAL DEFECTS BY PEDICLED FASCIAL FLAPS. Surgery, Gynecology & Obstetrics. Vol. 82, No. 2, pp. 144-150. February, 1946.

A method is described for increasing the range of utility of the iliotibial tract of fascia, pedicled on the tensor fascia femoris muscle in the repair of abdominal hernias. By employing the pedicled iliotibial tract as a replacement for a pedicled fascial flap swung up from the lower to the upper abdomen, any hernia of the abdominal wall becomes amenable to treatment by this method. Heretofore, incisional hernias with large defects in the upper abdomen have been difficult problems to resolve by any of the available methods. The procedure herein described gives promise of constituting a means of dealing satisfactorily with large defects of the upper abdominal wall. The method possesses the advantage over free fascial grafts of insuring satisfactory wound healing.

The instance of a patient having a defect 24 centimeters long and 18 centimeters in width in the upper abdomen, following excision of a large desmoid tumor of the abdominal wall is reported. A good firm abdominal wall resulted. A nonirritative, nonabsorbable suture such as fine silk is the suture material of choice for anchoring the pedicled grafts.

An instance is cited also in which the iliotibial tract of fascia pedicled upon the tensor fascia femoris muscle

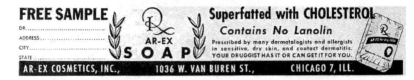

FREE SAMPLE   **AR-EX SOAP**   **Superfatted with CHOLESTEROL**
Contains No Lanolin
Prescribed by many dermatologists and allergists in sensitive, dry skin, and contact dermatitis. YOUR DRUGGIST HAS IT OR CAN GET IT FOR YOU.

DR.
ADDRESS
CITY
STATE

AR-EX COSMETICS, INC.,   1036 W. VAN BUREN ST.,   CHICAGO 7, ILL.

THE WILLIE CLINIC AND HOSPITAL

A private hospital for the diagnosis, study and treatment of all types of neurological and psychiatric cases. Equipped to give all forms of recognized therapy, including hyperpyrexia, insulin and metrazol treatments, when indicated. Consultation by appointment.

JAMES A. WILLIE, B.A., M.D.
Attending Neuro-psychiatrist

218 N. W. 7th St.—Okla. City, Okla.   Telephones: 2-6944 and 3-6071

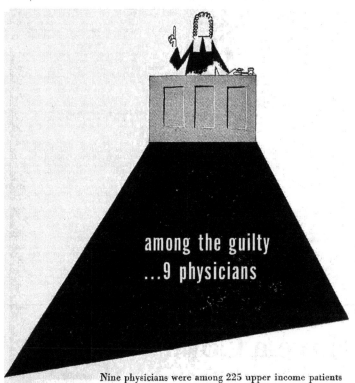

among the guilty
...9 physicians

Nine physicians were among 225 upper income patients found guilty of diets wanting in one or more vitamins. Low-vitamin diets are not restricted by income or by intelligence.[2] Greater assurance of adequate vitamin maintenance is available in potent, easy to take, and reasonably priced Upjohn vitamin preparations.

1. New England J. Med. 228:118 (Jan. 28) 1943.
2 J.A.M.A. 129:615 (Oct. 27) 1945.

FINE PHARMACEUTICALS SINCE 1886

U P J O H N   V I T A M I N S

was employed to replace the larger part of the musculo-fascial portion of the abdominal wall below the umbilicus attending excision of a large desmoid tumor weighing 1500 grams. The defect was 15 centimeters in length and 13 centimeters in width. A single pedicled graft of the iliotibial tract supplemented by its lateral extensions of fascia lata sufficed to fill the defect.

Removal of such large fascial flaps from the thigh does not impair its function and is not followed by untoward effects.—J.F.B., M.D.

NUTRITION IN NEWFOUNDLAND. The Canadian Medical Association Journal. Vol. 52, pp. 227-250. 1945.

As has been noted frequently and in many places the quantity and quality of man's life, other variables being equal, is determined by the adequacy of his food.

The findings of a medical mission to Newfoundland, here reported, again attests to the truth of this conclusion.

Two-thirds of the population of Newfoundland is descended from rugged fishermen of Devenshire and the Channel Islands: the other third is of no less rugged Irish stock. The poor fertility of the land and inadequacy of transportation facilities have led to food habits which are distinctly bad. In keeping with this poor average diet, a large proportion of the population was found with dry skin, staring hair, lustreless eyes, edema of the tongue, swollen gums, and other abnormalities of the skin and mucus membranes which have come to be regarded as indications of malnutrition.

The total food supply in Newfoundland provides per capita less than a third of the amounts recommended of vitamin A, and ascorbic acid, less than half the calcium and riboflavin, and less than two-thirds of the thiamine.

The matter of malnutrition is of vital interest to the physician. Poor nutrition retards convalescence and a poorly nourished patient is a poor surgical risk.

The purpose of this survey was to examine a sample of the people of Newfoundland for clinical and bio-chemical evidences of abnormalities relating to nutrition. The subjects of the study were 868 people in St. John's and several outports who voluntarily submitted to examination. The clinical examination was limited to a search for abnormalities of the scalp, hair, eyes, skin, lips, gums, tongue, and peripheral nervous system which are known to occur in states of malnutrition. A serverity rating was applied in only a few cases.

It is worthy of note that this survey was undertaken during the month of August, the season of the year during which the diet is most superior in that country.

Newfoundland, to a large extent, is a one-crop area with all the regretable consequences that this imposes. It owed its original settlement to cod fishing which makes up a large part of the diet. In addition to cod fish, the diet is supplemented with small amounts of meat and eggs, a moderate yield of garden produce and an extremely small amount of milk. The small amount of vegetables used are much reduced in dietary value by over-cooking.

The people's health in Newfoundland is far from satisfactory as evidenced from the death rate which is 12.5 per 100 population. The prevalence of tuberculosis is high. Roentgen evidence of active tuberculosis was obtained in 7.2 per cent of unselected individuals, while calcified lesions were detected in an additional 13.7 per cent. These figures indicate that death from this disease is more than three times as common as is the case in the United States.

Further evidence of improper dietary conditions were manifested in such conditions as flatulence, chronic constipation, and mild pains after eating. Goitre was observed but once. Pediculosis was encountered in 7.6 per cent of persons examined.

From assays it would appear that the food available is adequate with respect to calories and protein. The calcium available is inadequate by approximately 1/3 of the recommended amount, and the calcium-phosphate ratio was extremely low. The most severe deficiency seemed to be in the supply of ascorbic acid. The chief

Have a Coke

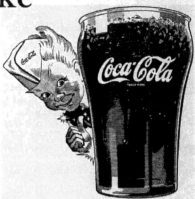

When you laugh, the world laughs with you, as they say—and when you enjoy *the pause that refreshes* with ice-cold Coca-Cola, your friends enjoy it with you, too. Everybody enjoys the friendly hospitality that goes with the invitation *Have a Coke.* Those three words mean *Friend, you belong —I'm glad to be with you.* Good company is better company over a Coca-Cola.

There is no substitute for ACCURACY in manufacturing and standardizing PHARMACEUTICALS

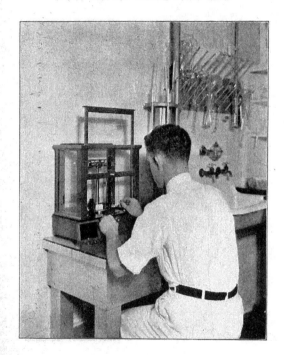

We Have Supplied The Profession With *Ethical Products* For More Than 45 Years.

"We Appreciate Your Preference"

FIRST TEXAS CHEMICAL MFG. CO.
Dallas, Texas

source of ascorbic acid is potatoes, and the cooking methods unfortunately result in a loss of almost 100 per cent of this protective substance. The amount of vitamin A in the available food supply is markedly below the recommended allowances, the amount of vitamin A supplied probably not exceeding 1400 I.U. compared with the recommended 4500.

The amount of niacin, 15 mgm, closely approximates the recommended allowance. It should be borne in mind that a significant loss of much of the mineral and vitamin content of these foods occurs in cooking.

Clinical examinations revealed lustreless hair in about 10 per cent of the cases. Further evidence of perifolliculosis, a condition characterized by a proliferation and engorgement of the capillaries around the hair follicles, was observed in about half of the cases. There also was found frequent occurance of blepharitis and suborbital pigmentation. Even the skin of the younger children exhibited a xerosis. Atrophy of the papillae of the tongue was noted in a large number of instances. Multiple fissuring and slight thinning of the tongue was noted, as well as many cases of hypertrophy of the papillae with an accompanying thickening of the tongue. Cheilosis and angular scars about the lips were noted in numerous cases. Circumcorneal injection was quite obvious in most cases, accompanied by some conjectival injection. Loss of interdental papillae was common from adolescence on. Redness and swelling of gingival tissue was not uncommon. Loss of teeth was quite frequently observed. In a large number of cases, patients reported their teeth loose enough so as to be pulled easily by themselves. Dental caries was wide spread and very prevelant. Malocclusion of a gross character was observed in 20 per cent of all people seen.

Evidence of rickets was encountered relatively infrequently. This may be due in part to the fact that for the past ten years a limited amount of evaporated milk has been imported for infants. Another possible factor is the vigorous education effort in promoting the use of cod-liver oil.

All of the deficiencies associated with a lack of vitamin A, riboflavin, and ascorbic acid were the most frequently encountered. While no cases of pellagra were seen, there was high prevalence of conditions which are known to respond to prolonged administration of niacin. No cases of beri-beri were seen although clinical symptoms resulting from a lack of thiamine were encountered. A study of the food supply in Newfoundland correlates quite closely with the prevalence of clinical signs of nutritional deficiency.

SUMMARY

1. Clinical examinations were conducted on 868 people of Newfoundland.

2. Evidence of nutritional deficiency due to lack of vitamin A, riboflavin, and ascorbic acid were seen with great frequency.

3. The clinical findings indicate an unsatisfactory intake of these nutrients in a high percentage of the population.

4. On the whole, a close correlation was found between the food deficiency and the chemical and clinical signs of malnutrition.

5. The infant mortality rate and the death rate from tuberculosis were quite high compared with rates for other groups of people of similar ancestry.

6. The poor nutritional status of the people in Newfoundland may wel be in large part responsible for their impaired health and efficiency.—H.J., M.D.

KEY TO ABSTRACTORS

J.F.B., M.D. ....John F. Burton, M.D.
E.D.M., M.D. ....Earl D. McBride, M.D.
H.J., M.D. ....Hugh Jeter, M.D.

(Continued from Page 132)

Kuhn, John F. ....Okla. City
Locheon, E. L. ....Frederick
Lusk, Earl M. ....915 S. Cinncinnati, Tulsa
Lytle, Wm. R. ....Okla. City
Martin, James D. ....Cushing
Matt, John G. ....1001 Med. Arts Bldg., Tulsa
McInnis, J. T. ....2609 N. W. 14, Okla. City
McIntosh, R. K. ....Tahlequah
Morton, R. W. ....Sulphur
Muntz, Earl R. ....525 S. Highland, Ada
Myers, Jack ....108½ S. Bickford, El Reno
Neely, Shade ....Comm. Nat'l Bldg., Muskogee
Newell, Waldo B. ....Broadway Tower, Enid
Ohl, Charles W. ....Chickasha
Orr, Herbert ....1307 S. Main, Tulsa
Padberg, E. D. ....Ada
Parker, D. F. ....Pawnee
Paulson, A. W. ....Clinton
Perry, Daniel L. ....804 Atlas Life, Tulsa
Pickhardt, W. L. ....Muskogee
Pierson, Dwight ....Buffalo
Pinholster, John H. ....Okla. City
Prosser, Moorman ....Box 151, Norman
Puckett, H. L. ....Stillwater
Ray, R. G. ....Tulsa
Reynolds, John H. ....1st Nat'l Bldg., Muskogee
Ricks, James R. ....1005 W. Hill, Okla. City
Rippy, O. M. ....418 Blakely, Stillwater
Ritan, Andrew ....Tahlequah
Ross, George T. ....1st Nat'l Bldg. Enid
Nadler, Leroy H. ....Med. Arts Bldg., Okla. City
Salkeld, Phil L. ....Vinita
Scott, George W. ....Tishomingo
Sewell, Dan R. ....400 N. W. 10, Okla. City
Shaw, James F. ....Wetumka
Shepard, S. C. ....807 Med. Arts Bldg., Tulsa
Shipp, J. D. ....Tulsa
Shofstall, Wm. H. ....1445 N. Main, Tulsa
Smith, Charles A. ....Okla. City
Smith, Roy L. ....Bryan, Texas
Spann, Logan A. ....203 Braniff Bldg., Tulsa
Speed, H. K., Jr. ....Sayre
Stokes, Lowell ....1008 Sunset Drive, Tulsa
Stoner, Raymond W. ....Checotah
Stotts, Charles S. ....Fairfax
Stout, Hugh A. ....809 N. Beard, Shawnee
Strecker, W. E. ....1601 Pennington Way, Okla. City
Swan, Joseph J. ....Chickasha
Terry, John B. ....307 Salomon Bldg., Helena, Ark.
Van Matre, R. M. ....640 S. Kingshighway, St. Louis, Mo.
Watson, Issac N. ....439 E. Ayers, Edmond
White, Eric M. ....312 Med. Arts Bldg., Tulsa
Williams, Gordon D. ....Weatherford
Word, Benjamin W. ....820 Wright Bldg., Tulsa
Word, Lee B. ....Union Nat'l Bldg., Bartlesville
Yeary, Edwin C. ....Clinton

Classified Advertisements

FOR SALE: Short wave diathermy, portable Garfield, to be used with coils. For information write J. M. Postelle, 303 Medical Arts Bldg., Oklahoma City.

FOR SALE—Hospital equipment, including Fischer 60-88 X-ray with tilt table and fluoroscope; Sanborn Metabolor; obstetric table; ultra-violet lamp, incubator, etc. Dr. Pierre Redman, Mena, Arkansas.

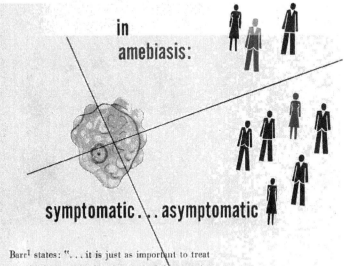

in
amebiasis:

symptomatic . . . asymptomatic

Barr[1] states: ". . . it is just as important to treat properly the symptomless 'carrier' of the parasite as to treat the patient suffering from amebic dysentery."

Stitt, Clough and Clough[2] report, "The disease may be symptomless . . . These mild or symptomless cases have been shown to outnumber greatly the cases with clinical dysentery. They constitute the carriers or 'cyst-passers'."

DIODOQUIN (5, 7-diiodo-8-hydroxyquinoline) is safe to use even in suspected cases of amebiasis. Nonirritating, nontoxic—Diodoquin has been found promptly destructive to protozoa in amebiasis and Trichomonas hominis (intestinalis).

DIODOQUIN

1. Barr, D. P.: Modern Medical Therapy in General Practice, 2:1830, Baltimore, Williams & Wilkins Company, 1940.

2. Stitt, E. R.; Clough, P. W., and Clough, M. C.: Practical Bacteriology, Haematology and Animal Parasitology, ed. 9, Philadelphia, P. Blakiston's Son & Co., 1938, pp. 410-412.

is the registered trademark of G. D. Searle & Co. Chicago 80, Ill.

SEARLE Research in the Service of Medicine

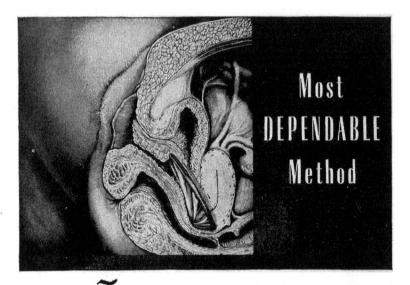

Most DEPENDABLE Method

The combined use of an occlusive diaphragm and vaginal jelly remains, in the published opinions of competent clinicians, the most dependable method of conception control.

Dickinson[1] has long held that the use of jellies alone cannot be relied upon for complete protection. It is noteworthy that in the series of patients studied by Eastman and Scott[2], an occlusive diaphragm was employed in conjunction with a spermicidal jelly for effective results. Warner[3], in a carefully controlled study of 500 patients, emphasized the value of a diaphragm.

In view of the preponderant clinical evidence in its favor, we suggest that physicians will afford their patients a high degree of protection by prescribing the diaphragm and jelly technique.

You assure quality when you specify a product bearing the "RAMSES"* trademark.

1. Dickinson, R. L.: Techniques of Conception Control. Baltimore, Williams and Wilkins Co., 1942.
2. Eastman, N. J., and Scott, A. B.: Human Fertility 9:33 (June) 1944.
3. Warner, M. P.: J. A. M. A. 115:279 (July 27) 1940.

gynecological division

JULIUS SCHMID, INC.

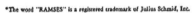

Quality First Since 1883

423 West 55 Street   New York 19, N. Y.

*The word "RAMSES" is a registered trademark of Julius Schmid, Inc.

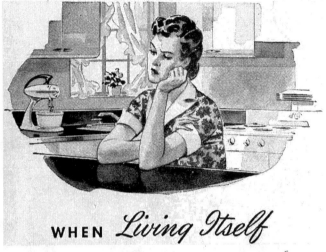

WHEN *Living Itself*
PROVES DIFFICULT

Stamina and strength, essential to a joyous, optimistic outlook, are vitally linked to the nutritional status, and will quickly wane if undernutrition is allowed to develop. Zestful living and boundless energy are hardly compatible with nutritional deficiencies.

For the below-par patient whose inadequate nutritional intake is the responsible factor, Ovaltine as a dietary supplement can make a real contribution toward assuring nutritional balance. A good source of high-quality protein, readily utilized carbohydrate, well-emulsified fat, and essential vitamins and minerals, Ovaltine can prove a significant factor in restoring the desired state of optimal nutrition. Three glassfuls daily, made with milk as directed, provide appreciable amounts of essential nutrients as indicated by the table. The low curd tension of Ovaltine assures rapid gastric emptying, hence the appetite for regular meals is not impaired. Ovaltine is enjoyed as a beverage and between meals.

THE WANDER COMPANY, 360 N. MICHIGAN AVE., CHICAGO 1, ILL.

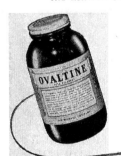

Ovaltine

Three daily servings of Ovaltine, each made of
½ oz. of Ovaltine and 8 oz. of whole milk,* provide:

CALORIES	669	VITAMIN A	3000 I.U.
PROTEIN	32.1 Gm.	VITAMIN B₁	1.16 mg.
FAT	31.5 Gm.	RIBOFLAVIN	1.50 mg.
CARBOHYDRATE	64.8 Gm.	NIACIN	6.81 mg.
CALCIUM	1.12 Gm.	VITAMIN C	39.6 mg.
PHOSPHORUS	0.939 Gm.	VITAMIN D	417 I.U.
IRON	12.0 mg.	COPPER	0.75 mg.

*Based on average reported values for milk.

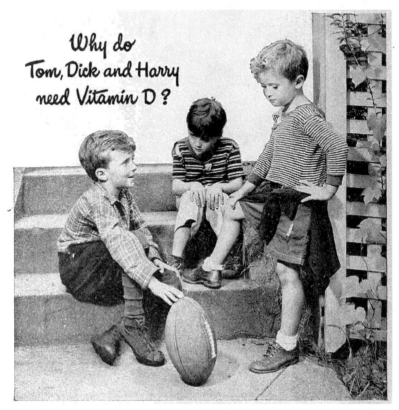

Why do Tom, Dick and Harry need Vitamin D?

Growing children require vitamin D mainly to prevent rickets. They also need vitamin D, though to a lesser degree, to insure optimal development of muscles and other soft tissues containing considerable amounts of phosphorus . . . Milk is the logical menstruum for administering vitamin D to growing children, as well as to infants, pregnant women and lactating mothers. This suggests the use of Drisdol in Propylene Glycol, which diffuses uniformly in milk, fruit juices and other fluids.

DRISDOL IN PROPYLENE GLYCOL
TRADEMARK REG U S. PAT. OFF & CANADA
Brand of Crystalline Vitamin D_2 (calciferol) from ergosterol
MILK DIFFUSIBLE VITAMIN D PREPARATION

Odorless
Tasteless
Economical

Average daily dose for infants 2 drops, for children and adults 4 to 6 drops, in milk.

Available in bottles of 5, 10 and 50 cc. with special dropper delivering 250 U.S.P. units per drop.

WINTHROP CHEMICAL COMPANY, INC.
Pharmaceuticals of merit for the physician • New York 13, N.Y. • Windsor, Ont.

"don't smoke"...

IS ADVICE HARD FOR PATIENTS TO SWALLOW!

May we suggest, instead, SMOKE "PHILIP MORRIS"? Tests* showed 3 out of every 4 cases of smokers' cough cleared on changing to PHILIP MORRIS. Why not observe the results for yourself?

*Laryngoscope, Feb. 1935, Vol. XLV, No. 2, 149-154

TO THE PHYSICIAN WHO SMOKES A PIPE: We suggest an unusually fine new blend—COUNTRY DOCTOR PIPE MIXTURE. Made by the same process as used in the manufacture of Philip Morris Cigarettes.

OFFICERS OF COUNTY SOCIETIES, 1946

★

COUNTY	PRESIDENT	SECRETARY	MEETING TIME
Alfalfa	W. G. Dunnington, Cherokee	L. T. Lancaster, Cherokee	Last Tues. each Second Month
Atoka-Coal	J. B. Clark, Coalgate	J. S. Fulton, Atoka	
Beckham	P. J. DeVanney, Sayre	J. E. Levick, Elk City	Second Tuesday
Blaine			
Bryan	W. K. Huynie, Durant	Jonah Nichols, Durant	Second Tuesday
Caddo	Preston E. Wright, Anadarko	Edward T. Cook, Jr., Anadarko	
Canadian	G. L. Goodman, Yukon	W. P. Lawton, El Reno	Subject to call
Carter	J. Hobson Veazey, Ardmore	H. A. Higgins, Ardmore	Second Tuesday
Cherokee	P. H. Medeais, Tahlequah	R. K. McIntosh, Jr., Tahlequah	First Tuesday
Choctaw	Floyd L. Waters, Hugo	O. R. Gregg, Hugo	
Cleveland	James O. Hood, Norman	Phil Huddock, Norman	Thursday nights
Comanche			
Cotton	G. W. Baker, Walters	Mollie Seism, Walters	Third Friday
Craig	Lloyd H. McPike, Vinita	J. M. McMillan, Vinita	
Creek	W. P. Longmire, Sapulpa	Philip Joseph, Sapulpa	Second Tuesday
Custer	Ross Deputy, Clinton	A. W. Paulson, Clinton	Third Thursday
Garfield	Bruce Hinson, Enid	John R. Walker, Enid	Fourth Thursday
Garvin	M. E. Robberson, Jr., Wynnewood	John R. Callaway, Pauls Valley	Wednesday before Third Thursday
Grady	Roy Emanuel, Chickasha	Rebecca H. Mason, Chickasha	Third Thursday
Grant	I. V. Hardy, Medford	F. P. Robinson, Pond Creek	
Greer	J. B. Lansden, Granite	J. B. Hollis, Mangum	
Harmon	W. G. Husband, Hollis	R. H. Lynch, Hollis	First Wednesday
Haskell	Wm. S. Carson, Keotah	N. K. Williams, McCurtain	
Hughes			First Friday
Jackson	E. W. Mabry, Altus	J. P. Irby, Altus	Last Monday
Jefferson	F. M. Edwards, Ringling	J. A. Dillard, Waurika	Second Monday
Kay	L. G. Neal, Ponca City	J. C. Wagner, Ponca City	Second Thursday
Kingfisher	John W. Pendleton, Kingfisher	H. Violet Sturgeon, Hennessey	
Kiowa	Wm. Bernell, Hobart	J. Wm. Finch, Hobart	
LeFlore			
Lincoln	J. S. Rollins, Prague	Ned Burleson, Prague	First Wednesday
Logan	James Petty, Guthrie	J. E. Souter, Guthrie	Last Tuesday
Marshall			
Mayes			
McClain	S. C. Davis, Blanchard	W. C. McCurdy, Purcell	
McCurtain	J. T. Moreland, Idabel	R. H. Sherrill, Broken bow	Fourth Tuesday
McIntosh	F. R. First, Checotah	W. A. Tolleson, Eufaula	First Thursday
Muskogee-Sequoyah			
Wagoner	R. N. Holcombe, Muskogee	William N. Weaver, Muskogee	First Tuesday
Noble	A. M. Evans, Perry	Jesse W. Driver, Perry	
Okfuskee	W. P. Jenkins, Okemah	M. L. Whitney, Okemah	Second Monday
Oklahoma	W. F. Keller, Okla. City		Fourth Tuesday
Okmulgee	F. S. Watson, Okmulgee	C. E. Smith, Okmulgee	Second Monday
Osage	Paul H. Hemphill, Pawhuska	Vincent Mazzarella, Hominy	Third Monday
Ottawa	C. F. Walker, Grove	W. Jackson Sayles, Miami	Second Thursday
Pawnee			
Payne	F. Keith Oehlschlager, Yale	C. W. Moore, Stillwater	Third Thursday
Pittsburg	Millard L. Henry, McAlester	Edward D. Greenberger, McAlester	Third Friday
Pontotoc-Murray	John Morey, Ada	R. H. Mayes, Ada	First Wednesday
Pottawatomie	F. P. Newlin, Shawnee	Clinton Gallaher, Shawnee	First and Third Saturday
Pushmataha	John S. Lawson, Clayton	B. M. Huckabay, Antler	
Rogers	W. A. Howard, Chelsea	P. S. Anderson, Claremore	Third Wednesday
Seminole	Clifton Felts, Seminole	Mack I. Shanholz, Seminole	Third Wednesday
Stephens	Evert King, Duncan	Fred L. Patterson, Duncan	
Texas	Daniel S. Lee, Guymon	E. L. Buford, Guymon	
Tillman	H. A. Calvert, Frederick	O. G. Bacon, Frederick	
Tulsa	John C. Perry, Tulsa	John E. McDonald, Tulsa	Second and Fourth Monday
Washington-Nowata	Ralph W. Rucker, Bartlesville	L. B. Word, Bartlesville	Second Wednesday
Washita	L. G. Livingston, Cordell	Roy W. Anderson, Clinton	
Woods	John F. Simon, Alva	O. E. Templin, Alva	Last Tuesday Odd Months
Woodward	T. C. Leachman, Woodward	C. W. Tedrowe, Woodward	Second Thursday

*(Serving in Armed Forces)

THE JOURNAL
of the
OKLAHOMA STATE MEDICAL ASSOCIATION

VOLUME XXXIX	OKLAHOMA CITY, OKLAHOMA, APRIL, 1946	NUMBER 4

The Management of Common Skin Diseases*

LOUIS A. BRUNSTING, M.D.

*Section on Dermatology and Syphilology,
Mayo Clinic,*

ROCHESTER, MINNESOTA

The patient with disease of the skin is in the unique and unenviable position of having his disorder exposed to the view of himself and others. He is not only embarrassed and concerned about the disfigurement, but worried over what he sees but cannot comprehend. He fears complications, contagion, malignancy or other systemic implications. Moreover, he suffers disability and, at times, extreme discomfort from pain and pruritus. He is first of all his own physician and in no other field of medicine is there so much self-medication as in dermatology. Under such conditions, the first question in treatment that confronts the practitioner is not *"what* to do" but rather *"what not* to do". Standard texts on dermatology are full of prescriptions, the druggist displays many sorts of proprietary creams and lotions and the journals and radio programs tell of new and guaranteed cure-alls. Rather than burden you, therefore, with additional formulas, I shall discuss the where, when and how of their application and reconsider for a moment some principles of undergraduate days.

We are not concerned about niceties of dermatologic nomenclature; we may leave that to the specialists; however, a good deal can be learned from a careful examination of the entire skin in a good light, not by hasty inspection of an exposed foot or hand, or of the V of the chest. Perhaps the scalp, or mouth, or genitalia, or palpable lymph nodes will provide collateral information. The disease may be limited to the skin itself and may be an irritation, infection, infestation, nevus, keratosis, or even a malignant lesion. There may be characteristic signs of such disorders as psoriasis, lichen planus, pityriasis rosea or eczema, and one may sus-

pect internal relationship but cannot prove it. The skin frequently reflects significant constitutional disturbances by means of changes in pigment, signs of deficiency states or metabolic diseases, or the eruptive forms of infectious granuloma. The skin is not merely a protective covering or an inert hide, but is actually an important, functioning organ of the body, a reactive membrane which is sensitive to influences within and without.

The most common of all skin diseases is eczema. The term denotes a state of sensitization and the reaction affects the epidermis in contact dermatitis, or the cutis in atopic dermatitis of an allergic diathesis. However, the distinctions, are not sufficiently clearcut, and there are other varieties of dermatitis to confuse the picture. Our knowledge of the mechanics of sensitization is still elementary and most discussions of it are oversimplified. Often there are contributing factors, such as stasis, mechanical or physical trauma, nutritional lack, vasomotor instability and pyogenic or fungus infections, which complicate the process.

CONTACT DERMATITIS

The irritants that may cause contact dermatitis are legion; in connection with the trades, the loss of man hours of work and the medicolegal problems that arise are considerable. In the course of treatment of patients with minor disorders of the skin, there may arise reactions that aggravate an already irritated skin, particularly in relation to the use of adhesive tape and local applications containing resorcinol, mercurial salts, sulfur, sulfonamide drugs and the local anesthetics such as ethyl aminobenzoate. Such reactions may develop suddenly after a long period of apparent tolerance and benefit.

*Delivered at the Oklahoma City Clinical Society, November 26, 1945.

Of course, first of all, it is desirable to separate the patient from the source of his irritation. Nevertheless, it is more important to relieve the distress in the skin than to prove an academic point. Patch tests should not be done during the acute stage of dermatitis because the adhesive tape and the irritant may provoke an unexpected exacerbation and generalization of the process. There is no internal medication that is effective in the treatment of acute dermatitis, although intramuscular autohemotherapy is widely used and the administration of acetyl salicylic acid by mouth reduces the degree of pruritus. Sedatives of the barbiturate type should be avoided. In cases of dermatitis due to poison ivy, ragweed or other plants, it is not wise to use injections of antigenic oils during the acute phase of dermatitis, for such agents often lead to a generalized flare. In some circles, there is enthusiasm concerning the value of such antigenic extracts in the prevention of plant dermatitis by immunization, but the beneficial effects are still debatable.

In the treatment of acute dermatitis which affects much of the body, the skin can be cleansed and pruritus relieved by immersing the patient once or twice a day for a half to two hours at a time, in a colloid bath of boiled cornstarch-soda paste or in a bath containing boiled oatmeal-soda gruel in a bag. In the acute stages, there is nothing better than the application of wet dressings to the affected parts. Several layers of loose gauze are saturated and squeezed partly dry; if the dressings are too wet, the skin becomes soggy; if they are too dry, the gauze adheres to the surface and the dried exudate prevents contact of the medicine with the skin. It is not advisable to cover the bandage with oiled silk or rubber-dam, for such impermeable membranes interfere with proper ventilation. It is best to wet and replace dressings at intervals of approximately four hours, allowing a short period between changes for drying of the skin. The most common preparations in general use are: a 0.5 per cent solution of aluminum subacetate, a saturated solution of boric acid, a 1:1,000 solution of silver nitrate and a 1:10,000 solution of potassium permanganate. If secondary infection is present, the best preparation is a solution of potassium permanganate or one of penicillin (250 units per cc), or Alibour's solution (copper sulfate 1.2; zinc sulfate 2.4; camphor water to make 120.0). For use, one ounce (30 cc) of this solution is diluted to one pint (500 cc) with water. If the hands or feet are affected, they should be immersed in a basin of the solution morning and evening for twenty to thirty minutes at a time. In cases in which the legs and feet are involved, edema usually is present. In such cases, there is no substitute for complete rest in bed with elevation of the affected parts.

As the acute phase subsides, the application of wet dressings may gradually be reduced to two applications or less each day, while switching to drying lotions and emollients in the intervals. There is no universal remedy that will soothe the sensitive skin; there is a wide variance among individuals with respect to tolerance and this changes from time to time. Some of the milder preparations that may be used for this purpose are calamine lotion plus an added film of cold cream, zinc oxide ointment containing 3 per cent of ichthyol and an oily lotion such as the following: menthol 0.6, phenol 4.0, olive oil 120.0, lime water 120.0 and zinc oxide 20.0.

ATOPIC DERMATITIS

A familial form of eczema called atopic dermatitis is recognized as a common phase of the allergic diathesis and is seen in infancy, childhood, adolescence and, at intervals, in adults. Often, there are associated allergic symptoms such as hayfever or asthma in the patient or members of his family. At first, the involvement is on the face and the flexural folds of the extremities, and although one recognizes the signs in the skin, the underlying biologic alterations are difficult to understand and, for the present, the treatment must be symptomatic.

There has been a great deal of discussion about the value of skin tests in cases of atopic dermatitis. Positive reactions are obtained by the scratch or intradermal technic in a high percentage of instances, and on the basis of such information there have been proposed many procedures of elimination and desensitization, on the whole with unsatisfactory results and often not without detriment to the general health of the patient. There is usually a poor degree of correlation between positive skin tests, experience of the patient and his cutaneous symptoms, and the patterns of the positive reactions are often changing, conflicting and confusing. In the study of such patients, one appreciates the response of the skin to other factors, including emotional, endocrine and climatic influences, and the interpretation of these phenomena is colored by the personal bias of the observer. When the disorder occurs in childhood, one can predict a long course of ups and downs, and it often is more important to treat the parents than the little patient himself. Affected children and adolescents are usually overstimulated and overambitious, and the management involves more than the care of the skin itself; of course, the obvious external and dietary irritants should be removed but, at the same time, it is necessary to reduce the internal conflicts to a minimum. In some instances, it is advisable to recommend a decided change of environment to a climate which is at all times sunny and equable.

In the treatment of forms of chronic eczema it is well known that stimulating remedies are well tolerated in most instances, and the use of tars such as pine tar (pine tar 2, salicylic acid 2 and zinc oxide ointment 96), and White's crude coal tar ointment are quite useful. Ultraviolet irradiation and sunlight are most valuable aids. Until we learn more about the underlying mechanism which leads to sensitivities, we must proceed by trial and error toward the relief of symptoms.

OTHER TYPES OF DERMATOLOGIC TREATMENT

Sulfonamides and penicillin: One does not need to be a pharmaceutical manufacturer to appreciate how the introduction of antibiotics, especially penicillin, has affected the use of sulfonamides. For a time, sulfathiazole and sulfadiazine, by topical or internal use, proved to be the most effective remedies available for the treatment of superficial pyogenic infections of the skin, such as infected ulcers and eczema, impetigo, furunculosis, carbuncle, and even lymphangitis, cellulitis and erysipelas. Gradually, it was realized that these drugs were potent sensitizers without and within; the hazards of their systemic use have become too well known to need emphasis.

Notwithstanding, there are certain conditions in which the sulfonamides are indispensable. Sulfathiazole is without peer in the control of chancroid and is useful in the early stage of lymphopathia venereum. Sulfapyridine relieves the symptoms and signs of dermatitis herpetiformis when administered orally in doses of 1.0 to 3.0 gm. daily. Untoward reactions may occur and should be anticipated, but they usually appear within the first few weeks of treatment, if at all. Urinary calculi do not occur if a liberal intake of fluid is maintained. The milder sulfonamides, sulfasuxidine, sulfaguanidine and neoprontosil have a limited field of usefulness in certain cases of pyoderma associated with infection of the bowel, but these drugs too will probably be rendered obsolete when streptomycin becomes available.

Penicillin, in the form of wet dressings of water or physiologic solution containing 250 units of penicillin per cubic centimeter is highly effective in the treatment of pyogenic infections of the skin. It can also be used as an ointment containing 200 to 1,000 units per gram of water-soluble base. These preparations deteriorate slowly under refrigeration. However, they are not without sensitizing properties and dermatitis may occur, although present experience is too limited to indicate the relative index of reaction.

In the treatment of systemic infection, frequent intramuscular injections of penicillin are required to maintain a satisfactory concentration of the drug in the blood, but this disadvantage will soon be overcome by the use of beeswax in peanut oil as a vehicle for a single massive daily dose.

The most common reaction to penicillin is urticaria which affects 5 per cent or more individuals who are undergoing systemic treatment. Vesicular eruptions occasionally occur, and they resemble dermatophytids. I have observed two instances in which penicillin provoked exfoliative dermatitis.

Benadryl: It is supposed that in anaphylactic shock in animals and in the allergic phenomena of human beings there is released a histamine-like substance which accounts for the clinical signs and symptoms. Various anti-histamine substances have been developed, some of them too toxic for general use, but one will hear a good deal of a recently developed benzhydryl compound which has been named benadryl. When administered orally in doses of 50 to 100 mg. three to five times daily, it is highly effective in controlling the symptoms of acute and chronic urticaria and angioneurotic edema, although the relief is purely palliative.[1][2] Side effects are not serious; drowsiness, dizziness, dryness of the mouth and dilated pupils may be noted. The drug is given by mouth or by the intravenous or intramuscular route. Preliminary investigations indicate that benadryl relieves pruritus in certain dermatologic conditions besides urticaria; therefore, extensive use of the drug may be anticipated.

Vitamins: There are few, if any, common skin disorders which are benefited by vitamin therapy. While it is true that the skin reflects characteristic signs of such deficiency states as pellagra, scurvy, starvation and experimental avitaminosis, this does not justify the indiscriminate abuse of vitamin therapy in skin diseases in general. In Darier's disease and pityriasis rubra pilaris, there is evidence of an inability of the patient to assimilate and store vitamin A properly; nevertheless, the results of treatment in such cases have been disappointing. It is not conceded that vitamin A is beneficial in acne vulgaris. On the other hand, if there is fulminating acne with pyoderma and associated cachexia, the constitutional disorder calls for complete fortification including the use of B complex plus crude liver extract. Certain patients with seborrhea have dermatitis of the nasolabial folds and the angles of the mouth as in ariboflavinosis, but there is no specific benefit in such cases from the administration of riboflavin by itself. Some years ago, it seemed that administration of massive doses of vitamin D was beneficial in psoriasis, but subsequent experience has shown such therapy is worthless. In general, I wish to emphasize that vitamin therapy in dermatology is indicated only when there is evidence of constitutional deficiency.

BIBLIOGRAPHY

1. Curtis, A. C. and Owens, B. B.: Beta-dimethylamino-ethyl benzhydryl ether hydrochloride (benadryl) in treatment of acute and chronic urticaria. Univ. Hosp. Bull., Ann Arbor. Vol. 2, pp. 25-26. April, 1945.

2. O'Leary, P. A. and Farber, E. M.: Benadryl in the treatment of urticaria. Proc. Staff Meet., Mayo Clinic. Vol. 20, pp. 429-432. November 14, 1945.

Dr. Puckett Taking Post-Graduate Course In South America

H. L. Puckett, M.D., plans to attend the Assembly of the International College of Surgeons at Lima, Peru, from March 18 to 31. He will give a lecture on traumatic surgery and show a color movie on the subject.

During his stay in Lima, Dr. Puckett will visit with an old schoolmate from the University of Michigan, Oscar Sarzola Tellez, who is Ministerio de Salud Publica of Lima.

Dr. Puckett, a graduate of the University of Michigan, now resides in Stillwater, Oklahoma.

Herpes Simplex

JOHN LAMB, M.D.

OKLAHOMA CITY, OKLAHOMA

Herpes simplex, commonly known as "fever blister" or "fever sore", is one of the most common skin lesions encountered. Their recurrence is both painful and unsightly but little attention is paid to their prevention or to the dangers of inoculation to other eczematous or irritated areas. Since there has been a great deal of study done in recent years a review of the newer ideas is believed warranted.

Sulzberger[1] in a recent discussion states that there are many forms of herpes simplex infection in addition to the classic "cold sore". There is the recurrent herpetic paronychia and the recurrent bullous herpes simplex of the finger which resembles an eczematous eruption. There is the follicular herpes simplex of the bearded areas with minute, discrete vesicles and crusts often accompanied by severe itching. There is the zosteriform herpes simplex simulating herpes zoster in its arrangement along the course of the nerves.

Aphthous stomatitis[2] particularly in children, has been proved to be a herpetic infection. The symptoms are those of the local lesion plus general symptoms of toxicity.

The mouth lesion commences as a reddened area with a vesicular center, which may spread and become purulent. Sometimes the vesicles spread and produce extensive membranous lesions, the breath is offensive and the regional lymph glands are enlarged. There may be a fever accompanying the infection which subsides in from seven to fourteen days.

Roberts[3] reports a case that developed peculiar verruciform plaques three weeks after a herpes simplex eruption had appeared on the right cheek. Histologic examination revealed a striking resemblance to spinocellular carcinoma but the lesions did not recur after removal. Other cases of herpes vegetans have

been described but were localized on the oral mucosa or in the anogenital region.

Anderson[4] suggests that there is an etiologic relationship of the herpes simplex virus in erythema multiforme. He concludes that in a considerable percentage of cases in which herpes simplex is an immediate preceding lesion of recurrent erythema multiforme, he found that repeated vaccinations with smallpox vaccine appeared to be of value in the prevention of recurrent erythema multiforme associated with a preceding herpes simplex.

Ebert[5] states that since the herpes simplex virus is neurotrophic in animals that it is not only dermatotrophic in human beings but is at times neurotrophic and that it was believed to be the cause of some cases of von Economo's encephalitis which appeared in epidemic form during World War I. The question of the relationship of the herpes virus to this disease is still unsettled.

In the past year several reports[6][7][8][9] have been given of generalized varicelliform eruptions, some of which have complicated cases of infantile eczema. Serum from several of these cases transferred from an unruptured vesicle to the cornea of rabbits produced a herpetic keratitis. The herpes simplex virus was also isolated from one of Lane's[8] generalized cases and was inoculated on the choriollantoic membrane of chick embryos, where it produced numerous small pocket-like lesions.

The splendid work of these authors confirmed a suggestion made by Wise and Sulzberger in Year Book of Dermatology and Syphilology for 1942 in which they stated that varicelliform eruptions were not uncommon in severe types of eczema and expressed the opinion that the disease might have been due to a generalized or rather widespread external inoculation or hematogenous distribution and fixation of herpes simplex virus in the open and scratched areas abounding in these patients.

ETIOLOGY

The etiological factors concerning herpes simplex infections are still of great interest. It must now be assumed that there are latent resident viruses present on the skin and that various factors seem to incite these viruses to an active infection or there is some decrease in local tissue immunity allowing the virus to become activated.

During the course of febrile reactions from pneumonia, malaria, and other infections, the herpes simplex virus is activated. Artifically produced fever by means of typhoid vaccine also produce a certain percentage of herpes labialis. Immunity to the virus is finally produced so that the latter fevers in the course fail to produce fever blisters.

The eruptions may recur independently of febrile attacks constituting the so-called recurrent herpes simplex.

Recurrence of facial herpes, especially the lip, follows exposure to sunshine and wind. In our study[10] of cancer of the lower lip a high percentage of the patients gave a history of a recurrent fever blister from sunlight appearing in the same site at which the epithelioma finally appeared.

Becker[11] reports herpes simplex has occurred with each menstrual period.

A cause of herpes simplex which is important is that of traumatism.

Herpes progenitalis is one example of this type of recurrence. There can be do doubt that the traumatism undergone in the sexual act is a factor in the recurrence of penile herpes. I do not recall having seen a case of herpes progenitalis in the young male before puberty.

In the literature there is mention of Vitiligo[12] of the lip caused by playing some type of horn in the band but no mention is made to herpes simplex produced by the trauma of horn playing.

Three such cases have been observed:

Case No. 1. G. Y. a white male 26 years of age, came to the office with herpes labialis in several groups in the upper lip and one large lesion on the lower lip. He was a French horn played in the Oklahoma Symphony Orchestra and he gave the history that in the past week he had been rehearsing several hours extra each day as he had some special solos in one symphony which was to be presented in concert for the following week. He said he had had previous herpes labialis but only of a mild type. Examination revealed three elevated vesicular lesions on the upper lip with erythema and edema of the lip and one solitary lesion of similar type on the lower lip. Treatment consisted of moist calomine packs to which 4 per cent

spirits of camphor was added. This cleared up promptly with no recurrence to date.

Case No. 2. V. C. a white male, 28 years of age, a French horn player in the same orchestra gave the history of recurrent herpes labialis following bouts of intense practicing. This time the lesions were more severe and he felt that exposure to the sun during a golf game had greatly exaggerated the symptoms. Examination revealed several herpetic lesions on the upper and lower lip only in the areas contacted by the mouthpiece of the French horn which was metal. Metal filings from the mouthpiece were applied for 72 hours to the chin and the forearm but no reaction was elicited. Treatment consisted of the 4 per cent spirts of camphor in calomine lotion and the lesions healed promptly.

Case No. 3. G. P. a white male, age 9 years, came into the hospital complaining of inability to eat because of sore lips and mouth. His parents gave the history that he

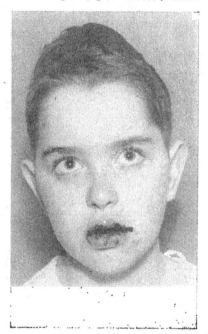

was a trombone player in the school orchestra and that during the previous six months he had had recurrent herpes labialis. The last previous attack was very severe but only involved the lips. This attack started with several groups of vesicles on the upper and lower lips and spread to the tongue. Treatment had consisted of sulfanilamide by mouth and sulfathiazole 5 per cent ointment on the lips, tongue and buccal muscosa. Examination revealed an acutely sick boy with reddened, swollen, fissured upper and lower lips. The sides of the tongue, the gum margins and buccal mucosa of the cheeks were covered with ulcers, some the size of an English pea others larger and coalescent into large ulcerated areas. The margins of the ulcers were white and the inner surfaces were grayish in color. The mucosa was reddened and swollen. There were several discrete erythematous lesions on the right forearm the size of a pea. The lesions were vesicular with a slight umbilication and an erythermatous base. The blood count showed 3,970,000 RBC, 6,950 WBC. Differential white count showed neutrophiles 61 per cent, 44 filamented, 17 non-filamented, 33 lymphocytes and 6 monocytes. Urinalysis showed specific gravity 1.0102, reaction was alkaline, albumin and globulin were negative. The temperature ranged from 101° to 102° F. but was not of a septic type. Material from several ulcers were inoculated in the cornea of a rabbit but no fresh clear vesicles could be found for the purpose. There was no reaction in the rabbit's cornea after 72 hours observation. The patient was given intravenous glucose, 5 cc calcium thiosulfate intravenously for several doses; 500 cc of whole citrated blood; 10 units of intramuscular liver daily and filtered x-ray 50 R units to each side of face and neck. Recovery was slow but in five days time the entire process had subsided. Since recovery he has not yet been vaccinated with smallpox virus because of the marked reaction both febrile and dissimenated from the herpetic infection and there was fear of causing a generalized vaccinia.

This patient has had two slight recurrences; the first after playing the trombone. The second relapse was after a sun and wind exposure and consisted of one large vesicle in the center of the lower lip. This unruptured vesicle was punctured under sterile conditions and the tip of a sterile applicator was soaked with the vesicle fluid. This was scarified on the left cornea of a rabbit, the right cornea was scarified with a sterile applicator without any vesicle fluid. In 48 hours the rabbit had a complete paralysis of the hind legs.

The left cornea was highly injected and on examination by Dr. T. O. Coston with the slit lamp showed a typical dendritic ulcer of the cornea characterized by fine multiple branches and identical with the dendritic ulcers of herpetic origin seen in humans.

The right cornea used as a control showed no reaction from the scarification without the vesicle fluid.

DISCUSSION

These three cases; two of a mild type; the third rather acute, present a new type of trauma in causation of herpes labialis. Metal irritation possibly of nickel in the mouthpiece might be an explanation of the irritating factor in these cases, but patch tests of the metal from the mouthpiece in one case failed to elicit any reaction in 72 hours on the skin of the forearm. The suggestion was made that these players should experiment with plastic type mouthpieces to allay the suspicion that the exacerbation came from metal irritation.

The local treatment of herpes simplex consisted of the application of calomine lotion with the addition of 4 per cent spirits of camphor. In the acute stage as in Case No. 3 filtered x-rays, calcium and whole blood seemed to be of some value. Repeated inoculation of smallpox virus has been the most successful method in preventing recurrences of herpes labialis and herpes progenitalis. Urbach[13] suggests that the internal administration of methenamine shortens the course of herpes labialis.

The last case presented seems to substantiate the statement of Burnett and Williams[2] that apthous stomatitis in children is due to the herpes simplex virus. However in adults this probably is not true. An adult with recurrent apthous stomatitis has been studied with tests on the cornea of rabbit from fresh vesicles on the lip. The rabbit developed a keratitis in the inoculated eye but it was not herpetic in type. This leads us to the suspicion that another unknown virus may be the causative organism in apthous stomatitis in adults.

SUMMARY

The importance of the herpes virus as a causative organism in skin eruptions other than herpes labialis is stressed.

Apthous stomatitis in children is probably due to the herpes simplex virus.

Three cases of recurrent herpes labialis in players of percussion instruments have been recorded, one of acute and extensive nature.

BIBLIOGRAPHY

1. Sulzberger; Arch. D. & S. Vol. 51, Page 136. February, 1945.
2. Burnett and Williams; Med. Jour., Australia. Vol. 1, pp. 637-642. April, 1939.
3. Roberts; Dermatologica, Edition 3. Vol. 79, pp. 73-79. February, 1939.
4. Anderson; Arch. D. & S. Vol. 51, pp. 10-15. January, 1945.
5. Ebert; Discussion Arch. D. & S. Vol. 51, Page 15. January, 1945.
6. Wenner, H. A.; Am. Jr. Dis. of Children. April, 1944.
7. Borton, R. L.; Brunsting, Louis A.; et al; Arch. D. & S. Vol. 50, pp. 99-105. August, 1944.
8. Lane, Clinton W.; Arch. D. & S. December, 1944.
9. Lynch, Francis; et al; Arch. D. & S. Vol. 51, pp. 129-138. February, 1945.
10. Lamb and Eastland; Jr. A.M.A. Vol. 117. August, 1941.
11. Becker; Textbook of Dermatology and Syphilology.
12. Freeman, C. Wendell and Vitiligo, H. H.; Hazen of the Upper Lip in Players of Wind Instruments. Arch. D. & S. Vol. 48, Page 605. December, 1943.
13. Urbach; Arch. D. & S. Vol. 51, Page 228. March, 1945.

Poliomyelitis: Failure of Intrauterine Fetal Transmission *

E. MALCOLM STOKES, M.D.

TULSA, OKLAHOMA

The effect of the virus of anterior poliomyelitis on the fetus assumes a great deal of importance if one agrees with Fox and Sennett[1] that the pregnant woman is more susceptible to poliomyelitis than the nonpregnant. In analyzing four cases of their own and six of others,[2] these authors found a total of ten pregnant women among 32 adult females with poliomyelitis. On the other hand it is generally agreed,[3] [4] that acute poliomyelitis is rarely associated with pregnancy. Aycock[5] estimates that it occurs once in every fifty thousand pregnancies. Most observers[1] [7] [8] [9] [10] [11] agree that; there is apparently no transmission of virus to the fetus; the disease has no effect on pregnancy, and; pregnancy does not affect the course of the disease.

The following case report is presented to offer additional evidence that anterior poliomyelitis, in any form, has no effect on pregnancy.

CASE REPORT

F. M., (W-9210), a 29 year old, white, graxida III, page II, in the last month of pregnancy was admitted to Parkland Hospital on September 19, 1943. Eight days previously the present illness began with lower abdominal pain. Four days before admission the patient began to have headaches and a high temperature. The following day she became weak and complained of backache and stiff neck. On the day before admission she lost complete control of her legs. On the day of admission a spinal puncture was performed, confirming the diagnosis of acute poliomyelitis.

By menstrual history the patient was at term. Previous pregnancies were perfectly normal. There was no serious illness prior to the present and no history of contact with any known cases of poliomyelitis during the prenatal course.

On admission the patient was acutely ill with a temperature of 100 degrees F. and had a marked cyanosis, especially of the lips. The respirations were shallow, labored, and fast with extension of the neck at each inspiration. The chest was relatively immobile, the diaphragm moved only slightly with respiration, and the accessory muscles of respiration were overly active. The heart sounds were weak and the rhythm irregular. A fetus distended the uterus to the xyphoid process, and a fetal heart beat with a rate of 140 beats per minute was audible.

A diagnosis of acute bulbar poliomyelitis with extensive involvement of the entire body was made. There was little abdominal breathing at this time. The chest was packed every fifteen minutes by the Kinney method, and the excursions improved slightly. The color of the patient did not improve despite administration of oxygen, and the pulse was weak, thready, and irregular. The day after admission the cyanosis increased and respiration became more labored. The pulse was rapid and the blood pressure dropped to 70/30. At this time the fetal heart rate was 150 per minute. Immediately a Cesarean section was done, and a normal female infant removed from the uterus three minutes after maternal death. After fifteen seconds the baby breathed spontaneously. It was not cyanotic and had no difficulty with respiration. Three months later it appeared to be a normal healthy infant.

Autopsy revealed microscopic evidence of anterior horn involvement of the cord and marked degenerative changes in the anterior portion of the medulla. Death was thought to be due to the bulbar lesion.

This case report is presented to illustrate the nontransmissability of the poliomyelitis virus to the fetus even with acute bulbar poliomyelitis. It is believed that the pregnancy had no effect on the poliomyelitis nor did the disease affect the pregnancy. There is no attempt to discuss the merits or demerits of post-mortem Cesarean section as most obstetricians[12] [13] [14] already have fixed ideas on this question.

BIBLIOGRAPHY

1. Fox, M. J. and Sennett, L: Poliomyelitis in Pregnancy. American Journal of Medical Science, Vol. 209, pp. 383-387. March, 1945.
2. Brahdy, M. D., and Lenarsky, M.: Acute Epidemic Poliomyelitis Complicating Pregnancy. Journal of A.M.A., Vol. 101, page 195. July 15, 1933.
3. Editorial: The Question of Intrauterine Poliomyelitis. J.A.M.A., Vol. 123, pp. 210-211. September 25, 1943.
4. McGeogan, L. S.: Acute Anterior Poliomyelitis Complicating Pregnancy. Amer. Jour. Obst. & Gynec., Vol. 24, pp. 215-224. August, 1932.
5. Aycock, W. L.: The Frequency of Poliomyelitis in Pregnancy, New England Jour. Med., Vol. 225, pp. 405-408. September, 1941.

*From Parkland Hospital and the Department of Obstetrics and Gynecology of the Southwestern Medical College, Dallas, Texas.

6. Harmon, P. M., and Hoyne, A : Poliomyelitis and Pregnancy, J.A.M.A., Vol. 123, page 185. September 25, 1943.
Kleinberg, S., and Horwitz, T.: The Obstetric Experiences of Women Paralyzed by Acute Anterior Poliomyelitis. Surg. Gynec. & Obst , Vol. 72, page 58. January, 1941.
8. Peelen, J. W.: Pregnancy Complicated by Acute Anterior Poliomyelitis Jour. Michigan Med Soc., Vol. 42, pp. 30-35. January, 1943.
9. Miller, M. F.: Anterior Poliomyelitis Complicating Pregnancy, with Report of Two Cases. Jour. Michigan Med. Soc., Vol. 23, pp. 58-60. February, 1924.
10. Klein. P., and Sittig. O : A Case of Acute Poliomyelitis During Pregnancy, with Delivery of a Healthy Baby, Schweiz. Med. Woch., Vol. 68, page 1228. November, 1938.
11. Spishakoff, M. M , Golenternek, K., and Bower, A. G.: Premature Obstetrical Delivery Due to Poliomyelitis, California and Western Med., Vol. 54, page 121. March, 1941.
12. Campbell, A. M., and Miller, J. D : Post-mortem Cesarean Section, Jour. Mich. Med. Society, Vol. 30, page 923. December, 1931.
13. Ryder, F. D.: Post-mortem Cesarean Section with a Living Child, Nebraska Med. Jour., Vol. 16, pp. 474-475. December, 1931.
14. Yule, G. W.: Note on a Case of Post-mortem Cesarean Section in Twin Pregnancy, with Survival of One Child, Trans. Edinbr. Obst. Soc., Vol. 45, pp. 49-51. 1925-1926.

Recent vistors on the Medical School campus were: Dr. D. A. Ward, member of the class of 1931, and who is now in the Navy; Dr. O. L. Tefertiller, member of the class of 1942, who is now stationed at Naval Ammunition Depot at McAlester; Captain Trzaska, class of 1943. Dr. Trzaska is a member of the Medical Corps on his way to California preparatory to going overseas.

The 6th Annual meeting of the Oklahoma City Internists Association was held at the School of Medicine, University of Oklahoma, on February 22, 1946. Dr. Bert Keltz, as president of the Association, arranged the program which consisted of eight papers concerning primarily the diagnosis and therapy of various medical diseases. Luncheon was held at the University Hospitals for the doctors in attendance. In addition to those physicians from Oklahoma City, approximately sixty doctors attended from other towns and cities over the state.

Caffeine*

VERN H. MUSICK, M.D.; HOWARD C. HOPPS, M.D.; HARRY T. AVEY, M.D.;
ARTHUR A. HELLBAUM, M.D.*

OKLAHOMA CITY, OKLAHOMA

For centuries uncivilized peoples throughout different parts of the world have used extracts of plants containing the xanthine compounds, caffeine, theophylline, and theobromine as a beverage. Since plants containing these drugs possess neither a peculiar odor or taste, nor is their effect on the human mechanism startling, it is of interest that natives were able to select them with such uncanny accuracy. It may be that they noted the soothing carminative effect of the hot beverage or perhaps the brightening of the intellect, or relief from fatigue. The use of coffee in Abyssinia was recorded in the 15th century. It is said that a sheperd, observing his flocks grazing upon Coffea arabica during the season when the berries were ripe, noticed that they became restless, friskly, and had undue energy. He gathered some of the berries and took them to a nearby monastery where a monk prepared coffee as a beverage for the first time.

The physiologic action of coffee in dissipating drowsiness and preventing sleep was used to advantage in connection with the prolonged religious services of the Mohammedans. This stirred up fierce opposition on the part of the strictly orthodox and conservative section of the priests since coffee, by then, was held to be an intoxicating beverage, and therefore prohibited by the Koran. In spite of threats of devine retribution and

other devices, the coffee drinking habit spread rapidly among the Arabian Mohammedans.

The appreciation of coffee as a beverage in Europe dates from the 17th century. "Coffee houses" were instituted in England, Germany, France, Sweden and other countries at about the same time. In Europe, as in Arabia, coffee at first made its way into favor in the face of various adverse and even prohibitive restrictions. In England, Charles II endeavored to suppress coffee houses on the ground that they were centers of political agitation.

This coffee bean, now so extensively used, contains from 1 to 2 per cent caffeine. It also contains volatile substances such as furalcohol, produced by the very delicate process of roasting, which is important in developing a proper flavor. These aromatic substances resemble in their action the volatile oils in producing a mild carminative effect.

Tea is a decoction of the leaves of Thea chinensis, a plant containing caffeine as well as theophylline. Both green and black tea contain volatile substances (Theon) and, in addition, approximately 7 per cent tannic acid, which can be tasted as a bitter substance if the tea has been steeped too long.

Cacao, cocoa or chocolate are made from the seeds of Theobroma cacao found in Brazil and Central America. They contain no caffeine, and the principal drug is theobro-

*Departments of Medicine, Pathology and Pharmacology. The School of Medicine, University of Oklahoma.

mine, 0.5-1 per cent. Theobromine does not possess the marked antisoporific action of caffeine, so that chocolate may be taken instead of coffee before retiring without the risk of sleeplessness. Theobromine may, however, exert a toxic effect upon the gastric mucosa if taken too frequently.

The Kola nut is grown in Central Africa. It contains both caffeine and theobromine and is used in the preparation of various cola beverages. Brazil produces Paullinia sorbilis, the seeds of which contain caffeine. In the Argentine, Yerba mate or Paraguay tea is used as a beverage which also contains caffeine.

It has been wisely noted that no civilization has ever existed wherein the complexities of that system could be tolerated by the people without stimulants and narcotics. The common beverages used in this country with their approximate amount of caffeine per unit or usual container are:

Coffee	1½-2 gr.
Pepsi Cola	1 1/5 gr.
Spur	⅞ gr.
Coca Cola	½ gr.
Tea	¼-½ gr.
Sanka	⅛-¼ gr.[1 2 3 4]

For many years we have considered caffeine containing beverages as harmless when taken in moderate quantities. During the strain of war, however, it has not been uncommon to see patients who drink from 18 to 25 cups of coffee a day. From such large doses of caffeine, headaches and confusion may occur. There may be ringing in the ears, flashes of light and pounding of the heart. Mild precordial pain is often observed, and tremor is common. Since caffeine is a stimulant to the cerebral cortex, it follows naturally that many sleepless nights occur from the ingestion of coffee or caffeine containing beverages late in the evening. The marked variations in insomnia in response to such stimuli is rather difficult to explain, but may be accountable by variations in the threshold of excitement.

Another group of patients who should avoid caffeine containing beverages even in small quantities are those who have burning in the pit of the stomach and "indigestion" following a cup of coffee, tea or cola drink. Among these individuals are those who have previously experienced or who are actually suffering from peptic ulcer. It includes also those who have the so-called ulcer personality or "pre-ulcer" state or those who exhibit persistent gastric hypersecretion of hydrochloric acid as determined by fractional gastric analysis following various test meals.

Recently[5] by measuring the total gastric secretion of hydrochloric acid, we have demonstrated (confirming the work of Ivy[6]) that normal patients secrete increased amounts of hydrochloric acid when the gastric mucosa is stimulated with caffeine. We have demonstrated also that in active duodenal and gastric ulcers there is a high prolonged secretory phase of gastric activity following stimulation with caffeine. Furthermore, it has been shown (unpublished data) that in duodenal ulcer in remission, a prolonged high secretory response to the caffeine test meal persists for many months even though there is complete freedom from symptoms.

Ivy has shown that 5 per cent of "normal" people exhibit a prolonged high gastric secretory response to caffeine stimulation, and that a considerable proportion of this "normal" 5 per cent develop duodenal ulcer within a year or two.

It is believed that, in this approximately 5 per cent of susceptible individuals, caffeine exerts its deleterious effects in the following manner: (a) caffeine produces a toxic irritating effect upon the parietal gastric glands so that (b) histamine is released by such action, which in turn causes (c) hypersecretion of acid with resultant (d) corrosive destruction of the gastric mucosa.

In conclusion it may be said that:

1. Caffeine, in excessive doses, may produce a variety of untoward effects principally as a result of stimulation of the higher nervous centers.

2. Caffeine, in relatively small doses, stimulates gastric secretion in normal individuals.

3. In approximately 5 per cent of "normal" persons and in those suffering from peptic ulcer (10 per cent of the male adult population in the United States), caffeine produces an excessive prolonged gastric secretion of hydrochloric acid.

4. Part of the gastric hypersecretion which results from stimulation by caffeine may be due to an abnormal humoral mechanism.

5. Patients with active or latent peptic ulcer should not drink coffee, cola or other beverages which contain caffeine.

BIBLIOGRAPHY

1. Sollman, T.; A Manual of Pharmacology, Philadelphia, W. B. Saunders Company, 1943.
2. Bethea, O. W.; Caffeine Beverages, Internal M. Digest, Vol. 27, Page 46, July, 1935.
3. Pepsi Cola, Spur and Coca-Cola; New Hampshire Health News, Vol. 19, July, 1941.
4. Sanka; Examination of Three Caffeine Reduced (So Called Decaffeinated) Coffees, Report of the Clinical Laboratory, J.A.M.A. Vol. 91, Page 880. September 22, 1928.
5. Musick, Vern H.; Hopps, Howard C.; Avery, Harry T.; Hellbaum, Arthur A.; The Effect of Caffeine on Gastric Secretion. Read before the Gastroenterological Section of Southern Medical Meeting, Cincinnatti. 1945.
6. Roth, J. A.; Ivy, A. C.; Atkinson, A. J.; Caffeine and Peptic Ulcer. The J.A.M.A, Vol. 126, pp. 814-820. November 25, 1944.
Judd, E. S.; Experimental Production of Peptic Ulcers with Caffeine. Bull. A. M. Coll. Surg, Vol. 28, Page 46, August, 1943.
Roth, J. A. and Ivy, A. C.; The Experimental Production of Acute and Subacute Gastric Ulcers in Cats by the Intramuscular Injection of Caffeine in Beeswax. Gastroenterology, Vol. 2, Page 274, April, 1944.
Goodwin, L. and Gilman, A.; The pharmacological Basis of Therapeutics. Macmillan Company, 1941.
Gastro Enterology, Bockus, Vol. 1, pp. 198-230. W. B. Saunders and Company, Philadelphia, 1943.

Clinical Pathological Conference

University of Oklahoma School of Medicine

Presented by the Departments of Pathology and Surgery

J. MOORE CAMPBELL, M.D.—BELA HALPERT, M.D.

OKLAHOMA CITY, OKLAHOMA

DOCTOR HALPERT: The patient whose story we are to discuss today presented a number of possibilities and was for quite a while a a diagnostic problem. By the time the correct diagnosis was arrived at the patient had arrived at the end of his journey. We have Dr. Campbell to present and analyze the clinical data.

PROTOCOL

Patient: R. R., white male, age 52; admitted October 24, 1946; died November 23, 1946.

Chief Complaint: Dyspnea, productive cough, and swelling of epigastrium.

Present Illness: The patient, a 50-year-old farmer, was seen in the Outpatient Department on October 23, 1945, and admitted to University Hospitals on October 24, 1945. He stated that about the first part of March he noticed a mild pain in the precordial region. He used hot packs and other home remedies. By April the pain was in the left side of the chest, and by June it was low on the left, still not severe, but not relieved by any method. By the first of October he noticed swelling of the epigastrium and localization of pain in this area. On October 4, 1945, he began coughing and expectorating a "cream-blue" sputum. Coughing increased the epigastric pain. About the same time he noticed swelling of the feet and ankles at night, less in the mornings. He became increasingly weaker after the first of October and since October 20, 1945, he has been forced to sleep with his head elevated because of "smothering spells".

Past and Familty History: The patient was treated for "stomach trouble" in 1940 at University Hospitals' Outpatient Department with good results. A nonproductive cough has been present for several years. He has never had hemoptysis, fever, pleurisy or weight loss. Family history is noncontributory.

Physical Examination: On admission he was well developed, fairly well nourished and appeared to be of the stated age. He had loss of hearing in the left ear, pyorrhea, dental caries, and partial edentia. The pharynx was red. The P. M. I. was at the anterior auxillary line, and a systolic murmur was heard over the mitral valve area. The blood pressure was 150/90. Sonorous rales were heard over most of the chest, louder over the left base. Dullness was noted over the right chest. The liver was palpable to the umbilicus. Tenderness was noted in the epigastrium, and a nodule 2 cm. in diameter was felt in that region on the surface of the liver. The spleen was questionably palpable. A bilateral herniorrhaphy scar was present, with recurrence on the left side. The reflexes were physiological. There was 1+ edema of the legs.

Laboratory Data: On repeated examinations of the urine the specific gravity varied from 1.014 to 1.016; it was acid only once and the albumin was 0, 1+, 2+, and 0. Glucose was reported as a trace on the first examination, negative on three others. Occasional white blood cells were seen on one occasion, and many on another. On October 25, 1945, the hemoglobin was 13.5 Gm., the red blood cell count 5.3 million, the white blood cell count 15,200 with 89 per cent neutrophils (7 per cent non-filamented), 1 per cent eosinophils, 2 per cent basophils, 6 per cent lymphocytes and 2 per cent monocytes. On November 1, 1945, the white blood cell count was 18,900 with 89 per cent neutrophils (22 per cent stabs) and 11 per cent lymphocites. On November 21, 1945, the icteric index was 16. The sulfonamide blood level was 11.6 mg. per cent on November 5, 1945. The Mazzini test was negative. The ascitic fluid cell count on November 5, 1945, was: 100,000 fresh red blood cells and 75 white blood cells. On October 31, 1945, the cephalin flocculation test was negative at 24 hours and 1+ at 48 hours. No acid fast bacilli were found on repeated examinations of the sputum; pyocyaneous was cultured from it. Type 16 pneumococcus was reported from the sputum on November 13, 1945. On October 25, 1945, the total protein was 5.5 per cent, and on November 6, 1945, 5.1 per cent. The A/G ratio was 3.8/1.3. A chest plate was reported as chronic fibrous tuberculosis on October 23, 1945. On review, in conjunction with gastric studies, on November 9, 1945, the impression was carcinoma of lung with metastases. On October 10, 1945, roentgenographically, intestinal obstruction was suggested.

Clinical Course: Peritoneoscopy on October 29, 1945, revealed an enlarged, nodular liver, with no distortion of the omentum over the stomach or pancreas. The nodules were firmer and lighter than the rest of the liver; about 500 cc. of cloudy amber fluid was removed. The patient was given codeine q 3 h. p.r.n., seconal for rest, and hykinone, 1 ampule on two occasions. On November 5, 1945, paracentesis was again done and a bloody fluid was obtained, with some relief. On November 7, 1945, the patient complained of pain in the right side of the abdomen, radiating from the umbilicus to the right flank. Morphine sulfate gr. 1/6 stat and q 4 h. p.r.n. was given. The abdomen became more distended, and paracentesis was repeated on November 10, 1945, but distention was marked the next day. A Wangensteen apparatus was inserted, with little relief. Ileus was suspected. Distention persisted and on November 12, 1945, sodium sulfadiazene was given, and potassium iodide gtt xv t.i.d. On November 17, 1945, syrup of hydriotic acid zi q 3-4 h. was given for the cough. Morphine was necessary at times for pain. On November 20, 1945, bronchial breathing was noticed. The abdomen became more distended, and 4 to 6 pints of clear amber fluid was obtained by paracentesis. Breathing became progressively more difficult and the patient died on November 23, 1945.

CLINICAL DIAGNOSIS

DOCTOR CAMPBELL: It is the prime purpose of a conference of this sort to discuss a particular clinical problem with the pathologists; to study a disease process from a diagnostic standpoint as accurately as possible and then predict the necropsy findings from the data obtained while the patient was still alive.

The mark of a good clinician is found best of all in the manner in which he orders his laboratory, radiologic and consultation studies. After the patient is interviewed and his story recorded, after the physical examination is completed and recorded, the first step for the careful diagnostician is to check all of his positive findings by requestioning the patient and re-examining all points of positive or nearly positive physical patholgy. You will find that you can interrogate a patient more to the point after you have collected all the clinical data. Furthermore, the patient invariably remembers some details that he is anxious to tell you about. More important still is the re-examination; invariably the positive physical signs are a little clearer, and some of the questionably positive physical changes cannot now be found. The first clinical study that you order for the patient then is a recheck of significant findings. Now you are ready to classify his problem with a tentative diagnosis. In surveying hospital charts, I get the feeling that it is your object in recording the diagnosis of impression, to enumerate a series of diseases to which you honestly believe that the patient is eligible, and you hope that the final diagnosis will reside somewhere within the listing, preferably, I might add, near the top.

This tentative diagnosis should be used as a starting point from which the correct management of the case begins. You decide whether the patient should be kept in bed, what he should be fed, what immediate therapy he needs, and how to make him comfortable and at ease in his hospital surroundings. Particularly, from your summary and estimate, you determine the logical sequence of laboratory, radiologic and therapeutic studies necessary to arrive at an exact anatomic and functional diagnosis. The accuracy of your diagnosis will decide the accuracy of your effective treatment in no small measure. This should be the purpose of the diagnosis rather than its confirmation at necropsy.

You will notice that the studies carried out in our case for the morning are pointed in their requisition. Each was ordered for a specific purpose; nothing was done at random or to delay for time. Two omissions are striking: the electrocardiogram and a bronchoscopic examination. For completeness, these should have been done. In the absence of more focal cardiac symptoms, the electrocardiogram was probably deemed a luxury. Bronchoscopic examination, however, should have been seriously considered in view of the reports given after x-ray of the chest. Perhaps the hazards of bronchoscopy were taken into consideration, and rightly so. I have seen two deaths directly attributable to the bronchoscope, and two deaths directly caused by the esophagoscope. It should be the province of the bronchoscopist to decide the question of how much danger is entailed in the examination, and the diagnostician should not necessarily protect his patient from the bronchoscopist any more than he shields him from the surgeon.

If you have already tried to integrate all of the supplementary diagnostic procedures in this case, you are confused and discouraged. The patient has no particular anemia. You can feel tumor nodules in or near the liver, so there ought to be an anemia. Perhaps the patient is dehydrated and the blood count artificially high. Urinary specific gravity of 1015 doesn't concur with this impression, so you have two alternatives at this point: order another blood count and hope for an anemia, or accept the probable fact that anemia is absent. Moderate leucocytosis can be accounted for on the basis of his cough alone. One test for syphilis is negative, and you know that if the liver nodules were gummata, that test should be positive. Hoping for a massive lesion of the stomach to account for the primary site of the tumor, you are confounded by a radiologic impression of partial intestinal obstruction and no masses seen. This adds, rather than subtracts from confusion.

Peritoneoscopic examination was of some help: the nodules were in the liver and not in the transverse mesocolon. A biopsy was not taken probably because of fear of hemorrhage from the liver. In that connection the peritoneoscope, it seems to me, is an instrument of little value, used by doctors for a curious poking around in the surgeon's field. A small incision over the tumor nodule, under local anesthesia, and a big piece of tissue could have been secured for Dr. Halpert. Resorting to that long narrow tube, you can only look forward while you may be macerating tissue, causing perforations and hemorrhage in all directions.

Positive information finally arrived at for correlation include: 1. Seven months of productive cough, accompanied by lower chest pain, especially on the left side, the pain aggravated very much by the cough. 2. Epigastric soreness and swelling of two months duration with progression of swelling and progression of loss of appetite. 3. Radiologic impression of carcinoma and/or tuberculosis of the lungs. 4. Visible and palpable tumor nodules on an enlarged, non-cirrhotic liver. 5. Moderate ascites. 6. A suggestion of partial intestinal obstruction by the radiologist. 7. No systemic effect that cannot be accounted for by the pathologic changes in the chest and abdomen.

With no sign of any tumor tissue except in the liver and possibly the lung, until the patient's death; in the absence of more diffuse hepatic involvement of tumor tissue, and with none central enough to cause obstructive jaundice and obstructive cirrhosis or hepatic necrosis with sweating and fever; since the symptoms were primarily pulmonary, secondarily epigastric; since carcinoma of the lung is more than ten times as frequent as primary carcinoma of the liver; since the tumor was evidently the cause of death rather than a relighting of pulmonary tuberculosis, I would say that the patient has a primary carcinoma of the left upper bronchus, with extension into the posterior mediastinum, liver, and probably the left posterior parietal pleura. I believe that pulmonary tuberculosis was also present with some evidence of activity in the old tubercles at the apex of the left upper lobe and mediastinum.

CLINICAL DISCUSSION

QUESTION: What did you think was the precipitating cause of death?

DOCTOR CAMPBELL: I was primarily concerned with surgical observations so that I did not look over the medical list very carefully. In spite of sulfonamide therapy, the patient had, terminally, a high fever. This means that he had a terminal infection. There was edema evident over the trunk and lower extremities and, on account of dyspnea, one would assume that there was pulmonary edema also. This plus an obstructive bronchial lesion, probably caused bronchopneumonia.

QUESTION: How do you account for the initial RBC of 5.3 million?

DOCTOR CAMPBELL: This was probably due to dehydration but at the time one can never be sure. Dehydration can be very deceptive when interpreting the blood count.

DOCTOR HOPPS: In patients such as this, an evaluation of the color index may be very helpful. If the blood picture is actually normal, the color index should be approximately one. In most surgical cases, if anemia is present it will be of the microcytic, hypochromic type so that even if dehydration produces a hemoconcentration and renders the number of RBCs/cu.mm. 5.0 million or more, the Hb will still be less than normal since the cells are hyperchromic. In this particular case the color index was approximately 0.85 which should have suggested that the red blood cell count was elevated as a result of hemoconcentration.

ANATOMIC DIAGNOSIS

DOCTOR HALPERT: At necropsy we found this patient to be somewhat emaciated. There was a decubital ulcer about 6 x 4 cm. over the sacral promontory and there was pitting edema of the extremities and the scrotum. The peritoneal cavity contained about three liters of dark amber fluid and each pleural cavity contained about 50 cc. of fluid. The liver was markedly enlarged as had been observed clinically; its weight was about four times the normal (5,000 gms.). The surface was densely studded with firm white-yellow nodules presented a slight umbilication. Cut surfaces revealed extensive metastases throughout the liver, quite sufficient to explain the marked increase in weight. The liver was dark green. Although extrahepatic bile ducts were widely patent it was evident that the numerous metastic nodules within the liver were responsible for some obstruction of intra-hepatic bile ducts. This would explain the slight increase in icteric index, the greenish discoloration of the liver and the mild jaundice observed at necropsy. The primary neoplasm was located in the left lung; it was a carcinoma. This lung weighed 1525 gms. (5 x normal). Almost the entire upper lobe was involved by the tumor and, distal to its origin in a secondary bronchus, there were several bronchiectatic abscesses, a common sequel of carcinoma of the lung. Regional lymph nodes were extensively involved. There was also metastasis to the left suprarenal gland. In addition there was in the lower lobe of the left lung, an old inactive calcified tubercle, 1.5 cm. in diameter. The right lung weighed 775 gms. (2 x normal). Particularly the dependent 1/3 exhibited a lumpy induration and was subcrepitant (bronchopneumonia). Histologically, this neoplasm is the type that occurs in about 30 per cent of all carcinomas of the lung—a reserve cell carcinoma. This is a rather undifferentiated type of neoplasm which does not present any particular pattern. All of the cells look alike and tend to lie in sheets or nests with a rather scanty, connective tissue stroma. This is the type of tumor which used to be called "round cell sarcoma".

DISCUSSION

QUESTION: How do you explain the rather peculiar pain of which this patient complained?

DOCTOR HALPERT: There were old pleural adhesions, left, which would have allowed for metastatic spread of the neoplasm into paravertebral nervous structures.

QUESTION: Did the patient have dysphagia?

DOCTOR CAMPBELL: When he had epigastric pain—not before.

QUESTION: At what time in this patient's course would pneumonectomy still have been curative?

DOCTOR CAMPBELL: I can not answer that question. The rate of growth of these tumors is quite variable and one cannot, on the basis of initial symptoms, determine the extent of the tumor even at that time.

NEUROLOGICAL HOSPITAL

Twenty-Seventh and The Paseo
Kansas City, Missouri

Modern   Hospitalization   of Nervous   and   Mental   Illnesses, Alcoholism and Drug Addiction.

THE ROBINSON CLINIC
G. WILSE ROBINSON, M.D.
G. WILSE ROBINSON, Jr., M.D.

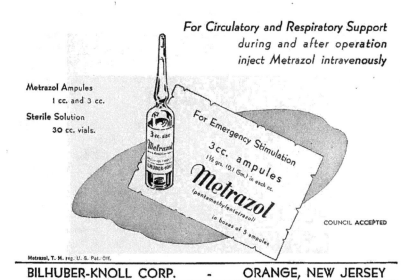

For Circulatory and Respiratory Support during and after operation inject Metrazol intravenously

Metrazol Ampules
1 cc. and 3 cc.

Sterile Solution
30 cc. vials.

For Emergency Stimulation

3cc. ampules
1½ grs. (0.1 Gm.) in each cc.

Metrazol
(pentamethylenetetrazol)
in boxes of 5 ampules

COUNCIL ACCEPTED

Metrazol, T. M. reg. U. S. Pat. Off.

BILHUBER-KNOLL CORP.   -   ORANGE, NEW JERSEY

THE PRESIDENT'S PAGE

Hearing on the Wagner-Murray-Dingell Bill will start about the 1st of April and there are 400 proponents of the bill to be heard. Oklahoma State Medical Association will have representation at the hearing consisting of the most able talent available. Every councilor's district in the state will be appraised of the happenings and the content of the bill is being discussed in every county medical society in the state and we are enlisting and getting the enthusiastic support of the allied professions.

If every person in the state knew that there would be approximately $40.00 deducted from each thousand dollars earned; that it makes no difference as to your belief in the regular form of practicing medicine or if you are Christian Scientist or any of the other members of the healing art. Under regimentation you will have to pay the tax whether you use it not not; that not all the doctors will be regimented; that the people can not have free choice of doctors unless their doctor is willing to participate in the regimentation. That if all countries where regimentation is practiced there is a limitation on the number of patients that any chosen doctor can service during a day; that more money is spent in administering the plan than is paid for medical and hospital services.

We mention these radical changes to show you that there will be a round-about-face in our way of securing medical service and it behooves the doctors of our profession to honestly and truthfully give to their patients the facts contained in this bill of compulsory medical service and assure them that it is not our desire to deny the public of a better system for better health care in our great nation. Every interested and working member of the State Association is requested to acquaint themselves with the true facts and conscientiously and intelligently give this information to the people of our state.

President.

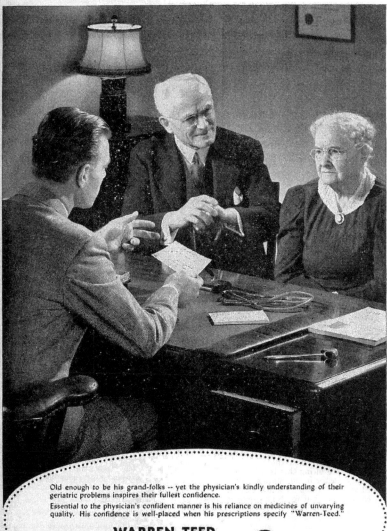

Old enough to be his grand-folks -- yet the physician's kindly understanding of their geriatric problems inspires their fullest confidence.

Essential to the physician's confident manner is his reliance on medicines of unvarying quality. His confidence is well-placed when his prescriptions specify "Warren-Teed."

WARREN-TEED

Medicaments of Exacting Quality Since 1920

THE WARREN-TEED PRODUCTS COMPANY, COLUMBUS 8, OHIO

Warren-Teed Ethical Pharmaceuticals: capsules, elixirs, ointments, sterilized solutions, syrups, tablets. Write for literature.

The JOURNAL Of The
OKLAHOMA STATE MEDICAL ASSOCIATION

EDITORIAL BOARD
L. J. MOORMAN, Oklahoma City, Editor-in-Chief
E. EUGENE RICE, Shawnee
BEN H. NICHOLSON, Oklahoma City
MR. DICK GRAHAM, Oklahoma City, Business Manager
JANE FIRRELL TUCKER, Editorial Assistant

CONTRIBUTIONS: Articles accepted by this Journal for publication including those read at the annual meetings of the State Association are the sole property of this Journal.

The Editorial Department is not responsible for the opinions expressed in the original articles of contributors.

Manuscripts may be withdrawn by authors for publication elsewhere only upon the approval of the Editorial Board.

MANUSCRIPTS: Manuscripts should be typewritten, double-spaced, on white paper 8½ x 11 inches. The original copy, not the carbon copy, should be submitted.

Footnotes, bibliographies and legends for cuts should be typed on separate sheets in double space. Bibliography listing should follow this order: Name of author, title of article, name of periodical with volume, page and date of publication.

Manuscripts are accepted subject to the usual editorial revisions and with the understanding that they have not been published elsewhere.

NEWS: Local news of interest to the medical profession, changes of address, births, deaths and weddings will be gratefully received.

ADVERTISING: Advertising of articles, drugs or compounds unapproved by the Council on Pharmacy of the A.M.A. will not be accepted. Advertising rates will be supplied on application.

It is suggested that members of the State Association patronize our advertisers in preference to others.

SUBSCRIPTIONS: Failure to receive The Journal should call for immediate notification.

REPRINTS: Reprints of original articles will be supplied at actual cost provided request for them is attached to manuscripts or made in sufficient time before publication. Checks for reprints should be made payable to Industrial Printing Company, Oklahoma City.

Address all communications to THE JOURNAL OF THE OKLAHOMA STATE MEDICAL ASSOCIATION,
210 Plaza Court, Oklahoma City 3

OFFICIAL PUBLICATION OF THE OKLAHOMA STATE MEDICAL ASSOCIATION
Copyrighted April, 1946

EDITORIALS

OKLAHOMA COUNTY MEDICAL SOCIETY GOES ON RECORD

Through a well-planned educational program the Oklahoma County Medical Society is serving the people of the State at a critical time in their existence. This service consists of a series of full-page statements in the Sunday Oklahoman presenting pertinent facts about compulsory taxation for political medicine. The members of the medical society believe the people should know the truth about the proposed government plan embodied in the Wagner Bill. With the senate committee hearings on the Wagner Bill in the immediate offing this is a timely movement. Every doctor in the State should be interested and every county and district medical society should put forth an organized effort to make this publicity effective. It is to be hoped that some of the larger county societies may initiate similar programs. Regardless of what organized medicine may do, now is the time for every doctor who cherishes the welfare of his people to sit down and write his representatives in Washington urging them to protect their constituency against further government medicine in any form.

THE OMINOUS WEB

Over the breadth and length of this great country where the currents of freedom and liberty have moved in the clear atmosphere of constitutional protection, we envision an intricate web of concentric weave. At the center we see sitting "spider-like" the Social Security administrator awaiting the hopeless entanglement of 130,000,000 people who must pay a price for the loss of liberty. This imprisoning web is to be reinforced by the Wagner-Murray-Dingle Bill if the people concerned do not protest. If you love your country and want to save it you should see that your friends and patrons write to their senators and representatives immediately.*

Senator Elmer Thomas, Senate Office Building, Washington, D. C.

Senator E. H. Moore, Senate Office Building, Washington, D. C.

Rep. A. S. "Mike." Monroney, House Office Building, Washington, D. C.

Rep. Lyle H. Boren, House Office Building, Washington, D. C.

Rep. George B. Schwabe, House Office Building, Washington, D. C.

Rep. Wm. G. Stigler, House Office Building, Washington, D. C.

Rep. Victor Wickersham, House Office Building, Washington, D. C.

Rep. Jed Johnson, House Office Building, Washington, D. C.

Rep. Paul Stewart, House Office Building, Washington, D. C.

Rep. Ross Rizley, House Office Building, Washington, D. C.

FRESH AIR

Of all the states in the Union, Oklahoma has the most stimulating atmospheric conditions. It has much more fresh air than many states and less hot air than some. But even in Oklahoma many people must still learn the importance of proper ventilation and the value of outdoor living.

Victor Robinson has said that Benjamin Franklin preaching the gospel of fresh air, opened the windows of America. In truth, the windows of America were really opened by a more militant apostle of fresh air, Edward Livingston Trudeau, who literally prepared the way for wide open windows with a definite purpose and a well founded hope.

But fifty years before Trudeau demonstarted the value of fresh air we find Florence Nightingale making the following appeal: "The extraordinary confusion between cold and ventilation, even in the minds of well educated people, illustrates this. To make a room cold is by no means necessarily to ventilate it. Nor is it at all necessary, in order to ventilate a room, to chill it. Yet, if a nurse finds a room close, she will let out the fire, thereby making it closer, or she will open the door into a cold room, without a fire, or an open window in it, by way of improving ventilation. The safest atmosphere of all for a patient is a good fire and an open window, excepting in extremes of temperature. (Yet no nurse can ever be made to understand this.) To ventilate a small room without draughts of course requires more care than to ventilate a large one.

"Another extraordinary fallacy is the dread of night air. What air can we breathe at night but night air? The choice is between pure night air from without and foul night air from within. . . . An open window most nights in the year can never hurt any one."

We have profited little by the report of the New York Commission on ventilation and heating which took its place on dusty bookshelves twelve or fifteen years ago. The experimental studies of this Commission revealed that the ideal room temperature is $68\frac{1}{2}°$ and that susceptibility to respiratory infection increased as the temperature rose above this point. It was proven that on the whole, open window ventilation was more healthful than circulating currents of air through the fan system with closed windows. Capacity for work, both physical and mental was demonstrably lowered as the temperature passed above the ideal point of $68\frac{1}{2}°$. These are facts that doctors should utilize in their daily practice. Houses and particularly living rooms, should be equipped with thermometers and mothers should be instructed with reference to the desirable temperature and the value of open window ventilation.

PRESCRIPTION WRITING

The best medical treatment is that fitted to the individual patient. Drug theraphy, highly significant in most medical treatment, is secured by the prescription. As Sollmann aptly says, a prescription is "an order for medicine sent by a physician to a pharmacist". Some of the practical requirements for writing an effective and correct prescription are often neglected. The instructions for the pharmacist and patient must be legible and intelligible; this is why English is now preferred to Latin. The prescriber should use correct, descriptive names for the ingredients and not just their trade names; such description insures fewer misunderstandings. If an ingredient is official or otherwise open to manufacture by several firms, a firm name should be placed adjacent to the ingredient if the physician wishes to show his confidence in any one manufacturer; otherwise any brand may be used to fill the prescription. The use of English abbreviations and numbers as designations for drugs should be avoided. Complex mixtures should not be ordered if simple ones will suffice. Unrelated substances such as purgatives and hypnotics are not properly included in a single prescription. They are best prescribed separately and timed in their administration to be most effective. The physician should be mindful of the frequency with which prescriptions are refilled without his knowledge. Thus he may limit the number of doses to the actual needs of the patient and state specifically on the prescription whether it can be refilled and, if so, how often. The importance of such directions, for example when barbituric acid compounds are prescribed, is obvious. Of course the pharmacist bears the responsibility of filling the prescription; when he is in doubt concerning the ingredients or directions, it is his moral responsibility to call the prescribing physician; to do otherwise invites disastrous results.

THE OKLAHOMA DIVISION OF THE AMERICAN CANCER SOCIETY

The Oklahoma Division of the American Cancer Society is composed of a number of illustrious lay people who are individually interested in the cancer problem, and the Cancer Committee of your State Medical Association. It has been fully realized that any program dealing with the subject of cancer must be executed with the complete cooperation of the medical profession, not only as to the State Medical Organization, but also in conjunction with the County Societies.

The aims and objects of the Society are three-fold. These are: Education, Detection Clinics and Research. Under *Education* Speakers Bureaus have been established, the Women's Field Army has been fostered and many newspaper articles and radio talks have been given. It has been suggested that each local medical society in the State have one monthly program each year devoted entirely to cancer. A traveling *Detection Clinic* truck has been purchased and is available at the invitation of any County Medical Society. Several clinics have been held and it is the feeling of the participating doctors that much good has been done; not only has it served those who have appeared for examination, but also those who, through the publicity, have been incited to apply to their personal physicians for examination. It is the hope of this Society that a clinic of this type be held in every County of the State every year. The Detection Clinic truck can be obtained by the asking. These clinics will not be in any locality unless they are invited by the local association. Under *Research* we have several projects now under consideration.

The patient with cancer must be educated to consul a doctor *early*. The patient's doctor must make an *early* diagnosis. *Then* at least one out of every three patients dying of cancer can be saved.—P.B.C., M.D.

MEDICAL SCIENCE AND ANIMAL EXPERIMENTATION

In five successive decades hardly a year has passed without a fight against animal experimentation for the benefit of medical science. Recently it required the combined efforts of the New York State Medical Society, the New York Academy of Medicine and County Medical Societies, Medical Schools and other agencies to defeat a bill designed to destroy the effectiveness of medical research through the prohibition of animal experimentation.

As indicated above, there is nothing new about New York's experience. In 1900, when the Yellow Fever Commission was working in Havana, Osler, Welch, General Sternberg, W. W. Keen and others were before the 56th Congress to testify against Senate Bill 34, championed by Senator Gallinger. As early as 1894 Alfred L. Loomis, President of the Tri Annual Congress of American Physicians and Surgeons devoted his presidential address before this Congress to animal experimentation and William H. Welch introduced a resolution protesting any legislation tending to interfere with the advancement of medical science. During this period, Welch was before many medical and scientific bodies for the purpose of introducing similar resolutions. No doubt Welch's untiring efforts and his active campaign resulted in defeat of the successive legislative proposals to prohibit animal experimentation. Osler, through his association with Welch, was well

prepared when, in November, 1907, he was called to testify before the Royal Commission on Vivisection at the British Parliamentary Hearing.

Though medical science has successfully stemmed the tide, storms are still ahead and eternal vigilance is necessary to avert disaster. In truth, the seriousness of the New York situation caused medical authorities to arrange for planned opposition on a national level. This decision led to the organization of the National Society for Medical Research on February 11, last with H. K. Carlson as Chairman of this organization.

We may expect an alert and active educational campaign and prompt aid wherever and whenever needed. The purpose of this editorial is to suggest the advisability of action on the part of the State Medical Association pledging moral support and financial aid, if necessary. County Medical Societies should consider following suit. The Alumni Association of the University of Oklahoma School of Medicine is now launching a campaign for funds in anticipation of a Research Institute. Think what it would mean if we were suddenly faced with legislation to prohibit animal experimentation. We cannot afford to withhold our support from any national movement which offers protection.

BISMARCK AND HITLER

Through government paternalism (social security) Bismarck placed the German people under obligation to the government. Through government power (Facism) Hitler placed the people under the whip with the purge for those who failed to respond. Under Bismarck's social security and compulsory health insurance program the progress of medicine and the effectiveness of scientific endeavor gradually declined. Under Hitler's regime there was rapid deterioration in both medical practice and medical education. In the New England Journal of Medicine March 7, 1946, Col. Robert M. Zollinger, M. C., A. U. S., discusses Medical Education and Practice in Germany during the War. After visiting the clinics of the professors of medicine and surgery in three prominent German medical schools Col. Zollinger lifts the veil of secrecy which had enshrouded German medicine during the past five years. His report shows what Facism has done to both teachers and students of medicine.

In the editorial columns of the Oklahoma State Medical Association Journal, the evil effects of the governments accelerated program in medical schools has been discussed repeatedly with the suggestion that it may take fifty years to recover our losses. If this is true in the United States what must be the situation in Germany. After indicating the low level to which medical education and practice have descended in Germany the author enumerates the converging causes and places the blame on government control. In support of the above brief statement Col. Zollinger's closing paragraphs are quoted.

"During the recent conflict little was known of the German medical profession, and many have though that because of its past ingenuity and skill it might have made many valuable discoveries. It is now apparent that the myth of German superiority in the medical profession is as much a fallacy as it was found to be in other forms of German endeavor. This deterioration has been due in part to the curtailments resulting from a long war, but prolonged interference and regulation by the State in the selection and activities of the students, as well as of the teaching staffs, did irreparable damage to the German medical profession. Although political intereference and State control have been carried to extremes in Germany, the tendency for such influences to stifle high professional standards in any country must not be overlooked.

"That any significant new developments have been made in Germany, either in medicine or in surgery, in recent years is doubtful. The practices of therapy there are in most instances antiquated as judged by our standards, and it will unquestionably be years before the German medical profession regains, if it does so at all, the high position that it held twenty or thirty years ago."

OUR STATE MEETING

Fifty-two times the Oklahoma State Medical Association has called its members in for contact, companionship, counsel and scientific discourse. On the fifty-third anniversary of the Association the members and guests will gather in Oklahoma City for a social and scientific feast which stems from the first meeting held fifty-two years ago when hardy medical pioneers came from their respective homes "on the range" to initiate and sponsor organized medicine. Though we may have fifty-three times as much scientific knowledge, it is doubtful if in the sum of our membership we can match the courage, the ambition, the good will and the fortitude that rode into town on the first meeting day. As a tribute to those who laid the foundation for the super structure which houses our professional aspirations and ideals, let us attend this meeting with profound humility and eager acquisitiveness. This is the fifty-third meeting. It is time to take stock and live up to our obligations and opportunities. Don't miss it.

THE SPIRIT OF MEDICINE

The true spirit of medicine is perpetually striving for higher ground, forever moving toward commendable goals. It enters the realm of the unknown in search of new truths, often revealing the cause of disease, the prevention and cure. Thus the blessings of medical science have been realized for the benefit of humanity. Medicine, animated by this spirit, seeks no reward other than freedom from bureaucratic directives, fine print bulletins, stereotyped records, incomprehensible blanks and the annoying necessity of political rating. .

James Stevenson, M.D.
108 West Sixth Street
Tulsa, Oklahoma
My dear Doctor Stevenson:
　Taking advantage of my very first opportunity since the adjournment of our House of Delegates, I am writing to convey to you and through you to members of the Oklahoma State Medical Association who so signally honored me in the presentation of the fine painting that was presented by you at the dinner for the House of Delegates in Chicago on the evening of December 4, 1945.
　I was deeply touched by the expression of friendship from members of the Oklahoma State Medical Association. Having had no information that the presentation would be made, I was totally unprepared and my emotions were so deeply stirred that it was not possible to give utterance to my feeling of gratitude for the kindly remembrance and the heartening encouragement that it brought to me.
　Mrs. West and I will always consider the painting to be one of our most treasured objects and will always remember with humble and heartfelt gratitude the kindness of our Oklahoma friends.
　With all good wishes for you and for the Oklahoma State Medical Association and all of its members, I am
　　　　　Very sincerely yours,
　　　　　　Olin West, M. D.

Southwest Medical Meeting Held in Hobart
The Southwest Medical Society held their annual meeting for the election of officers at the Country Club in Hobart on March 19.
　Dr. James Stevenson of Tulsa and Mr. Dick Graham presented a "Mock Senate Hearing" on the Wagner-Murray-Dingle Bill, patterned after a similar type of program put on recently by the National Physicians Committee in St. Louis.
　Newly elected officers of the Society are: D. D. Pearson, M.D., President, Mangum, Oklahoma; A. W. Paulson, M.D., Vice-President, Clinton, Oklahoma, and W. A. Starkey, Secretary and Treasurer, Altus, Oklahoma.
　These newly elected officers are all veterans of World War II.

Muskogee, Sequoyah, Wagoner County Medical Society Approves O. P. S.
Dr. L. S. McAlister, acting Secretary of the Muskogee, Sequoyah, Wagoner County Medical Society has advised the Executive Office that the March 5th meeting of the society approved Oklahoma Physicians Service.
　This approval brings to 13 the number of county medical societies that have approved the plan and made its services available to the people in these areas.
　County medical societies desiring to include this service to the people and their surrounding communities should contact Mr. N. D. Heland, Executive Director, Oklahoma Blue Cross Plan, 910 South Boston, Tulsa, Oklahoma, and invite him to present the plan before the county society as it will not be offered unless approved by the physicians.

Councilor Reports

Annual Report of Councilor, District No. 1

To the Council of Oklahoma State Medical Association:
Gentlemen:

During the past year I have attended three Council Meetings at Oklahoma City on May 30, 1946; November 25, 1946; and March 10, 1946. I missed one meeting in October, 1945, because of the death of my wife.

I have attended the Woods County Medical Society Meetings May 29, 1945; December 14, 1946; January 29, 1946. I have attended the Alfalfa County Medical Society Meetings on September 25, 1945, and March 26, 1946. I have visited the Woodward County Medical Society at Supply, June 8, 1945, December 14, 1945, and February 27, 1946. I participated in a Crippled Childrens' Clinic at Alva, December 17, 1945, and a Cancer Clinic at Alva, March 26, 1946. I have made public speeches on Socialized Medicine to the Kiwanis Club of Alva on February 13, 1946, to the Alva Rotary Club on February 18, 1946, and to the Business and Professional Women's Club on February 19, 1946.

I attended the Kansas City Southwest Society on October 1-3, 1945, and the Aero Medical Association of America at Chicago, April 7-9, -946.

I have been especially active in my district on the work against Socialized Medicine in distributing literature and getting letters to senators and representatives. I have distributed approximately 4,000 pieces of literature and secured about 2,000 letters to be mailed to Congressmen.

I assisted in the registration of the doctors of Alva and vicinity in the post-graduate course which is now going on.

I also rendered what services I could in the collection of annual dues for the year. I have visited all parts of my district except the Panhandle Region. As this region is remote and there are few doctors I have made no visits during the year.

Respectfully submitted,
O. E. Templin, M.D.
Councilor, District No. 1

Annual Report of Councilor, District No. 3

To the Council of Oklahoma State Medical Association:
Gentlemen:

As Councilor of the Third District, in accordance with the By-Laws of the State Association, I herewith submit my annual report.

I have visited the Garfield, Kay and Payne County Societies, and have kept in contact by telephone and letter with the other inactive counties.

Some of the highlights of the year are: On June 13, 1945 a district meeting was held in Enid, with representatives from most all of the counties. An interesting program was presented to the laity in the afternoon, with Dr. V. C. Tisdal present representing the Oklahoma State Medical Association and presented its objective and recommended programs. Dr. E. N. Smith of Oklahoma City spoke on Maternity Mortality. The Prepaid Surgical, Obstetrical and Hospital plan was presented by me. That evening the County Society met at a dinner meeting, at which time the same subjects were presented in a more detailed and scientific manner. About forty-five members were present and the program well received.

On September 26, 1945, a district meeting was held at the Jens-Marie Hotel in Ponca City, with approximately thirty-five members present. We had seven guest speakers on this occasion, including Dr. V. C. Tisdal, President of the Association from Elk City; Dr. C. R. Rountree, Dr. Tom Lowry and Dr. Joseph Kelso all of Oklahoma City. The above speakers stressed state health problems and the methods which are being employed by

the State Association in meeting these problems. Concluding the program was an address by Dr. A. S. Risser, who spoke on the Blue Cross Plan.

A joint society meeting was held in Billings on November 15, 1945 to honor Dr. T. F. Renfro upon his completion of fifty years of practice. This meeting was well attended by members of the Kay and Garfield Societies, and. there were some doctors attending from other counties in northern Oklahoma. We were particularly happy that Dr. Tom Lowry could bring the eulogy on this occasion.

A well attended cancer detection clinic was held in Tonkawa February 14, 1946, with the educational program recommended by the Association being presented to the laity in the afternoon. Dr. Paul Champlin of Enid and Dr. Everett S. Lain, Oklahoma City, discussed the disease and its symptoms. Dr. A. S. Risser, Blackwell, introduced visiting specialists. Specialists staffing the clinic were Dr. Everett S. Lain, Dr. Wendell Long, Dr. C. P. Bondurant, Dr. Howard Hopps, Professor of Pathology at the University Medical School, Dr. R. G. Goodwin and Dr. Joseph Kelso, all of Oklahoma City. The County Society dinner meeting was held that evening at the Tonkawa Hotel and a well attended and interesting program presented by Dr. Paul Champlin of Enid, Dr. Wendell Long, Dr. C. P. Bondurant and Dr. Floyd Moorman.

I have made every effort to convey to the medical profession in this district the action taken by the Council at their meetings, and encouraged their participation in carrying out the recommended programs as outlined at the Council meetings.

There has been some preliminary work done toward consolidating some of the less active and smaller counties with the larger ones. This matter is being given attention, and the decision will come only after consideration by the societies and the State Association.

It has been a sincere pleasure to represent the profession of the Third District as Councilor during the past year.

Respectfully submitted,
C. E. Northcutt, M.D.,
Councilor, District No. 3

Report of Councilor District No. 5

Your Councilor has attended all county meetings throughout the District. A District Meeting was held in Duncan in the early fall and a public meeting was held on the same date. These meetings were well attended. The doctors were very enthusiastic about our president's program and all expressed a desire to help put it over.

Cotton and Jefferson County Medical Societies have not been active in the past several years and because of this they have been invited to join with the Stephens County Society. Some have done so and others will do so in the near future.

A previous report of this District was made at the meeting on October 7, 1945.

Respectfully submitted,
J. L. Patterson, M.D., Councilor

Report of District No. 6

I realize that my report is not as complete as it should be and can only plead that family illness has prevented my visiting all the Societies in this District. From reports received from officers of the various Societies I think that they have been carrying on very faithfully during the past year.

The Osage County Society did not have as many meetings as usual, but these were made entertaining by scientific papers and medical films. This Society had, for ten weeks during the summer, the State postgraduate lectures on surgical diagnosis given by Dr. Patrick Wu. These lectures were well attended and well received. Several members of the Washington-Nowata Society attended them faithfully.

Creek County Society carried on their meetings regularly throughout the year, alternating between Bristow and Sapulpa. They had several speakers from the Speakers' Bureau initiated by President Tisdal, and report that these were greatly appreciated. Medical films were shown also.

As always, Tulsa County Society has had more activities than the others. It would be very surprising if this were not so, because of their larger membership. This Society, in addition to having many out of County or out of State speakers for its regular meetings, has functioned in many respects as a civic club, getting into and boosting worthy community projects. This is a mark for other Societies to shoot at.

The Rogers County Society, though small, has carried on with fairly regular meetings and has had some help from the State Speakers' Bureau.

The Washington-Nowata County Society has held all its regular meetings with fair attendance, averaging about 60 per cent of its membership, and has had several men from the Speakers' Bureau. It expects to have a "Cancer Day" on March 13, when the mobile cancer unit and its personnel will be present for diagnostic examinations.

It is to be regretted that there is not more interest taken in the defeat of the very vicious compulsory insurance bill for medical care.

A majority of the men who have been in the armed services from this District are home again, most of them taking up their former practices, a few finding new locations.

Respectfully submitted,
J. V. Athey, M.D.,
Councilor, 6th District.

Annual Report of Councilor, District No. 7
To the Council of Oklahoma State Medical Association:
Gentlemen:

In accordance with the custom established in the By-Laws, the Councilor of the Seventh District now submits a report of activities during the fiscal year 1945-46.

The outstanding medical event of the year was the post-graduate course in surgery arranged by the committee of the Oklahoma State Medical Association and directed by Dr. Patrick Wu. Attendance and interest were very satisfactory.

We have attempted to encourage the activities of the Crippled Children's Commission, particularly through the Rotary Clubs of this district, several of which have enrolled their entire membership in the Crippled Children's Society.

The councilor has attempted at all times to keep each of the county medical societies informed of various legislative items having to do with public health welfare. Members have been encouraged to maintain a high degree of interest in political activities in order that they may become more articulate in the interest of medical legislation. Much satisfaction is expressed in regard to the attitude of the Representative from the Fourth Congressional District, the Honorable Lyle Boren, who in no uncertain terms opposes the regimentation of doctors and patients.

During this year the Councilor of the Seventh District has resigned as the Chairman of the Medical Advisory Committee to the Department of Public Welfare and Dr. Mack I. Shanholtz of Wewoka has been elected to fill that vacancy.

The Councilor of the Seventh District has functioned as Chairman of the Medical Advisory Committee to the Vocational Rehabilitation Division of the State Board of Education.

The Councilor of the Seventh District has attended District Meetings in various parts of the state, including meetings at Sayre, McAlester, Hobart, Muskogee and Durant. County meetings attended one or more times, include Pontotoc, Lincoln, Okfuskee-Okmulgee and Garvin. The Councilor has maintained close contact with the various secretaries of the counties in the Seventh District by telephone and in writing. A serious attempt has been made to convey all information regarding activities of the State Association to all physicians in the Seventh District.

Much encouragement has been given to the prepaid medical plans now sponsored by the State Medical Association. Most of the counties in the district have approved the Oklahoma Physicians Service and several important industrial organizations have been enrolled in the Blue Cross and the Oklahoma Physicians Service. With the assistance of Mr. Glen Leslie, Chairman of the Board of Trustees of the Oklahoma Physicians Service and Mr. N. D. Helland, State Manager of the Blue Cross, plans are being made to have meetings of the important business and civic persons in the very near future. The purpose is of course to still further advance enrollment in prepaid plans.

It has been a genuine pleasure to represent the Seventh District and I am deeply grateful for the privilege of the many happy associations.

Respectfully submitted,
C. Gallaher, M.D.
Councilor, District No. 7

Annual Report of Councilor, District No. 8
To the Council of Oklahoma State Medical Association:
Gentlemen:

Two very fine Councilor meetings were held in the late summer and fall of 1945 of the Eighth Councilor District.

The first of these two Councilor meetings was held at Vinita in the Eastern State Hospital. All the phy-

WILLIAM E. EASTLAND, M.D.
F. A. C. R.

RADIUM AND X-RAY THERAPY
DERMATOLOGY

405 Medical Arts Bldg.

Oklahoma City, Oklahoma   Phone 3-1446

sicians living in the north half of the Eighth District were invited to be at this meeting. A good turn out and an interesting meeting and discussion was held. Dr. Tisdal, President of Oklahoma State Medical Association was present, and many other representatives of the State Medical Association.

The second Councilor meeting was held at Muskogee at Dr. Ed. White's ranch. This was a very fine meeting and was attended by some 25 physicians from different parts of Oklahoma. Later in the evening—when almost time for the barbecue, some other physicians arrived. All business was then adjourned and a good time was had by all physicians attending.

I have not been able to attend any other Councilor meeting since that time. However, I have reports from almost every District in the Eighth Councilor District.

Respectfully submitted,
J. G. Edwards, M.D.
Councilor, District No. 8

Annual Report of Councilor, District No. 9

To the Council of Oklahoma State Medical Association:

Gentlemen:

I wish at this time to give you a report of the Ninth Councilor's District.

As your files will reveal, the ninth district is composed of Pittsburgh, LeFlore, Haskell, McIntosh, and Latimer Counties.

For the year 1946, Pittsburgh County is by far the most active county in our district, both in membership and in activity. Also Pittsburgh County can boast of having our good friend, the president-elect, Dr. L. C. Kuyrkendall. This county has the most comprehensive program of any county in this district, possibly because of its membership which is approximately twenty-five members. The society is under the able leadership of Dr. M. L. Henry, president, and Dr. Greenberger, secretary. This society has in view a program which is threefold; (1) Social, (2) Economic, (3) Scientific; therefore, it is plainly evident that the men in this group are seeking to hold the interest of all the membership. Regular meetings for this group are the third Friday evening of each month.

LeFlore County has ten members paid for 1946, with regular officers duly elected. This county plans to have an active society for this year, and the regular meeting dates are the second Thursday evening of each month.

Haskell County, with our good friends, Dr. W. S. Carson as president, and Dr. N. K. Williams as secretary, has only four members, but these men have decided among themselves that it is not worth while to attempt to have regular meetings, but call meetings instead.

McIntosh County has only five members for this year, and the old reliable Dr. Tolleson keeps the membership up the best he can, but is handicapped by the fact that most of these men are in advanced years. The McIntosh Medical Society meets regularly, and frequently visits the society meetings in Muskogee and in McAlester.

Latimer County has no medical society, and there are only four active practicing physicians in this county. Only one of these men is active in Medical Society work, and he belongs to the LeFlore County Medical Society. The other three men belong to no county society, and have not for years.

Our president's four point program is very popular with the physicians over the Ninth Councilor's District, and it is heartily approved by all the county societies in our district.

It has been this councilor's idea for several months that the counties comprising this district should be joined. In other words, two or more counties should be joined for the purpose of becoming more active, for the purpose of a larger membership, and for the purpose of interest, but after talking to the men or a representative body of the men in the counties involved, I do not now believe that the members of the above counties would desire this arrangement.

Respectfully submitted,
Earl M. Woodson, M.D.
Councilor, District No. 9

Committee Reports

Report of the Insurance Committee

During the year 1945-46 the Insurance Committee has continued to interest the profession as much as possible in the malpractice policy. We have seen many men returning from the Army, some of these men kept their policies during military service, some have renewed their policies promptly upon return. In addition a number of young men have returned from the service and for the first time are in practice.

Most of these men have been eager to get the malpractice policy. Several suits have been handled out of court. For the past 18 months or more the Committee has worked to get a health and accident policy for the members of the Oklahoma State Medical Association. The desire of the Committee was to get a policy with a cost that would be in the reach of all members and at the same time give as broad a coverage as possible. An excellent policy was worked out with the North American Accident Insurance Company. This has been presented to approximately twenty-five counties throughout the state and in each instance it has been very heavily subscribed to.

We feel that this program has been very successful up to this time and feel sure that it will continue to succeed.

Respectfully submitted,
V. K. Allen, M.D., Chairman

Report of the Committee on Medical Education And Hospitals

Undergraduate Teaching: The School of Medicine graduated a class of sixty-nine on March 22, 1946. This marks the end of the accellerated program of the School of Medicine. The next session will begin as before the war in September. The School thereby reverts to the normal schedule of nine months with three months vacation.

Graduate Teaching: Graduate medical training received a great impetus at the ending of hostilities. The School of Medicine has given refresher courses, one in medicine and one in surgery of one month each, and these are to be repeated in April and May. Since the doctors have been returning home there has been a great demand by the younger group of physicians for graduate training in the form of residences of a quality that will meet the requirements of the Specialty Boards. To meet this demand the University Hospitals have expanded their residencies to twice the normal, and other hospitals also have cooperated. In this way a very considerable number of veteran young physicians are being given the training necessary to qualify them for the Specialty Boards. Hospitals over the State are interested in working some affiliation with the University whereby they can also help, and be helped, by this program. This is especially true of Orthopedic Surgery, since to qualify for this board it is necessary to have a certain amount of children's orthopedics.

A new Veterans Administration Hospital is in process of organizing in cooperation with the School of Medicine. It is planned to offer residency training here to meet the requirements of the various boards.

A program of Basic Science training is also being worked out at the Medical School. This is primarily intended for the residents in this institution, but will also be able to care for a certain number of residents from other hospitals.

It will be noted from the above that great emphasis is being placed upon Specialty Board Certification. Your writer is of the opinion that too much emphasis is being placed upon this unless a Specialty Board of General Practice can be set up to train Specialists in this, the largest field of practice.

Respectfully submitted,
Wann Langston, M.D.

The First Year

THE SUCCESSFUL NUTRITIONAL history of S-M-A babies is due to the remarkable similarity of S-M-A to mother's milk. It is essentially the same as human milk in percentage of protein, fat, carbohydrate and ash, in chemical constants of the fat and in physical properties.

S-M-A* IS RECOMMENDED for normal, full term infants in the early weeks of life when a supplementary food is required for the breast-fed infant. It may be given to infants of any age whenever the mother's milk is unavailable, of poor quality or insufficient quantity.

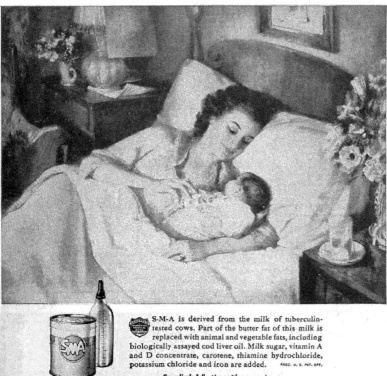

S-M-A is derived from the milk of tuberculin-tested cows. Part of the butter fat of this milk is replaced with animal and vegetable fats, including biologically assayed cod liver oil. Milk sugar, vitamin A and D concentrate, carotene, thiamine hydrochloride, potassium chloride and iron are added.   *REG. U. S. PAT. OFF.

Supplied: 1 lb. tins with measuring cup.

REG. U. S. PAT. OFF.

S. M. A. DIVISION · WYETH INCORPORATED · PHILADELPHIA 3, PA.

Report of the Committee on Cancer

The Cancer Committee of your Association has been very active during the past year. This Committee, with several illustrious lay people, has formed the Oklahoma Division of the American Cancer Society. Mr. L. C. Griffith was elected President; Everett S. Lain, M.D., Vice-President; Fred L. Dunn, Treasurer; and Ralph McGill, M.D., Secretary. Mrs. E. Lee Osbirn was also included in the organization due to her position as Commander of the Field Army for the State of Oklahoma. Mr. Hugh Payne was employed as Executive Director and an office was established in the Braniff Building in Oklahoma City. Policy, Procedure and Operation of Mobile Cancer Detection Clinics were adopted by the Cancer Medical Committee. For details in this regard, see the February issue of the Journal. A truck was purchased for the Mobile Detection Clinic. Equipment for this truck was purchased by money contributed by the Oklahoma Federation of Women's Clubs. We have had three clinics to date. Others are scheduled several weeks in advance.

The first clinic was held in Tonkawa with twenty-two patients seen and seven active cancer patients were found and referred to their local physicians. A medical society meeting was held that night at which three papers were given to the medical profession of Kay County in regard to cancer.

The second Clinic was held in Tulsa at which time both a white and colored clinic was held and one-hundred patients were examined and thirty-seven cancer patients were seen. Several were found who had not been accurately diagnosed. Mr. Ralph Talbot, member of the Board of Directors of the Oklahoma Division of the American Cancer Society invited the members of the Detection Clinic staff, and other interested parties, to a banquet at the Southern Hills County Club and the cancer problem was thoroughly discussed.

A third Clinic was held at Bartlesville at which thirty-seven patients were seen and seventeen active cancers were discovered. Papers were given before the Washington County Medical Society by Doctor A. S. Risser of Blackwell and Doctor C. E. Northcutt of Ponca City.

An attempt is being made to encourage every local medical unit in the state to invite this Clinic to their locality at least once a year and in this way the people of the state will have brought before them the tremendous importance of periodic examinations and made aware of the danger signs of cancer.

The newspaper editors of the state, through the Oklahoma Press Association, have formed a Press Relations Committee to work with the Executive Director in publicizing the Cancer Program and presenting to the people educational articles in relation to cancer. Educational articles consisting of an eight week's series are now appearing in practically all Oklahoma papers.

A study course has been arranged through the County Home Demonstration Agents on cancer for 25,000 Home Demonstration club members.

The Annual Drive for funds is to be held again this year in April. We have a very ambitious program outlined for the coming year. We have a full-time Executive Director. We have our Mobile Detection Clinic and a workable organization. We are working in direct conjunction with the State and local medical societies and we feel that we are deserving of the support of every member of the Society.

Respectfully submitted,

Paul B. Champlin, M.D., Chairman
Ralph McGill, M.D.
I. A. Nelson, M.D.
Joseph W. Kelso, M.D.
Wendell Long, M.D.
C. P. Bondurant, M.D.
E. H. Fite, M.D.
T. H. McCarley, M.D.
Roy E. Newman, M.D.
W. Floyd Keller, M.D.

Report of the Medical Advisory Committee to the Vocational Rehabilitation Division

The Medical Advisory Committee on Vocational Rehabilitation to the State Board of Education submits the following report of activities during the fiscal year 1945-46.

The Committee membership is composed of representatives from the Oklahoma State Hospital Association, the Oklahoma State Dental Society and the Oklahoma State Medical Association. With few exceptions the Committee has met regularly on the first Sunday of each month in Oklahoma City. Many problems in general have been discussed and policies interpreted and attempt has been made to answer two specific questions.

The first of these has to do with a fee schedule. The Vocational Rehabilitation Division has asked what fees shall be paid for various types of medical and surgical care. Since your Committee is attempting to represent the wishes of the physicians of the Oklahoma State Medical Association this question has been submitted to various physicians and surgeons throughout the state. Eight hundred eighty-six letters were written and three hundred sixty-five replies were received. From these answers we have compiled a list of medical and surgical procedures and fees recommended. In most instances the physician replying felt that the suggested fee schedule was reasonable. A few felt that certain fees were somewhat excessive and others felt that some of the fees were too low. With but two or three exceptions to the hundred of items considered the recommended fee has been in excess of the amount which the majority of physicians considered reasonable. This fee schedule in its present status has been referred to the Vocational Rehabilitation Division for their approval.

It is the considered opinion of the Medical Advisory Committee that it is our mission to interpret the wishes of physicians to the Vocational Rehabilitation Division and to inform the physicians of the activities and the policies of the Vocational Rehabilitation Division. We have assumed no authority and no responsibility except that of the advisory capacity to which we are appointed, the liaison function which we are asked to assume.

The second specific task of the Committee has been the establishment of a panel, a list of physicians and surgeons with special qualifications who may be asked to act as consultants and in some instances to perform special surgical procedures for which they have special training. In this panel are included the names of all physicians and surgeons who are members of the Oklahoma State Medical Association, who are certified by the several American Boards, and those who are fellows in the American College of Surgeons and the American College of Physicians. The further extension of this panel has been considered but no definite action has been taken except in the case of a few individuals. In each case where a physician has been named to a panel outside the regular channels as above outlined, this has been accomplished by referring to outstanding physicians who have been living in the community where this physician is practicing and well acquainted with him.

It has been our thought that it might be possible to so organize the various sections of the Association so that membership in those sections might likewise be used as a means of qualification to certain specialty functions. Thus far, however, we have been unable to find any precedent for this method or to arrive at any conclusion as to the manner in which it might be accomplished to your satisfaction. Although we would like to have the facility of a definite sectional organization and membership within the various sections, we conceive that this is not a function of the Advisory Committee and leave it for the consideration of the officers of the section. We ask that the various sections consider this suggestion but we have no plan to offer for its accomplishment at present.

Respectfully submitted,

Clinton Gallaher, M.D., Chairman

J. O. Asher, M.D.   Fred O. Pitney, D.D.S.
Bert F. Keltz, M.D.   Mr. Harry Smith
John Perry, M.D.

Report of the Committee on Study and Control Of Tuberculosis

The Committee for Study and Control of Tuberculosis makes recommendation as program for 1946, the following:

1. Urgently recommends taking measures to reactivate the 200 beds in the State Tuberculosis Sanatoria which have been closed during the war.

2. Persons receiving Aid for Dependent Children should be compelled to carry out recommended hospital treatment in order, to receive such benefit.

3. Provide adequate facilities for proper isolation of the tuberculosis inmates of the state mental hospitals, state prisons, corrective institutions and orphanages; and furthermore, recommends that on admission routine chest X-rays should be taken.

4. We favor the present policy of the State Health Department in conducting mass X-ray surveys throughout the state where such surveys are indicated.

5. Recommend that County Medical Societies have a committee on Tuberculosis for the purpose of stimulating a broader interest in Tuberculosis case finding.

6. More adequate facilities in the field of vocational rehabilitation for the Tuberculous.

The Committee further recommends that a copy of this program be sent to the Governor, and to the Chairman of the State Board of Public Affairs.

Respectfully submitted,

James F. McMurry, M.D., Chairman
E. M. Woodson, M.D.
C. W. Tedrowe, M.D.
F. P. Baker, M.D.
R. M. Shepard, M.D.

CREDIT SERVICE

330 American National Building

Oklahoma City, Oklahoma

(Operators of Medical-Dental Credit Bureau)

We offer a dignified and effective collection service for doctors and hospitals located anywhere in the State. Write for information.

28 YEARS
Experience In Credit and Collection Work

Robt. R. Sesline, Owner and Manager

SATISFACTORY RESULTS WITH Safety

Estrogen Therapy

Schieffelin BENZESTROL
(2, 4-di (p-hydroxyphenyl) -3-ethyl hexane)

Relief of menopausal and other symptoms arising from the hypo-ovarian state comes promptly and comfortably under the influence of Schieffelin BENZESTROL.

The exceptionally low incidence of untoward side effects, as well as the high degree of potency, merit the physician's confidence in Schieffelin BENZESTROL as a safe and satisfactory synthetic estrogen.

Literature and sample on request

Schieffelin BENZESTROL Tablets:
Potencies of 0.5, 1.0, 2.0 and 5.0 mg.
Bottles of 50, 100 and 1000.
Schieffelin BENZESTROL Solution:
Potency of 5.0 mg. per cc. in 10 cc.
Rubber Capped Multiple Dose Vials
Schieffelin BENZESTROL Vaginal Tablets:
Potency of 0.5 mg. Bottles of 100

Schieffelin & Co.
Pharmaceutical and Research Laboratories
20 COOPER SQUARE   NEW YORK 3, N. Y.

Honorary Membership Application

A. C. Lucas, M.D. ....Castle, Oklahoma

Okfuskee County Medical Society

Obituaries

W. E. Floyd, M.D.
1880-1946

On January 22, 1946, Dr. W. E. Floyd, Holdenville, passed away at his farm home near Lincoln, Arkansas, where he had gone for rest and recuperation from virus pneumonia with which he was stricken late in October.

Dr. Floyd was born in Shubuta, Mississippi in 1880. He took his premedic work at Tulane University in New Orleans but completed his medical education at Vanderbilt University School of Medicine, Nashville, receiving his degree in 1903. In 1904 he moved to Oklahoma, practicing in Coweta and Muskogee before going to Holdenville in 1926.

Throughout his long career as a physician and surgeon, Dr. Floyd was a crusader for public health improvement especially among children of school age. He gave liberally of his time and talents to public health improvement.

Surviving Dr. Floyd are his wife, Mrs. Adelicia Floyd, a son, John E. Floyd of Houston, Texas, his mother, Mrs. Octavia Floyd of Holdenville and his grandson, John E. Floyd Jr., Houston, Texas.

C. M. Fullenwider, M.D.
1878-1946

Dr. C. M. Fullenwider, eye, ear, nose and throat specialist in Muskogee, died on January 26 from a heart ailment.

Dr. Fullenwider was born in Mechanicsburg, Ill. but lived in Kansas where he began his education as an electrical engineer. After two years he decided upon a medical career and enrolled in the University of Kansas

for a pre-medical course. He received his medical degree from Rush Medical School in Chicago in 1903. Dr. Fullenwider then moved to Muskogee where he married. Shortly afterward he went to Vienna where he studied under leading European specialists in his field. He returned to open his practice in Muskogee in 1910.

Prominent in Masonic bodies for more than a quarter of a century, Dr. Fullenwider was a member of Oriental lodge No. 403, Royal Arch Masons, Muskogee Commandery, Knights Templar and Bedouin Shrine Temple. Dr. Fullenwider was a member of the Muskogee County Medical Society, the Oklahoma State Medical Association and the American Medical Association.

Surviving Dr. Fullenwider are his wife, two daughters and one son.

A. L. Davenport, M.D.
1873-1945

Dr. A. L. Davenport, Holdenville, died on December 10 following a brief illness. He had practiced in Holdenville for forty years and was a member of the Hughes County Medical Society whose members were honorary bearers. Dr. Davenport had been active in the Society since its inception and was also active in the State Association.

Survivors include his wife, six daughters, ten grandchildren and one great-grandchild.

The Riggs Optical Company of Chicago, through their Manager Mr. J. E. Bohle, presented the School of Medicine with a slit lamp for the eye clinic. Dr. Lamb acknowledged the gift on behalf of the Oklahoma University of Medicine. The School of Medicine is most appreciative of the valuable contribution from the Riggs Optical Company.

DIAGNOSTIC CLINIC OF INTERNAL MEDICINE AND ALLERGY

Phiilp M. McNeill, M. D. ,F. A. C. P.

General Diagnosis

CONSULTATION BY APPOINTMENT

Special Attention to Cardiac, Pulmonary and Allergic Diseases

Electrocardiograph, X-Ray, Laboratory
and Complete Allergic Surveys Available.

1107 Medical Arts Bldg.
Oklahoma City, Okla.   Phone 2-0277

the norm and standard...

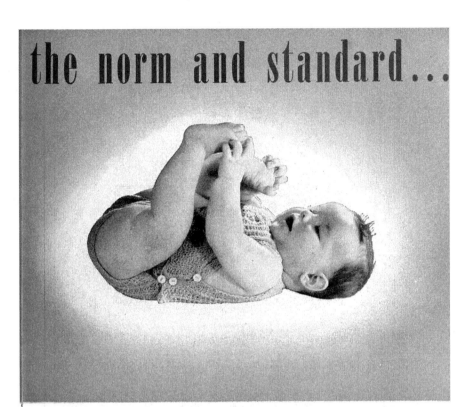

by which all infant antirachitic agents are measured...

... is cod liver oil, the natural vitamin D of which is unsurpassed as a means of prevention or treatment of rickets.

This *ne plus ultra* of antirachitics, together with vitamin A as provided by time-honored cod liver oil, is supplied in three stable convenient, palatable dosage forms by White's Cod Liver Oil Concentrate ... at a cost-to-patient of *less than a* *penny a day* for prophylactic antirachitic infant dosage.

In *Liquid* form for drop dosage to infants; *Tablets* for growing children or adults; *Capsules* where larger dosage may be required. Council Accepted. Ethically promoted—not advertised to the laity.

White Laboratories, Inc., Pharmaceutical Manufacturers, Newark 7, N. J.

White's COD LIVER OIL CONCENTRATE—LIQUID, TABLETS, CAPSULES

From here ... to here

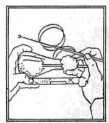 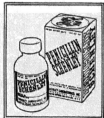

CONTROL
... ALL THE WAY

FROM the initial culture to the end product, an extraordinarily comprehensive program of control characterizes the production of Penicillin Schenley.

At every single step, the most extreme care is exer- cised, to insure for Penicillin Schenley a maximum degree of purity...potency... freedom-from-pyrogens.

This system of control is your assurance that you can specify Penicillin Schenley with the greatest confidence.

SCHENLEY LABORATORIES, INC.
Executive Offices: 350 Fifth Avenue, N. Y. C.
Producers of

PENICILLIN SCHENLEY

Your Local Distributor for **PENICILLIN** SCHENLEY *is:*

Caviness-Melton Surgical Company
OKLAHOMA CITY

TO ALL OKLAHOMA PHYSICIANS

You Are Cordially Invited To Visit The MAICO Exhibit — Space No. 22 At The State Meeting May 1, 2 & 3. There Will Be Displayed

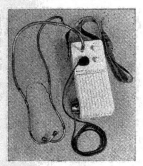

PURE-TONE AUDIOMETERS
AMPLIFIED STETHOSCOPES
INDIVIDUAL HEARING AIDS

If you cannot attend the State Meeting please write and one of our Technicians will call on you by appointment.

MAICO HEARING SERVICE

ROSS McDOWELL, MANAGER
EXCLUSIVE OKLAHOMA DISTRIBUTERS
627 1ST NATIONAL BLDG., OKLAHOMA CITY
PHONE 3-0911

AVAILABLE SURPLUS PROPERTY
INSTRUCTIONS FOR PUBLIC HEALTH CLAIMANTS

Surplus Property Administration Regulation 14 provides for a 40 per cent discount on sales to public health claimants. The discount is allowed from the "fair value" (defined as the lowest prevailing at any trade level at the time of the transaction). The following groups of claimants are eligible:

1. State, county and local health and sanitation departments and units (including publicly owned and operated services such as water works, sewerage systems, garbage and refuse disposal units).
2. Hospitals operated by (non-Federal) governmental agencies.
3. Nonprofit hospitals, clinics and public health research organizations.
4. Schools of nursing, medicine, public health, dentistry and pharmacy.
5. Miscellaneous nonprofit groups organize primarily to promote the public health.

If you are in doubt as to your status you should check with the Special Representative, Public Health Service, Office of Surplus Property Utilization, 609 Neil P. Anderson Building, Ft. Worth 2, Texas. To obtain a list of available consumer goods, contact the Agency Manager, War Assets Corporation, 609 Neil P. Anderson Building, Ft. Worth 2, Texas. For information and lists of capital goods, get in touch with the Public Health Service, Office of Surplus Property Utilization, Cotton Exhange Building, Oklahoma City 2, Oklahoma.

"Consumer goods" includes finished products ordinarily used by individuals or commercial establishments, as well as construction machinery, farm machinery, and motor vehicles. "Capital goods" includes items used in industry and manufacture such as machinery, machine tools, raw materials (except agricultural), semi-fabricated items, together with transportation and communication property.

To buy "consumer goods" listed as available by the disposal agency, the claimant should use his usual purchase order form in quadruplicate drawn to the office of the disposal agency listing the property, stating on the order that "Funds are available for the purchase of these items at fair value less 40 per cent". In an emergency the disposal agency will accept a "letter of intent", indicating that the applicant is willing to purchase items requested, to be followed by a formal purchase order.

For the purchase of capital goods, the claimant's usual purchase order form in quadruplicate may be used as outlined above. However, the disposal agency will accept a "letter of intent" in lieu of the purchase order form. It is not essential that capital goods requested be contained in a published list of available property.

Application for discount in duplicate to accompany the order should be addressed to the Office of Surplus Property Utilization, United States Public Health Service and should comprise the following parts:

1. A request that a 40 per cent discount be approved for the accompanying purchase order.
2. Statement: "The applicant represents and warrants that: It is an (instrumentality)* or a (nonprofit institution)*, that the property is required for its own use and to fill its own existing need for carrying on medical, public health, or sanitation activity; that the property will not be resold within 3 years of the date of purchase without written consent of the disposal agency."
3. A statement to show how and to what extent the volume or quality of service will be increased and why the area served needs such an increase.
4. Signature and title of a responsible official.

If on the basis of eligibility and need, the discount is authorized, the Public Health Service will send the order directly to the disposal agency to be filled. If it should be advisable for the buyer to make an inspection of property and present the approved order in person at time of sale, the approved order will be returned to the claimant at his request.

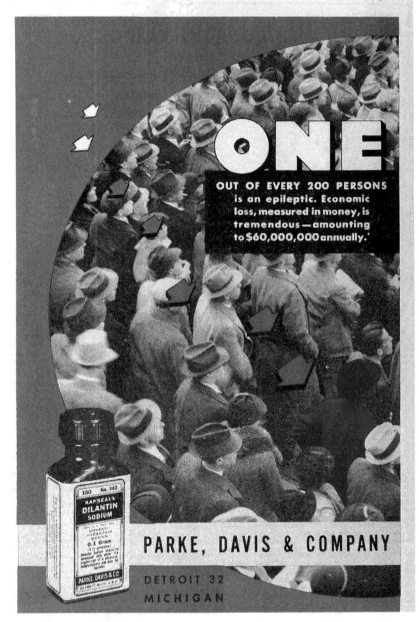

ONE OUT OF EVERY 200 PERSONS is an epileptic. Economic loss, measured in money, is tremendous — amounting to $60,000,000 annually.

KAPSEALS DILANTIN SODIUM

PARKE, DAVIS & COMPANY

DETROIT 32 MICHIGAN

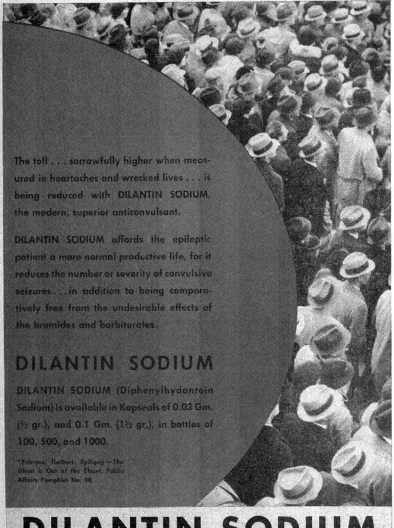

The toll . . . sorrowfully higher when measured in heartaches and wrecked lives . . . is
being reduced with DILANTIN SODIUM,
the modern, superior anticonvulsant.

DILANTIN SODIUM affords the epileptic
patient a more normal productive life, for it
reduces the number or severity of convulsive
seizures. . . in addition to being comparatively free from the undesirable effects of
the bromides and barbiturates.

DILANTIN SODIUM

DILANTIN SODIUM (Diphenylhydantoin
Sodium) is available in Kapseals of 0.03 Gm.
(½ gr.), and 0.1 Gm. (1½ gr.), in bottles of
100, 500, and 1000.

*Yahraes, Herbert: Epilepsy—The
Ghost Is Out of the Closet, Public
Affairs Pamphlet No. 98.

DILANTIN SODIUM

DELEGATES AND ALTERNATES SELECTED FOR ANNUAL MEETING

In compliance with the By-Laws of the Oklahoma State Medical Association, the following listed delegates and alternates have been certified to the Executive Office as representatives of their respective counties at the Annual Meeting.

Credential cards have been mailed to the delegates and alternates, who in turn must present their credentials to the Credentials Committee prior to the first meeting of the House of Delegates on Tuesday evening, April 30.

County	Delegate	Alternate
Alfalfa	L. R. Kirby, Cherokee	Jack F. Parsons, Cherokee
Atoka-Coal	J. S. Fulton, Atoka	W. W. Cotton, Atoka
	J. J. Hipes, Coalgate	J. B. Clark, Coalgate
Beckham	P. J. Devanney, Sayre	J. E. Levick, Elk City
Blaine	W. F. Bohlman, Watonga	
Bryan	John A. Haynie, Durant	O. J. Colwick, Durant
Caddo	Preston E. Wright, Anadarko	P. H. Anderson, Anadarko
Canadian	J. T. Phelps, El Reno	M. E. Phelps, El Reno
Carter	F. W. Boadway, Ardmore	J. Hoyle Carlock, Ardmore
	H. A. Higgins, Ardmore	R. C. Sullivan, Ardmore
Cherokee	R. K. McIntosh, Jr., Tahlequah	H. A. Masters, Tahlequah
Choctaw	Edgar A. Johnson, Hugo	Fred D. Switzer, Hugo
Cleveland	James O. Hood, Norman	Phil Haddock, Norman
Comanche	F. M. Adams, Vinita	J. M. McMillan, Vinita
Cotton	G. W. Baker, Walters	Mollie Seism, Walters
Craig		
Creek	P. K. Lewis, Sapulpa	J. E. Hollis, Bristow
*Custer	McLain Rogers, Clinton	Gordon Williams, Weatherford
	Ellis Lamb, Clinton	J. D. Wood, Weatherford
Garfield	Julian Feild, Enid	
	P. W. Hopkins, Enid	
Garvin	Carl T. Steen, Pauls Valley	Galvin L. Johnson, Pauls Valley
Grady	H. M. McClure, Chickasha	
Grant	F. P. Robinson, Nash	I. V. Hardy, Medford
Greer	J. B. Hollis, Mangum	R. W. Lewis, Granite
Harmon	R. H. Lynch, Hollis	W. G. Husband, Hollis
Haskell	N. K. Williams, McCurtain	W. S. Carson, Keota
Hughes	Casper A. Hicks, Holdenville	Paul Kernek, Holdenville
Jackson	J. R. Reid, Altus	E. A. Abernathy, Altus
Jefferson	W. T. Andreskowski, Ryan	
Kay	Dewey Mathews, Tonkawa	L. H. Becker, Blackwell
	C. W. Arrendell, Ponca City	E. C. Mohler, Ponca City
Kingfisher	F. C. Lattimore, Kingfisher	A. O. Meredith, Kingfisher
Kiowa	J. P. Braun, Hobart	
LeFlore	F. P. Baker, Talihina	
Lincoln	Ned Burleson, Prague	Carl H. Bailey, Stroud
Logan	L. H. Ritzhaupt, Guthrie	James Petty, Guthrie
Marshall		
Mayes		
McClain	R. L. Royster, Purcell	
McCurtain	W. W. Williams, Idabel	E. A. Kelleam, Wright City
McIntosh	F. R. First, Jr., Checotah	F. R. First, Sr., Checotah
Muskogee-Sequoyah-Wagoner	R. N. Holcombe, Muskogee	George L. Kaiser, Muskogee
	Finis W. Ewing, Muskogee	L. S. McAlister, Muskogee
	H. K. Riddle, Coweta	John H. Plunkett, Wagoner
	John A. Morrow, Sallisaw	N. H. Newlin, Sallisaw
Noble	C. H. Cooke, Perry	J. W. Francis, Perry
Okfuskee	A. S. Melton, Okemah	M. L. Whitney, Okemah
Oklahoma	L. C. McHenry, Oklahoma City	J. F. Kuhn, Oklahoma City
	W. Floyd Keller, Oklahoma City	Paul Vickers, Oklahoma City
	R. Q. Goodwin, Oklahoma City	J. P. Wolff, Oklahoma City
	R. H. Akin, Oklahoma City	Meredith Appleton, Oklahoma City
	C. M. O'Leary, Oklahoma City	W. E. Eastland, Oklahoma City
	John H. Lamb, Oklahoma City	F. Redding Hood, Oklahoma City
	James R. Reed, Oklahoma City	Ben H. Nicholson, Oklahoma City
	John F. Burton, Oklahoma City	Bert E. Mulvey, Oklahoma City

J. E. HANGER, Inc.

ARTIFICIAL LIMBS, BRACES, AND CRUTCHES

Phone: 2-8500

612 N. Hudson

L. T. Lewis, Mgr.

BRANCHES AND AGENCIES IN PRINCIPAL CITIES　Oklahoma City 3, Okla.

	Onis G. Hazel, Oklahoma City	T. O. Coston, Oklahoma City
	W. W. Rucks, Jr., Oklahoma City	Bert F. Keltz, Oklahoma City
	George H. Kimball, Oklahoma City	O. A. Watson, Oklahoma City
	Lee K. Emenhiser, Oklahoma City	Jim M. Taylor, Oklahoma City
Okmulgee	J. C. Matheney, Okmulgee	E. D. Rodda, Okmulgee
	G. Y. McKinney, Henryetta	S. B. Leslie, Okmulgee
Osage	Roscoe Walker, Pawhuska	M. Karasck, Shidler
Ottawa	Matt Connell, Miami	C. F. Walker, Grove
	W. Jackson Sayles, Miami	L. P. Hetherington, Miami
Pawnee	H. B. Spalding, Ralston	M. L. Saddoris, Cleveland
Payne	Haskell Smith, Stillwater	L. R. Wilhite, Perkins
*Pittsburg	Elbert H. Shuller, McAlester	C. E. Lively, McAlester
	L. S. Willour, McAlester	F. J. Baum, McAlester
*Pontotoc-Murray	Ollie McBride, Ada	Sam A. McKeel, Ada
	Alfred R. Sugg, Ada	F. E. Sadler, Sulphur
	W. P. Rudell, Sulphur	M. M. Webster, Ada
Pottawatomie	W. M. Gallaher, Shawnee	C. C. Young, Shawnee
	E. E. Rice, Shawnee	G. S. Baxter, Shawnee
Pushmataha	E. S. Patterson, Antlers	J. S. Lawson, Clayton
Rogers	W. A. Howard, Chelsea	P. S. Anderson, Claremore
Seminole	Claude S. Chambers, Seminole	A. N. Deaton, Wewoka
Stephens	W. K. Walker, Marlow	C. N. Talley, Marlow
Texas	Daniel S. Lee, Guymon	L. G. Blackmer, Hooker
Tillman	J. D. Osborn, Frederick	T. F. Spurgeon, Frederick
Tulsa	Ralph A. McGill, Tulsa	Horace H. Porter, Tulsa
	Marvin D. Henley, Tulsa	W. A. Walker, Tulsa
	John C. Perry, Tulsa	Earl M. Lusk, Tulsa
	L. C. Northrup, Tulsa	M. O. Hart, Tulsa
	Walter S. Larrabee, Tulsa	R. Q. Atchley, Tulsa
	H. B. Stewart, Tulsa	W. J. Trainor, Tulsa
	M. V. Stanley, Tulsa	C. A. Pigford, Tulsa
	H. A. Ruprecht, Tulsa	W. R. Turnbow, Tulsa
	W. A. Showman, Tulsa	D. O. Smith, Tulsa
Washington-Nowata	S. A. Lang, Nowata	S. P. Roberts, Nowata
	H. C. Weber, Bartlesville	E. E. Beechwood, Bartlesville
	L. B. Word, Bartlesville	
Washita	Aubrey E. Stowers, Sentinel	A. H. Bungardt, Cordell
Woods	D. B. Ensor, Alva	John F. Simon, Alva
Woodward	John L. Day, Supply	Myron England, Woodward
	O. C. Newman, Shattuck	Roy Newman, Shattuck
	Hardin Walker, Buffalo	F. Z. Winchell, Buffalo

*—Final statistics not available at this printing.

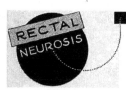

YOUNG'S Rectal Dilators

Rectal disturbance is never trivial. Young's Rectal Dilators afford mechanical correction for bowel sluggishness when due to tight sphincter muscles. Effective elimination relieves nervous tension, permitting normal nerve reaction. Sold only by prescription. Obtainable at your surgical supply house; available for patients at ethical drug stores. Adults and children's sizes, in sets of 4 dilators. Write for Brochure.

F. E. YOUNG & CO. 424 E. 75TH STREET, CHICAGO 19, ILLINOIS

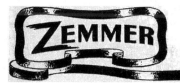

Prescribe or Dispense

Zemmer Pharmaceuticals

A complete line of laboratory controlled
ethical pharmaceuticals.   OK 4-46

Chemists to the Medical Profession for 44 years.

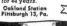

The Zemmer Company   Oakland Station
Pittsburgh 13, Pa.

Annual Audit Report

March 21, 1946

V. C. Tisdal, M.D., President
Oklahoma State Medical Association
210 Plaza Court
Oklahoma City, Oklahoma
Dear Sir:
    We have completed the audit of the financial records of:

THE OKLAHOMA STATE MEDICAL ASSOCIATION
OKLAHOMA CITY, OKLAHOMA

for the period from January 1, 1945. to December 31, 1945, and submit herewith the following Exhibits:
    EXHIBIT "1"—Balance Sheet
    EXHIBIT "2"—Statement of Cash Receipts and Disbursements
    EXHIBIT "3"—Operating Statement
    EXHIBIT "4"—Bank Reconciliation
We wish to thank you for this audit, and if we can be of further service, please feel free to call upon us.
Respectfully Submitted,
H. E. COLE COMPANY
By: H. E. Cole

OKLAHOMA STATE MEDICAL ASSOCIATION
Oklahoma City, Oklahoma

EXHIBIT "1"
BALANCE SHEET
December 31, 1945

	Total	Membership Fund	Journal Fund	Medical Defense Fund	Annual Meeting	State Fair Fund
ASSETS						
Petty Cash	$ 11.13	$ 11.13	$............	$............	$............	$............
Liberty National Bank	7,248.37	3,919.01	2,411.55	619.34	236.60	61.87
United States Defense Bonds	2,220.00	2,220.00				
United States Savings Bonds	4,000.00	4,000.00				
United States Treasury Bonds	6,178.88	6,178.88				
TOTAL ASSETS	$19,658.38	$16,329.02	$ 2,411.55	$ 619.34	$ 236.60	$ 61.87
LIABILITIES						
Withholding Tax Reserve	$ .50	$ .50	$............	$............	$............	$............
Operating Reserve	19,657.88	16,328.52	2,411.55	619.34	236.60	61.87
TOTAL LIABILITIES	$19 658.38	$16,329.02	$ 2,411.55	$ 619.34	$ 236.60	$ 61.87

OKLAHOMA STATE MEDICAL ASSOCIATION
Oklahoma City, Oklahoma

EXHIBIT "2"
STATEMENT OF CASH RECEIPTS AND DISBURSEMENTS
January 1, 1945 to December 31, 1945

	Total	Membership Fund	Journal Fund	Medical Defense Fund	Annual Meeting	State Fair Fund
Cash Balance, January 1, 1945	$11,407.49	$ 9,433.51	$ 846.17	$ 619.34	$ 446.60	$ 61.87
Petty Cash Balance, January 1, 1945	11.09	11.09				
RECEIPTS						
Membership Dues — 1945	13,781.00	13,781.00				
Journal Advertising and Subscriptions	14,139.35		14,139.35			
Government Bond Interest	197.50	197.50				
Annual Meeting Income	1,425.00	690.00			735.00	
Miscellaneous Income	4.91	3.50	1.41			
Year Book Income	74.00		74.00			
Total Cash to be Accounted for	$41,040.34	$24,116.60	$15,060.93	$ 619.34	$ 1,181.60	$ 61.87
DISBURSEMENTS						
Expenses for 1945	$31,781.34	$18,186.96	$12,649.38	$............	$ 945.00	$............
United States Bonds — Series "G"	2,000.00	2,000.00				
	$33,781.34	$20,186.96	$12,649.38		$ 945.00	
Balance, December 31, 1945	$ 7,259.00	$ 3,929.64	$ 2,411.55	$ 619.34	$ 236.60	$ 61.87
Withholding Tax Reserve	.50	.50				
	$ 7,259.50	$ 3,930.14	$ 2,411.55	$ 619.34	$ 236.60	$ 61.87
Bank Balance 12-31-45	$ 7,248.37	$ 3,919.01	$ 2,411.55	$ 619.34	$ 236.60	$ 61.87
Petty Cash on Hand	11.13	11.13				
	$ 7,259.50	$ 3,930.14	$ 2,411.55	$ 619.34	$ 236.60	$ 61.87

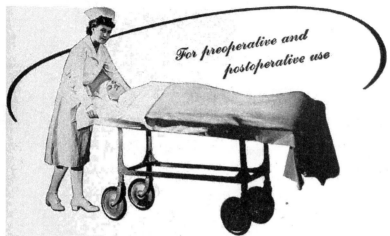

For preoperative and postoperative use

Demerol hydrochloride, administered from thirty to ninety minutes pre-operatively, relieves much of the surgical patient's apprehension and reduces the amount of anesthetic agent required to obtain a given depth of narcosis. The average preoperative dose for adults is 100 mg. injected intramuscularly, which may be combined with scopolamine or a barbiturate to assure amnesia.

Compared with morphine, Demerol causes considerably less nausea and vomiting, and the danger of respiratory depression is greatly reduced. Unlike morphine, Demerol does not interfere with the cough reflex or the reflexes and size of the pupil. It does not cause constipation, and urinary retention is less than with morphine.

Postoperatively, Demerol is a reliable analgesic in the majority of cases, regardless of the type of surgery or the severity of pain. Patients in the older age group, in particular, respond most favorably to this drug. The average postoperative dose for adults varies from 50 to 100 mg., administered by intramuscular injection or by mouth.

Demerol

Trademark Reg. U. S. Pat. Off. & Canada

H Y D R O C H L O R I D E

Brand of Meperidine Hydrochloride (Isonipecaine)

Synthetic ANALGESIC • SPASMOLYTIC • SEDATIVE

Available for *injection*, ampuls of 2 cc. (100 mg.), in boxes of 6, 25 and 100; also vials of 30 cc. (50 mg. per cubic centimeter). For *oral use* in tablets of 50 mg., bottles of 25, 100 and 1000.

Subject to regulations of the Federal Bureau of Narcotics

W R I T E   F O R   D E T A I L E D   L I T E R A T U R E

Winthrop CHEMICAL COMPANY, INC.

Pharmaceuticals of merit for the physician   •   New York 13, N. Y.   •   Windsor, Ont.

OKLAHOMA STATE MEDICAL ASSOCIATION
Oklahoma City, Oklahoma

EXHIBIT "3"

OPERATING STATEMENT
1945

	Total	Membership Fund	Journal Fund	Medical Defense Fund	Annual Meeting	State Fair Fund
REVENUES						
Membership Dues — 1945	$ 3,781.00	$13,781.00	$............	$............	$............	$............
Journal Advertising and Subscriptions	14,139.35	....	14,139.35	....	....	....
Government Bond Interest	197.50	197.50	....	....	....	....
Annual Meeting Income	1,425.00	690.00	....	....	735.00	....
Miscellaneous Income	4.91	3.50	1.41	....	....	....
Year Book Income	74.00	....	74.00	....	....	....
TOTAL REVENUES	$29,217.76	$14,672.00	$14,214.76	$............	$ 735.00	$............
EXPENSES						
Salaries	$10,051.14	$ 4,551.14	$ 5,500.00	$............	$............	$............
Telephone and Telegraph	605.15	605.15	....	....	....	....
Postage	747.41	559.43	187.98	....	....	....
Rent	600.00	300.00	300.00	....	....	....
Stationery and Printing	373.04	351.15	21.89	....	....	....
Office Supplies	557.66	557.66	....	....	....	....
Traveling	720.14	720.14	....	....	....	....
Journal Printing and Mailing	6,227.46	....	6,227.46	....	....	....
Journal Engraving	164.35	....	164.35	....	....	....
Auditing and Legal	477.50	377.50	100.00	....	....	....
Express	11.38	11.38	....	....	....	....
Post Graduate Committee	2,000.00	2,000.00	....	....	....	....
Sundry	316.88	296.38	20.50	....	....	....
Office Equipment	648.13	648.13	....	....	....	....
Chamber of Commerce	25.00	25.00	....	....	....	....
Council and Committee Expense	310.34	310.34	....	....	....	....
Flowers	67.69	67.69	....	....	....	....
Annual Secretaries Conference	199.72	199.72	....	....	....	....
Books and Magazines for Library	5.00	5.00	....	....	....	....
Annual Meeting Expense	1,375.32	1,375.32	....	....	....	....
Surety Bond	56.25	56.25	....	....	....	....
Annual Meeting Refunds	945.00	....	....	....	945.00	....
Press Clipping Service	127.20	....	127.20	....	....	....
Pictures of Past Presidents	2.55	2.55	....	....	....	....
Refunds of Dues	12.00	12.00	....	....	....	....
Year Book Expense	1,474.72	1,474.72	....	....	....	....
Public Policy Committee	2,389.93	2,389.93	....	....	....	....
American Society for Cancer Control	750.00	750.00	....	....	....	....
A.M.A. Delegates Expense	503.34	503.34	....	....	....	....
Typewriter Repair	37.04	37.04	....	....	....	....
TOTAL EXPENSES	$31,781.34	$18,186.96	$12,649.38	$............	$ 945.00	$............
TOTAL REVENUE OVER EXPENSES	—$2,159.58	—$3,514.96	$ 1,565.38	$............	—$ 210.00	$............

UNSCENTED COSMETICS

FOR THE ALLERGIC PATIENT

AR-EX Cosmetics are the only complete line of unscented cosmetics regularly stocked by pharmacies. To be certain that your perfume sensitive patients do not get scented cosmetics, prescribe AR-EX Unscented Cosmetics. SEND FOR FREE FORMULARY.

AR-EX

FREE FORMULARY

DR._____
ADDRESS_____
CITY_____
STATE_____

AR-EX COSMETICS, INC.,   1036 W. VAN BUREN ST.,   CHICAGO 7, ILL.

THE WILLIE CLINIC AND HOSPITAL

A private hospital for the diagnosis, study and treatment of all types of neurological and psychiatric cases. Equipped to give all forms of recognized therapy, including hyperpyrexia, insulin and metrazol treatments, when indicated. Consultation by appointment.

JAMES A. WILLIE, B.A., M.D.
Attending Neuro-psychiatrist

218 N. W. 7th St.—Okla. City, Okla.   Telephones: 2-6944 and 3-6071

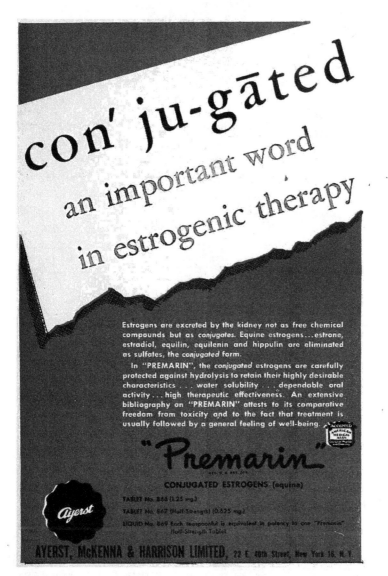

con' ju-gāted

an important word

in estrogenic therapy

Estrogens are excreted by the kidney not as free chemical compounds but as conjugates. Equine estrogens...estrone, estradiol, equilin, equilenin and hippulin are eliminated as sulfates, the conjugated form.

In "PREMARIN", the conjugated estrogens are carefully protected against hydrolysis to retain their highly desirable characteristics . . . water solubility . . . dependable oral activity . . . high therapeutic effectiveness. An extensive bibliography on "PREMARIN" attests to its comparative freedom from toxicity and to the fact that treatment is usually followed by a general feeling of well-being.

"Premarin"

CONJUGATED ESTROGENS (equina)

TABLET No. 866 (1.25 mg.)
TABLET No. 867 (Half-Strength) (0.625 mg.)
LIQUID No. 869 Each teaspoonful is equivalent in potency to one "Premarin" Half-Strength Tablet

AYERST, McKENNA & HARRISON LIMITED, 22 E. 40th Street, New York 16, N. Y.

OKLAHOMA STATE MEDICAL ASSOCIATION

Oklahoma City, Oklahoma

EXHIBIT "4"

BANK RECONCILIATION

December 31, 1945

LIBERTY NATIONAL BANK

MEMBERSHIP FUND

Balance per Bank Statement, December 24, 1945		$ 3,892.64
Add: Deposit, December 29, 1945		570.00
		$ 4,462.64
Outstanding Checks		
Voucher No. 1802 R. H. Graham	$190.40	
Voucher No. 1806 R. H. Graham	62.33	
Voucher No. 1807 Mary Jo Taylor	12.90	
Voucher No. 1808 Jane Firrell Tucker	28.20	
Voucher No. 1809 Jane Firrell Tucker	10.00	
Voucher No. 1810 Mary Jo Taylor	10.00	
Voucher No. 1811 Dick Graham	101.09	
Voucher No. 1812 Collector of Internal Revenue	128.30	
Voucher No. 1859 Addressograph-Multigraph	.41	
		543.63
Balance per Books		$ 3,919.01
JOURNAL FUND		
Balance per Bank Statement, December 29, 1945		$ 2,821.00
Add: Deposit, December 29, 1945		79.45
		$ 2,900.45
Outstanding Checks		
Voucher No. 1803 R. H. Graham	$190.40	
Voucher No. 1804 Lewis J. Moorman	88.50	
Voucher No. 1813 Collector of Internal Revenue	210.00	
		488.90
Balance per Books		$ 2,411.55
ANNUAL MEETING FUND		
Balance per Bank Statement, December 31, 1945		$ 236.60
Balance per Books		$ 236.60
MEDICAL DEFENSE FUND		
Balance per Bank Statement, December 31, 1945		$ 619.34
Balance per Books		$ 619.34
STATE FAIR FUND		
Balance per Bank Statement, December 31, 1945		$ 61.87
Balance per Books		$ 61.87
TOTAL MONEY ON DEPOSIT PER BOOKS		$ 7,248.37

Classified Advertisements

FOR SALE: Surgical instruments and general office equipment. May be seen at Anadarko. Mrs. J. W. Henry, 408 W. Central, Anadarko, Oklahoma.

FOR SALE: Complete office setup including examining tables, sterilizers, surgical E.N.T., a few bone instruments and an instrument cabinet. Nearly all equipment in A-1 condition. Will sell reasonable. Address Box R c/o Journal, Oklahoma State Medical Association, 210 Plaza Court, Oklahoma City 3, Oklahoma.

Announcement

The Wm. T. Stover Co., Inc., of Oklahoma announce the opening of their store located at 610 South Boston, Tulsa, Oklahoma. The Stover Company will handle hospital and physicians' equipment and supplies including Keleket X-Ray Equipment and will maintain a complete service department. Mr. Lamar Massie is manager of the Tulsa store.

Program

FIFTY-THIRD ANNUAL SESSION OF THE OKLAHOMA

STATE MEDICAL ASSOCIATION

OKLAHOMA CITY, MAY 1, 2 AND 3, 1946

GREETINGS FROM THE OKLAHOMA COUNTY MEDICAL SOCIETY

This year it is the privilege of the Oklahoma County Medical Society to be host at the Fifty-Third Annual Meeting of the Oklahoma State Medical Association. In 1945, due to the ruling of the Office of Defense Transportation, the Fifty-Third Meeting was not held. Although it has been the policy, in the past, to alternate the meeting each year between Oklahoma City and Tulsa, and Oklahoma City was to be host in 1945, it was the decision of the House of Delegates that Oklahoma City be given the privilege of being host in 1946.

Attendance for the Meeting this year is expected to exceed that of past meetings. The excellent program is justification of the expenditure of time of the busy physician. The Oklahoma County Medical Society is also pleased to provide, through enjoyable social events, a much-needed relaxation.

You are invited to attend a Buffet Dinner at 6:30 P.M. on Tuesday night, April 30, the night before the opening of the Scientific Program. The Dinner will be in the Skirvin Hotel and will be complimentary. This event will be for members of the Association, out-of-state physicians and military personnel and is presented by the Oklahoma County Medical Society.

The Ladies Auxiliary of the Oklahoma County Medical Society has planned a full program for the wives of attending physicians. Make your plans to bring your wife with you.

We hope that you can make arrangements to attend the Fifty-Third Annual Meeting and assure you that you will find a well-filled, interesting program.

W. Floyd Keller, M.D., President
Oklahoma County Medical Society

General Information

HEADQUARTERS

Skirvin Tower Hotel

ROOM RESERVATIONS

Adequate housing facilities at the leading hotels have been arranged. However, it will not be possible to house everyone in the Skirvin-Skirvin Tower Hotels. It is suggested that all those planning on attending the Annual Meeting make their hotel reservations either direct with the hotel of their choice or through the Executive Office of the Association, 210 Plaza Court, Oklahoma City 3, Oklahoma, at the earliest possible date.

In making your reservations, please be certain that you advise the date of your arrival, the approximate time you expect to register into the hotel and the date you will leave. Room reservations are canceled at 7:00 P.M. unless a later arrival time is specified and guaranteed.

REGISTRATION

Lobby, Skirvin Tower Hotel

Registration will be in the Lobby of the Skirvin Tower Hotel, in front of the elevators. All physicians except those from outside the state, visiting guests, and those on military assignment, must present membership cards for 1946 before registering. Dues will not be accepted at the Registration Desk except from County Secretaries.

Registration will be from 10:00 A.M. to 4:00 P.M., Tuesday, April 30 and will open at 8:00 A.M., Wednesday, May 1.

GENERAL SESSIONS

The General Sessions will be held at 2:00 P.M. on Wednesday, May 1; Thursday, May 2; and Friday, May 3, in Room No. 2 in the Silver Glade Room, Third Floor, Skirvin Tower Hotel.

SECTION MEETINGS

All Section Meetings will be held on Wednesday, Thursday and Friday, May 1, 2, and 3, beginning at 9 00 A.M. for morning sessions. All meeting rooms will be in the Silver Glade Room in the Skirvin Tower Hotel.

SYMPOSIUM

On Thursday evening at 8:00 P.M. in the Rose Room of the Skirvin Hotel there will be a Symposium on "Penicillin" in which all guest speakers will participate.

HOUSE OF DELEGATES

The House of Delegates will meet on Tuesday, April 30, the day preceding the opening of the Scientific Program in order that the business may be completed in time for the Delegates to be able to enjoy the Scientific Program. All Meetings of the House of Delegates will be in Parlor A, Mezzanine of the Skirvin Tower Hotel, the first meeting to be held at 2.00 P.M. and the second immediately after the Buffet Supper. Other meetings at call of the Speaker of the House.

COUNCIL

The Council will convene at 9:30 A.M., Tuesday, April 30, in the Green Room of the Skirvin Htoel.

RESOLUTIONS

Resolutions to be submitted to the House of Delegates should be prepared in triplicate and presented at the first meeting of the House of Delegates.

WOMAN'S AUXILIARY

Registration will be on the Mezzanine Floor of the Skirvin Tower Hotel. The completed Program will be found elsewhere in this Program.

TECHNICAL EXHIBITS

The exhibits will be displayed in the Silver Glade Room of the Skirvin Tower Hotel.

SOCIAL EVENTS

Oklahoma County Medical Society Buffet Dinner

The complimentary Buffet Dinner of the Oklahoma County Medical Society will be Tuesday evening, April 30, at 6:30 P.M. at the Skirvin Hotel. This event will be for members of the Association, out-of-state physicians and military personnel.

Oklahoma University Medical Alumni Dinner

The Dinner will be at the Skirvin Hotel Wednesday, May 1, in the Rose Room, 6:30 P.M. The complete program appears elsewhere in this Program. Tickets will be on sale at the Registration Desk.

Roundtable Luncheons

On Wednesday, Thursday and Friday at 12 15 P.M., Roundtable Luncheons will be held in the Empire Room of the Skirvin Hotel. Those participating in the roundtable discussions will be those sections participating in the Scientific Program for the day. Tickets will be on sale at the registration desk.

President's Inaugural Dinner Dance

The President's Inaugural Dinner Dance will be held in the Venetian Room of the Skirvin Hotel at 7:30 P.M., Friday, May 3. Governor Robert S. Kerr will be guest speaker. Ticket reservations must be made at the time of registering.

Woman's Auxiliary

OKLAHOMA STATE MEDICAL ASSOCIATION
State Auxiliary Officers

President	Secretary
Mrs. J. W. Rogers	Mrs. Walter S. Larrabee
Tulsa	Tulsa
President-Elect	Treasurer
Mrs. Ollie McBride	Mrs. Frank J. Nelson
Ada	Tulsa
Vice-President	Historian
Mrs. Charles Rayburn	Mrs. Walker Morledge
Norman	Oklahoma City

Parliamentarian
Mrs. C. C. Young
Shawnee

CONVENTION PROGRAM
Mrs. C. P. Bondurant, Oklahoma City, Convention Chairman

WEDNESDAY, MAY 1, 1946

9 00 A.M. Registration ....Mezzanine, Skirvin Tower Hotel
7:00 P.M. Buffet Supper. Pre-convention Executive Board meeting in the home of Mrs. C. P. Bondurant, 253 N. W. 35th St., Oklahoma City. Hostesses; Mrs. Gerald Rogers, Mrs. Gregory Stanbro, Mrs. Floyd Keller, Mrs. Walker Morledge, Mrs. Neil Woodward and Mrs. C. P. Bondurant.

THURSDAY, MAY 2, 1946

9:00 A.M. Registration ....Mezzanine, Skirvin Tower Hotel
10:00 A.M. Annual Meeting ....Library, Y. W. C. A.
1:00 P.M. Luncheon—Empire Room, Y. W. C. A., $1.50. All visiting ladies invited. Tickets may be secured at the Registration Desk.
3:00 P.M. Post-convention Executive Board Meeting ....Library, Y. W. C. A.

Officers of
Oklahoma State Medical Association

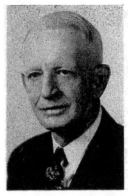

L. C. Kuyrkendall, McAlester
President-Elect

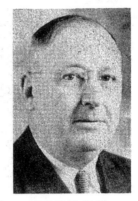

V. C. Tisdal, Elk City
President

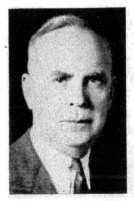

Lewis J. Moorman, Oklahoma City
Secretary-Treasurer

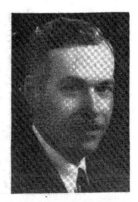

George H. Garrison, Oklahoma City
Speaker of the House of Delegates

Scientific Program

All Sections will meet in the Silver Glade Room, Skirvin Tower Hotel

GENERAL SESSIONS

The General Sessions will meet in the Silver Glade Room, Skirvin Tower Hotel

SECTIONS

Section on Public Health—Room No. 1, Thursday, May 2, 9:00 A.M.-12:00.
Section on Eye, Ear, Nose & Throat—Room No. 1, Wednesday, May 1, 9:00 A.M.-12:00; Room No. 1, Friday, May 3, 9:00 A.M.-12:00.
Section on Urology and Syphilology—Room No. 3, Wednesday, May 1, 9:00 A.M.-12:00.
Section on Pediatrics—Room No. 3, Friday, May 3, 9:00 A.M.-12:00.
Section on Obstetrics & Gynecology—Room No. 2, Wednesday, May 1, 9:00 A.M.-12:00; Room No. 2, Thursday, May 2, 9:00 A.M.-12:00.
Section on General Medicine—Room No. 4, Friday, May 3, 9:00 A.M.-12:00.
Section on Dermatology & Radiology—Room No. 4, Wednesday, May 1, 9:00 A.M.-12:00; Room No. 4, Thursday, May 2, 9:00 A.M.-12:00.
Section on General Surgery—Room No. 5, Thursday, May 2, 9:00 A.M.-12:00; Room No. 5 Friday, May 3, 9:00 A.M.-12:00.
Section on Neurology, Psychiatry and Endocrinology—Room No. 6, Thursday, May 2, 9:00 A.M.-12:00.

Scientific Program

OKLAHOMA STATE MEDICAL ASSOCIATION

May 1, 2 and 3, 1946

Silver Glade Room, Skirvin Tower Hotel
Oklahoma City

WEDNESDAY, MAY 1, 1946

General Chairman, V. C. Tisdal, M.D., Elk City

ROOM NO. 1
Silver Glade Room, Skirvin Tower

SECTION ON EYE, EAR, NOSE & THROAT
Clinton Gallaher, M.D., Shawnee, Chairman
James P. Luton, M.D., Oklahoma City, Secretary

9:00   "The Mastoid, An Anatomic and Clinical Study"—J. D. Singleton, M.D., Dallas, Texas.
9:30   "Nasal Fractures, New and Old"—O. Alton Watson, M.D., Oklahoma City.
9:50   "Fenestration"—Wm. L. Bonham, M.D., Oklahoma City.
10:20 "Adenoids in Adults"—R. R. Coates, M.D., Oklahoma City.
10:50 "Endocrine Complaints in the E.E.N.T. Area"—E. H. Coachman, M.D., Muskogee.
11:10 General Discussion.

ROOM NO. 2
Silver Glade Room, Skirvin Tower

SECTION ON OBSTETRICS AND GYNECOLOGY
Roy Emanuel, M.D., Chickasha, Chairman
Ed N. Smith, M.D., Oklahoma City, Secretary

9:00   "Cervicitis"—Kenneth Wilson, M.D., Oklahoma City.
9:30   Discussion—Henry G. Bennett, M.D., Oklahoma City.
9:40   "Low Spinal Anesthesia in Obstetrics"—Phil Risser, M.D., Blackwell.
10:20 Discussion—E. G. Wolff, M.D., Tulsa.
10:30 "R. H. Factor in Obstetrics"—Gordon Livingston, M.D., Cordell.
11:00 Discussion—F. R. Hassler, M.D., Oklahoma City.

Guest Speakers

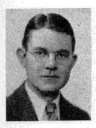

Paul Padget, M.D., Baltimore, Maryland. Assistant Professor of Medicine, Johns Hopkins University School of Medicine; Assistant Visiting Physician, John Hopkins Hospital.

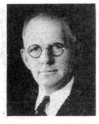

Russell L. Haden, M.D., F.A.C.P., Internist, Cleveland, Ohio. Chief of the Medical Division of the Cleveland Clinic.

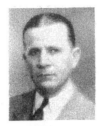

J. Dudley Singleton, M.D., Otolaryngologist, Dallas, Texas. Associate Professor of Otolaryngology at Southwestern Medical College.

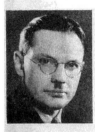

Michael L. Mason, M.D., F.A.C.S., Surgeon, Chicago, Ill. Associate Professor of Surgery, Northwestern University Medical School.

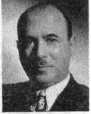

M. Edward Davis, M.D., F.A.C.S., Obstetrician and Gynecologist, Chicago, Ill. Professor of Obstetrics and Gynecology, University of Chicago. Obstetrician and Gynecologist, Chicago Lying-In Hospital.

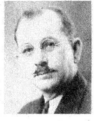

George B. Fletcher, M.D., F.A.C.P., Neurologist, Hot Springs, Arkansas.

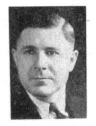

Herbert J. Rinkel, M.D., F.A.C.P., Allergist, Kansas City, Missouri.

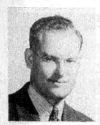

Harry Hauser, M.D., Radiologist, Cleveland Ohio. Assistant Professor of Radiology, Western Reserve University Medical School and Director of Radiology University Hospitals of Cleveland and City Hospital.

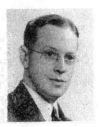

H. Rommel Hildreth, M.D., Ophthalmologist, St. Louis, Mo. Assistant Professor of Ophthalmology at Washington University.

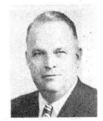

Honorable Robert S. Kerr, Governor of Oklahoma.

A. I. Folsom, M.D., Urologist, Dallas, Texas. Professor of Urology, Baylor University College of Medicine, Dallas, Texas. (Photograph of Dr. Folsom not available).

ROOM NO. 3
Silver Glade Room, Skirvin Tower

SECTION ON UROLOGY AND SYPHILOLOGY
J. W. Rogers, M.D., Tulsa, Chairman
W. F. Lewis, M.D., Lawton, Secretary

9:00 "Syphilis in Private Practice"—J. W. Rogers, M.D., Tulsa.
9:20 "Institutional Treatment of Early Syphilis"—A. B. Colyar, M.D., Oklahoma City (By Invitation).
9:40 Discussion—A. M. Young, III, M.D., Oklahoma City.
9:50 "Sulfonamide Anuria"—Don Branham, M.D., Oklahoma City.
10:10 Discussion—C. B. Taylor, M.D., Oklahoma City.
10:20 "Traumatic Urology"—Berget Blockson, M.D., Tulsa.
10:40 Discussion—Henry S. Browne, M.D., Tulsa.
10:50 "Ureteral Strictures"—W. F. Lewis, M.D., Lawton.
11:10 Discussion—Robert H. Aikin, M.D., Oklahoma City.
11:20 "Unusual Pyelograms"—Joseph Fulcher, M.D., Tulsa.
11:40 General Discussion—A. I. Folsom, M.D., Dallas, Texas.

ROOM NO. 4
Silver Glade Room, Skirvin Tower

SECTION ON DERMATOLOGY AND RADIOLOGY
John Heatley, M.D., Oklahoma City, Chairman
Peter E. Russo, M.D., Oklahoma City, Secretary

9:00 "Typhoid Vaccine for Induction of Fever in Neurosyphilis"—Phyllis Jones, M.D., Oklahoma City and John Lamb, M.D., Oklahoma City.
9:30 Discussion—Marque O. Nelson, M.D., Tulsa.
9:50 "Vesicular Diseases of the Hand"—Onis Hazel, M.D., Oklahoma City.
10:20 Discussion—Carl Brundage, M.D., Oklahoma City.
10:30 "Unusual Manifestation of Erythema Multiforme"—James Stevenson, M.D., Tulsa.
11:00 Discussion.
11:15 Election of Officers.

ROOM NO. 6
Silver Glade Room, Skirvin Tower

SECTION ON NEUROLOGY, PSYCHIATRY AND ENDOCRINOLOGY
John L. Day, M.D., Supply, Chairman
Arnold H. Ungerman, M.D., Tulsa, Secretary

9:00 "Modern Treatment of Epilepsy"—Carl Steen, M.D., Pauls Valley.
9:30 Discussion—C. R. Rayburn, M.D., Norman.
9:40 "Myanthenia Gravis"—T. R. Turner, M.D., Tulsa.
10:10 Discussion—J. Moore Campbell, M.D., Oklahoma City.
10:20 "Fatigue States Associated with Endocrine Disorders"—Henry H. Turner, M.D., Oklahoma City.
10:50 Discussion—Wendell Long, M.D., Oklahoma City.
11:00 "Electroencephalograph Studies in Neuropsychiatric Diagnosis" — Charles Leonard, M.D., Oklahoma City.
11:30 Discussion—Jess Herrman, M.D., Oklahoma City.

Empire Room, Skirvin Hotel

12:15 Roundtable Luncheon—Section on Eye, Ear, Nose & Throat; Section on Obstetrics and Gynecology; Section on Urology and Syphilology; Section on Derlatology and Radiology; Section on Neurology, Psychiatry and Endocrinology.

GENERAL SESSION
Room No. 2, Silver Glade Room

2:00 "Paralysis Agitant"—George B. Fletcher, M.D., Hot Springs, Ark.
2:30 General Discussion.
2:40 "Acute Otitis Media: It's Management by the General Practitioner and Pediatrician" —J. D. Singleton, M.D., Dallas, Texas.
3:10 General Discussion.
3:20 "Minor Urological Procedures of Value to the General Practitioner and General Surgeon"—A. I. Folsom, M.D., Dallas, Texas.
3:50 General Discussion.

GENERAL ASSEMBLY
Room No. 2, Silver Glade Room

4:00   Oklahoma Physicians Service—John F. Burton, M.D., Oklahoma City, Vice-President of the Oklahoma Physicians Service.. . . . .

ENTERTAINMENT PROGRAM
Annual Spring Meeting of the Oklahoma University Medical School Alumni
Rose Room, Skirvin Hotel
6:30 P.M.
Lee K. Emenhiser, M.D., President, Oklahoma City, Presiding
John H. Lamb, M.D., Oklahoma City, Secretary

Business Meeting
Class of 1916—Introduction by Wann Langston, M.D., Oklahoma City.
Class of 1926—Introduction by George Kimball, M.D., Oklahoma City.
Class of 1936—Introduction by Harry Deupree, M.D., Oklahoma City.
Class of 1946—Introduction by David Lowery, M.D., Oklahoma City.
In Honor of Lea A. Riely, M.D., Emeritus Professor of Clinical Medicine—Phillip McNeil, M.D., Oklahoma City.
In Honor of William Taylor, M.D., Emeritus Professor of Pediatrics—Carroll Pounders, M.D., Oklahoma City.
Introduction of Guest Speaker—Dean Wann Langston, M.D., Oklahoma City.
"Research—Its Place in the Advancement of the Medical Sciences"—M. Edward Davis, M.D., Chicago, Ill.

THURSDAY, MAY 2, 1946
General Chairman, L. C. Kuyrkendall, M.D., McAlester
ROOM NO. 1
Silver Glade Room, Skirvin Tower
SECTION ON PUBLIC HEALTH
Charles W. Haygood, M.D., Shawnee, Chairman
Gertrude Neilson, M.D., Oklahoma City, Secretary

9:00   "Penicillin in the Treatment of Syphilis"—Paul Padget, M.D., Baltimore, Md.
9:30   "The RH Factor"—H. F. Marsh, M.D., Oklahoma City (By Invitation).
9:50   Discussion—Carroll Pounders, M.D., Oklahoma City.
10:00   "Recent Development in the Diagnosis and Treatment of Tuberculosis"—David M. Gould, M.D., Dallas, Texas. (By Invitation).
10:30   "Present Status of Immunization Procedures"—J. S. Hackler, M.D., Oklahoma City.
10:50   Discussion—F. R. Hassler, M.D., Oklahoma City.
11:00   General Discussion.
11:20   Election of Officers.

ROOM NO. 2
Silver Glade Room, Skirvin Tower
SECTION ON OBSTETRICS AND GYNECOLOGY
Roy Emanuel, M.D., Chickasha, Chairman
Ed N. Smith, M.D., Oklahoma City, Secretary

9:00   "The Obstetrician's Responsibility to the Newborn with Particular Reference to Asphyxia"—Roy Emanuel, M.D., Chickasha.
9:30   "The Overweight Patient with Special Reference to Use of Dexedrine Sulfate"—J. Wm. Finch, M.D., Hobart.
10:00   "The Heart in Pregnancy"—F. Redding Hood, M.D., Oklahoma City.
10:30   Discussion—J. B. Eskridge, Jr., M.D., Oklahoma City.
10:40   "Intravenous Clotting As Applies to Obstetrics"—Reynold Patzer, M.D., Oklahoma City (By Invitation).
11:10   "Management of Uterine Fibroids"—E. O. Johnson, M.D., Tulsa.
11:40   General Discussion—M. Edward Davis, M.D., Chicago, Ill.

ROOM NO. 4
Silver Glade Room, Skirvin Tower
SECTION ON DERMATOLOGY AND RADIOLOGY
John W. Heatley, M.D., Oklahoma City, Chairman
Peter E. Russo, M.D., Oklahoma City, Secretary

9:00   "Pioneers in the Use of X-Ray in Oklahoma"—John Heatley, M.D., and Peter E. Russo, M.D., Oklahoma City.
9:30   "X-Ray in Evacuation Hospitals"—E. D. Greenberger, M.D., McAlester.
10:00   "Pulmonary Complications of Hodgkins Disease and the Treatment"—Leland F. Shryrock, M.D., Oklahoma City.

10:30 "Value of A-P Lordotic Film of the Chest"—John R. Danstrum, M.D., Oklahoma City
         (By Invitation).
11:00 General Discussion—Harry Hauser, M.D., Cleveland, Ohio.

ROOM NO. 5
Silver Glade Room, Skirvin Tower

SECTION ON GENERAL SURGERY
Ralph A. McGill, M.D., Tulsa, Chairman
Neil Woodward, M.D., Oklahoma City, Secretary

9:00   "Injuries of the Hand, with Particular Reference to Indications for Primary and Sec-
         ondary Nerve and Tendon Repair"—Michael L. Mason, M.D., Chicago, Ill.
9:30   "Surgical Lesions of the Intestines in Children"—D. L. Garrett, M.D., Tulsa.
10:00 Discussion—E. Eugene Rice, M.D., Shawnee.
10:15 "Pre and Post Operative Surgical Care"—A. B. Smith, M.D., Stillwater.
10:45 Discussion—A. S. Risser, M.D., Blackwell.
11:00 "Carcinoma of the Corpus Uteri"—Ralph McGill, M.D., Tulsa.
11:30 Election of Officers.

ROOM NO. 6

SECTION ON NEUROLOGY, PSYCHIATRY AND ENDOCRINOLOGY
John L. Day, M.D., Supply, Chairman
Arnold H. Ungerman, M.D., Tulsa, Secretary

9:00   "Post-War Psychiatry in Oklahoma"—John L. Day, M.D., Supply.
9:30   "Prefrontal Lobotomy"—Coyne Campbell, M.D., Oklahoma City.
10:00 Discussion—Harry Wilkins, M.D., Oklahoma City.
10:15 "Practical Treatment of the Neuroses"—Moorman Prosser, M.D., Oklahoma City.
10:45 Discussion—Hugh Galbraith, M.D., Oklahoma City.
11:00 General Discussion—George B. Fletcher, M.D., Hot Springs, Ark.
11:30 Election of Officers.

Empire Room, Skirvin Hotel
12:15 Roundtable Luncheon—Section on Public Health; Section on Obstetrics and Gynecolo-
         gy; Section on Dermatology and Radiology; Section on General Surgery, and Sec-
         tion on Neurology, Psychiatry and Endocrinology.

GENERAL ASSEMBLY
Room No. 2, Silver Glade Room
4:00   "Veterans Administration's Program for Care of Military Personnel"—Dick Graham,
         Oklahoma City.

SYMPOSIUM

Rose Room, Skirvin Hotel
Walker Morledge, M.D., Oklahoma City
Moderator
8:00 P.M.   Symposium on Penicillin—all guest speakers participating.

FRIDAY, MAY 3, 1946
General Chairman, Ralph McGill, M.D., Tulsa

ROOM NO. 1
Silver Glade Room, Skirvin Tower Hotel

SECTION ON EYE, EAR, NOSE & THROAT
Clinton Gallaher, M.D., Shawnee, Chairman

James P. Luton, M.D., Oklahoma City, Secretary
9:00   "Chronic Rhinitis"—R. W. Rucker, M.D., Bartlesville.
9:30   "Sympathetic Ophthalmology with Case Reports"—J. R. Reed, M.D., Oklahoma City.
10:00 "Army Squints"—W. W. Sanger, M.D., Oklahoma City.
10:30 "Myopia"—C. A. Royer, M.D., Alva.
11:00 "Staphylococcic Ulcer of the Cornea"—W. W. Mall, M.D., Ponca City.
11:30 "Ophthalmology"—H. Rommel Hildreth, M.D., St. Louis, Mo.

ROOM NO. 3

Silver Glade Room, Skirvin Tower Hotel

SECTION ON PEDIATRICS

G. R. Russell, M.D., Tulsa, Chairman

9:00   "Brucelosis in Children"—G. R. Russell, M.D., Tulsa.
9:20   "Epidemic Diarrhea in Children"—Harold Buchner, M.D., Oklahoma City (By Invitation).
9:40   Discussion—J. B. Snow, M.D., Oklahoma City.
9:50   "Infectious Mononucleosis"—W. H. Kaeiser, M.D., McAlester.
10:10   Discussion—T. H. McCarley, M.D., McAlester.
10:20   "Perennial Nasal Allergy in Children"—C. W. Arrendell, M.D., Ponca City.
10:40   Discussion—Carroll M. Pounders, M.D., Oklahoma City.
10:50   "Choice of Carbohydrates Used in Artificial Feeding of Infants"—C. J. Alexander, M.D., Clinton.
11:10   Discussion—George H. Garrison, M.D., Oklahoma City.
11:20   General Discussion—Herbert J. Rinkel, M.D., Kansas City, Mo.
11:40   Election of Officers.

ROOM NO. 4

Silver Glade Room, Skirvin Tower Hotel

SECTION ON GENERAL MEDICINE

Samuel R. Goodman, M.D., Tulsa, Chairman

Walker Morledge, M.D., Oklahoma City, Secretary

9:00   "Survey of the Pneumonias"—Samuel R. Goodman, M.D., Tulsa.
9:20   "Rheumatic Fever"—Wm. Bailey, M.D., Oklahoma City.
9:40   "Gall Bladder Patient After Surgery"—Fred T. Perry, M.D., Okeene.
10:00   "Periarteritis Nodosa; Recent Advances in the Pathogenesis and Therapeutic Implications"—E. Rankin Denny, M.D., Tulsa.
10:20   Discussion—Wm. K. Ishmael, M.D., Oklahoma City.
10:30   "Small Town Practice"—Carl Bailey, M.D., Stroud.
10:50   "Penicillin in Endocarditis"—R. Q. Goodwin, M.D., Oklahoma City.
11:10   "The Diagnosis and Treatment of Cardiac Emergencies" — Felix M. Parke, M.D., Tulsa.
11:30   Discussion—Homer A. Ruprecht, M.D., Tulsa.
11:40   General Discussion—Russel Haden M.D., Cleveland, Ohio.

ROOM NO. 5

Silver Glade Room, Skirvin Tower Hotel

SECTION ON GENERAL SURGERY

H. M. McClure, M.D., Chickasha, Vice-Chairman

Neil Woodward, M.D., Oklahoma City, Secretary

9:00   "Kronlein Technique in Gastric Resection of Carcinoma of the Stomach"—Andre B. Carney, M.D., Tulsa.
9:30   Discussion—Joe Parker, M.D., Oklahoma City.
9:45   "Surgery in the Treatment of Diseases of the Stomach and Duodenum"—C. C. Fulton, M.D., Oklahoma City.
10:15   Discussion—Maynard Jacobs, M.D., Oklahoma City.
10:30   "Treatment of Pilonidal Cysts"—Byron Cordonnier, M.D., Enid.
10:50   Discussion—Malcolm Phelps, M.D., El Reno.
11:00   "Amputation of the Lower Extremities in Peripheral Vascular Disease"—Pat Fite, M.D., Muskogee.
11:20   Discussion—Captain Chester K. Mengel, M.C., Muskogee.
11:30   General Discussion—Michael Mason, M.D., Chicago, Ill.

Empire Room, Skirvin Hotel

12:15   Roundtable Luncheon—Section on Eye, Ear, Nose & Throat; Section on Pediatrics; Section on General Medicine; Section on General Surgery.

GENERAL SESSION
ROOM NO. 2
Silver Glade Room, Skirvin Tower Hotel

2:00 "Treatment of Pernicious Anemia"—Russell Haden, M.D., Cleveland, Ohio.
2:30 General Discussion.
2:40 "Pulmonary Sarcoidosis"—Harry Hauser, M.D., Cleveland, Ohio.
3:10 General Discussion.
3:20 "Public Health Aspects in the Treatment of Syphilis"—Paul Padget, M.D., Baltimore, Md.
3:50 General Discussion.

GENERAL ASSEMBLY
Room No. 2
Silver Glade Room, Skirvin Tower Hotel

4:00 Mock Senate Hearing on Wagner-Murray-Dingell Bill—James Stevenson, M.D., Tulsa and Dick Graham, Oklahoma City.

ENTERTAINMENT PROGRAM
7:30 P.M.

PRESIDENT'S INAUGURAL DINNER DANCE
Venetian Room
Skirvin Hotel, Oklahoma City
J. H. Robinson, M.D., General Chairman, Presiding

PROGRAM

Introduction of Guests ....J. H. Robinson, M.D., Oklahoma City
Address of Welcome—W. Floyd Keller, M.D., President, Oklahoma County Medical Society.
Response and Introduction of President-Elect—V. C. Tisdal, M.D., Elk City, President, Oklahoma State Medical Association.
President's Response—and Introduction of President's Guest Speaker — L. C. Kuyrkendall, M.D., McAlester.

Guest Speaker's Address
Robert S. Kerr, Governor of Oklahoma.
(Tickets must be purchased at time of registration.)

MAKE IT A POINT TO VISIT THE TECHNICAL EXHIBITS
AT THE 53RD ANNUAL MEETING

The following companies will exhibit at the 53rd Annual Meeting of the Oklahoma State Medical Association. Plans have been made for well arranged, helpful booths. Please make it a point to visit your technical exhibits and see what the various companies are offering the profession.

Eli Lilly & Company
The Zemmer Company
Mead Johnson Company
E. R. Squibb and Sons
Holland-Rantos Company, Inc.
Credit Service
Burroughs Wellcome & Co., Inc.
Sharp and Dohme
Philip Morris and Co.
G. D. Searle & Co.
Producers Creamery
Ortho Pharmaceutical Corp.
The Maltine Company
The C. V. Mosby Company
The Coca-Cola Company
Merkle X-Ray Company
Caviness-Melton Surgical Supply Co.
J. A. Majors Company
Maico Hearing Aid Company
The Smith-Dorsey Company
The Mid-West Surgical Supply Company, Inc.
A. S. Aloe Company

White Laboratories, Inc.
The Warren-Teed Products Co.
Lederle Laboratories, Inc.
Frederick Stearns & Company
Physicians Service
C. B. Fleet Company, Inc.
U. S. Vitamin Corporation
The Borden Company
The Gilbert X-Ray Company
Greb X-Ray Company
Cameron Heartometer Company
Pet Milk Sales Corp.
Parke-Davis Company
General Electric X-Ray Corp.
F. E. Young & Company
United Medical Equipment Co.
Lea & Febiger Publishing Company
Wm. T. Stover Company, Inc.
J. B. Lippincott Co.
The Ediphone Company
Roach Drug Company
Connie Prescription Shop

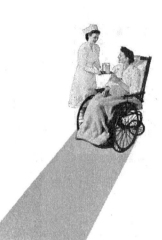

"SMOOTHAGE" FOR THE CONVALESCENT

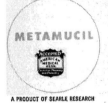

METAMUCIL

A PRODUCT OF SEARLE RESEARCH

*By promoting normal peristalsis
without irritating the delicate mucosa,
Metamucil is particularly desirable for treating
the constipation of hospital patients.*

*Metamucil provides "smoothage" . . . a modern concept
for the treatment of constipation. It does not
interfere with digestion or absorb oil-soluble vitamins.
It is rapidly miscible, pleasantly palatable.*

*Metamucil is the highly-purified, nonirritating extract
of the seed of the psyllium, Plantago ovata (50%),
combined with dextrose (50%). In 1-lb., 8-oz. and 4-oz. containers.*

Metamucil is the registered trade-mark of G. D. Searle & Co.

SEARLE RESEARCH IN THE SERVICE OF MEDICINE.

OFFICERS OF COUNTY SOCIETIES, 1946

COUNTY	PRESIDENT	SECRETARY	MEETING TIME
Alfalfa	W. G. Dinnlugton, Cherokee	L. T. Lancaster, Cherokee	Last Tues. each Second Month
Atoka-Coal	J. B. Clark, Coalgate	J. S. Fulton, Atoka	
Beckham	P. J. DeVanney, Sayre	J. E. Levick, Elk City	Second Tuesday
Blaine	W. F. Bohlman, Watonga	Virginia Curtain, Watonga	Third Thursday
Bryan	W. K. Haynie, Durant	Jonah Nichols, Durant	Second Tuesday
Caddo	Preston E. Wright, Anadarko	Edward T. Cook, Jr., Anadarko	
Canadian	G. L. Goodman, Yukon	W. P. Lawton, El Reno	Subject to call
Carter	J. Hobson Venzey, Ardmore	H. A. Higgins, Ardmore	Second Tuesday
Cherokee	P. H. Medearis, Tahlequah	R. K. McIntosh, Jr., Tahlequah	First Tuesday
Choctaw	Floyd L. Waters, Hugo	O. R. Gregg, Hugo	
Cleveland	James O. Hood, Norman	Phil Haddock, Norman	Thursday nights
Comanche			
Cotton	G. W. Baker, Walters	Mollie Seism, Walters	Third Friday
Craig	Lloyd H. McPike, Vinita	J. M. McMillan, Vinita	
Creek	W. P. Longmire, Sapulpa	Philip Joseph, Sapulpa	Second Tuesday
Custer	Ross Deputy, Clinton	A. W. Paulson, Clinton	Third Thursday
Garfield	Bruce Hinson, Enid	John R. Walker, Enid	Fourth Thursday
Garvin	M. E. Robberson, Jr., Wynnewood	John R. Callaway, Pauls Valley	Wednesday before Third Thursday
Grady	Roy Emanuel, Chickasha	Rebecca H. Mason, Chickasha	Third Thursday
Grant	I. V. Hardy, Medford	F. P. Robinson, Pond Creek	
Greer	J. B. Lansden, Granite	J. B. Hollis, Mangum	
Harmon	W. G. Husband, Hollis	R. H. Lynch, Hollis	First Wednesday
Haskell	Wm. S. Carson, Keotah	N. K. Williams, McCurtain	
Hughes	Victor W. Pryor, Holdenville	L. A. S. Johnson, Holdenville	First Friday
Jackson	E. W. Mabry, Altus	J. P. Irby, Altus	Last Monday
Jefferson	F. M. Edwards, Ringling	J. A. Dillard, Waurika	Second Monday
Kay	L. G. Neal, Ponca City	J. C. Wagner, Ponca City	Second Thursday
Kingfisher	John W. Pendleton, Kingfisher	H. Violet Sturgeon, Hennessey	
Kiowa	Wm. Bernell, Hobart	J. Wm. Finch, Hobart	
LeFlore	S. D. Bevill, Poteau	Rush L. Wright, Poteau	
Lincoln	J. S. Rollins, Prague	Ned Burleson, Prague	First Wednesday
Logan	James Petty, Guthrie	J. E. Souter, Guthrie	Last Tuesday
Marshall			
Mayes	L. C. White	V. D. Herrington, Pryor	
McClain	S. C. Davis, Blanchard	W. C. McCurdy, Purcell	
McCurtain	J. T. Moreland, Idabel	R. H. Sherrill, Broken bow	Fourth Tuesday
McIntosh	F. R. First, Checotah	W. A. Tolleson, Eufaula	First Thursday
Muskogee-Sequoyah			
Wagoner	R. N. Holcombe, Muskogee	William N. Weaver, Muskogee	First Tuesday
Noble	A. M. Evans, Perry	Jesse W. Driver, Perry	
Okfuskee	W. P. Jenkins, Okemah	M. L. Whitney, Okemah	Second Monday
Oklahoma	W. F. Keller, Okla. City		Fourth Tuesday
Okmulgee	F. S. Watson, Okmulgee	C. E. Smith, Okmulgee	Second Monday
Osage	Paul H. Hemphill, Pawhuska	Vincent Mazzarella, Hominy	Third Monday
Ottawa	C. F. Walker, Grove	W. Jackson Sayles, Miami	Second Thursday
Pawnee	H. B. Spalding, Ralston	R. L. Browning, Pawnee	
Payne	F. Keith Oehlschlager, Yale	C. W. Moore, Stillwater	Third Thursday
Pittsburg	Millard L. Henry, McAlester	Edward D. Greenberger, McAlester	Third Friday
Pontotoc-Murray	John Morey, Ada	R. H. Mayes, Ada	First Wednesday
Pottawatomie	F. P. Newlin, Shawnee	Clinton Gallaher, Shawnee	First and Third Saturday
Pushmataha	John S. Lawson, Clayton	B. M. Huckabay, Antler	
Rogers	W. A. Howard, Chelsea	P. S. Anderson, Claremore	Third Wednesday
Seminole	Clifton Felts, Seminole	Mack I. Shanholz, Seminole	Third Wednesday
Stephens	Evert King, Duncan	Fred L. Patterson, Duncan	
Texas	Daniel S. Lee, Guymon	E. L. Buford, Guymon	
Tillman	H. A. Calvert, Frederick	O. G. Bacon, Frederick	
Tulsa	John C. Perry, Tulsa	John E. McDonald, Tulsa	Second and Fourth Monday
Washington-Nowata	Ralph W. Rucker, Bartlesville	L. B. Word, Bartlesville	Second Wednesday
Washita	L. G. Livingston, Cordell	Roy W. Anderson, Clinton	
Woods	John F. Simon, Alva	O. E. Templin, Alva	Last Tuesday Odd Months
Woodward	T. C. Leachman, Woodward	C. W. Tedrowe, Woodward	Second Thursday

THE JOURNAL

of the

OKLAHOMA STATE MEDICAL ASSOCIATION

| VOLUME XXXIX | OKLAHOMA CITY, OKLAHOMA, MAY, 1946 | NUMBER 5 |

Surgical Treatment of Bronchietasis

J. MOORE CAMPRELL, M.D.

OKLAHOMA CITY, OKLAHOMA

Bronchiectasis is present in from two to three per cent of all autopsies performed, and its incidence in patients as a whole is estimated variously from two to seven per cent. This occurrence rate should be recognized in both private and clinical practice, and every patient with persistent coughing, either continuously or intermittently, should be suspected of having bronchiectasis. If the sputum is purulent in type, the diagnosis may often be strongly suspected. When pus in the respiratory tract is investigated carefully, most patients with the disease can be diagnosed, treated and relieved before the stage of foul smelling sputum, clubbed fingers, and the general pathologic changes that occur with any chronic septic disease.

Anatomic and pathologic diagnosis can be extremely accurate, and hinges upon the findings of x-rays of the chest, the bronchogram, sputum examinations for acid-fast bacilli, and bronchoscopic examination. The bronchoscope is particularly valuable because direct visualization of the tracheo-bronchial tree will sometimes explain the reason for unusual types of bronchial dilitation, particularly when a bronchial tumor or foreign body complicates the picture.

Radiologic findings on routine chest films may be negligible, and a bronchogram may be necessitated by the clinical aspect of the cough alone: if it is persistent, the quantity of the sputum is large, and if the systemic effect of the pulmonary process is profound. Minimal x-ray markings are apt to be quite significant, and the cardiac silhouette may obscure the principal involvement of the left lower lobe. If the pulmonary markings at the base of the lungs are prominent, if stelectatic areas are suspected, or if there is any sign of slowly resolving broncho-pneumonia, the x-ray studies of the patient's lungs are incomplete without a bronchogram[1].

The presence of tubercle bacilli is unusual in patients with typical bronchiectasis, but their presence does not rule out the disease. Tuberculous infections can be superimposed upon bronchiectatic lesions, and conversely, an acid-fast process may lead to secondary bronchial dilitation. Bronchographiic and bronchoscopic procedures are not necessarily contra-indicated in pulmonary tuberculosis, and the results of these studies may determine the proper management of the patient. Hemoptosis frequently occurs in bronchiectasis, and for that reason blood-streaked sputum may of itself, be an idication for a bronchogram. This is especially true if no acid-fast bacilli are found after careful search in repeated sputum specimens.

A bronchogram will often show bronchiectasis in children and adults who have been subject to repeated colds, recurrent "influenzal attacks", or chronic "bronchitis". Purulent sinusitis is the rule, and persons with sinusitis and a chronic cough, especially in the younger age group, should always be suspected of having pathologic bronchial ectasia.

THE BRONCHOGRAM

By direct introduction of Lipiodol into the lumen of the trachea and directing its course by gravity into dependent bronchi, every portion of the tracheo-bronchial tree can be visualized with surprising detail under the fluoroscope and on x-ray film. A simple technique consists of giving the patient a moderate dose of barbituric acid type of sedative and a grain or half-grain of codeine by mouth to suppress the cough reflex. Thirty minutes or more should elapse, and then a small bore catheter is passed through the nose, down to the opening of the larynx. The patient holds his tongue forward to assist him suppress swallowing and coughing, using a piece of gauze to prevent it from slipping from his fingers. A 20 cc. syringe filled with Lipiodol that has been warmed to 85 or 90 degrees Farenheit, is connected to the catheter and the oil is slowly introduced with the patient in the upright position, leaning somewhat to the left. Forcibly holding the tongue forward will tend to prevent swallowing, and the patient is instructed to breathe slowly and not to cough. After five or ten cc. of the oil has been inserted, the left lung tree should be sufficiently delineated, and the patient now leans toward the right so that the radiopaque substance can pass into the opposite lung.

This simple technique will serve to visualize both lower lobes fairly well, and bronchiectasis occurs most frequently at the lower extremes of pulmonary tissue. For a detailed description of bronchography of the entire lung fields, the reader is referred to an excellent article by Adams and Davenport[2].

MEDICAL MANAGEMENT

Careful medical attention of the patient as a whole, adequate nutrition, postural drainage, fortification of his immune processes with chemo-therapy and penicillin, have made surgical excision of diseased pulmonary tissue a relatively safe procedure. From a statistical point of view, medical treatment alone will neither prolong the life of the patient, nor will it prevent him from the hazards of recurrent pneumonitis, or metastitic abscesses in the lungs, brain and elsewhere. Since no return to normal physiologic state in the bronchial ectasis and sac formation, occurs under medical therapy alone, surgery should be advised in all children and young adults who can be brought into operable condition[3]. This can also be said of the older age adult group, because their operative risk is scarcely greater than in the young if they are given careful pre-operative study and preparation. Severely bronchiectatic persons, however, do not usually live beyond the early adult age.

SURGICAL MANAGEMENT

In estimating a patient for pulmonary resection, the general background of the patient, his nutritional status, systemic effects that chronic pulmonary sepsis has engendered, and the present acuteness of the process are carefully recorded. By integrating the past and present status of the disease with the physical examination of the patient, his bronchograms and his laboratory findings, the safety and the necessity of segmental pulmonectomy can be arrived at with a fair degree of accuracy. The optimal time for operation and the number of broncho-pul-

monary segments that should be removed are tentatively decided upon. At operation, it may be found that more or less pulmonary tissue should be excised than originally planned, but this is not usually the case.

Since spread of the ectatic bronchial changes rarely occurs after the process has delineated itself, removal of all diseased tissue on one side of the chest is usually accomplished at one operation, although this is not absolutely necessary. Surgery is not limited to patients with unilateral disease; the most severely involved lobe or lobes on a particular side are resected first, and at a later date, the contralateral disease can be eradicated if, after re-estimating his status carefully as before his first operation, this is desirable.

TYPICAL TYPES OF INVOLVEMENT

Here presented are five of the common types of bronchiectasis that show clear-cut surgical indication.

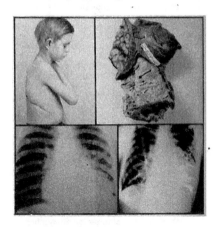

1. *Severe bronchiectasis left lower lobe.* (Fig. 1). Boy, age 14, with cough productive of three to eight ounces of thick, foul smelling purulent sputum daily; onset nineteen months prior to admission and following a severe pneumonia for which he was hospitalized. Loss of strength, shortness of breath on minimal exertion, eighteen pounds weight loss, marked bulbing of fingers. After complete removal bronchiectatic tissue, cessation of productive cough 48 hours after operation, restoration of weight loss six weeks post operative, absence of clubbed fingers four weeks post operative, return to normal exercise tolerance two months after operation.

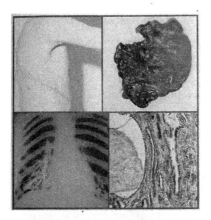

2. *Moderately severe bronchiectasis, right lower lobe.* (Fig. 2). Male, age 24, with cough productive of about two to fourteen ounces of thick, yellow grey sputum daily with onset after severe pneumonia three years prior to admission, while in active duty in the army. Loss of strength, always tired, 28 pounds weight loss. Occasional hemoptosis. After removal of the right lower lobe, immediate cessation of purulent sputum. Marked personality change bordering on euphoria, on relief of cough. Returned to college classes third post operative week.

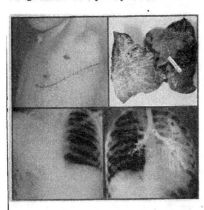

3. *Unilateral Complete Bronchiectasis.* (Fig. 3). Girl, age 9, marked stunting in growth, appears to be age five. Continual hacking cough since age one, and follwing a

severe pneumonia and croup. Swallows sputum, and quantity difficult to estimate. Frequent attacks of broncho-pneumonia, with high fever each time. Marked clubbing of fingers. After removal of the entire left lung, productive cough ceased within one week after operation, and patient changed from morose, timid type to jovial person interested in playing with other children by three weeks post operative. Absence of clubbed fingers except thumbs, four weeks post operative. Excellent exercise tolerence, skipping rope and playing ball, four weeks post operative. Weight gain pronounced.

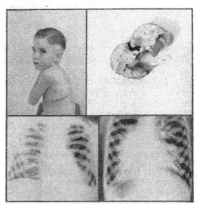

4. *Bilateral Bronchiectasis, Severe on Left.* (Fig. 4). Boy, age seven, with productive cough since severe whooping cough at age two. For the past year prior to admission, slept in mother's lap while she slept in chair, because his productive cough during the night would cause severe attacks of cyanosis, relieved only by her helping patient in postural drainage. Estimated four to eight ounces of thick yellow sputum daily for past six months. Shortness of breath on minimal exertion, frequent attacks of broncho-pneumonia in past two years, unable to attend school regularly. After removal of the left lower lobe, cough changed to a dry, infrequent hack for first post-operative month, and then disappeared nearly completely. Exercise markedly improved, weight gain pronounced. Will be followed closely, and if symptoms recur, he will be re-studied to determine the need for removal of the right lower lobe. At the present time (eight months post-operative) the patient shows no clinical evidence of pulmonary disease, the ectasis on the right entirely quiescent.

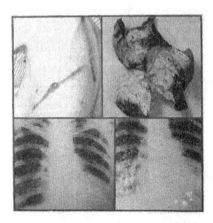

5. *Bronchiectasis Left Lower Lobe, with associated Abscesses.* (Fig. 5). Young lady, age 18. Cough productive of four to about 16 ounces of purulent sputum, at intermittent intervals since pneumonia 5 years prior to admission. Progressive weakness and occasional hemoptosis. One year prior to admission, weakness and cough so severe that she spent most of her time in bed. Admitted to tuberculosis sanatorium for 4 months, where diagnosis of bronchiectasis was made. Foul smelling sputum, marked clubbing of all fingers, fever 103 degrees or more if out of bed for a day. After removal of severely bronchiectatic left lower lobe, which showed in addition multiple abscesses, two of which were 1½ inches in diameter, patient made quick recovery, but complicated by the development of a moderate empyema of the left lower chest, with associated wound infection. Two months following surgery, cough absent, wound well healed, no evidence of empyema or pleural fluid on x-ray, and clubbed fingers gone. Improvement in weight general strength and mental attitude very pronounced.

DISCUSSION

Recent advancements in operative anesthetic techniques, careful pre-operative preparation and accurate antomical diagnosis have reduced the operative mortality from pulmonary excision in bronchiectasis to less than five per cent. Involved broncho-pulmonary segments are now removed, depending upon the exact location of the ectatic bronchi and making it unnecessary to sacrifice normal respiratory tissue. Convalescence is comparatively rapid; patients often sit up the day after operation, and are usually out of bed in four or five days in the absence of a complication; they may get out of bed sooner if they so desire.

Shortly or immediately after bronchiectatic segments have been removed, the productive cough disappears. If the disease is bilateral, reduction in the quantity of sputum is striking after removal of the pathology on the more severe side, and some patients are completely symptom free, even through demonstrable pathology remains on the opposite side.

The results of excision should be directly in proportion to the amount of disease process removed. If all demonstrable bronchiectatic segments are excised, the patient should be permanently symptom free, for progression to new segments is extremely rare. A patient with minimal disease on one side, may be completely symptom free after removal of his more severe contralateral disease, and during careful follow-up over a period of years, it may never be necessary to remove this remaining, minimal bronchiectasis if the process remains quiescent. If necessary, however, remaining pathology can be removed two months to a year or more after the first operation, depending upon whether it is thought that his disease has completely delineated itself. The patient's general condition and his ability to carry on his needed daily activities are to be considered.

After the full convalescent period no restrictions are placed on physical activity. One of our patients is now on his high school baseball and basketball teams. Most of our patients overcompensate for their previously restricted physical activities.

In a follow-up of 400 patients treated medically alone, Perry and King[4] found the mortality rate in the group was 26 per cent over a period of twelve years. Of 59 patients who lived beyond the age of 40, only 15 per cent had the onset of the disease before the age of ten. The morbidity of inter-current infections, the danger of recurrent pneumonia, hemorrhages, metastatic abscesses, and the hazards of chronic invalidism are to be considered worth relieving even if fatal termination is not considered as a probability.

SUMMARY

1. Bronchiectasis should be seriously considered in all patients with persistent or recurrent productive cough.

2. Bronchograms can easily be done on out-patients, and should always follow routine chest films that show (a) persistent pulmonary markings at the lung bases, (b) slowly resolving or recurrent broncho-pneumonia, (c) areas of suspected atelectasis.

3. All patients with bronchiectasis deserve surgical consideration, since medical

management alone is ineffective and does not protect the patient from fatal termination or purulent complications of the disease.

4. Resection of all bronchiectatic broncho-pulmonary segments can clinically and pathologically relieve a patient of his bronchiectasis.

BIBLIOGRAPHY

1. W. A. Evans, Jr. and L. J. Galinsky: American Journal of Roentgenology, Volume No. 51, page 587; May, 1944.

2. Ralph Adams and L. F. Davenport: Technique of Bronchography: Journal American Medical Association, Volume No. 118, page 11; January 10, 1942.

3. S. Diamond and E. L. van Loon: Bronchiectasis in Childhood: Journal American Medical Association, Volume No. 118, page 771; March 7, 1942.

4. K. M. A. Perry and D. S. King: Bronchiectasis, Study of Prognosis: American Review of Tuberculosis, Volume No. 41, page 531; May, 1940.

Announcement

A luncheon and meeting was held at the Huckins Hotel at 12:00 noon, April 6, of a group of professional service representatives, representing pharmaceutical manufacturers to discuss and organize the Oklahoma City chapter of the Medical Service Society of America.

The purpose of this organization is to establish better relationship between ourselves and our allied professions.

By secret ballot and a majority vote the following officers were elected:

President ....William K. Golden
First Vice-President ....Jack Murray
Second Vice-President ....Frank R. Cotton
Secretary ....William A. Cates
Treasurer ....Herman B. Fry

The President made the following appointments:

Business Manager ....Grear W. Shilling
Publicity Committee ....H. H. Huff
                                                           Cecil C. Cornutt
                                                           T. F. Spigener

Psychosomatic Problems in an Army General Hospital

MAX E. JOHNSON, CAPTAIN, M.C., A.U.S.

The term "psychosomatic medicine" has come into use in recent years to designate a certain group of morbid conditions as well as a viewpoint, or method of approach, toward all illness. A psychosomatic disease has been well defined as follows: "A bodily disorder whose nature can be appreciated only when emotional disturbances (i.e. psychological happenings) are investigated in addition to physical disturbances (i.e. somatic happenings)'". While this term has come into vogue comparatively recently, the importance of mental and emotional factors in illness has been recognized explicitly and implicitly since the very beginnings of medicine. This concept has always been recognized, though not formally expressed, by laymen as is evidenced by expressions current in everyday language. Such phrases as "I felt a lump in my throat", "my heart jumped", "I can't stomach that", etc., indicate that there is nothing new about the idea of a connection between emotions and certain organs. The vast progress made by medicine during the past 140 years along lines of purely organic investigation has led to a predominantly organic orientation of medical thought which is only recently undergoing some change. The enormous task of developing and assimilating the advances of organic and laboratory medicine has consumed the energies of the researcher and the practitioner alike and tended to discourage attention to less tangible aspects of illness[13]. During the past generation or so the once extremely narrow specialty of psychiatry has grown rapidly and spread

beyond the bounds of its former restriction to the study of the psychoses, has passed beyond the walls of the mental hospital and has acquired a closer relationship with other branches of medicine. This broadening of the field of psychiatry has brought about in recent years a resurgence of interest in emotional aspects of illness and deliberate scientific investigations of this inter-relation which previously had been merely conjectured or implied. The extent of present day interest in this subject may be realized by a glance at the already quite considerable literature, and the number of papers on these problems presented both by psychiatrists and other specialists before medical societies, and the ever expanding volume of research activities. Interest in the matter has been particularly stimulated by medical experiences in the armed services[5].

The basic concept of modern psychiatry and of psychosomatic medicine is that of the oneness and inseparability of body and mind, i.e., the concept of the total personality. We believe that body and mind cannot be separated from each other, but are rather two different aspects of an individual and unitary organism. The age old idea of cleavage between the somatic and psychic is felt by many to be an expression of the limitations of our investigative methods and not to represent a real division. The person may be studied from the somatic standpoint on the one hand, or from the emotional or psychic on the other, and his reactions described accordingly, but he nevertheless remains the same individual. The psychosomatic viewpoint is that there is a constant and intimate relation between body and mind; and that consequently a study of an individual's reactions cannot be complete where either of these aspects is inadequately considered[4][6][7][13]. The sick person is to be regarded as an individual reacting with his whole personality and not simply as a case of this or that nosological entity. This attitude toward illness is not at all foreign to medical practice and has traditionally been expressed as "the art of medicine". The practitioner has long known that medicines alone did not always cure his patients and has acted accordingly, although often perhaps being unaware of the implications of his actions.

The psychosomatic approach to illness obviously requires the giving of equal attention to emotional factors and to physical factors in arriving at a diagnosis and in carrying out treatment. This entails the taking of a much fuller and more detailed history than is ordinarily obtained, which will include far more than the bare facts of symptom development. The life history and emotional development of the individual must be gone into with greater or lesser thoroughness in order that his personality and emotional reactions may be understood. Of particular importance in this connection are those environmental influences operating during the first few years of life, which include the family history, personality of the parents, relations with brothers and sisters and other relatives, sexual development, family attitude toward illness, etc. The growth and development of the personality through later years to maturity must also be investigated and will indicate general personality trends and tendencies toward certain types of reactions characteristic of the individual. Emotional and mental states and influences operating shortly before or at the time of onset of the patient's complaints and the relation of such factors to the varying course of the condition must be carefully considered. A bird's eye view of the patient's general life adjustment in all its aspects is to be sought[2][13][14].

The intimate relationship between emotions and the body may be readily demonstrated by common and everyday examples. We may select such everyday experiences as blushing, stage fright, physical signs of fear and anxiety, grief, and the like, to indicate the very obvious and even dramatic physical changes which occur as the result, purely, of emotional actions. Anyone may add numerous examples from the normal by observation of others or of himself. Consideration of this fact, that there is emotional control over body functions, at once leads to an interest in the anatomic and physiologic mechanisms by which this control is mediated. A large

body of evidence has been accumulated pointing to the great, and probably paramount, importance of the autonomic nervous system and the endocrine system in this mediation[1].

It has been repeatedly demonstrated that not only do these obvious and relatively superficial mind-body reactions occur, but also that a more deep-seated and chronic, even unconscious, emotional disturbance may, in the same manner, bring about or be accompanied by chronic somatic symptoms and physical changes. The causative emotional or psychic factors operating in a particular instance may not at first glance be apparent but may be found on careful investigation into the patient's personality and emotional life. The person himself is, of course, very often incompletely or not at all aware of the presence or importance of such factors. Some evidence has been produced to indicate the possibility that chronic emotional disturbances may eventuate, in time, in irreversible pathological changes[1][13]. At the present time this idea is, in large part, speculative. However, the concept is not as grotesque and magical as it may first appear to one trained from the organic viewpoint when the pathogenesis of such conditions as essential hypertension and peptic ulcer are considered. In these conditions, particularly, it would appear that chronic emotional disturbance and tension may produce, in the former condition, chronic arterial constriction in the body generally with resultant increase in blood pressure, and in the latter instance local ischemia in the duodenal mucosa which, if continued long enough, may lead to devitalization of tissues and acutal ulcer formation. The final elucidation of this particular problem must await further study.

What illnesses are psychosomatic? The broad viewpoint may be taken that actually all disease is psychosomatic, i.e., that in all illness, or rather, in every sick person, there are emotional and psychic factors as well as organic. In this sense the term may be applied even to such characteristically organic diseases as the neoplastic and infectious. Not only do emotions cause physical changes, but also the presence of organic illness has its influence on the person's emotional state. However, the use of the term at the present time is ordinarily restricted to a rather large and heterogenous group of disorders in which the emotional aspect is of particular importance. In this sense psychosomatic disorders may be segregated into two groups, one in which this relationship is rather well defined and understood, and the other in which such a relationship is probable but has not been so well demonstrated[7]. In the first group (those conditions in which there seems little doubt that emotional influences are of great or even sole importance) we may mention the following:

in the gastro-intestinal system, duodenal ulcer, mucous colitis, visceroptosis, and some cases of constipation; in the cardio-vascular system, essential hyptertension and what has been called neuro-circulatory asthenia; in the respiratory system, bronchial asthma; in the genito-urinary system, nocturnal enuresis, some instances of menstrual disturbance and leukorrhea, impotence and frigidity; in the musculo-skeletal system, many cases of so-called fibrositis, neuritis, sciatica; in the endocrine system, exophthalmic goiter and hyper-thyroidism; in the nervous system, migraine, chorea, and perhaps some cases of epilepsy; among dermatological conditions, many cases of eczema, dermatitis, psoriasis, urticaria; in the eyes, some cases of chronic conjunctivitis, and miner's nystagmus. The large group of psychoneuroses also, obviously are psychosomatic. Among those conditions which probably are psychosomatic may be mentioned gall-bladder disease, angina pectoris, allergic conditions such as hay-fever and sinusitis, prostatism, rheumatoid arthritis, diabetes, obesity, paralysis agitans, and hypochromic anemia. Certain criteria for the consideration of a condition as being psychosomatic may be presented[7]. Important among these are the following: first, emotion as a precipitating factor; second, association with a certain personality type; third, in most cases a disproportion in sex incidence; fourth, frequent association of these disorders with each other in the same case; fifth, high incidence of positive family history for the same or similar conditions; and sixth, a tendency of these illnesses to be phasic, i.e., to show characteristically periods of exacerbation and remission. Another feature may be mentioned: all of these conditions will be noted to be those in which the etiology is regarded as "non-specific". We are concerned here with the great host of widely prevalent chronic diseases which are, in the main, non-fatal, but productive of untold ilness, misery, and incapacity, which have been poorly understood and have resisted the best therapeutic efforts of physicians. Modern medical science and the great advances in the laboratory have provided us with a means of controlling or even eradicating many of the time honored scourges of humanity, but has not provided us with much in the way of therapeutic measures for these conditions. This same reduction in morbidity and mortality due to the infectious and traumatic diseases has served to bring into greater prominence the helplessness of modern medicine in the face of these chronic disorders productive of so much illness and unhappiness. It is here that the psychosomatic approach to medical practice may in the future be of very great benefit[11][12].

The prevalence of psychosomatic disorders is very great. It has been estimated by many observers that at least 30 per cent of the patients in an average medical practice fall into this group. This fact has long been recognized, though perhaps expressed somewhat differently, and it is quite common for the professor of medicine to inform his students that they can expect a goodly proportion of their practice to consist of "functional" illnesses. Certainly these conditions are of great frequency in the armed services[3][5][9][12]. Complete and precise statistics in this respect are not available, but it would appear that the incidence is not out of line with that in civil practice. This is notwithstanding the fact that in the military service we are dealing with a quite restricted and in many ways selected segment of the population. The writer's experience has led him to believe that there may be a somewhat wider recognition of these problems in military service than in outside practice. There are a number of factors which may contribute to this occurrence. One of considerable importance is the close relationship of the psychiatrist in an army hospital to medical officers of other specialties. The daily contacts and necessity for close cooperation and joint study of cases have led to a greater awareness on the part of non-psychiatric medical officers of the importance of emotion in illness, and, not less importantly, to a considerable broadening of the psychiatrist's understanding of general medical problems. Opportunity exists in an army hospital for full study of patients from all aspects, and has produced, I believe, in the medical officer a willingness to consider illness from a broader viewpoint than that of his own specialty. A high incidence of psychosomatic affections among soldiers is not surprising when one considers the emotional upheaval which occurs to a greater or lesser degree in every person in his transition from civil to military life[9]. Most individuals, of course, make this transition without too great difficulty and without the development of illness. However, a great many do not, and they react in various ways to the maladjustment. These emotional reactions include development of psychoneuroses with predominantly psychic symptoms, the occurence of frank psychoses, psychopathic reactions which become disciplinary problems, and a great number of psychosomatic conditions. These reactions may occur at any point in the person's army career and are related to the emotional traumata inevitable in military life. On induction into the service the individual is suddenly placed in an environment totally foreign, in most instances, to his previous experience, and at the same time he is bereft of the emotional support and security afforded by his family, his friends and associates, and his occupation in civil life. He is subjected to regimentation and routine, which is particularly disturbing to persons reared in our individualistic society. The lack of privacy in barracks life, the loss of individuality and often of recognition of accomplishment, is difficult for many to accept without protest. The very existance of an army is dependent upon authority and obedience; the soldier finds himself in one or the other of these situations, either of which may be, depending upon his personality, productive of tension and emotional discomfort. Also, in military life there are a number of obvious incentives to illness, so that what may be called secondary gain from illness becomes of considerable importance. In other words, the individual may consciously or unconsciously become ill for a purpose, either that of avoiding arduous duties or combat, or of attaining the eventual objective of separation for the service. These previously mentioned factors are common to military life as a whole. To them may be added special situations, such as overseas service and combat duty, which naturally increase the problems of adjustment for the individual. Here we are concerned with actual threat to life and limb, actual physical danger and insecurity, as well as the inestimable hardships, deprivations, and chronic unremitting fatigue experienced by combat soldiers. Much has been said and written about combat neuroses which develop under such circumstances. It is widely recognized that such reactions may take the form not only of purely psychic phenomena, but may be expressed in the form of physical, i e., psychosomatic, illness. It has been noted repeatedly that during the course of recovery of a patient from an acute battle anxiety state, relief of the anxiety may be coincident with the appearance of physical complaints of one sort or another. Some of these may be in the form of purely hysterical conversion symptoms, but at times there may be physical illness such as gastro-intestinal disturbance, flare-up of an old sinusitis, and what-not[12].

A number of cases have been selected for presentation from the writer's personal experience at an army general hospital. They have been chosen, so far as possible, to illustrate some of the different types of disorders as previously listed.

CASE NO. 1. A 21-year-old Corporal was admitted to the hospital with complaints of pain in the lower back, left hip and thigh, and headaches of three months duration. Headaches began during the time the patient was hospitalized soon after he reached a new station, because of a boil in his right leg. He had become anxious and worried for fear that he would not pass an examination for air cadet training and might be placed in a ground crew which he would not like. The patient himself attributed onset of his headaches to this situation. Soon after that he was engaged in "rough and tumble" play in physical training, during which he was thrown to the ground, landing on his back. There were no immediate symptoms, but three days later there was severe pain over the sacroiliac region with radiation to the left hip and thigh which persisted. The patient's past history revealed that his mother had always been ill after his birth and had had numerous operations. The patient had always been an individual who was restless and wanted to "be on the go", was intolerant toward routine, had changed jobs frequently, liked to "be his own boss", and had little tolerance for authority. He was quite active in athletics. Examination found that severe pain was produced by flexion of either thigh, and that there was an indefinite small area of sensory reduction over the dorsum of the left foot. X-ray studies of the spine were negative. In this case the diagnostic possibility of herniation of a nucleus pulposus was strongly considered in view of the onset following trauma and the physical signs. It was felt that the patient's personality and emotional reaction were of great importance, and he was accordingly treated from that standpoint. It was felt that in view of the emotional factor further diagnostic measures, such as lumbar puncture, to determine the presence or absence of disc herniation were not warranted. Discussion with the patient of emotional factors and explanation and encouragement with placing of the patient in the reconditioning program enabled him to return to duty, though still with some complaints. The presence of a disc herniation, at any rate at the time of onset of the complaints, was considered entirely possible, but it was felt that the larger part of the patient's actual disability was due to the associated emotional factors. Experience has shown, at least in the army situation, that elective operations such as that for this condition, in the presence of associated personality disorders, are quite often unsuccessful so far as relieving symptoms is concerned and may even be productive of further disability, new symptoms appearing in the wake of surgery. Army directives have recognized this fact and have stipulated that patients considered for such measures should, where feasible, have neuropsychiatric appraisal beforehand. While the patient was by no means cured, rather simple psychotherapeutic measures were sufficient to return him to further service. This case illustrates that the patient's condition could not be adequately understood, appreciated, or treated without considering both the organic and emotional factors.

CASE NO. 2. A 27-year-old sergeant was admitted to the hospital complaining of productive cough, nervousness, and weakness. He had first developed symptoms about a year previously when he was in a desert training unit, and had begun to complain of nasal congestion and discomfort, which were ascribed to dust. During the months following his unit was broken up and he was transferred first from one unit, then to another, had some periods of boring inactivity, and began to become increasingly dissatisfied with his lot. He also began to have some difficulties with his superiors and associates and noted increasing nasal symptoms which, he had been told, were due to sinusitis. He had received orders to a cadet training center when he became ill with a productive cough, some fever, and general weakness, so that he was hospitalized. A diagnosis of atypical pneumonia was made, and subsequently on persistence of productive cough, a diagnosis of bronchiectasis. Physical examination found bronchiectasis of the lower lobes confirmed by bronchogram. The condition itself was not considered incapacitating. After a period in the rehabilitation program and therapeutic discussions, the patient improved both in his general symptoms of nervousness and weakness and in decrease of cough and was able to return to duty. The patient had previously been well, except for chorea at the age of ten. His parents were quite strict and rigid in their attitude toward their children, requiring strict obedience and discouraging any show of affection. The parents had been divorced when he was four year of age. He had always been somewhat seclusive, a "lone-wolf" type of individual, stubborn, with a high sense of duty, and a perfectionist with intolerance toward lower ideals and inefficiency in others. It was felt that these personality traits contributed definitely toward his dissatisfaction and maladjustment in his assignments, which in turn led to the development of increased emotional tension and this, in addition to the development of the organic change of bronchiectasis, produced his disability. Studies of cases of bronchial asthma have shown that the bronchial musculature is under emotional control through the autonomic nervous system. That such smooth muscle spasm may influence the symptoms and degree of disability due to an actual organic process such as bronchiectasis is illustrated by this case. There was a rather direct relationship between the patient's emotional adjustment and the degree of cough during the onset of the condition and during the course of his improvement.

CASE NO. 3. This 21-year-old soldier was seen as an out-patient. About one and one half years previously while in a training camp he had first noted a papular and vesicular eruption first appearing on his leg and spreading within a month or so to involve all regions of his body. The condition was extremely pruritic, the source of much discomfort and annoyance, so that he was hospitalized and for many months received various and sundry local treatments, had been given adrenalin, and was found to be allergic to penicillin. There was some improvement, and he returned to duty where he remained, but continued to have periods of exacerbation of the eruption which continued to itch excessively. The patient's mother had died when he was 11 year of age, and he had become very closely attached to his father and had in some ways taken his mother's place in the home. He was a seclusive individual with difficulty in making friends or personal contacts, was very religious, and had conflict and dissatisfaction regarding the coarseness and vulgarity, as he considered it, of barracks life in the army. These factors had caused continual dissatisfaction with his assignments and difficulty in his general adjustment. The patient had noted that increase in severity of his eruptions coincided with periods of increased anxiety and adjustment difficulties. The condition had been diagnosed as a dermatitis herpetiformis. It was felt that in this case there was very definite emotional relation to the physical condition and that this factor was of etiological importance in the onset of the complaints. This patient's personality type and degree of emotional immaturity made him quite vulnerable to the impact of the army situation, giving rise to this type of reaction. There seemed to be also an allergic factor operating in the case. The close relation of personality type and emotional condition to allergic states has been well recognized and appears to explain why, in many cases, an individual may be sensitive to a certain substance and yet present no allergic symptoms while another sensitive individual will have some manifestations of allergy clinically. This individual through encouragement and discussion has thus far been able to remain on duty[s].

CASE NO. 4. A 29-year-old soldier was hospitalized because he complained of general weakness, low afternoon fever, pains in his extremities on exertion, and occasional testicular pains. This soldier had been stationed for many months in the Cook Islands in the South Pacific. After a time many soldiers in his unit including himself came down with an affection which was diagnosed as filariasis. The patient's symptoms at onset consisted of swelling and pain in the testicles, a little swelling of the legs, some burning on urination, and some cloudiness of the urine. He was hospitalized and returned to the United States and eventually to duty, although he continued to complain of general aching and weakness, reduced stamina, and dragging pains in the testicles. The complaints had continued so that he was again hospitalized. Rather extensive and repeated laboratory examinations were performed but no parasites were demonstrated. Physical examination was also essentially negative. The patient had previously been in good health, was a somewhat seclusive person with few friends, had not been married, and had had frequent job changes in civil life. The patient had remained convinced that he still suffered from filariasis, feared that exertion of any kind would bring a recrudescence of the symptoms, and that his sexual potency and fertility would suffer. Repeated assurances to the contrary and explanations of his condition were entirely without effect, and the amount of resentment which developed necessitated his separation from the service. It could not be definitely ascertained in this particular case whether or not acutal infection with filariasis had occured, although that seemed probable. It was definitely felt, however, that in the absence of any present clinical and laboratory indications of the disease, his symptoms were emotional and psychic in origin. It is not uncommon for such attitudes and obsessions regarding obscure chronic illnesses to arise. Difficulty in caring for these situations is increased by our ignorance concerning the disease and by the fact that it apparently may remain latent for long periods of time. However, little is gained by contributing to invalidism and incapacity on the remote possibility that recurrence of the condition might occur. Experience so far in the war with filariasis has indicated that the disease apparently dies out of itself when the individual is removed from an endemic area and that the chronic and particularly frightening symptoms, especially elephantiasis, occur only when there is such exposure to the infection for many years. The main effort in situations of this sort is obviously one of prevention of development of the defective attitude toward the illness. Treatment of such deep-seated obsessive ideas, once developed, is exceedingly difficult[10].

CASE NO. 5. This 24-year-old soldier had been returned from overseas as a patient because of fracture dislocation of the hip sustained in a jeep accident. He had also had a head injury at that time and had headaches for about two months thereafter. The fracture healed properly, and he became ambulatory, but began to complain of "stomach trouble" in the form of continued feeling of discomfort and fullness in the epigastrium and at times sharp burning pain related to meals. He also complained of severe pruritus ani accompanied by constant scratching. These complaints had become manifest during recovery from his accident. Previous health had been good, and the background was unremarkable except for the fact that the patient considered himself to have always been a "nervous person". He had been in combat for about four months in Germany. He states that he was quite nervous at first but after that adjusted well without undue discomfort. Medical investigation disclosed no organic disease of the gastro-intestinal tract; there were no changes except some anal excoriation due to scratching. This individual, although giving evidence of mild nervousness previously, had adjusted to prolonged combat duty quite well, had not had unusual difficulties until after his accident. This traumatic event and the subsequent hospitalization had, it is believed, disturbed his adjustment and emotional equilibrium and resulted in the expression of emotional tension in the form of gastro-intestinal complaints and pruritus ani. It is interesting also that the patient had considered himself constipated for some years. A similar chain of events has been noted in other individuals to result in the appearance of a definite anxiety state with dreams of combat, reaction to loud noises, etc., which this patient did not present. It seems likely that this patient's anxiety and tension was converted or drained off into the formation of these somatic symptoms. A contributory factor, doubtless, had been prolonged hospitalization and invalidism due to his fracture with inactivity which provides a fertile ground for emergence of emotional conflicts. Psychogenic involvement of the gastro-intestinal tract is particularly common since this system is so closely under emotional influences[15][16].

The remarks about the above cases have indicated some aspects of treatment in these disorders. In the planning of treatment of such conditions neither the organic nor psychic aspect should be neglected, but both should receive adequate attention. In pursuing strictly organic measures of therapy in an individual with a definite emotional factor, reasons for such therapy should be carefully explained to the patient and the fact emphasized that such is not the whole treatment and that the emotional causes also must receive attention. In dealing with emotional factors in illness the physician should avoid an attitude of therapeutic nihilism. Although in many instances it may not be possible to do much toward changing the patient's personality or general mode of reaction or to do much about important situational influences, nevertheless, usually much can be done toward help-

ing the patient live with his illness and become better adjusted within the limitations of his personality and his environment. An attitude of hopeful encouragement should be maintained by the physician, but the patient should be made to see that most of the effort must be on his own part. The majority of these conditions not only can, but should be, cared for by the general practitioner or internist and do not require profound psychiatric knowledge or special techniques. Correct therapy presupposes that an adequate history has been taken and the personality of the patient, as well as his present life situation, evaluated. On this basis the patient's total adjustment is discussed with him in simple terms and necessary explanations given about his illness. The ways in which emotions can influence the body can be explained simply, using examples from the normal. The importance of any actual disease present should be carefully explained to the patient. Definite reassurance and knowledge on this point may be of very great benefit to him. The very experience of discussing with a sympathetic listener personal worries and problems is the essential part of psychotherapy and in itself has the effect of relieving anxiety and tension. Worries and fears that have been kept hidden and mulled over tend to lose much of their importance and seriousness to the patient when talked about and looked over in the light of day. In many instances the efforts of the physician ought to be along the lines of encouraging the patient and helping him form the ability to live in spite of symptoms and disabilities, to go along even though he does have discomfort and aches and pains. Sometimes etiological factors in the environment, such as unsuitable type of work, incompatible marriages, family differences and the like may be subject to alteration. Usually, however, not a great deal can be done from this standpoint, and in the end the patient should acquire the ability to get along regardless of the environmental influences. The patient should be encouraged to develop various means of draining off emotional tension and of increasing his range of interests with suitable hobbies and avocations. Knowledge of the patient's personality type and inclinations will be of help in suggesting such activities. There will be cases in which such rather superficial measures will be unavailing, and which may have to be referred to a psychiatrist for more prolonged treatment and the use of special therapeutic measures[4]
5 13 16

The psychosomatic viewpoint of illness is valuable in the treatment of almost all sickness. Regardless of what the disease is that a person has, he remains a person who is sick, and the rapidity and degree of his recovery from any illness may depend on factors other than purely physical ones, i.e., on his attitudes and emotional state. Rest has long been, and will always remain, one of the prime forms of therapeusis. However, it is beginning to be recognized that there are instances in which this measure, as a good many other things, can be carried too far. A number of writers recently have expressed the view that too long a period of convalescence has heretofore been considered necessary following surgical operations or serious illnesses. Experiences in the army have confirmed this idea. The dangers of prolonged convalescence are of course greater in a situation where there is a premium placed on illness, where there are important motives for the patient not to get well. The army has recognized this, and as a result convalescence from surgical procedures has been shortened considerably; the patient is got out of bed sooner and more quickly returned to duty. Not only has there been apparently no increase in morbidity because of this, but some organic complications of surgery have been felt to have been avoided. It is important in the military service as well as in many situations in civil life to avoid the inculcation of an attitude of invalidism on the part of the patient and to return him to his normal activity as rapidly as possible, consistent with the patient's good. The army has set up rather elaborate facilities in all hospitals for this very purpose. The reconditioning and rehabilitation units have been of enormous value in shortening the period of hospitalization and returning the soldier to duty in much better condition than was previously possible. There is a graduated program of increasing activity, both physical and intellectual, so that the patient is not overtaxed and is not given the opportunity to feel that he will be injured by exertion. The fact that the soldier is well and fit for duty when he returns to his unit and is not out of condition due to prolonged hospital stay and inactivity reduces materially the number of relapses and rehospitalizations. It is felt that such an attitude toward convalescence and return to normal activity is equally applicable to civil practice and might be productive of equally good results. Centers for the purpose, such as the army has, may of course not be feasible, but the general viewpoint is. We are all familiar with individuals who "enjoy ill health" during a long life and who may be encouraged in such an attitude by well-intentioned relatives and not infrequently by their physicians.

Many internists and practitioners have interested themselves particularly in problems of psychosomatic medicine so that it may be that a definite specialty of psychosomatic medicine will appear. This may, in a sense, be unfortunate in view of what many consider the present over-specialization of medicine. The psychosomatic viewpoint is one which should permeate all medical practice. As was previously suggested, psychosomatic medicine may in the future offer hope of solving the problems of the great category of obscure, chronic diseases which have such high morbidity and for which so little could previously be done. It may be instrumental in increasing the happiness and efficiency of many people and enable an even higher level of medical care to be given. Such hopes may, it is true, be over-enthusiastic and even visionary. However, the present degree of progress has provided us with a method of approach toward treatment which has already demonstrated its usefulness and practicality.

SUMMARY

General remarks concerning the concept of psychosomatic disease and the importance of emotion in illness have been made. The various psychosomatic affections have been mentioned and described. Cases from an army general hospital experience have been presented, illustrating some of these concepts. The important psychological factors in adjustment to army life have been mentioned. Treatment of these conditions has been discussed, with stress on the importance of adequate history—taking, and recognition of emotional and psychic influences in illness.

BIBLIOGRAPHY

1. F. Dunbar: Emotions and Bodily Changes: New York, Columbia University Press; 1938.

2. F. Dunbar: Psychosomatic Diagnosis, New York: Paul B. Hoeber; 1943.

3. F. Dunbar: Medical Aspects of Accidents and Mistakes in the Industrial Army and in the Armed Forces: War Medicine, Volume No. 2, page 161; August, 1943.

4. Jack R Ewalt: Psychosomatic Problems: Journal American Medical Association, Volume No. 126, page 150; September 16, 1944.

5. D. N. W. Grant: The Medical Direction of Human Drives in War and Peace: Journal American Medical Association, Volume No. 126, page 607; November 4, 1944.

6. J L. Halliday: Principles of Aetiology: British Journal of Medical Psychology, Volume No. 19, page 367; 1943.

7. J. L. Halliday: Concept of a Psychosomatic Affection: The Lancet, page 692; December 4, 1943.

8. F. F. Heller: The Relation of Dermatology to Psychiatry: Britain Medical Journal, page 583; April 29, 1944.

9. M. H. Maskin and L L. Altman: Military Psycho-dynamics: Psychiatry, Volume No. 6, page 263; August, 1943.

10. H. P Rome and R H. Fogel. The Psychosomatic Manifestations of Filariasis: Journal American Medical Association, Volume No. 15, page 123; December 11, 1943.

11. Edward O. Strecker: The Leaven of Psychosomatic Medicine: Annals of Internal Medicine, Volume No. 18, page 735; May, 1943.

12. Alfred Torrie: Psychosomatic Casualties in the Middle East: Lancet; January 29, 1944.

13 Edward Weiss and O. S. English: Psychosomatic Medicine: Philadelphia, Saunders; 1943.

14. John C. Whitehorn: Guide to Interviewing and Clinical Personality Study: Archives of Neurology and Psychiatry, Volume No. 42, page 197; September, 1944.

15. H. G. Wolf: Disturbances of Gastro-Intestinal Function in Relation to Personality Disorders: Annals of New York Academy of Science, Volume No. 44, page 567; December 22, 1943.

16. J. C. Yaskin: The Treatment of Functional Gastro-Intestinal Disturbances of Neuropsychiatric Origin: Annals of Internal Medicine, Volume No. 18, page 949; June, 1943.

Medical Aspect of Peptic Ulcer

S. G. MOLLICA, M.D. AND
WILLIAM G. HARTNETT, M.D.

Veterans Hospital,

MUSKOGEE, OKLAHOMA

INTRODUCTION

Peptic ulcers are chronic, benign ulcerations of the digestive tract. They occur only in areas which are exposed to active gastric juice. An acute loss of mucosa in a healthy stomach is rapidly repaired; an acute ulcer of the stomach usually gets well rapidly. A chronic ulcer behaves differently, indicating that there is some complicating factor to keep it from healing. A gastric ulcer is an oval crater in the stomach lining. Similar lesions occur in the lower portion of the esophagus, in the duodenal bulb which receives the gastric juice from the pylorus. After gastro-enterostomy gastric juice flowing directly upon small intestinal mucosa may produce the anastomotic or jejunal ulcer.

INCIDENCE

Peptic ulcer may occur at any age, but it is principally a disease of young adults. The onset is most frequent in the third and fourth decades when the responsibilities of life are mounting[1]. The exact incidence is unknown[2]. Autopsy and x-ray studies have shown that from 10 to 12 per cent of all persons suffer at some time in their lives from a chronic gastric or duodenal ulcer[3]. In recent years post mortem studies have shown that duodenal ulcers and scars occur much more frequently than gastric lesions. Duodenal ulcer is more prevalent in the male 4 to 1. For gastric ulcer the male to female ratio is 3 or 4 to 1. In the Mayo Clinic one encounters 9 duodenal ulcers to 1 gastric ulcer, the patients representing the average cross section of the American population. Reeser and Guthrie[3], in February issue, 1946, Military Surgeon, report a ratio of 14 duodenal to 1 gastric ulcer in a series of 40,000 Army Hospital admissions.

The increasing importance of dyspepsia

and particularly peptic ulcer as causes of disability in both civilian and military life has been stressed in many recent reports from England[4], Canada[5], Germany[6] and the United States[7]. In England it proved high during air raid periods and in forces having military reverses. In Germany, disability was prevalent in war workers and in mimlitary personnel before or immediately on going into front lines. In the United States the greatest increase in incidence of these disorders is noted in civilians and in the army. Hurst concluded that dyspepsia was the largest single disease in the British Army and the most important medical problem of this war. The incidence of peptic ulcer among all gastro-intestinal diseases in England is reported as from 35 to 58 per cent[8], in Canadian soldiers invalided at home 21 per cent[9], in United States Army Hospitals from 7.2 per cent to 3 per cent[10]. In a South Pacific Combat Zone Hospital 19 per cent. In England it has been estimated that 90 per cent of the patients had the condition before enlisting[11] while in the United States from 50 to 93 per cent[12] had it before enlisting. The ratio of gastric to duodenal ulcers in the British Army is quoted as 1 to 3.6[13]; in the Army Hospitals of the United States it varies from 1 to 8, to 1 to 49[14]. In the Naval Personnel the proportion was 1 to 9[15]. Bockus concludes that well over 10 per cent of all adults of the male sex, have or have had an ulcer.

PATHOGENESIS

Exact knowledge of the cause of chronic peptic ulcer is lacking and it must be admitted that we may not know anything of the real fundamentals involved. It has been thought that chronic ulcer may develop from acute erosions. Acute ulcerations of the mucosa membrane are thought to be fairly common, but ordinarily are healed promptly.

The one factor which may change an acute erosion to a chronic ulcer and about which we are most certain, is the digestive action of the gastric juice. Normal gastric and duodenal mucous membrane is resistant to gastric digestion. If, however, a localized area becomes devitalized or injured, it may lose this resistance and on exposure to strongly active juice a portion of tissue is digested away with the formation of an ulcer. Chronicity results from the continuous digestive action on the lesion.

Several theories have been advanced to explain the pre-disposing constitutional factor or ulcer diastesis which ulcer patients seem to have; among them may be mentioned the bacterial inflammation theory, the traumatic theory, the non-bacterial inflammation theory of Konjetzny[16]; disturbance of blood supply, chemical inflammation theory and the theories implicating the nervous system and metabolic conditions such as hyperth-

roidism, diabetes mellitus; Vitamin and endocrine dificiencies have also been incriminated. The association of ulcer with pulmonary T. B., syphilis, cirrhosis of the liver, acute appendicitis, duodenal stasis, polycythemia, thromboagiitis obliterans, heart disease, arterial hypertension and other infections seem to be purely a coincidence. The pathogenesis of ulcer is unsettled and none of the hypothesis adequately expained the complete course of the lesion. The following observations are worthy of note. Peptic ulcer occurs only in those portions of the digestive tract exposed to the action of acid gastric juice. Chronic peptic ulcer does not occur in the complete absence of acid gastric juice. Approximately 10 per cent of the population is achlorhydric and is not susceptible to ulcer. The failure of various authors to find active chronic ulcer in the presence of pernicious anemia is striking and significant. Acute superficial lesions can apparently occur, however, with achlorhydria, but they heal rapidly and do not become chronic. The experimental evidence on the importance of acid gastric juice[17] is fully conclusive. Artificially produced ulcers heal rapidly if protected from further action of acid gastric juice. The clinical and experimental evidence confirms the dictum of Schwarz enunciated in 1910 "no acid-no ulcer". But the question, as to why ulcer occurs in some persons with acid gastric juice and not in others with equally acid gastric juice, remains unanswered.

That a functional disturbance of an organ may in time lead to structural (organic) tissue changes, is an etiologic fact of primary importance, which might be the solution for many etiologic riddles of modern medicine.

Bon Bergman and Westphal came to the conclusion that most peptic ulcers may be considered as complications of functional stomach neurosis of long standing. The etiologic problem is then to establish the origin of the chronic functional disturbance, and here is where the significance of the emotional factors become obvious. Different authors found that certain types of persons are more inclined than others to peptic ulcers. Alvarez[18] spoke of the efficient, active Jewish business man, the go-getter type, as being particularly disposed to peptic ulcer. Jones and Pollack[19] say "the man with duodenal ulcer is usually of special value to industry, for he is over-conscientious, with plenty of drive and a sense of good standard of work". Hartman[20] claimed that the Indians of Latin America and the Chinese Coolies never have ulcers and explained this as the result of the stoic almost pathetic attitude, the lack of strain and ambition, characteristic of these races. According to him ulcer is a disease of the civilized world and afflicts chiefly the striving and ambitious men of western civilization.

The extensive nerve supply through the vagus, connecting the stomach with the higher centers, has led many to incriminate the autonomic nervous system in the neurogenic theory of the causation of ulcer. In theory, nerve impulses travel down the vagus and spread to branches supplying the duodenal and gastric wall. This causes spasm of arterioles, possibly by the formation of acetylcholine at the nerve endings. Constriction of the vessels by spastic contraction of the muscularis is another theoretical mechanism.

There results an ischemic infarction of the mucosa which eventually is digested to form an ulcer. Again these suggested mechanisms are only theoretical. In the intestinal tract the para-sympathetic system is motor and the sympathetic system is inhibitory. The sphincters are, however, inervated in opposite fashion. In gastric secretion there is a vagus phase and a chemical phase. In the latter a hormone called gastrin acts directly on the fundus cells of the stomach without nervous intervention. Histamine acts this way. There is an inhibitory factor present in the duodenum and jejunum called enterogastrone which has recently been tried in an effort to accelerate the healing of gastric ulcer. The true dysfunction behind this autonomic physiology remains unknown. We do know, however, that in gastric and duodenal ulcer hyper-secretion of acid is an almost constant concomitant finding which is indirect evidence of a parasympathetic preponderance. The effect of acetylcholine secretion as a result of anxiety, if continued long enough may lower the resistance of the gastro-intestinal tract preparing the way for secondary invasion of bacteria, their toxins or other substances. This lowered resistance may also predispose portions of the G. I. tract to the effects of certain deficiency states. Kogan-Yansy[21] defines peptic ulcer as a disease of the neurohumoral mechanism in which the vegetative nervous system and the glandular apparatus of the stomach plays a special part[22].

DIAGNOSIS

In uncomplicated peptic ulcer the clinical history is remarkably constant. The patient complains of chronic indigestion with recurring spells which last from one to several weeks and yet having normal digestion between attacks. The outstanding symptom is pain which is always localized and distressing. This pain has been described as hunger pain, heart burn, gnawing, and occurring with regular periodicity. Berkley Moyihan[23] have described the rhythm of gastric ulcer pain as follows: Food, comfort, pain, comfort and then again food, comfort, pain, comfort; of duodenal ulcer it is food, comfort,

pain and then again food, comfort, pain. The pain is usually relieved by antacid or a glass of milk. Occasionally the distress induces vomiting and this always relieves. Pain is believed to be caused by abnormal peristalsis and pylorospasm which are relieved when the acid is neutralized. Hyper-secretion after meals and at night is characteristic of peptic ulcer and it is as much a part of the disease as the ulcer itself. Consequently a knowledge of the acid secretion in the individual case is of value and the gastric analysis is important in the diagnosis and treatment. In the typical duodenal ulcer the acidity curve after test meal, in comparison with normal, is much higher and more sustained. Gastric acidity readings alone are not diagnostic.

Duodenal ulcer may occur in the normal range of gastric acidity between 20 and 50 and gastric ulcers occur frequently without hyperacidity. Free acid values above 50 indicate hyperchlorhydria. It is in this level that duodenal ulcers occur frequently and gastric ulcers may occur. But even with hyperacidity, ulcer may be absent. If the free acidity remains below 20, hypochlorhydria exists and duodenal ulcer is improbable. Gastric ulcers may occur at this level. If free acid is consistently absent from the gastric juice, ulcer does not occur. If correctly evaluated, the gastric analysis then is an important diagnostic aid without which a diagnosis of ulcer is not sound.

The x-ray is the most important single procedure in diagnosis[24]. It should include both fluoroscopy and films; with a small amount of barium the mucosa pattern is studied first and the wavy parallel longitudinal folds of gastric mucosa are visualized. With the stomach filled with barium the gastric outlines are studied fluoroscopically for projections and areas of rigidity or fixation. The diagnosis of peptic ulcer is practically certain when a characteristic crater is demonstrated. Gastric ulcers tend to occur along the lesser curvature so it is usually not difficult to bring the profile of the barium filled niche into view. With small amounts of barium the enlarged rugae may be seen radiating from the city of the ulcer. The demonstration of an ulcer crater in the duodenum is more difficult but has the same diagnostic significance. The use of the pressure cone or spot film technique makes it possible in some instances to demonstrate craters which are not seen in the routine examinations.

The demonstration of occult bleeding is at times of diagnostic value, but it is not essential for the diagnosis of active ulcer, indeed occult blood is usually absent from the stool. Not infrequently, however, marked anemia is seen in patients who have not vomited blood or observed passage of tarry stools. Thus the value of feces examinations and blood count.

TREATMENT

The management of a patient with simple uncomplicated peptic ulcer whether gastric or duodenal must by necessity be treated on an empirical rather than on a rational basis, the etiology and pathogenesis of the affection being unknown. Many programs have been evolved but until the disturbances responsible for its occurrence and until its pathological physiology are determined, none of the procedures can be regarded as on a truly scientific basis. The principles of therapy are based on results and varied experiences.

Rest is the primary principle of treatment. Three to six weeks period of hospital care is desirable. This improves the patient's general health, promotes healing and the patient learns to follow a regime. The physical and nervous relaxation obtained with bed rest, in congenial surroundings, is the important factor which promotes a return to normal gastric physiology. The outdoors, fresh air and sunshine are helpful measures.

The second principle is a diet which does not mechanically injure new formed mucosa, stimulate gastric secretion or interfere with motility and yet supply an adequate amount of protein, vitamins and minerals.

The third principle is the neutralization of acid and gastric juice. If this is kept neutralized or at a low level, healing of the ulcer is promoted. Hourly milk and cream, supplies protein which neutralizes acid, and fat, which depresses gastric secretion. The Sippy diet consisting of additional feeding of albuminous foods, largely milk and egg dishes, at two hour intervals supplies calories and furnishes constant neutralization of acid. Rest and diet will relieve symptoms for many patients without any supplementary measures to control acidity. Complete neutralization is not necessary for healing in many cases, but there are some that require antacid drugs for relief of distress and for healing of the ulcer. For efficient neutralization a non-absorbable antacid like aluminum hydroxide gel can be prescribed. The usual dose is 2 teaspoonsful. Neutralization therapy in the hospital is based upon the chemical reaction of the acid juice. Frequent stomach aspiration may be used to determine the effectiveness of the treatment and serve as a guide for adequate dosage. The amount of night secretion of acid should be estimated and controlled. Before the patient is discharged the regime is changed to three meals a day, the menu is quite liberal. For breakfast there may be orange juice, eggs, bacon, toast, butter, jelly and coffee. For main meal at noon, creamed soup, lamb chop, bread, butter, baked potato, puree vegetables, pudding and milk. The evening meal should be lighter: Milk-toast, gelatin or cooked fruits, sponge cake and milk. The regime of milk and cream with raw eggs or antacid is continued between meals for six months to a year. In a year's time milk only is used between meals and an antacid at bedtime. Alcoholic beverages are taboo, alcohol is a strong stimulant to acid secretion. As to tobacco it is said that after smoking the average acidity is definitely higher. Theoretically nicotine may also cause capillary spasm in the ulcer bearing area. Recurrent flare ups of ulcer activity are often associated with acute infections. Ulcer patients should then be put to bed and maintain complete ulcer regime for the duration of any acute illness. Rest and recreation are important and the psychological factors should not be neglected for at present time, great emphasis is being placed on the psycho-somatic medicine, in general. Briefly then we should strive to obtain relief from pain, relief from physical, mental, emotional strain and adequate nutrition[25]. Lt. Col Garnett Cheney[26] outlined a new type of ulcer diet on the basis of a deficiency of an anti-ulcer factor designated as vitamin U, known to be effective in preventing or curing gastric ulcer in experimental animals. The special dietary regime was based on the usual convalescent or gastric ulcer diet with the addition of certain specific substances known to contain the anti-ulcer factor. The diet included six eggs daily, two soft boiled eggs for breakfast and four uncooked in egg nog as shown in the sample diet. 50 grams of butter, 30 grams of peanut butter, 30 cc. of olive oil and certain fresh greens were also included. In addition to these specific foods the patient also received one helping of tender meat and orange juice and tomato juice daily and soft vegetables were not pureed. The diet consisted of protein 150 grams, carbohydrates 50 grams, and fat 200 grams for a total of 4200 calories. With this diet were administered special medications: Cerophyl tablets, made from green grass stalks and rich in anti-ulcer factor, were given daily; stomach extract in the form of ventriculin was also given. Bile salts were given not only to promote the absorption of the fat soluble factor, but also because it possibly has an anti-ulcer factor similar to cerophyl and ventriculin. No other medical therapy was given except an occasional alkaline powder and a mild sedative at bedtime. This type of treatment was used on individuals with a diagnosis of gastric or duodenal ulcer who have not responded satisfactorily to previous conventional anti-ulcer therapy of restricted diet, antacids, anti-spasmodics and sedatives. Eighty-seven per cent of the patients treated with the above regime of Cheney were clearly benefitted and the author concluded that the result suggests a disturbance in nutrition may be a factor in percipitating symptoms or in retarding healing in certain cases of peptic ulcer.

PATHOLOGY

The clinical course and complications of peptic ulcer are inherently associated with the pathologic anatomy of the lesion. A section through an acute ulcer shows the destruction of the mucous membrane with formation of a shallow crater. The base is covered by a fibrinopurulent exudate. The muscle layer is not involved. In a chronic ulcer, a deep crater is found involving the mucous membrane and extending down through the muscularis. Over-hanging edges and a large amount of blue staining connective tissue about the lesion are characteristic. Healing of an ulcer begins with epithelialization of the floor of the crater. Connective tissue fills in beneath and around the ulcer which decreases in size and depth until only a depression in the mucosal surface remains. This marked scar tissue reaction is responsible for the anatomical distortion associated with chronic ulcer. The development of a chronic callous ulcer begins with a devitalized area which is eroded to form a crater. The contraction of scar tissue causes a drawing in of the duodenal wall.

MANAGEMENT OF COMPLICATIONS

The clinically important complications of peptic ulcer are: Perforation, hemorrhage, stenosis and malignant degeneration. Of these, perforation is primarily surgical, but the internist must make the diagnosis promptly before referring the patient to a competent surgeon. Crile and Crile noted the incidence of perforation in 8 per cent of their series of cases of ulcer, 59 per cent are duodenal perforations, 26 per cent gastric and pyloric 15 per cent. If the ulcer is on the posterior wall there is extension into the pancreas. A large majority of acute perforations occur while the patient is at work, it rarely happens while at rest or while the patient is following treatment. If the gastric ulcer perforates posteriorly or into the gastro-hepatic omentum a localized abscess connecting with the stomach results. Pain which is not controlled by the usual therapeutic measures, tenderness, fever and leukocytosis are common manifestations. Perforation of an anterior wall ulcer permits sudden outburst of gastric contents into the free abdominal cavity. There is sudden agonizing pain, profound shock, characteristic board-like rigidity of the abdomen. The diagnosis is supported by history of indigestion and by x-ray of the abdomen in the upright position, which shows free gas under the diaphragm. Immediate operation is indicated.

OBSTRUCTION

Pyloric obstruction is one of the complications that result from chronic ulcer with cicatrix formation. The outstanding symptom of this condition is vomiting of large quantities of stomach content at fairly regular intervals. The stomach may retain food for several days and become markedly dilated. When this difficulty is of long standing and is the result of rigid scarring of the chronic ulcer, surgical relief is necessary.

HEMORRHAGE

According to T. Grier Miller[27], hemorrhage is as strictly a medical problem as is perforation a surgical one. The results from medical management of bleeding peptic ulcer are now so satisfactory, that only in the rarest instances is there any justification for an immediate surgical consultation and that when some additional complication is suspected. Later when the bleeding has ceased operation is frequently indicated, especially if more than one hemorrhage has occurred. From 20 to 25 per cent of all patients with ulcer experience massive bleeding at some period. The prompt feeding regime for the treatment of bleeding ulcer, advocated by Lenhartz, by Adresen and in 1934 by Meulengracht, has been adopted in many clinics throughout this country. Soper of St. Louis has condemned the procedure as unscientific and yet reliable statistics by Miller, Elsom, Finsterer, Kirshner and Palmer show a much lowered death rate from hemorrhage. Fatal hemorrhage is practically always arterial in origin. It is inevitable that death will occur in a few cases of bleeding ulcer, usually those older people who have a large open sclerotic vessel in the base of the ulcer. But on the basis of analogy it would seem that the number is exceedingly small, surely far less than would result if surgery were employed in all of these severe cases. Furthermore, it would seem possible to explain the lessened mortality in promptly fed cases, as compared to those treated by starvation, on the basis of an adequate diet which maintains nutrition throughout the period of shock, of a sufficient fluid intake, which also combats shock and a freedom from anxiety which has been a marked characteristic of all the cases treated by prompt feeding. When the patient is fed, it is rarely necessary to use morphine which has a tendency to keep the gastric duodenal musculature relaxed. Whatever the explanation the present results seem definitely to justify the so-called Meulengracht regime[28]. In addition to the prompt feeding, blood transfusions, blood plasma, amigen, ferrous sulfate and sodium luminal are used as indicated; the latter is preferred instead of morphine. In such a program the bleeding may continue for some days, but since the patient is comfortable, is not in shock and the blood loss can be cared for by transfusions, one should not lose confidence in the regime. Eventually in almost all cases the hemorrhage ceases. In order to detect continued or repeated hemorrhage, the blood pressure and pulse rate are recorded every half hour. A fall in blood pressure and rise in pulse rate occur coincident with a hemorrhage. If there is no further bleeding normal levels are gradually restored. Persistent hemorrhage in spite of treatment is extremely serious. The high risk of surgery under these circumstances must be accepted when the ligation of the bleeding vessel becomes of the utmost urgency.

MALIGNANCY

The complication of malignant degeneration in a peptic ulcer deserves appropriate emphasis, since the mere suspicion of such a change is always an indication for prompt surgical removal of the affected area. Fortunately only gastric ulcers become malignant and a relatively small percentage of them, perhaps not more than 5 to 10 per cent. Palmer[29] doubts if any peptic ulcer, primarily benign, ever develops this complication, believing that the malignant ones are so from the beginning. In any event, malignant ulcer of the stomach with roentgenological findings that cannot be differentiated from those of a benign lesion, does occur and so in treating every gastric ulcerative lesion, the possibility of malignancy of the gastric ulcer must be different from that of the duodenal one. Every such gastric case should be re-examined roentgenologically after two or three weeks and, unless all the indications are then favorable, the patient should be hospitalized for another short period of medical therapy on a stricter basis and for a complete examination. Unless the latter investigation and a third x-ray study clearly suggest that the lesion is benign, he should be subjected to surgery. Additional x-ray and gastroscopic follow-up should be had from time to time, until the lesion has healed.

From this general review of the medical aspect of peptic ulcer it is hoped that certain important features have been adequately emphasized, namely: The increasing incidence, the unsettled pathogenesis, the basis for adequate and effective treatment and the early recognition of the more serious complications.

BIBLIOGRAPHY

1. Bockus: Gastro-Enterology; Volume No. 1, page 318.
2. H. Tidy: Increase of Peptic Ulcer in 20 Years: British Medical Journal, pp. 473-477; October, 1943; A.J.D D., pp. 15-22; January, 1944; British Medical Journal, Volume No. 1, pp. 319-324; March 10, 1945.
3. Portis: Disease of the Digestive System, page 478; 1941.
   R. Reeser and M. Guthrie: Management of Army Personnel with Peptic Ulcer, pp. 125-126; Military Surgeon, February, 1946.
4. P. H. Wilcox: Gastric Distress in the Services: British Medical Journal, Volume No. 1, pp. 1008-1012; June 22, 1940.
   D. N. Stewart and D. M. Wisener: Incidence of Perforated Peptic Ulcer: Effect of Heavy Air Raids: Lancet, Volume No. 1, page 259; February 28, 1942.

H. Tidy (See 2), F. A. Jones and H. Pollak: Civilian Dyspepsia: British Medical Journal, Volume No. 1, pp. 797-800; June 9, 1945.
5. W. R. Feasley. Peptic Ulcer in the Canadian Army 1940-44: War Medicine, Volume No. 6, page 300; November, 1944
6. E. Miller: The Neuroses in War: New York McMillan Company; 1940.
7. J. W. Hinton: Incidence of Peptic Ulcer and Its Complications: American Journal Surgery, Volume No. 20, page 102; April, 1933.
   A. Hurst: American Journal of Digestive Diseases, Volume No. 8, page 321; September, 1941
   William Brockbank: The Dyspeptic Soldider: Lancet, Volume No. 1, pp. 30-42; Year Book of Medicine, page 707; January 10, 1942.
8. J. L. Kantor: Digestive Diseases and Military Medicine: Journal American Medical Association, Volume No 5, page 391; November, 1941; Volume No. 120, page 254; September 26, 192.
9. R. W. Urquart: Peptic Ulcer Problem: Canadian Medical Journal, Volume No. 43, page 391; November, 1941.
10 D. T. Chamberlin and W. C. Wallace: Perforated Peptic Ulcer in an Army General Hospital. Military Surgeon, Volume No. 92, page 193; February, 1943
    W. L. Palmer: The Stomach and Military Service: Journal American Medical Association, Volume No. 119, page 1155; August 3, 1942.
11 H Tidy: (See 2)
12. R. C. Kirk: Peptic Ulcer at Fort Sill: American Journal of Digestive Diseases, Volume No. 10, page 411; November, 1943.
    D. T. Chamberlin: Peptic Ulcers and Irritable Colon in the Army: American Journal of Digestive Diseases, Volume No. 9, pp. 245-248; August, 1942.
    A. Rush: Gastro Intestinal Disturbances in Combat Area: Journal American Medical Association, Volume No. 123, page 389; October 16, 1943.
    H. Schildkrant: Management of the Dyspeptic Soldier in a Staging Area: War Medicine, Volume No. 6, page 151; September, 1941.
    L. Setzel: Experience with Peptic Ulcer in an Army Station Hospital: Gastro-Enterology, Volume No. 3, page 472; December, 1944.
    Lt. Col. J. W. Hall, Jr.: Benign Peptic Ulcer as a Diagnostic Problem: Military Surgeon, Volume No. 120; February, 1946.
13. H. Tidy: (See 2)
1. J. E. Berk and A. W. Frediani: Peptic Ulcer Problem in the Army: Gastro-Enterology, Volume No. 3, page 435; December, 1944. (See 3)
15. W. Walters and H. R. Butt: Management of Peptic Ulcers Among Naval Personnel: Annals of Surgery, Volume No. 118, page 489; October, 1943.
16. Portis: Disease of Digestive System, page 482; 1941.
    Brockus: Gastro-Enterology, Volume No. 1, page 328.
17. A. C. Ivy: The Prevention and Recurrance of Peptic Ulcer, An Experimental Study: Gastro-Enterology, Volume No. 3, pp. 443-449; December, 1944.
    L. J. Hay, R. L. Varco, C. F. Code and O. H. Wagensteen: Experimental Production of Gastric and Duodenal Ulcers: Surgery, Gynecology and Obstetrics, Volume No. 75, pp. 170-182; August, 1942. (Year Book of Medicine, page 681; 1942)
18. W. C. Alveres: Ways in Which Emotions Can Affect the Digestive Tract: Journal American Medical Association, Volume No. 92, page 1231; April 13, 1929.
19. F. A. Jones and H. Pollak: Civilian Dyspepsia: Year Book of General Medicine, page 624; 1945.
20. H. R. Hartman: Neurogenic Factors in Peptic Ulcer: Medical Clinics of North America, Volume No. 16, page 1357; May, 1933.
    Portis: Page 215; 1941.
    Ensterman: Year Book, General Medicine, page 625; 1944.
21. Kogan and V. M. Yanay: Klinicheskaya Meditsina, Volume No. 22, pp. 12-15; 1944 American Review of Soviet Medicine, Volume No. 2, pp. 233-287; February, 1945. Year Book of Medicine, page 676; 1944.
22. Harry Shay: Pathologic Physiology of Gastric and Duodenal Ulcer: Bulletin of New York Academy of Medicine, Volume No. 20, pp. 264-291; May, 1944. Year Book of Medicine, page 676; 1944.
23. Bockus: Gastro-Enterology: Vlume No. 1, page 374.
24. Ibid: Page 384.
25. T. Grier Miller: Medical Clinics of North America, Volume No. 403; March, 1944.
26. Lt. Col. Garnett Cheney: Peptic Ulcer and Nutrition: Military Surgeon, Volume No. 446; December, 1944.
    V. J. Gianelli and V. Bellofiore: Medical Clinics of North America, Volume No. 20, pp. 706-713; May, 1945 (Quarterly). Revista de Medecine, page 113; November, 1945.
27. T. G. Miller and K. A. Elsom: The Management of Massive Hemorrhage from Peptic Ulcer: Medical Clinics of North America, Volume No. 22, pp. 1711-1783; November, 1938.
28. Bockus: Gastro-Enterology, Special Procedures in the Management of Massive Hemorrhage, Volume No. 1, page 603.
29. W. L. Palmer: Benign and Malignant Gastric Ulcer: Annals of Internal Medicine, Volume No. 13, page 317; August, 1939.
    W. L. Palmer and E. M. Humphrey: Gastric Carcinoma:

Clinical Pathological Conference

University of Oklahoma School of Medicine.

Presented by the Departments of Pathology and Urology

ROBERT AKIN, M.D.—HOWARD C. HOPPS, M.D.

OKLAHOMA CITY, OKLAHOMA

DOCTOR HOPPS: The case for consideration this morning illustrates some of the difficulties which the urologist frequently encounters in his patients. The primary disease from which this man suffered is obvious to us all after studying the protocol. Our primary concern here is to determine the various complications which arose in this case, the mechanicism of their development and, in retrospect, to see what might have been done to save this man's life. Dr. Akin will present the clinical aspects of the case.

PROTOCOL

Patient: T.F.T., white male, age 59; admitted May 22, 1945, died June 11, 1945.

Chief Complaint: Bilateral costovertebral pain, nocturia and "interrupted urinary stream".

Present Illness: The patient stated that for the last ten years he had had intermittent attacks of costovertebral pain. These were mild, early, but in the last three years they had become much more severe. They were sharp and cutting, lasting a few minutes and followed by dull pain for a day or more in the costovertebral angles. An x-ray examination made in Tulsa, Oklahoma, one month before admission had revealed kidney stones, and the patient was referred to the University Hospitals.

Past and Family History: Noncontributory except for past history related above.

Physical Examination: This well developed, well nourished man appeared to be of the stated age of 59 years. He did not appear acutely ill. The head, chest, and heart were negative. The blood pressure was 115/70, pulse rate 70 and regular. The abdomen was negative. There was no tenderness in the C-V angles. The prostate was of normal size. The genitalia were normal.

Laboratory Data: The urine had a specific gravity of 1.022 and was acid. There was no albumin nor glucose. The sediment contained many white blood cells and an occasional red blood cell, but no casts. The hemoglobin was 11 Gm. with 4,100,000 red blood cells and 11,-600 white blood cells with 78 per cent neutrophils. A roentgenogram on May 23, 1945 revealed bilateral urinary calculi.

Clinical Course: After an uneventful period, the patient underwent a left nephrolithotomy on June 6, 1945. He went into shock during the operation, but recovered following supportive therapy. Penicillin therapy was begun. On June 8, 1945 he vomited his lunch and developed abdominal distention. A Wangensteen apparatus was inserted and was kept in place. His condition was poor. On the afternoon of June 11, 1945 the patient suddenly became much worse. His temperature was 106 (R), his pulse rate 152 and his respiratory rate 56, with a blood pressure of 40/10. He was gasping and cyanotic, and complained of epigastric pain. Crepitant rales were heard over the right lung base. In spite of plasma and stumulants, he died seven hours later.

CLINICAL DIAGNOSIS

DOCTOR AKIN: This patient entered our hospital with a diagnosis of renal lithiasis, a diagnosis which was promptly confirmed by our roentgenographic studies. I should emphasize that we performed intravenous pyelograms and that we never seriously considered retrograde studies because so often, in cases of this sort, if ureteral catheters are introduced into the renal pelvis, one may dislodge small calculi which may then produce an acute ureteral obstruction, ureteral colic etc. A cystoscopic examination was done and we observed a moderate excretion of dye from the left ureter, but none from the right from which we concluded that the right kidney had little function. The patient had complained of more pain on the right side than on the left and our x-ray visualization indicated that stones were more numerous and more widely scattered on the right side. On the left side there were about nine stones contained, for the most part, in the lower portion of the pelvis and the calices at the lower pole. For these reasons a left nephrolithotomy was performed and nine stones were removed. It was necessary also to make an incision in the pelvis in order to remove a large stone present here. The major question in clinical management was whether or not to treat this man conservatively with various chemotherapeutic agents and with supportive therapy. If he had not had this severe pain it would have been our choice to have followed the conservative course. It was our opinion however that if we could remove the stones from that kidney with the best renal function we would provide some relief from pain and, at the same time, reduce the possibility of subsequent renal failure and death from uremia. I am quite sure that there was already established a severe infection of the right kidney, whereas on the left the infection complicating lithiasis was not so extensive. It was my feeling that removal of the stones would provide a much better opportunity for penicillin to alleviate this infection in the left kidney. Had the patient responded in the manner that we anticipated we would probably have done a right nephrectomy at some later date inasmuch as the only function of this kidney was in serving as a serious focus of infection.

CLINICAL DISCUSSION

QUESTION: What about the occurrence of hypertension in patients such as this?

DOCTOR AKIN: That's a problem that is very difficult to evaluate. Experimentally there is no question but that renal ischemia may cause hypertension and I see many instances of renal hypertension in my practice. The peculiar thing however is that we see patients, such as this one for instance, who certainly must have renal ischemia and yet there is no hypertension. On the other hand we see patients with what may appear to be an almost identical renal lesion which is associated with hypertension. I have concerned myself with this problem for some time and must admit that in the case of many types of renal disease I know of no criterion by which the renal lesion can be evaluated as to whether it will or will not cause hypertension. I should say about this particular case that approximately half of patients such as this will exhibit hypertension. I should like to hear more about this from Dr. Hopps.

DOCTOR HOPPS: The first thing we must consider in this problem is whether or not the lesion in question actually produces renal ischemia. This is a very difficult thing to evaluate clinically since the size and shape of the kidney or the extent of pelvic dilatation need not correlate directly with renal ischemia. Furthermore, it has been adequately demonstrated that biologic variation within a single species allows a wide variation in the *extent* of renal ischemia tolerated before hypertension complicates the picture. I believe that it is this latter consideration which explains the variation described by Dr. Akin. I should say that the renal physiologists have devised methods by which glomerular blood flow, tubular mass, etc. can be accurately evaluated. Such observations are of course clinical and give us very valuable information. They are too elaborate for general use however.

QUESTION: In regard to the origin of renal stones in this case, do you think that a primary metabolic disturbance was at fault?

DOCTOR AKIN: The serum calcium was 11 and the phosphorus 3 mg. per cent in this case. This is probably within the normal range and although it is rather a crude index to mineral metabolism it tends to eliminate such gross metabolic abnormalities as would result from an adenoma of the parathyroid gland etc. In most cases of this sort, obstruction and/or infection are important from a causative standpoint. Such causes, if they existed, were obscured at the time we saw this patient. We cannot rule out a metabolic factor.

ANATOMIC DIAGNOSIS

DOCTOR HOPPS: Our first objective was to find the thing that actually precipitated death. Terminally, there was a marked rise in temperature and, according to the clinical history, the terminal event was of short duration. From this data we anticipated the possibility of pulmonary embolism and we were not disappointed. Although the pulmonary artery proper was widely patent and contained only fluid blood, both the left and right major pulmonary branches were completely obstructed by thrombotic emboli. These were composed of several fragments which, when unfolded, represented a total length of 24 cm. with a maximum diameter of 1.5 cm. A 28 cm. thrombus of similar appearance was expressed from the right iliac and femoral veins. There was no evidence of phlebitis here, nor was the right leg edematous. Pulmonary embolism is much more often a complication of phlebothrombosis than of thrombophlebitis for two reasons: (1) the very fact that there is inflammation allows, as a rule, for more rapid fixation of the thrombus by fibrous tissue extending from the vein wall into the thrombus and (2) with thrombophlebitis there is pain and edema which allows early recognition of the lesion and treatment either by rigid mobilization of the part or ligation of the affected vein at a point above the site of thrombosis. In our clinical pathologic conferences we have presented a number of cases of fatal pulmonary embolism and I hope that it brings about a constant realization of the importance of this problem. Pulmonary embolism is, I believe, the most important complication following abdominal operations and yet there is a great deal which can be done to prevent such tragedies.

To turn our attention to the kidneys, exactly how much damage had resulted from the renal lithiasis and infection? How much renal ischemia had resulted? Is there a reason why this man should or should not have had hypertension? The one blood pressure of 115/78 given in the protocol may mean nothing in so far as previous history is concerned. A week or a month before his blood pressure might have been 250/130. We often see a dramatic reduction of blood pressure in patients who are acutely ill and who are suffering moderate cardiac or peripherovascular failure. From our necropsy findings we can state, with considerable assurance however, that this man did not have a significant degree of hypertension. His heart weighed 300 grams which is, if anything, slightly less than normal. Any time a person has hypertension which persists for at least a few months there will result either cardiac hypertrophy or dilatation and failure. Furthermore we have another valuable criterion for the postmortem diagnosis of hypertension in the development of a very characteristic hyperplastic "sclerosis" of arterioles and small arteries. Such changes were not exhibited by this patient. I emphasize the hypertensive aspect of this case because, in my mind, this is by far the most interesting problem here. Frankly, from an evaluation of the kidneys alone I would have been willing to make a sizeable wager (and give odds) that this man did have hypertension, and yet I am completely satisfied that such was not the case. The right kidney had been converted to a thin walled multilocular sac filled with stones. In many areas the parenchyma was thinned to 2 or 3 mm. The left kidney appeared markedly swollen and dark red. The bulk of this, however, was made up of clotted blood lying between the renal capsule and the parenchymal surface. I shall not give a detailed histopathological description. Suffice it to say that the right kidney was practically functionless as Dr. Akin had assumed and that the left exhibited considerable interstitial fibrosis with marked parenchymal damage—the result of old healed and chronic active pyelonephritis. There was every indication of rather severe renal ischemia in this single functioning kidney and by all the rules and regulations that I know, this man *should* have had hypertension.

DISCUSSION

DOCTOR AKIN: Why do you think this man developed thrombosis of the femoral vein?

DOCTOR HOPPS: I believe that we have pretty well ruled out an infectious basis. The patient was kept quiet in bed, he had had a major operation which involved trauma to a lot of tissue and he, during his operation, suffered a severe drop in blood pressure. This furnishes adequate basis for (a) slowed circulation and (b) increased clotting tendency of the blood. It was probably a combination of these two factors that allowed the phlebothrombosis which ultimately caused the patient's death.

DOCTOR HALPERT: Phlebothrombosis is considerably more common in the left iliac and femoral veins (as in this case) because the left common iliac vein runs behind the artery and is thus compressed. This favors a slowed circulation.

DOCTOR AKIN: It is becoming increasingly popular to use an anticoagulant such as dicoumarol to forestall such complications as this case illustrates. I have not used them in cases of this sort because of the great hazard of postoperative bleeding. This is especially true following transurethral resection of the prostate.

QUESTION: Have you used fibrin foam in these cases?

DOCTOR AKIN: No, I have not.

DOCTOR HOPPS: Regarding the use of anticoagulants in cases such as these, coagulation time does not have to be markedly elevated. Many reports indicate that a relatively slight increase, one that carries very little hazard in so far as postoperative hemorrhage is concerned, is usually enough to shift the balance against thrombus formation.

DOCTOR AKIN: This case poses a very important research problem and one that might well fall within the scope of the proposed research institute at the School of Medicine. That problem concerns the formation of urinary calculi. It is all very well to speak about the role of calcium, phosphates, urates etc. in such formation, but the matter is much more complex than that. Its solution probably lies in the field of colloidal chemistry in that it isn't so much what the stone is composed of as what holds it together and allows its continued growth as a solid constituent rather than the precipitation of fine particulate matter which could easily be swept out by the urine.

Former Gorham Man Stabed in Throat
Dr. Don D. Cornell, 39, a physician at Gorham from November, 1942, to June, 1943, was found dead on the highway at Milton, Mass., Friday, April 5, a stab wound in his throat, the Associated Press reported. Dr. George Dalton, Milton medical examiner, said a scalpel was found near the body and that he would perform an autopsy. Police at first believed Dr. Cornell was the victim of a hit-and-run driver.

Special Article

Improved Distribution of Medical Care [*]

VICTOR JOHNSON, PHD., M.D.,

Secretary, Council on Medical Education and Hospitals
American Medical Association
and
Professorial Lecturer in Physiology
University of Chicago

CHICAGO, ILLINOIS

Introduction: Mr. President, graduates of the University of Oklahoma School of Medicine, ladies and gentlemen: Probably few if any convocation statements addressed to graduates in medicine fail to link the concepts of high privilege on the one hand and heavy responsibility on the other. In this I too shall adhere to tradition although much of what I wish to discuss is controversial and too new to constitute tradition. Although you who are graduating encountered the difficulties of acceleration, increased enrollments under depleted faculties, and uncertainties regarding your immediate future, your privileges were several. You were judged qualified to enter professional studies in a field where the competition for places is unequalled elsewhere; for every two students admitted to medical schools in this country, three applicants are judged unqualified and fail to gain admission. Furthermore, you studied in a country whose medical education is unexcelled anywhere in the world. The destruction of educational facilities by the war is only partly responsible for this condition. Recently Dr. Wilburt C. Davidson, dean of Duke University School of Medicine, who has had wide experience in European medical schools over a period of years, stated[1] that in Germany, too long regarded as the mecca for graduate and postgraduate instruction, medical education has been static for over thirty years. Very few countries abroad provide even an approximation to what medical students, interns and residents in this country take for granted. In the war just finished, there was an extremely low death rate from disease and wounds in our armed forces. This is ascribed by Dr. Perrin Long[2] of Johns Hopkins University, not to sulfa drugs (the development of which has depended so much on Dr. Long's research) or to penicillin or plasma, but primarily it was due to the high caliber and excellent education of our medical

officers. Without belaboring this point of your privileges, I may also state that medical education in this country occupied an especially favorable position by comparison with the sciences generally. The army forces and the Selective Service System of this country, unlike England or Russia, for example, have unwisely prevented the training of science students generally, and for the past two years, of premedical students as well. Of all the peacetime educational pursuits, that of medicine (in addition to theology) was recognized even by the military, even in this country, as an indispensible educational program despite the waging of total war with its tremendous manpower demands.

The companion of your privilege, your responsibility, is equally great. The challenge you face is larger than that faced in past years, for you are responsible not only for the practice and advancement of the profession and science of medicine, but for the solution of a major social problem as well; an improved distribution of medical care, so that the services of hospitals and physicians will be available to all who need and want them.

Maldistribution of Medical Care: The war brought the maldistribution of medical care into sharp focus, since approximately half of the actively practicing physicians in the United States were employed in caring for the ten or eleven million men in the armed forces, leaving the other half, consisting mainly of older age groups and the physically less qualified or active physicians, to care for 120 million people, eleven or twelve times the numbers in the armed forces. The overall shortage of civilian physicians was aggravated by acute local deficiencies. Initially, the strong-arm recruiting policies of the Army and Navy left large areas with far too few or no physicians. It was easiest for the armed forces to recruit officers from economically ill-favored areas, where previous shortages

[*] Convocation address, University of Oklahoma School of Medicine, Oklahoma City, Oklahoma, March 22, 1946.

were most pronounced. Consequently, those states which could least spare physicians provided their quotas of medical officers earliest and exceeded them with alarming rapidity. This hand-to-mouth policy of the military was later checked by the Procurement and Assignment Service for Physicians, by curbing wholesale recruitment of medical officers from medically deficient areas and stimulating it in areas with higher physician-population ratios.

Although the maldistribution of physicians and medical care was accentuated by the war, it has always existed and will remain a problem to be solved even now when the war is over and physicians are returning to civilian life so rapidly that two-thirds of the medical officers will have been discharged in less than a year after V-E day.

The availability of physicians and medical care geographically is largely an economic problem; a listing of the states in the order of increasing ratios of hospital beds to population serves also as a listing of states in the order of increasing per capita income. The poorer states and counties have fewer physicians and hospitals than the richer, just as they have fewer cars, telephones and bathtubs. Similarly, the rural communities, in general, can support fewer physicians than the economically more favored urban centers, unless assisted financially.

This economic problem is much more complicated than simply that of physician income. The state, county or area unable to provide a physician with an adequate income is also unable to provide other things, some of which may be more important to the physician than income alone. Medically deficient areas are likely also to lack homes, schools and churches of good quality as well as good stores and roads; there is likely also to be a dearth of stimulating professional and intellectual contacts. It is important to remember that these factors may influence the location of a physician fully as much as the size of his income or even the presence or absence of hospitals and other facilities for the diagnosis and care of the sick.

Apart from these factors, the mere density of the population, rich or poor, influences the distribution of physicians especially in the case of specialists. A physician who has spent years of training in surgery will not locate in a region whose population is too sparse to provide sufficient cases requiring surgical attention. His surgical skill and judgment deteriorate unless they are employed constantly. Within the area served by the specialist there must be enough pregnant women to occupy an obstetrician and enough sick children to occupy the pediatrician.

The attack upon these problems, which you These generalities apply no matter how wealthy the iinhabitants of the area may be. as physicians must make, should be in more than one direction. Construction of hospitals, diagnostic facilities and public health units on the one hand, are the most important and most promising developments currently occupying the attention and efforts of physicians and others interested in improving the quality of medical care in this country.

Hospital Surveys and Construction: Representing the American Medical Association, its House of Delegates, its Board of Trustees and its membership of 125,700 physicians, I appeared before the Senate Committee on Education and Labor a year ago, and the House Committee on Interstate and Foreign Commerce two weeks ago in support of the Hill-Burton Hospital Survey and Construction Act. This measure has passed the Senate and may pass the House and become law. The bill provides for a program of federal-state collaboration to survey local hospital needs by the states, to develop comprehensive state plans for hospital construction to meet these needs, and to give financial assistance to the states to carry out the plans. The bill provides for the allotment of 375 millions of dollars over a five year period for the construction and equipment of hospitals and public health centers; this sum will be supplemented by state funds, on a sliding scale depending on the financial resources and the needs of the various states. In all, probably more than a half billion dollars will be expended in this program in the next five years should the measure become law. This figure may be compared with an estimated evaluation of five billions of dollars for the 6611 hospitals (with 1,729,945 beds) in this country listed as registered hospitals by the Council on Medical Education and Hospitals of the American Medical Association. It has further been estimated that these hospitals will spend at least a half billion dollars and perhaps a billion dollars for expansion and replacement when materials become available. No one knows the construction and equipment costs of entirely new hospitals now being planned independently of federal aid. Such funds from private sources will supplement the considerably smaller sum provided for construction of new hospitals under the program of the Hill-Burton Bill. There has been a criticism that the federal contributions under this bill are inadequate to meet the needs. The obvious answer to this belief is that no one knows now just what the needs are in the various states, counties and communities.

Fortunately the sponsors and supporters of the Hill-Burton bill recognize this important fact and there is incorporated into the measure the requirement that construction funds will be allocated to a state only after the state has surveyed its hospital needs and presented an acceptable state-wide construction program. This feature of the bill alone, for which five millions of dollars are provided by the federal government, makes the measure worth while and warrants its becoming law. Anticipating passage of the act, several states have already embarged on hospital surveys and more have authorized them. Such surveys and subsequent planning are recognized by physicians to be a scientific approach to the problem, without which effective action is unlikely. The survey and planning provisions of the Hill-Burton bill can well set a pattern for federal participation in solving other problems of medical care.

Because the program is experimental in nature, because the needs can be determined only by scientific surveys, the funds allotted should be reasonably restriced to prevent a vast program of construction of hospitals which are not needed or cannot be maintained. A major effort in this program must be exerted in the direction of inhibition. Already we have encountered an avalanche of local demands for new hospitals, dictated as often by local pride as by real need. There is a tendency for every community to think it should have its own small hospital, with complete disregard for the fact that three nearby communities would be better served by one hospital of 150 beds than by three separate hospitals of fifty beds, as is also true of schools, for example.

Insurance for Costs of Hospitalization: The insurance principal of spreading costs of emergencies over periods of time and numbers of people is as characteristic of our country as the Ford and the Frigidaire. We insure against death, old age, accident, fire, hail, wind, steam and water; theft, burglarly, and mysterious disappearance; injury to others, property damage, illness of livestock and malpractice suits; war, shipwreck, and sundry and assorted other so-called "acts of God". Hospitalization is now an important member of this growing list of life's undesirable and costly eventualities, and prepayment insurance to cover hospital costs has grown at a phenomenal rate. In 1937 only 700,000 people were enrolled in group hospitalization plans. Eight years later, in 1945, the Blue Cross plans alone had thirty times this number, or 20,000,000[3]. It is now estimated that 40,000,000 people in the United States, nearly one in every three, are covered by some form of health and accident insurance[4]. Most of these insured are covered for hospitalization only. But the rapid expansion of such insurance promises well for programs to extend hospital coverage to include at least the most expensive forms of medical care as well.

Prepaid Medical Care: The growth of medical care plans in recent years, as compared with hospitalization insurance, is equally phenomenal, although the total figures reached are not as large, since such prepayment plans are more recent in origin and present more complications in their operation. It is relatively easy to establish a plan of hospitalization insurance, since costs of hospitalization can be pretty well standardized and predicted. This is far more difficult in the case of physician's services since these may be as varied in nature as are the ailments to which man is heir. Furthermore, the relationship of the patient to the physician is more complex than that of the patient to the hospital. This means that medical care insurance necessarily must grow relatively slowly, with expansion of the services rendered and the numbers covered determined by experience. Experimentation, the accepted method of science, is also determining such problems as sound insurance rates, fair fee schedules for various types of services and acceptable methods of payments to physicians. At every stage in the development and operation of medical care insurance plans, the quality of the service rendered must be the primary consideration. The high quality of medical service now supplied by physicians must be preserved. A prepayment plan providing inferior medical services and care is worse than no plan at all.

Despite these and other numerous difficulties, the enrollment in state and other medical society sponsored plans had doubled in the three years following 1941, and multiplied a further 2½ times in the year following mid-1944[5]. There are now 63 plans in operation in 25 states. Active planning for prepaid medical insurance is going on in several other states. In addition, the American Medical Association is now developing a national voluntary insurance plan to operate in those counties and states not now offered such opportunities by local medical societies.

The total numbers involved are still small. About three million people are now insured in medical care plans sponsored by medical societies[5]. However, we have been shown what can and should be accomplished by observing what has happened in the state of Michigan, where one of the oldest statewide medical care plans in the United States is operating under the auspices of the state medical society. Although it is relatively old, the Michigan plan was started only in 1939, a mere seven years ago. After this brief existance, there is now a coverage in Michigan of more than one person in seven[6].

Since there are so many medical care insurance plans now under way and a national plan is also being formulated by the American Medical Association, it appears sound to translate the Michigan experience into national terms. We may anticipate that only a few years will see the enrollment of perhaps 20,000,000 people, about as many as are now covered by Blue Cross hospitalization insurance. In the extension of medical care insurance, the rural population must be included. Important developments in this direction include the current negotiations of the State Grange in California and the California Physicians Service, in which it is anticipated that some 30,000 farm families (about 120,000 individuals) in California will receive the benefits of this service by one of the largest insurance plans sponsored by a state medical society.

Role of the Federal Government: There is much discussion now under way regarding the role which ought to be played by the federal government in the extension of medical care, particularly as it applies to hospital construction (which has been discussed) and a wider coverage of the population in prepayment insurance against the costs of hospital and other medical care. Regarding the latter, there is virtually no disagreement regarding the desirability of extending such insurance to cover all who need and desire it, consistent with a high quality of hospital and medical care at costs which are not excessive. This end is desired by nearly everyone. The disagreement, too often amounting to open conflict in which emotions are more in evidence than scientific analysis, lies in which of the methods to be employed give most promise of meeting the desired ends.

In general there are two major schools of thought. There are those who believe that we can accomplish our aim by a universal compulsory insurance plan established by federal law, supported by payroll taxes upon the worker and the employee and regulated by an agency in Washington. Others are convinced that the desired insurance coverage of the population with a preservation of high quality care can best be effected by an evolutionary process, in which the numerous plans now operated will continue to afford valuable experience and information which can serve as a basis for greater and greater expansion. To many, the latter appears to be the scientific approach of experimentation, evaluation of results, followed by further experimentation on broader fronts until the problem is as near to solution as possible.

Experimentation of this kind is being conducted even in the field of compulsory medical care insurance. In Rhode Island employees in industry are insured through compulsory payroll deductions with contributions by the employees, employers and the state government[7]. After a relatively short experience, the following significant conclusions pertinent to this discussion were reached by

these three groups and the participating physicians: the administrative costs were higher than anticipated, red tape was excessive, and centralization of the administration in Providence was too great. This latter finding is especially revealing in a state as small as Rhode Island, involving a geographical area and a population relatively very small by comparison with the entire country. Experiments of this kind are indispensible in the development and expansion of medical care programs involving larger sections of the country.

In estimating the probable effectiveness of a nation wide, federally regulated system of compulsory insurance, it is legitimate to examine into the record of the federal government in its operation of health and medical care programs. Three such major medical care activities have been, first, the work of the United States Public Health Service; second, the medical research projects and the medical care of the armed forces in the war, and third, the medical care of veterans.

Public Health activities, as contrasted with the care of a patient by a physician, are concerned with broad programs of health and of disease prevention such as venereal disease control, surveys and detection of cases in tuberculosis, sewage disposal and typhoid control, inspections of water, milk and meat, and numerous other similar functions. In this field, government units at all levels, from municipal to federal, have contributed immensely to reducing disease and death. In this field, there should and must be a strengthening of the programs, and a dissemination of the benefits even more widely throughout the country. Public Health units and services are lacking in many areas. Areas needing these and unable to provide them, should be assisted by the federal government, as is provided in the pending Hill-Burton Hospital Survey and Construction Act. One goal of the act is to assist in the establishment of one public health unit for each 30,000 persons, with even more of them in sparsely populated areas. This measure has the widest support from the public and from the professions concerned with providing medical care.

A second important federal project in medical care was that of the war, involving both research and care of patients. Wartime, government-sponsored, experimentation and investigation in medicine, so ably summarized by Dr. Perrin Long of Johns Hopkins University[8], has lead to great progress in our understanding and control of disease in many fields. The medical care of our armed forces was such that a very small fraction of sickness or injury resulted fatally, by comparison with the last war. The great success of these two wartime government ventures, in medical care and in research was probably due more to the high calibre of the scientists and physicians participating, than to any other single factor. These men and women willingly gave their time, their best efforts, and some, even their lives to win the war. But there was widespread dissatisfaction with the conditions under which they had to work. The complaints of medical officers are not that they were away from home or even exposed to danger, but with the needless red tape, the rigid regimentation, the endless restraints. Some of these may be necessary in wartime, but the general opinion is that they militated against good work and were usually unnecessary. In research, the story is essentially the same. Scientists on nuclear research are bitterly critical of the government policies both during wartime and especially now. One instance which was recounted as a typical example was the disposition of a nuclear scientist's request to make a gadget, whose principles are generally known, which was employed somewhere along the line in atomic research. The physicist wished to use the instrument in a peacetime research project bearing no relation to atomic bombs or energy. His request was refused and his research program must be modified to suit the whims of the brass hats. Medical scientists in wartime research projects were constantly hampered by senseless regulations preventing free discussion by collaborators on the same project.

Dr. Paul Henshaw, biologist at the Oak Ridge, Tennessee, atom bomb project conducted studies on the effects of radiation on human beings, during the development of the bombs. A few days ago he described his recent experiences in this army-controlled work[9]. The people who worked on the atomic bomb provided a wealth of material for his studies, which were concerned mainly with radiation and cancer. Abstracts of his finds, prepared for presentation at the Atlantic City meetings of the Cancer Research Association earlier this month, were presented to the Army for routine clearance. The answer was no. "As a consequence of the Army's action", said Dr. Henshaw, "I shall attend the meetings and listen to other papers in a related field . . . the (army) rules are so inflexible that release of these studies cannot be made".

On Wednesday March 13, 1946 an Associated Press dispatch[10] described the Army's ban upon the scientific paper of Drs. H. J. Curtis and J. D. Teresi of Oak Ridge. They were refused permission to present their findings at Atlantic City. Stupidly enough, the Army did clear the abstract of this paper for publication last December. The abstract reads as follows:[11]

"Activation of tissue elements by slow neutron exposure. B. H. J. Curtis and J. D. Teresi (by invita-tion). From Clinton Laboratories, Oak Ridge, Tennessee. When tissue is exposed to slow neutrons, a nuclear reaction takes place between the neutrons and the various atoms of the tissue. This reaction will release energy within the tissue in the form of various types of radiation, and will also produce radioactive isotopes which slowly decay and release further energy within the tissues. The present study concerns itself with the isotope production. Phosphorus, sodium, potassium and chlorine are the most important body elements in this regard. Calculations can now be made of the quantities of these isotopes formed and their biological effects. These have been checked experimentally in two ways. In the first place mice were exposed to slow neutrons from the Clinton graphite pile, and the exposures monitored by means of copper or indium foils. The animals were sacrificed at some definite time after exposure and various tissues analyzed quantitatively for P32, Na24, K41, and Cl38. In all cases the predicted amount was found within experimental error. Next, rats were exposed to slow neutrons and the excreta examined for P32 and Na24. From an analysis of the diet, the radioactive sodium excretion was as predicted assuming the excretion to be a true aliquot of all the Na in the body. About one-third of the phosphorus activated in this way was excreted as aliquot of the total body phosphorus, about one-third was excreted only slowly and the remainder appeared to be immobile."

These instances are cited as examples of what may happen when medical research or medical practice is controlled by people in power whose authority is exceeded only by their ignorance of medicine, research and science.

During the war, medical officers in the armed forces and scientists in wartime research contributed everything they had to do a necessary job—to win the war. Now that the war is over, the doctors and scientists are free to assert that they have had enough; that they wish to return now to independent research and practice in medicine.

A third major federal project in medical care has been that of the Veterans Administration. The quality of medical care rendered in veterans hospitals can only be characterized as disgraceful, until the inauguration of the recent policies of Veterans Administrator Omar Bradley and Surgeon General Paul Hawley and their expert advisors. These policies involve the operation of veterans hospitals by the faculties of medical schools, the establishment of programs of medical education for the younger physicians in the veterans hospitals and adequate rewards for the quality of service rendered by the physicians. Whether these sound policies will survive in the onslaughts of tradition and reaction of those in power is still an open question. Generals Bradley and Hawley are battling nobly against tremendous pressures in Washington to ruin their medical care program. The outcome of this irrational struggle is still doubtful.

We can summarize these three major health activities of the federal government as follows: (1) Public health services have been invaluable and should be extended; (2)

scientific medical research and medical care under army and navy auspices were outstanding under wartime conditions but are not applicable to peacetime; (3) veterans may get a high quality of medical care if the present medical leadership in the Veterans Administration is allowed to exercise that leadership.

Future Promise of Improved Medical Care: Government units at all levels can and should assist in the extension of medical care to all the people, with federal financial aid when necessary. This can and should be done in a variety of ways:

Improve the general economic level cultural conditions and facilities for healthful living of the people. This will not only reduce the incidence of disease but will also improve the general quality of medical care by effecting a better distribution of physicians and health facilities.

Expand and extend public health activities in the prevention of disease and the education of the public. Public health units or health centers should be provided for all areas throughout the country, with federal financial assistance and local control of the facilities.

Conduct surveys of local needs for hospitals, diagnostic facilities, health centers and physicians with federal aid to states.

Provide funds at the state and federal level for the construction of hospitals, health centers and diagnostic facilities where the surveys reveal their need, and where their maintenance is assured. These facilities should be controlled locally.

Foster and support basic scientific research institutes, with a minimum of centralized control in Washington, and a determination of the problems to be undertaken and the methods to be employed, by the participating institutions and scientists. Further promote scientific advances by providing scholarships in the sciences. Such a program is incorporated in the Kilgore-Magnusen bill (S.1850) under the administration of a National Science Foundation.

Study the feasibility of providing medical care for the indigent through enrolling them in voluntary hospitalization and medical care plans with the local government units, assisted by the federal government when necessary, paying for medical services rendered under the fee schedule of the plan. Any such program must take into account certain problems such as the higher incidence of disease among the indigent and the special case of chronic illness, often associated with, and sometimes the cause of indigency.

Develop state-wide plans for the care of veterans, similar to that in effect in Michigan. In that state the Veterans Administration has contracted with Michigan Medical Service, the prepayment medical care program of the state Medical society, for the medical care of veterans. The medical society sponsored California Physicians Service and the Medical Service Administration of New Jersey are collaborating in a similar manner[12]. Other state medical societies and medical care plans should also participate in this manner.

The federal government should correlate, coordinate and integrate its many health activities, except for those of the Army, the Navy and the Veterans Administration, under one Department of Health whose executive officer is of cabinet rank. Before the war there were over forty agencies, offices and authorities in the federal government engaged in some health activities including divisions of the Department of Agriculture, Commerce, Interior, Justice, Labor, Navy, State, Treasury and War[13]. The number is probably greater now.

This summary outlines the proper spheres of action of government, especially at the federal level, in an improved distribution of medical care in this country. The medical profession, the physicians of the country, have supported strongly the government activities described, and they should and will continue to collaborate with all their resources. However, the medical profession, you as physicians, will continue to bear the chief responsibility and must play the major role.

First and foremost we doctors must jealously guard against any compromise with high standards of medical care. We must strive to improve those standards, by strengthening undergraduate medical education, increasing the quality of hospital training at the levels of the internship and residency training for the medical specialties, providing the patient with ever better care. Any plan for the extension of medical care must be measured by its probable or possible effect on these. When there is reasonable doubt concerning such effects, the experimental method of science should be employed.

It is incumbent upon us to continue and increase our efforts to expand our voluntary prepayment medical care plans, both in terms of numbers served and services rendered. Veterans, the indigent and the temporarily unemployed should be included, 'perhaps by contracts between government and medical societies, similar to that now in effect for veterans in Michigan.

An improved coordination of medical care plans is also essential and is now under way. Through its Council on Medical Service and Public Relations, the American Medical Association has organized the Associated Medical Care Plans, Inc. Standards of acceptance and approval of medical care plans have been developed, coordinated and reciprocity among the plans to permit transference of subscribers from one plan to another or one locality or state to another are being organized and a nation wide plan is being developed to provide insurance benefits in such areas and states as are not now served by local units of the American Medical Association[14].

In all of these efforts, it is necessary to continue a vigorous program of education of the public regarding medical care and health and the facilities available to the people. Unfortunately, too many hundreds of thousands of our people do not desire scientific medical care through ignorance and prejudice, or do not know how or where to obtain the many benefits now at the service of the public.

I charge you, the graduates of the medical school of this great state university with the responsibility not only for the care of your own patients but also that of improving the distribution of medical care of high quality, a responsibility which you must shoulder with courage and determination. I further charge you with the responsibility of apply-

ing in these endeavors the same spirit of science, of experimentation, of research, which you have learned so well in the work you have done at your alma mater.

BIBLIOGRAPHY

1. Medical Education in Europe: Address at Forty-second Annual Congress on Medical Education and Licensure: Chicago, Illinois; February 11, 1946. (In press).
2. Personal Communication.
3. Journal of American Medical Association, Volume No 128, page 1173; August 18, 1945.
4. Statistics of the Bureau of Medical Economics of the American Medical Association, and the Health and Accident Underwriters Conference.
5. Statistics of the Bureau of Medical Economics of the American Medical Association.
6. There were 77,104 members in 1945 in a population, 1940 census, of 5,256,106. The benefits include surgical, obstetric, diagnostic x-ray, anesthesia and emergency surgical services, at a monthly cost of $1.00 for two persons or $2.25 for a family: Journal of American Medical Association, Volume No. 128, page 1174; August 18, 1945.
7. Medical Care, Volume No. 4, page 128; 1944.
8. Address: Medical Progress During the War: Perrin Long, M.D., 42nd Annual Congress on Medical Education and Licensure, Chicago, Illinois, February 11, 1946. (To be published).
9. University of Chicago Round Table Broadcast: Atomic Energy and Freedom, N.B.C., Washington; March 10, 1946.
10. The Chicago Sun; March 13, 1946.
11. Federation Proceedings, Volume No. 5, page 20; 1946.
12. Journal of American Medical Association, Volume No. 130, page 415; February 16, 1946.
13. Journal if American Medical Association, Volume No. 119, page 512; August 5, 1939.
14. Journal of American Medical Association, Volume No. 130, page 494; February 23, 1946.

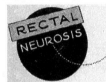

YOUNG'S Rectal Dilators

RECTAL NEUROSIS

Rectal disturbance is never trivial. Young's Rectal Dilators afford mechanical correction for bowel sluggishness when due to tight sphincter muscles. Effective elimination relieves nervous tension, permitting normal nerve reaction. Sold only by prescription. Obtainable at your surgical supply house; available for patients at ethical drug stores. Adults and children's sizes, in sets of 4 dilators. Write for Brochure.

F. E. YOUNG & CO. 424 E. 75TH STREET, CHICAGO 19, ILLINOIS

VON WEDEL CLINIC

610 N. W. Ninth Street

Oklahoma City, Oklahoma

PLASTIC and RECONSTRUCTION

CURT VON WEDEL, M.D.

C. A. GALLAGHER, M.D.

THE PRESIDENT'S PAGE

The Oklahoma State Medical Association is now recognized as one of the most progressive associations in the United States. This enviable position was gained only through the very fine cooperation of its members in all matters for the advancement of health and welfare of the people.

There is much to be done, and I am sure if you will continue to cooperate with your officers as you have in the past so we will be able to accomplish our objectives.

L. C. Kuykendall

President.

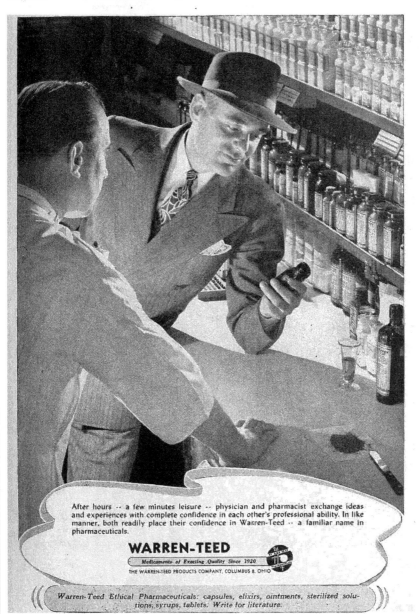

After hours -- a few minutes leisure -- physician and pharmacist exchange ideas and experiences with complete confidence in each other's professional ability. In like manner, both readily place their confidence in Warren-Teed -- a familiar name in pharmaceuticals.

WARREN-TEED

Medicaments of Exacting Quality Since 1920

THE WARREN-TEED PRODUCTS COMPANY, COLUMBUS 8, OHIO

Warren-Teed Ethical Pharmaceuticals: capsules, elixirs, ointments, sterilized solutions, syrups, tablets. Write for literature.

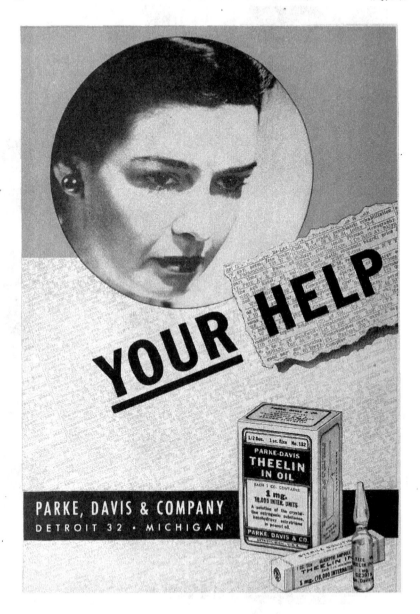

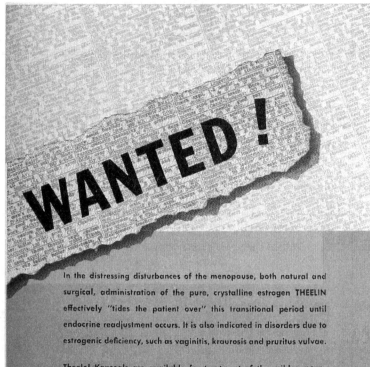

In the distressing disturbances of the menopause, both natural and surgical, administration of the pure, crystalline estrogen THEELIN effectively "tides the patient over" this transitional period until endocrine readjustment occurs. It is also indicated in disorders due to estrogenic deficiency, such as vaginitis, kraurosis and pruritus vulvae.

Theelol Kapseals are available for treatment of the milder menopausal symptoms and for maintenance between injections. Theelin Suppositories, Vaginal, are particularly well adapted for the treatment of gonorrheal vaginitis.

THEELIN

Theelin in Oil is available in ampoules of 0.1, 0.2, 0.5 and 1.0 mg., in boxes of 6 and 50. Theelin, Aqueous Suspension, in 2 mg. ampoules, in boxes of 6 and 25. Theelol Kapseals, 0.24 mg., in bottles of 20, 100 and 250. Theelin Suppositories, Vaginal, 0.2 mg., in boxes of 6 and 50.

The JOURNAL Of The
OKLAHOMA STATE MEDICAL ASSOCIATION

EDITORIAL BOARD

L. J. MOORMAN, Oklahoma City, Editor-in-Chief

E. EUGENE RICE, Shawnee   BEN H. NICHOLSON, Oklahoma City

MR. DICK GRAHAM, Oklahoma City, Business Manager

JANE FIRRELL TUCKER, Editorial Assistant

CONTRIBUTIONS: Articles accepted by this Journal for publication including those read at the annual meetings of the State Association are the sole property of this Journal.

The Editorial Department is not responsible for the opinions expressed in the original articles of contributors.

Manuscripts may be withdrawn by authors for publication elsewhere only upon the approval of the Editorial Board.

MANUSCRIPTS: Manuscripts should be typewritten, double-spaced, on white paper 8½ x 11 inches. The original copy, not the carbon copy, should be submitted.

Footnotes, bibliographies and legends for cuts should be typed on separate sheets in double space. Bibliography listing should follow this order: Name of author, title of article, name of periodical with volume, page and date of publication.

Manuscripts are accepted subject to the usual editorial revisions and with the understanding that they have not been published elsewhere.

NEWS: Local news of interest to the medical profession, changes of address, births, deaths and weddings will be gratefully received.

ADVERTISING: Advertising of articles, drugs or compounds unapproved by the Council on Pharmacy of the A.M.A. will not be accepted. Advertising rates will be supplied on application.

It is suggested that members of the State Association patronize our advertisers in preference to others.

SUBSCRIPTIONS: Failure to receive The Journal should call for immediate notification.

REPRINTS: Reprints of original articles will be supplied at actual cost provided request for them is attached to manuscripts or made in sufficient time before publication. Checks for reprints should be made payable to Industrial Printing Company, Oklahoma City.

Address all communications to THE JOURNAL OF THE OKLAHOMA STATE MEDICAL ASSOCIATION, 210 Plaza Court, Oklahoma City 3

OFFICIAL PUBLICATION OF THE OKLAHOMA STATE MEDICAL ASSOCIATION

Copyrighted May, 1946

EDITORIALS

OF INTEREST TO DOCTORS

Under the title "Volunteer Health Agencies", Gunn and Platt have written a book which seems to have been predicated upon the alleged need of unification of voluntary health agencies with one money raising campaign for the support of all. Apparently inspired by Albert Q. Maisel who has an article in the last issue of the McCall's Magazine; the April, 1946 Reader's Digest also carries a five page discussion of the Gunn-Platt report under the title "Urgently Needed, a National Health Fund". In this article it is stated "with funds from the Rockefeller Foundation, a three year study of voluntary health agencies has been conducted by two gifted and experienced workers in the health field".

To one who reads the book it is obvious that the authors are gifted in the art of confusing facts and fancies. Considering the contents of the book and the conclusions, one suspects that the authors started with a preconceived idea for which they should gather support. Space will not permit a general discussion, but since the Maisel article in McCall's directs its chief criticism at the National Tuberculosis Association and the National Foundation for Infantile Paralysis because they have had sufficient appeal to raise two-thirds of all the money made available for all the agencies, obviously someone should come to their defense.

The fact that these two agencies raise much more money than all of the others in the field consitutes no bonified reason for one money raising campaign and the arbitrary distribution of funds by a designated board. Neither does it justify the charge of greedy acquisition and careless spending. Over and against all of the criticisms of the National Tuberculosis Association there is an irrefutable record of accomplishment which cannot be gainsaid. The success of the Christmas seal sale is largely due to 40 years of faithful service and outstanding accomplishment.

The people know that the National Tuberculosis Association has cut the death rate from 200 per 100,000 to less than 45 per 100,000 in the past 40 years. They know that the National Association through its educational program has helped to provide more than 90,000 beds for the treatment of tuberculosis and that the Association's educational program and its various agencies continuously in operation have afforded protection against this dread disease and brought added safety to their own homes. And yet the people know the job has not been completed and they are glad to continue their support, with the hope that we may not only hold the protection we have gained, but ultimately eradicate the menace of Tuberculosis. Perhaps the people's judgment, supported by practically all of the doctors in the land, is better than that of the "two gifted" workers who surveyed the volunteer agencies.

Comparing the relative expenditures for Tuberculosis and Cancer and discussing their relative importance the authors do not point out the fact that Tuberculosis is an infectious disease, the specific cause of which is known and that while its killing power has been greatly reduced it still stands as the greatest killer in the most active period of life. The authors fail to point out the fact that with our present knowledge of Tuberculosis it should be possible to bring the disease under control if enough money is continuously available to keep up the fight against the disease. Admittedly money should be spent to acquire more knowledge concerning the cause of cancer and its control, but this need does not justify relaxation in the fight against a known disease with a specific cause rampant in the world because available scientific knowledge has not been freely applied.

The record of accomplishment, as shown by the history of the National Tuberculosis Association, justifies its independent existence. This is the only way it can hope to avoid the hazards of change and the handicaps of regimentation.

People who base their thinking upon public health experience cannot agree that a unified fund raising campaign will bring in more money than the individual campaign which affords them the privilege of giving through the Christmas seals because of personal interest and personal knowledge of special needs. In the last analysis and in line with present trends in the United States the authors of "Volunteer Health Agencies" recommend that the agencies accept regimentation and subject their experienced opinions to the mandates of an inexperienced Council.

YOUR VACATION

According to Osler, medicine is of the head, the heart and the purse. The head's long strain, augmented by the War, calls for a cooling period. There is grit in the gear, the calvarium grows heavy, it is time for relaxation and lubrication. The heart's response to sickness and suffering causes physical fatigue and coaxes the coronaries. Though the doctor's purse is of small concern and receives relatively little attention, whether lean or fat, it must sponsor a vaca-

tion. The cost need not be great. Webster says a vacation is "a period of intermission; rest, leisure".

To secure a real intermission with genuine rest and leisure, it is necessary to avoid all organized, standardized and commercialized forms of recreation. This means that fashionable clubs, lodges and dude ranches should be avoided. The switch on the motor should not be turned until the end of the road is reached. In search of the few remaining strong holds of God's great out-of-doors the companionship and common sense of pack horses is very iinvigorating. In the great open spaces under favorable conditions vitamins and viosterol may be forgotten. The subtle silence which settles about a beautiful camp, far removed from civilization, promptly calls into restorative action the primitive sources of physical and mental power which arise only from the soil. To see the sun rise and sun set striking across the rim of a vast untutored, unspoiled world; to witness the furtive movements of wild animals; to experience the shadowy mystery of the woodland waters; to enjoy the blessing of physical fatigue accompanied by mental relaxation; to sense the coming of night; to see the broken rays of silver stars falling through the branches of tall pines; finally to fall asleep under the mystic spell of the deep dark forest and to dream of the rhythmic race of wary trout in the black depts of mountain lakes is like having a transfusion.

Such experiences motivate the soul, move in the blood and abide in the very knot and center of our being. They refurbish the head, restore the heart and ignore the purse. Like an activating ferment, they change forever the chemistry of thought and upon the slightest provocation, throughout life, they call into service exhilerating moments which put to shame the spree of Arabic hay and hold you high above the hazardous vortex of a cockeyed world.

THE DANGER OF PROCRASTINATION

As your watch ticks the seconds away you are losing time and opportunity. Before another day passes you should write your representative that you want no more Washington made Social Security; that in your opinion charity begins at home and you want the blessing of personally participating in social reform and economic relief; that your contributions should be voluntary and directly applied full value; that they should not be compulsorily extracted and bureaucratically dissipated on the long journey to Washington and back; that you would take pride in the privilege of handling your own charity according to known needs rather than being coerced and unjustly penalized by government domination. he philosophy of Facism is incidiously invading the United States and it should be vigorously opposed.

The above general principles apply not only to Social Security in general, but to the threat of regimented medicine which for all who would fall into its clutches represents the most vicious phase of the Wagner-Murray-Dingell proposal. Isn't it strange that the proponents of this political scheme, including the Social Security administrator, should seek to invest more than four billion dollars in the very same medical service which they openly condemn. What an embarrassing paradox, especially when we take into account the fact that the people now are enjoying this medical service with freedom of choice at less than two billion dollars annually. Though there may be a prospect of some immediate political gain certainly there can be no postumous fame. There can be no inspiring mausoleam on the Potomac for the champions of this legislation. Such a monument on the Rhine might be appropriate, but the birth place of Social Security is now in ill-repute and there is little hope. Since we still have free speech in the United States somebody should play the good Samaritan and tell the proponents of this legislation the truth even though it becomes necessary to guarantee their lodging in the political inn.

Democrats and Republicans alike should remember that this is a national problem and too significant to be a party issue. Though the dreams of these ambitious politicians are bad their little lives will be rounded with a sleep. Let us hope that they may have their vacant hour of prattle and be forgotten.

QUESTION OF TODAY

How far will Public Welfare be extended is the question of the day.

During the past twelve years we have seen Public Welfare advance from a campaign promise to an expenditure of 35 million dollars a year for Public Welfare alone in Oklahoma, with the outlook of more to be added by the Federal Government.

A review of the figures just released by the Tax Commission reveals the following expenditures by the State for the fiscal year 1944-45:

Aid, Pensions and Assistance	$34,984,252.47
State Homes	293,563.98
Health and Hospitals	5,129,159.39
Penal Institutions	1,984,954.05
Employment and Unemployment	674,693.74
	$43,066,623.63

To this total must be added the expenditures by the counties for health and relief of at least $1,568,196 (1943) to say nothing of the community funds raised and spent by the cities and towns. The above $43,066,-623.63 is 46.13 per cent of the $93,356,642.29 accounted for in the Tax Commission report.

Figures indicate that 126,365 were being fed, housed, clothed or pensioned by the State in 1944 and an equal number in 1945. No figures are available showing the number of local cases of relief, but the expenditure of a million and a half dollars of public funds by the counties indicates at $200 per person another 7,500. These figures total some 150,000 out of our two million Oklahomans or 6.5 per cent of our population, excluding most of the children, who are unable to make a living or take care of themselves.

If the Wagner-Murray-Dingell bill becomes a law, thereby setting up a pure type of socialized medicine, these costs will take higher and higher percentages of the productive worker's income.

Some men are already asking the question, "What's the use"?—F. C. Harper.

NATIONAL HOSPITAL DAY MAY 12

Before this issue of the Journal reaches the doctors' desk, National Hospital Day will have passed. Presumably this day was set apart for the purpose of popularizing hospital service. Judging from local conditions this purpose has been fully realized. The people need many more days for the available hospital beds but since it is impossible to meet this need, we should have more beeds for the available days.

The increased demand for hospital beds has grown out of improved hospital service, and the progress of medical science. In addition the Blue Cross and other forms of hospital insurance have brought hospital care within the reach of many who otherwise would find it impossible. Considering these facts every hospital is faced with serious responsibilities and every community must appraise its hospital needs and try to meet its obligations.

OFF AGAIN ON AGAIN FOR SCIENCE AND SCENERY

Through the good offices of our own Dick Graham the doctors of Oklahoma are invited to travel via Special Train to the meeting of the American Medical Association in San Francisco with stopovers at all scenic points going and coming.

On June 27 all Oklahoma doctors and their traveling companions desiring this trip will converge in Newton, Kansas, where the Special Train will be assembled. Grand Canyon will be the principal point of interest on the way to San Francisco.

At the conclusion of the A.M.A. meeting all passengers will reassemble for a trip up the Pacific Coast to Portland and Seattle with side trips to Vancouver and Rainier National Park. From Seattle the Special Train will proceed to Yellow Stone National Park for a three-day sight seeing trip, after which it will return to Kansas City. The total time consumed will be sixteen days. The transportation arrangements will include all expenses except food, and even meals are included during the all American three days in Yellow Stone Park. Never were doctors offered so much for so little.

In the very near future each member of the Oklahoma State Medical Association will receive full particulars concerning the trip and it is suggested that those desiring reservations make them as soon as possible.

HEARINGS BEGIN ON HILL-BURTON BILL

The Hill-Burton Bill which would provide federal funds for assisting local communities in constructing non-profit hospitals and health facilities is being heard by the Committee on Interstate and Foreign Commerce of the House of Representatives.

This bill which would appropriate approximately $1,-732,000 per year to the State of Oklahoma on the basis of its per capita wealth has received the full endorsement of both the American Medical Association and the Oklahoma State Medical Association, but there is reason to believe that its early passage is not eminent.

Information coming from Washington indicates that while the bill will likely receive favorable consideration from the Committee on Interstate and Foreign Commerce it will not receive as favorable reception in the Committee on Appropriations where Representative Cannon, Chairman, has indicated his oposition.

The bill provides that the money would not be available to the various States until six months from the date of its passage and for this reason it is extremely unlikely that any community can benefit from the bill before 1947.

MID-WEST SURGICAL SUPPLY
CO., INC.

Kaufman Building
Wichita 2, Kansas

FRED R. COZART

2437 N. W. 36th Terrace

Phone 8-2561   Oklahoma City, Okla.

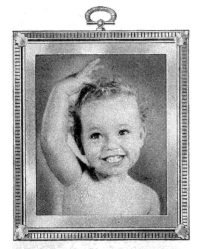

DOCTOR, MEET THE DARICRAFT BABY

Perhaps you are "meeting" the Daricraft Baby every day in your own practice. If not, may we call to your attention the following significant points of interest about Vitamin D increased Daricraft:

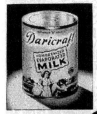

1. Produced from inspected herds; 2. Clarified; 3. Homogenized; 4. Sterilized; 5. Specially Processed; 6. Easily Digested; 7. High in Food Value; 8. Improved Flavor; 9. Uniform; 10. Dependable Source of Supply.

Producers Creamery Co.
Springfield, Mo.

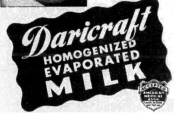

Daricraft HOMOGENIZED EVAPORATED MILK

ASSOCIATION COMMITTEE STUDYING MEDICAL CARE PROGRAM FOR VETERANS

The special Committee on Medical Care for Veterans, appointed by President Tisdal held its first meeting in Oklahoma City on Sunday, April 7. Present at the meeting were the following: John F. Burton, Oklahoma City; Ben Ward, Tulsa; E. G. King, Duncan; F. Redding Hood, Oklahoma City; Gordon Livingston, Cordell; Ralph W. Rucker, Bartlesville; Ned Burleson, Prague; E. H. Shuler, McAlester; J. B. Miles, Anadarko; W. P. Neilson, Enid.

Dr. W. P. Callahan of Wichita, Kansas, Chairman of the Committee of Kansas Medical Society which has placed in operation the Kansas Plan presented that state's organizational program and explained its various aspects.

The state programs which are now in operation are Michigan, Kansas, California, Oregan, Washington and New Jersey.

The basic principle of these plans is to enable a veteran to utilize local physicians in securing his physical examinations and out-patient care.

General Hawley of the Veterans Administration has made it very plain to organized medicine that the Veterans Administration expects the profession to participate in this program and it is refreshing to find an agency of government with this attitude.

Dr. John Burton, Chairman of the Committee, has announced that it is hoped his Committee will be in a position to make specific recommendations to the House of Delegates during the Annual Meeting.

HEARING ON WAGNER-MURRAY-DINGELL BILL BEGINS

The Senate Comittee on Education and Labor started hearings on the Wagner-Murray-Dingell Bill on April 6. In line with Senator Murray's previously announced policy the National organizations will be heard for and against the Bill. The medical and allied professions presentation of their testimony will begin April 16 at which time representatives of the American Medical Association will present their arguments against the Bill.

The first meeting of the Committee was punctuated by a verbal clash between Senators Murray and Taft which received wide publicity in the lay press.

The Oklahoma State Medical Association has placed itself on record with the Committee on Education and Labor as well as the individual members of Congress from this State opposing the Bill.

W-M-D Bill Would Regiment People

During recent months the general public has come to realize that the Wagner-Murray-Dingell Bill is not primarily a measure designed solely to put under government domination the medical profession, but that more particularly it is likely to regiment the vast majority of the people by placing upon them a compulsory tax for the financing of the program. Employers and employees are rapidly recognizing the fact that irrespective of the type of medical care they would receive it would be an extremely costly venture.

Members of the medical profession should call to the attention of their business associates that this legislation has many ramifications exclusive of the direct lowering of health standards. Every physician should follow the complete report of this hearing in the Journal of the American Medical Association.

A.M.A. ANNOUNCES NATIONAL HEALTH PROGRAM

Appearing elsewhere in this issue of the Journal is an announcement of the initial hearing of the Wagner-Murray-Dingell Bill before the Senate Committee on Education and Labor.

In the March 30 issue of its Journal, the American Medical Association announced a national health program for the United States, this health program having been adopted by the Board of Trustees and the Council on Medical Service, February 14, 1946.

National Health Program of A.M.A.

The following is a reprint of the National Health Program of the American Medical Association which appeared in the March 30 Journal of that association. Every physician should acquaint himself with this excellent and visionary program.

1. The American Medical Association urges a *Minimum Standard of Nutrition, Housing, Clothing and Recreation* as fundamental to good health and as an objective to be achieved in any suitable health program. The responsibility for attainment of this standard should be placed as far as possible on the individual, but the application of community effort, compatible with the maintenance of free enterprise, should be encouraged with governmental aid where needed.

2. The provision of *Preventive Medical Services* through professionally competent health departments with sufficient staff and equipment to meet community needs is recognized with the understanding that local areas shall control their own agencies as has been established in the field of education. Health departments should not assume the care of the sick as a function, since administration of medical care under such auspices tends to a deterioration in the quality of the service rendered. Medical care to those unable to provide for themselves is best administered by local and private agencies with the aid of public funds when needed. This program for national health should include the administration of *medical care, including hospitalization to all those needing it but unable to pay,* such medical care to be provided preferably by a physician of the patient's choice with funds provided by local agencies with the assistance of federal funds when necessary.

3. The procedures established by modern medicine for advice to the prospective Mother and for Adequate Care in Childbirth should be made available to all at a price that they can afford to pay. When local funds are lacking for the care of those unable to pay, federal aid should be supplied with the funds administered through local or state agencies.

4. The child should have throughout infancy *proper attention, including scientific nutrition, immunization against preventable disease and other services included in infant welfare.* Such services are best supplied by personal contact between the mother and the individual physician but may be provided through child care and infant welfare stations administered under local auspices with support by tax funds whenever the need can be shown.

5. The provision of *Health and Diagnostic Centers and Hospitals* necessary to community needs is an essential of good medical care. Such facilities are preferably supplied by local agencies, including the community, church and trade agencies which have been responsible for the fine development of facilities for medical care in most American communities up to this time. Where such facilities are unavailable and cannot be

J. E. HANGER, Inc.

ARTIFICIAL LIMBS, BRACES, AND CRUTCHES

Phone: 2-8500   612 N. Hudson

L. T. Lewis, Mgr.   BRANCHES AND AGENCIES IN PRINCIPAL CITIES   Oklahoma City 3, Okla.

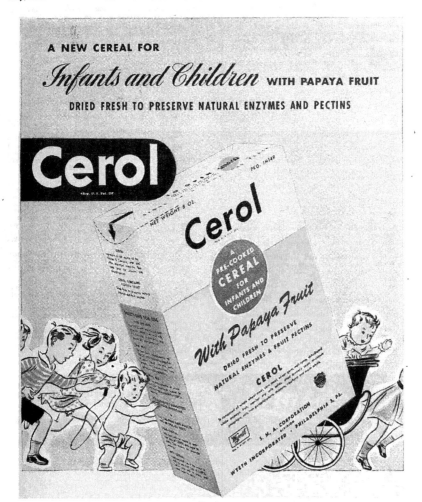

A NEW CEREAL FOR

Infants and Children WITH PAPAYA FRUIT

DRIED FRESH TO PRESERVE NATURAL ENZYMES AND PECTINS

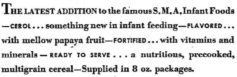

THE LATEST ADDITION to the famous S. M. A. Infant Foods —CEROL ... something new in infant feeding—FLAVORED ... with mellow papaya fruit—FORTIFIED ... with vitamins and minerals — READY TO SERVE . . . a nutritious, precooked, multigrain cereal—Supplied in 8 oz. packages.

S. M. A. DIVISION • WYETH INCORPORATED • PHILADELPHIA 3 • PA.

supplied through local or state agencies, the federal government may aid, preferably under a plan which requires that the need be shown and that the community prove its ability to maintain such institutions once they are established (Hill-Burton Bill).

6. A program for medical care within the American system of individual initiative and freedom of enterprise includes the establishment of *Voluntary nonprofit prepayment plans for the costs of hospitalization* (such as the Blue Cross plans) *for medical care* (such as those developed by many state and county medical societies. The principles of such insurance contracts should be acceptable to the Council on Medical Service of the American Medical Association and to the authoritative bodies of state medical associations. The evolution of voluntary prepayment insurance against the costs of sickness admits also the utilization of private sickness insurance plans which comply with state regulatory statutes and meet the standards of the Council on Medical Service of the American Medical Association.

7. A program for national health should include the administration of *medical care, including hospitalization, to all veterans*, such medical care to be provided preferably by a physician of the veteran's choice, with payment by the Veterans Administration through a plan mutually agreed on between the state medical association and the Veterans Administration.

8. *Research for the advancement of medical science* is fundamental in any national health program. The inclusion of medical research in a National Science Foundation, such as proposed in pending federal legislation, is endorsed.

9. The services rendered by *Volunteer Philanthropic Health Agencies* such as the American Cancer Society, the National Tuberculosis Association, the National Foundation for Infantile Paralysis, Inc., and by philanthropic agencies such as the Commonwealth Fund and the Rockefeller Foundation and similar bodies have been of vast benefit to the American people and are a natural outgrowth of the system of free enterprise and democracy that prevail in the United States. Their participation in a national health program should be encouraged, and the growth of such agencies when properly administered should be commended.

10. Fundamental to the promotion of the public health and alleviation of illness are *widespread education in* *the field of health* and the widest possible dissemination of information regarding the prevention of disease and its treatment by authoritative agencies. Health education should be considered a necessary function of all departments of public health, medical associations and school authorities.

OKLAHOMA COUNTY MEDICAL SOCIETY SPONSORS PUBLICITY CAMPAIGN

The Oklahoma County Medical Society in cooperation with other allied professions has just completed a series of full page ads in the Sunday Daily Oklahoman pointing out to the public the full import of the Wagner-Murray-Dingell Bill to the individual person.

This series of ads run by the Oklahoma County Medical Society stimulated great interest among the readers of the Daily Oklahoman and were instrumental in bringing about an awakening of public sentiment against this bill.

Oklahoma City Chamber of Commerce Protests Bill

The Oklahoma City Chamber of Commerce recognizing that the Wagner-Murray-Dingell Bill is not solely a problem of the medical profession, referred the study of this measure to its Medical Center and National Affairs Committees which two committees in turn reported to the Board of Directors of the Chamber recommending that the Board of Trustees go on record opposing this legislation. It is believed that this is the first instance in which a Chamber of Commerce in Oklahoma has taken this positive stand.

The Oklahoma County Medical Society should be congratulated for its visionary and militant advance into the field of advertising as a method of reaching the people.

In cooperation with the Oklahoma County Medical Society, the Junior Chamber of Commerce, State, County and City Health Departments, Radio Station WKY of Oklahoma City is sponsoring a series of 15 minute broadcasts on Venereal Disease to be heard each Friday evening at 9:45.

The program as announced by Mr. Tom Rucker of WKY will present in narrative form the importance of early treatment of Venereal Disease and its various public health aspects.

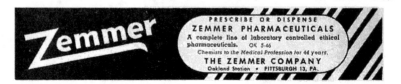

PRESCRIBE OR DISPENSE
ZEMMER PHARMACEUTICALS
A complete line of laboratory controlled ethical pharmaceuticals. OK 5-46
Chemists to the Medical Profession for 44 years.
THE ZEMMER COMPANY
Oakland Station • PITTSBURGH 13, PA.

WILLIAM E. EASTLAND, M.D.
F. A. C. R.

RADIUM AND X-RAY THERAPY
DERMATOLOGY

405 Medical Arts Bldg.

Oklahoma City, Oklahoma   Phone 3-1446

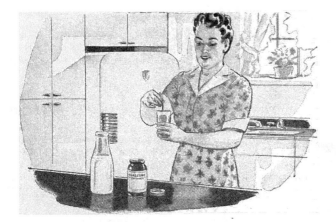

In the Nutrition Problems of
CHRONIC CHOLECYSTITIS

Because of the low fat intake which is frequently necessary, many foods and beverages are denied the patient with chronic gall bladder disease. If dietary curtailment becomes too drastic, however, nutritional deficiencies are apt to develop, adding further complications and physical discomfort.

The delicious food drink prepared by mixing Ovaltine with skim milk provides many of the nutrients considered essential in hepato-biliary disease, without appreciably increasing the fat intake. Its biologically adequate protein, readily utilized carbohydrate, B complex and other vitamins, as well as essential minerals aid in satisfying the need for these nutrients. This readily digested food supplement makes a nutritionally excellent as well as delicious component of the extra feedings which are frequently required in the management of chronic cholecystitis.

THE WANDER COMPANY, 360 N. MICHIGAN AVE., CHICAGO 1, ILL.

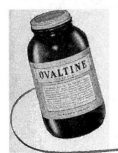

Ovaltine

Three servings daily of Ovaltine, each made of
½ oz. of Ovaltine and 8 oz. of skim milk*, provide:

CALORIES	426	VITAMIN A	2058 I.U.
PROTEIN	32.3 Gm.	VITAMIN B₁	1.16 mg.
FAT	2.5 Gm.	RIBOFLAVIN	1.55 mg.
CARBOHYDRATE	66.3 Gm.	NIACIN	6.81 mg.
CALCIUM	1.12 Gm.	VITAMIN C	39.5 mg.
PHOSPHORUS	0.939 Gm.	VITAMIN D	400 I.U.
IRON	12.0 mg.	COPPER	0.50 mg.

*Based on average reported values for skim milk.

**Postgraduate Course in Surgical Diagnosis
To Open in Tulsa, June 17**

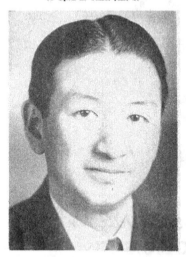

On Monday, June 17, the postgraduate course in Surgical Diagnosis will open in Tulsa. A lecture will be given each night for ten nights, excluding Saturday and Sunday. Dr. Patrick P. T. Wu, of Shanghai, China, will be the instructor.

Doctor Wu is a graduate of the University of Virginia, has had extensive training in New York, Chicago, Boston and several years at the Mayo Clinic, Rochester, Minnesota. He is an exceptionally well trained and capable surgeon. Doctor Wu is an excellent speaker, has a magnetic personality and has been very popular among the doctors with whom he has come in contact.

Due to the shortness of time that Doctor Wu will be in the United States it has been necessary to reduce the number of circuits.

Physicians in Tulsa County who desire to take advantage of this unusual opportunity, which is not primarily for the surgeon but for every practicing physician, should send in their enrollments promptly to the Postgraduate Committee, Oklahoma State Medical Association, 210-212 Plaza Court, Oklahoma City.

$85,000 ALLOCATED TO STATE REGENTS FOR UNIVERSITY HOSPITAL

Due to unforseen circumstances the appropriations for the University Hospital were found to be inadequate for the efficient conduct of its various services and functions.

During the early part of the fiscal year it was apparent that approximately $85,000 additional funds would be required to maintain the services of the University Hospital. Governor Kerr was apprised of the critical situation facing the Hospital and the Governor immediately requested an opinion from the Attorney General as to whether or not money from his contingent fund could be used to supplement the initial hospital appropriations. Attorney General Mac Q. Williamson immediately rendered an opinion favorable to the Governor's request and Governor Kerr has now allocated to the State Board of Regents the $85,000 requested by the Hospital and the usual services will be maintained.

Effective
Convenient
Economical

THE effectiveness of Mercurochrome has been demonstrated by more than twenty years of extensive clinical use. For professional convenience Mercurochrome is supplied in four forms—Aqueous Solution in Applicator Bottles for the treatment of minor wounds, Surgical Solution for preoperative skin disinfection, Tablets and Powder from which solutions of any desired concentration may readily be prepared.

Mercurochrome

(H. W. & D. brand of merbromin, dibromoxymercurifluorescein-sodium)

is economical because stock solutions may be dispensed quickly and at low cost. Stock solutions keep indefinitely.

Mercurochrome is antiseptic and relatively non-irritating and non-toxic in wounds.

Complete literature will be furnished on request.

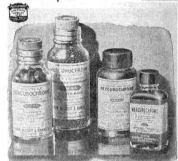

HYNSON, WESTCOTT
& DUNNING, INC.
BALTIMORE, MARYLAND

congestive heart failure

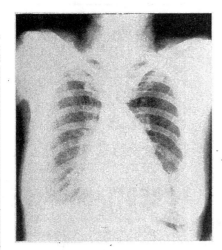

The de-edematizing action of Searle Aminophyllin decreases the cardiac burden, permitting the heart muscle to function more efficiently.

Searle Aminophyllin produces diuresis whether administered orally or parenterally, and thus has a field of usefulness covering emergencies and chronic congestive cardiac failure.

SEARLE AMINOPHYLLIN
contains at least 80% of anhydrous theophyllin.
G. D. Searle & Co., Chicago 80, Illinois

SEARLE

RESEARCH IN THE SERVICE OF MEDICINE

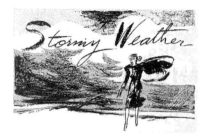

WHEN the menopausal storms set in—vaso-motor disturbances, mental depression, un-accountable pain and tension—physicians today can take prompt, positive action to alleviate symptoms.

By the administration of a reliable solution of estrogenic substances, you may exert a gratifying measure of control.

For control of menopausal symptoms, you may turn with confidence to Solution of Estrogenic Substances, Smith-Dorsey . . . manufactured in the fully equipped, capably staffed Smith-Dorsey Laboratories . . . meeting rigid standards of purity and potency.

With such a medicinal, you can indeed *do something* about "stormy weather."

SOLUTION OF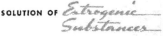

SMITH-DORSEY

Supplied in 1 cc. ampuls and 10 cc. ampul vials representing potencies of 5,000, 10,000 and 20,000 international units per cc.

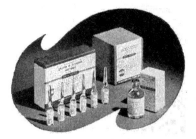

THE SMITH-DORSEY COMPANY
LINCOLN • NEBRASKA
Manufacturers of Pharmaceuticals to the Medical Profession Since 1908

RADIUM
(Including Radium Applicators)
FOR ALL MEDICAL PURPOSES
Est. 1919

Quincy X-Ray and Radium Laboratories
(Owned and directed by a Physician-Radiologist)

HAROLD SWANBERG, B.S., M.D., Director
W.C.U. Bldg.   Quincy, Illinois

NEUROLOGICAL HOSPITAL
Twenty-Seventh and The Paseo
Kansas City, Missouri

Modern Hospitalization of Nervous and Mental Illnesses, Alcoholism and Drug Addiction.

THE ROBINSON CLINIC
G. WILSE ROBINSON, M.D.
G. WILSE ROBINSON, Jr., M.D.

CREDIT SERVICE
330 American National Building
Oklahoma City, Oklahoma
(Operators of Medical-Dental Credit Bureau)

We offer a dignified and effective collection service for doctors and hospitals located anywhere in the State. Write for information.

28 YEARS
Experience In Credit and Collection Work
Robt. R. Sesline, Owner and Manager

IT IS

GOOD PRACTICE

... in judging the irritant properties of cigarette smoke... to base your evaluation on scientific research. In judging *research*, you *must* consider its *source**.

PHILIP MORRIS claims of superiority are based *not* on anonymous studies, but on research conducted only by competent and reliable authorities, research reported in leading journals in the medical field.

Clinical as well as laboratory tests have shown PHILIP MORRIS to be definitely and measurably less irritating to the sensitive tissues of the nose and throat. May we send you reprints of the studies?

PHILIP MORRIS

PHILIP MORRIS & CO., LTD., INC.,
119 FIFTH AVENUE, N. Y.

*Laryngoscope. Feb. 1935. Vol. XLV. No. 2. 149-154   Proc. Soc. Exp. Biol. and Med., 1934. 32. 241
Laryngoscope. Jan. 1937. Vol. XLVII, No. 1, 58-60   N. Y. State Journ. Med., Vol. 35, 6-1-35, No. 11, 590-592.

TO THE PHYSICIAN WHO SMOKES A PIPE: We suggest an unusually fine new blend—COUNTRY DOCTOR PIPE MIXTURE. Made by the same process as used in the manufacture of Philip Morris Cigarettes.

Have a Coke

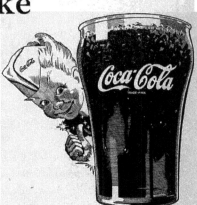

When you laugh, the world laughs with you, as they say—and when you enjoy *the pause that refreshes* with ice-cold Coca-Cola, your friends enjoy it with you, too. Everybody enjoys the friendly hospitality that goes with the invitation *Have a Coke*. Those three words mean *Friend, you belong —I'm glad to be with you.* Good company is better company over a Coca-Cola.

DIAGNOSTIC CLINIC OF INTERNAL MEDICINE AND ALLERGY

Phiilp M. McNeill, M. D., F. A. C. P.

General Diagnosis

CONSULTATION BY APPOINTMENT

Special Attention to Cardiac, Pulmonary and Allergic Diseases

Electrocardiograph, X-Ray, Laboratory
and Complete Allergic Surveys Available.

1107 Medical Arts Bldg.
Oklahoma City, Okla.   Phone 2-0277

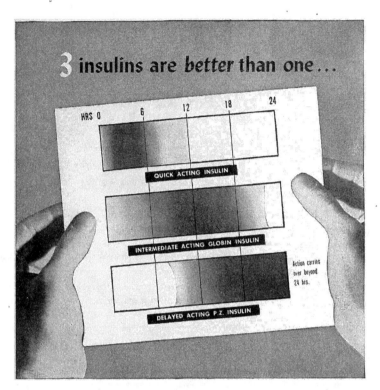

3 insulins are better than one...

HRS 0   6   12   18   24

QUICK ACTING INSULIN

INTERMEDIATE ACTING GLOBIN INSULIN

Action carries over beyond 24 hrs.

DELAYED ACTING P.Z. INSULIN

THE PHYSICIAN treating diabetes today has the choice of three types of insulin. One is rapid-acting but short-lived. Another is slow-to-start but prolonged. Intermediate between them is the new 'Wellcome' Globin Insulin with Zinc which starts fairly promptly and continues *for sixteen hours or more*. Action is maximal during the times of major carbohydrate intake but diminished toward bedtime so that the likelihood of nocturnal reactions is decreased. Today, the physician is wise to consider all *three* insulins.

'Wellcome' Globin Insulin with Zinc is a clear solution, comparable to regular insulin in its freedom from allergenic properties.

Accepted by the Council on Pharmacy and Chemistry, American Medical Association. Developed in the Wellcome Research Laboratories, Tuckahoe, New York. U.S. Patent No. 2,161,198. Available in vials of 10 cc., *80 units in 1 cc.* and vials of 10 cc., *40 units in 1 cc.* Literature on request.

'Wellcome' Trademark Registered

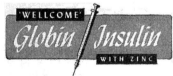

'WELLCOME'
Globin Insulin
WITH ZINC

BURROUGHS WELLCOME & CO. (U.S.A.) INC., 9 and 11 EAST 41ST STREET, NEW YORK 17

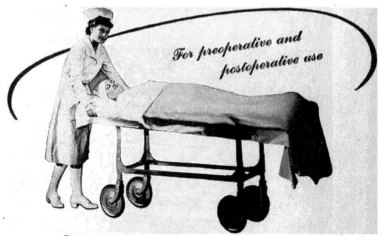

For preoperative and postoperative use

Demerol hydrochloride, administered from thirty to ninety minutes pre-operatively, relieves much of the surgical patient's apprehension and reduces the amount of anesthetic agent required to obtain a given depth of narcosis. The average preoperative dose for adults is 100 mg. injected intramuscularly, which may be combined with scopolamine or a barbiturate to assure amnesia.

Compared with morphine, Demerol causes considerably less nausea and vomiting, and the danger of respiratory depression is greatly reduced. Unlike morphine, Demerol does not interfere with the cough reflex or the reflexes and size of the pupil. It does not cause constipation, and urinary retention is less than with morphine.

Postoperatively, Demerol is a reliable analgesic in the majority of cases, regardless of the type of surgery or the severity of pain. Patients in the older age group, in particular, respond most favorably to this drug. The average postoperative dose for adults varies from 50 to 100 mg., administered by intramuscular injection or by mouth.

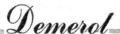

Demerol

Trademark Reg. U. S. Pat. Off. & Canada

H Y D R O C H L O R I D E

Brand of Meperidine Hydrochloride (Isonipecaine)

Synthetic ANALGESIC • SPASMOLYTIC • SEDATIVE

Available for *injection*, ampuls of 2 cc. (100 mg.), in boxes of 6, 25 and 100; also vials of 30 cc. (50 mg. per cubic centimeter). For *oral* use in tablets of 50 mg., bottles of 25, 100 and 1000.

Subject to regulations of the Federal Bureau of Narcotics

W R I T E   F O R   D E T A I L E D   L I T E R A T U R E

Winthrop CHEMICAL COMPANY, INC.

Pharmaceuticals of merit for the physician   •   New York 13, N. Y.   •   Windsor, Ont.

YOU CAN'T OVERRATE THE VALUE OF <u>CONTROL</u>

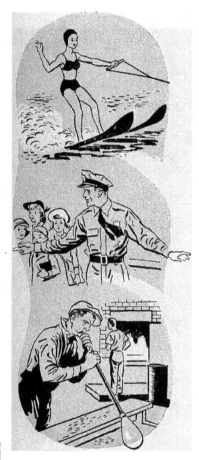

When you come to think of it, it's surprising how much control means. In various forms it adds enjoyment to sports—security to daily routine—satisfaction to work of skill.

And as *quality control* it assures safety in medicines. This is particularly well demonstrated in the development and production of U.D. pharmaceuticals. For throughout modern U.D. laboratories and plants a carefully conceived and remarkably efficient system of tests and checks results in products with an enviable reputation for consistent excellence.

Credit for maintenance of these high standards rests with a body of doctors, chemists and pharmacists, known as the Formula Control Committee. As the ultimate precaution, this group personally checks every finished product.

Such professional attention insures that your prescriptions are filled with finest ingredients when you specify U.D. pharmaceuticals. Your neighborhood Rexall Drug Store offers this service—together with complete facilities for meeting your patients' needs reliably and economically.

UNITED-REXALL DRUG CO.

U.D. products are available wherever you see *this* sign

PHARMACEUTICAL CHEMISTS FOR MORE THAN 43 YEARS
Los Angeles • Boston • St. Louis • Chicago • Atlanta • San Francisco
Portland • Pittsburgh • Ft. Worth • Nottingham • Toronto • So. Africa

UNITED-REXALL DRUG COMPANY AND YOUR REXALL DRUGGIST • *Your Partners in Health Service*

OFFICERS OF COUNTY SOCIETIES, 1946

★

COUNTY	PRESIDENT	SECRETARY	MEETING TIME
Alfalfa	W. G. Dunnington, Cherokee	L. T. Lancaster, Cherokee	Last Tues. each Second Month
Atoka-Coal	J. B. Clark, Coalgate	J. S. Fulton, Atoka	
Beckham	P. J. DeVanney, Sayre	J. E. Levick, Elk City	Second Tuesday
Blaine	W. F. Bohlman, Watonga	Virginia Curtain, Watonga	Third Thursday
Bryan	W. K. Haynie, Durant	Jonah Nichols, Durant	Second Tuesday
Caddo	Preston E. Wright, Anadarko	Edward T. Cook, Jr., Anadarko	
Canadian	G. L. Goodman, Yukon	W. P. Lawton, El Reno	Subject to call
Carter	J. Hobson Veazey, Ardmore	H. A. Higgins, Ardmore	Second Tuesday
Cherokee	P. H. Medearis, Tahlequah	R. K. McIntosh, Jr., Tahlequah	First Tuesday
Choctaw	Floyd L. Waters, Hugo	O. R. Gregg, Hugo	
Cleveland	James O. Hood, Norman	Phil Haddock, Norman	Thursday nights
Comanche	Wm. Cole, Lawton	E. P. Hathaway, Lawton	
Cotton	G. W. Baker, Walters	Mollie Seism, Walters	Third Friday
Craig	Lloyd H. McPike, Vinita	J. M. McMillan, Vinita	
Creek	W. P. Longmire, Sapulpa	Philip Joseph, Sapulpa	Second Tuesday
Custer	Ross Deputy, Clinton	A. W. Paulson, Clinton	Third Thursday
Garfield	Bruce Hinson, Enid	John R. Walker, Enid	Fourth Thursday
Garvin	M. E. Robberson, Jr., Wynnewood	John R. Callaway, Pauls Valley	Wednesday before Third Thursday
Grady	Roy Emanuel, Chickasha	Rebecca H. Mason, Chickasha	Third Thursday
Grant	I. V. Hardy, Medford	F. P. Robinson, Pond Creek	
Greer	J. B. Lansden, Granite	J. B. Hollis, Mangum	
Harmon	W. G. Husband, Hollis	R. H. Lynch, Hollis	First Wednesday
Haskell	Wm. S. Carson, Keotah	N. K. Williams, McCurtain	
Hughes	Victor W. Pryor, Holdenville	L. A. S. Johnson, Holdenville	First Friday
Jackson	E. W. Mabry, Altus	J. P. Irby, Altus	Last Monday
Jefferson	F. M. Edwards, Ringling	J. A. Dillard, Waurika	Second Monday
Kay	L. G. Neel, Ponca City	J. C. Wagner, Ponca City	Second Thursday
Kingfisher	John W. Pendleton, Kingfisher	H. Violet Sturgeon, Hennessey	
Kiowa	Wm. Bernell, Hobart	J. Wm. Finch, Hobart	
LeFlore	S. D. Bevill, Poteau	Rush L. Wright, Poteau	
Lincoln	J. S. Rollins, Prague	Ned Burleson, Prague	First Wednesday
Logan	James Petty, Guthrie	J. E. Souter, Guthrie	Last Tuesday
Marshall			
Mayes	L. C. White	V. D. Herrington, Pryor	
McClain	S. C. Davis, Blanchard	W. C. McCurdy, Purcell	
McCurtain	J. T. Moreland, Idabel	R. H. Sherrill, Broken Bow	Fourth Tuesday
McIntosh	F. R. First, Checotah	W. A. Tolleson, Eufaula	First Thursday
Muskogee-Sequoyah			
Wagoner	R. N. Holcombe, Muskogee	William N. Weaver, Muskogee	First Tuesday
Noble	A. M. Evans, Perry	Jesse W. Driver, Perry	
Okfuskee	W. P. Jenkins, Okemah	M. L. Whitney, Okemah	Second Monday
Oklahoma	W. F. Keller, Okla. City		Fourth Tuesday
Okmulgee	F. S. Watson, Okmulgee	C. E. Smith, Okmulgee	Second Monday
Osage	Paul H. Hemphill, Pawhuska	Vincent Mazzarella, Hominy	Third Monday
Ottawa	C. F. Walker, Grove	W. Jackson Sayles, Miami	Second Thursday
Pawnee	H. B. Spalding, Ralston	R. L. Browning, Pawnee	
Payne	F. Keith Oehlschlager, Yale	C. W. Moore, Stillwater	Third Thursday
Pittsburg	Millard L. Henry, McAlester	Edward D. Greenberger, McAlester	Third Friday
Pontotoc-Murray	John Morey, Ada	R. H. Mayes, Ada	First Wednesday
Pottawatomie	F. P. Newlin, Shawnee	Clinton Gallaher, Shawnee	First and Third Saturday
Pushmataha	John S. Lawson, Clayton	B. M. Huckabay, Antler	
Rogers	W. A. Howard, Chelsea	P. S. Anderson, Claremore	Third Wednesday
Seminole	Clifton Felts, Seminole	Mack I. Shanholz, Seminole	Third Wednesday
Stephens	Evert King, Duncan	Fred L. Patterson, Duncan	
Texas	Daniel S. Lee, Guymon	E. L. Buford, Guymon	
Tillman	H. A. Calvert, Frederick	O. G. Bacon, Frederick	
Tulsa	John C. Perry, Tulsa	John E. McDonald, Tulsa	Second and Fourth Monday
Washington-Nowata	Ralph W. Rucker, Bartlesville	L. B. Word, Bartlesville	Second Wednesday
Washita	L. G. Livingston, Cordell	Roy W. Anderson, Clinton	
Woods	John F. Simon, Alva	O. E. Templin, Alva	Last Tuesday Odd Months
Woodward	T. C. Leachman, Woodward	C. W. Tedrowe, Woodward	Second Thursday

THE JOURNAL
of the
OKLAHOMA STATE MEDICAL ASSOCIATION

VOLUME XXXIX   OKLAHOMA CITY, OKLAHOMA, JUNE, 1946   NUMBER 6

President's Inaugural Address

Compulsory Health Insurance

L. C. KUYRKENDALL, M.D.

Freedom of enterprise is America's guarantee to all and when this is taken away or restricted by acts of legislation or directives, and bureaucrats assume the role of dictating the acts and thoughts of the people, then the Constitution of the United States becomes a scrap of paper and "Life, Liberty and Pursuit of Happiness' is done away with.

Thomas Jefferson once said, "A wise and frugal government, which shall restrain men from injuring one another, which shall leave them otherwise free to regulate their own pursuits of industry and improvement and shall not take from the mouth of labor the bread it has earned, this is the sum of good government."

Ours is a Democracy and as such the individual makes the state and not the reverse as some in these United States would have us believe. The reverse can happen here unless we are on the alert at all times. Those who would reverse the order, do not come out in the open, but on the other hand dress their schemes up in terms such as "freedom from want and fear", "security" and many other terms which strike a sympathetic note in the hearts of the majority, but behind it all is the insiduous plan for the eventual subjugation of the individual to the State and we will have been duped into a state of false security.

Such is the case in the Compulsory Health Insurance plan as introduced in the United States Congress. The planners and proponents of this measure hold out to the people so called "security" in the form of health insurance, which is not "voluntary", but which amounts to "compulsory taxation" of the participants; this would include everyone earning up to $3,600.00 a year.

If one could believe the claims of the proponents of this proposed legislation we would indeed face a horrible situation, but despite conditions under which our physicians have had to labor, it is my sincere belief that very few if any have suffered or died for lack of medical attention because they were unable to pay.

The proponents of Compulsory Health Insurance make much of the high percentage of rejections for military service by our induction centers, in fact it seems to be their principle talking point. There were approximately 5,000,000 rejections for service in our armed forces because of physical conditions many, which they contend would not have existed had these had proper medical attention which they propose to supply by this Health Insurance.

Broken down into comprehensive figures we find over 700,000 rejected because of mental diseases, 580,000 because of mental deficiency, 280,000 because of syphilis, 445,000 as manifestly disqualified, 160,000 because of eyes or visual defects, 320,000 because of musculo skeletal defects and 220,000 because of hernia.

How by any stretch of the imagination could anyone expect medicine to prevent the mental disease or mental deficiencies found in these men. There are specific laws relative to syphilis and our Public Health Service is available for these cases and appropriate treatment is made available to all who apply. How could compulsory health insurance alter these figures. It is questionable whether health insurance would have altered the story of the deaf, blind and those who had lost an arm or a leg or prevented the rejection of any of those found to be disqualified because of eyes or visual defects since most of these were of hereditary origin.

LIBRARY OF THE
COLLEGE OF PHYSICIAN
OF PHI - ꞏꞏ ꞏꞏꞏꞏ

Of those with musculo-skeletal defects can anyone hazard a guess as to whether any of these defects could have been prevented? There is no medical care known that will prevent an inguinal or femonal hernia and its occurence is in no way considered as evidence of neglect on the part of medical men, they occur because of congenital defects. Of rejections from causes not listed above, there is a question as to whether any appreciable number of them had physical defects which were caused by lack of medical care or whether any medical plan would have prevented their occurence.

A measure which has been considered very favorably in Congress is one whereby health centers. and hospitals may be constructed and certain hospitals enlarged in areas where, after a survey has been made, the need is shown for construction or enlargement. This should be far reaching in benefits in most sections of the country. We feel it should pass and that work should be started as soon as possible in order that existing needs may be met. This has nothing to do with the compulsory health insurance bill spoken of in the beginning which if enacted into law will regiment the people who labor and exact a tax not only from them but from the employer as well. Even the self employed is not exempt.

Thomas Jefferson said, "The God who gave us life, gave us liberty." If freedom of enterprise as well as freedom of choice be limited, denied or circumvented then the good old American custom of being able to think for one's self will be done away with. Compulsory health insurance would be an entering wedge for measures of like character and further curtailment of our personal liberties.

Now let us see what the situation in two countries under compulsory health insurance at present can show us. Germany and England both have health insurance and yet our rate of rejections for military service was 38 per cent with extremely high standards of qualifications, while in England is was 50 per cent. Their requirements were very much less exacting than ours even after our exacting requirements were modified.

Malingering is universal, probably more in a free country than in one that is not free, but in Germany before the war among the insured the rate of sickness was 200 per cent while among the uninsured it was practically the same as the United States: viz. 10 per cent.

One would naturally suspect that the great difference in sickness rate of the insured over the uninsured was due to the fact that they were being paid while sick and this causes one to wonder if many of them were merely taking a rest at the government's expense.

The majority of the states have adopted and have in operation at this time some form of voluntary health insurance which is available to all and at a cost so very much less than the tax which would be enacted should the bill which is now under consideration in our National Capitol pass, that it is inconceivable that anyone would prefer to be regimented when they can be free, free to exercise the right under our Democracy of individual thought and action.

We have been subjected to undeserved criticism which would never have occurred had there been more cooperation on the part of the government with medical men in their endeavors to raise the standards of health and to prolong life's span.

The challenge has been made and while we stand ready to answer it, we must not rest our case on our accomplishments but continue as we have in the past to be alert to the needs of the people. If we do this then there will be no need for radical legislation such as has been proposed. It is up to us.

Injuries to The Hand--With Particular Reference to Indications For Primary and Secondary Nerve and Tendon Repair[*]

Michael L. Mason, M.D.

CHICAGO, ILLINOIS

In the management of an injury of the hand it is as necessary to know what not to do as it is what to do, since extensive ill advised surgery may produce irreparable damage. This is particularly true in cases of divided nerves and tendons. The temptation to repair these structures in wounds unsuitable for this type of surgical treatment will be avoided if the surgeon realizes that early secondary repair is highly successful and may be accomplished three to five weeks

[*]Delivered before the Section on General Surgery, Oklahoma State Medical Association, Annual Meeting, May 2, 1946.

after injury in a wound which has healed by primary intention.

The general principles upon which wounds are treated have been repeatedly stressed and the recent war has served to emphasize their importance. The first principle in the management of any wound is to protect it immediately from further trauma and contamination with a large sterile dressing bandaged on firmly. This dressing should be large enough to cover the wound and a good area beyond, and voluminous enough to permit snug bandaging. This firm resilient dressing controls bleeding and prevents edema, a particularly important function if much time elapses between first aid and definite care. This dressing should not be disturbed for inspection of the wound until the patient arrives in an emergency room where it can be inspected, if need be, under aseptic conditions. Preferably the wound is not exposed at all until the patient reaches the operating room when the dressing is removed by the surgeon who will prepare the hand for surgery. The importance of secondary contamination of wounds cannot be too strongly emphasized since it has been shown that the majority of wound infections are due to organisms introduced after, rather than at, the time of wounding. Diagnosis of nerve and tendon damage can usually be made without disturbing the dressings and certainly should not be made by probing and searching in the wound. If it seems necessary to look at the wound, the surgeon should be masked, and use aseptic technic. One very brief glance is usually enough to inform him if skin grafts or a flap may be necessary.

The transformation of the contaminated wound into a surgically clean wound is accomplished by careful washing with soap and water for 10 to 15 minutes or longer, followed by irrigation with large amounts of normal saline solution. Gentle but prolonged washing with plenty of suds prepares the wound for whatever surgery is indicated.

Excision of devitalized tissue rids the wound of one of the most, if not the most, serious handicaps to healing. This procedure is not intended to excise all the exposed tissues; it is not aimed at the removal of contaminated tissues but at removal of dead tissues which interfere with healing and which furnish foci for bacterial growth.

It should be understood of course that excision in cases of the hand must be done carefully. There must be no sacrifice of any living tissue, particularly muct nerves and tendons be avoided. Skin, too, must not be needlessly sacrificed. Many flaps may be saved by careful handling, and a resilient pressure afterwards to prevent venous congestion.

During cleansing and excision the surgeon makes a careful survey of the damage sustained and plans the subsequent steps of the operation. Repair of divided nerves and tendons is accomplished at the initial operation if satisfactory conditions obtain. If deep repair is not advisable the wound is closed and nerve and tendon suture planned at a later date after healing has occurred.

Closure of the wound should be done in all but the virulently contaminated, or old wounds. The majority of hand wounds may be closed but suture, care being taken to obtain accurate apposition of edges and avoidance of tension. In some instances closure is not possible by simple suture, and here skin grafts are indicated. In practically all cases split thickness grafts will serve the purpose. In some instances, however, pendunculated flaps are necessary, especially when bones, joints and tendons are exposed, since these structures will not support a free graft.

A pressure dressing is applied to the hand before the blood pressure cuff is released to control postoperative edema and oozing. My practice is to have the splint prepared ahead of time and sterilized. The splint is covered with several thicknesses of abdominal pads and the hand then laid upon it in the position in which the surgeon wishes it to be immobilized. It is then covered with large amounts of fluffed gauze; care should be taken to place gauze between the fingers and between any folds of skin where intertrigo may develop. Over the fluffed gauze are placed several more abdominal pads and then the whole is bandaged with elastic bandage to secure firm, even resilient pressure over the whole hand. After the pressure has been applied the blood pressure cuff is deflated.

It is usually advantageous to keep the hand elevated on pillows in the immediate postoperative period to favor circulation, since it is usually venous return which is compromised rather than the arterial supply.

Little need be said about general operating technic since this has been emphasized on many occasions. The necessity of a bloodless field secured by means of a blood pressure apparatus has been accepted by everyone who does this type of surgery. The need for fine sutures and small needles, for careful hemostasis, gentle handling of tissues, careful retraction and a minimum of tissue damage by the surgeon and his assistant are all well established principles. Some observations however still seem appropriate in the matter of incisions for enlargement of the wound in order properly to expose deep structures. Frequently the enlarging incision made at the primary operation is a source of major disability in itself and seriously handicaps the surgeon who must attempt secondary repair.

In so far as it is possible the original

wound should be enlarged in such a manner as to conform to the principles of incision on the hand. These principles are few: (1) Avoid midline incision. (2) Do not cross flexion creases. (3) Avoid longitudinal incision on flexor or extensor surfaces. (4) Plan incision so as to make flaps of skin and subcutaneous tissues to overlie areas of deep repair. Since accidental wounds do not conform to these principles, the surgeon must use a good deal of ingenuity in enlarging them to conform to the correct lines. The surgeon should first visualize the probable amount of deep repair necessary and then enlarge the wound in such a way as to secure adequate exposure and leave well vascularibed flaps. In no case should the wound be crossed by a second incision, leading to a cruciate scar. It is usually possible to prolong one or both ends of the original wound. Longitudinal wounds across flexor or extensor surfaces may be enlarged by a curving incision passing toward radial or ulnar borders of the forearm or fingers. In the case of oblique or transverse wounds over flexor or extensor surfaces one or both ends may be prolonged toward the radial or ulnar borders of the forearm and then carried as a longitudinal incision along the side of the forearm to permit as wide exposure as the case demands. Enlargements must be individualized for each case, but if made along the general lines as indicated above they permit adequate exposure and do not increase whatever disabling scar may follow the wound itself.

Under what conditions is the surgeon justified in performing primary nerve and tendon suture? The decision as to immediate suture depends upon whether or not the surgeon anticipates healing of the wound by primary intention. One condition essential to satisfactory functional restoration is primary reactionless healing. If this be absent and if wound disturbance occurs secondary repair will be rendered extremely difficult, if not impossible. The factors upon which judgment is based have to do with the possibility or probability of serious contamination, interval since injury and associated tissue damage.

The interval of time between injury and surgical care is an important factor. Tendon wounds over four hours old when first seen are seldom amenable to immediate repair, and in case of wounds involving the flexor tendons in the digital sheaths a two hour limit is best. One might occasionally suture a tendon on the dorsum of the hand five or six hours after injury, since these tendons do not retract so much as do sheath-enclosed tendons and little tissue need be exposed to mobilize the stumps. Probably nerves may be repaired up to six or eight hours after

wounding since here retraction of stumps is not so great as in the case of tendons and the surgeon does not need to open up extensive areas of uninvolved tissue to expose freshly divided nerves.

The amount and nature of exposure to contaminants to which the wound was subjected prior to surgical intervention is very important. This exposure may have taken place at the time of injury, i.e., the divided extensor tendon over the knuckles which occurs in fist fight injuries or the autopsy knife injury. In these, as in certain other rarer injuries, the immediate inoculation of virulent pathogens produces a seriously contaminated wound in which deep repair of nerves and tendons is contraindicated. Serious initial contamination of a wound is, however, very rare; in practically all instances serious contamination is a secondary affair and *not* primary, and occurs usually from avoidable exposure to droplet contamination, fingers, unsterile dressings, etc., during first-aid care or during inspections made elsewhere previous to the time the patient reached surgery. If a serious primary contamination is present or seems likely to have taken place, or if the wound has been exposed to inquiring fingers, nasal droplets and unsurgical dressing technic, a decision must be made to forego primary tendon and nerve repair.

A previous unsuccessful attempt to perform nerve and tendon repair, say in an emergency room or aid station, by unskilled or unprepared hands, under questionable conditions of asepsis, precludes primary nerve and tendon repair. Even if the patient can be brought immediately to an operating room under ideal conditions, discretion is the better part of valor. The surgeon may very seriously regret having performed tendon repair under these conditions.

In certain instances great loss of skin and other covering tissue may necessitate the use of free grafts or pedunculated flaps in order to secure primary closure, and under such circumstances it is unwise to expose and isolate nerves and tendons and attempt their primary suture. Here too a secondary repair is to be done after suitable skin covering has been obtained.

The presence of compound fractures within the hand, particularly when the site of these fractures coincides with the site of tendon injury, is contraindicative to tendon repair. It may be permissable to bring nerve ends together under such circumstances, since their isolation does not ordinarily entail wide exposure in the immediate injury and since they may often be protected from involvement in the callus. Tendons on the other hand are apt to be incorporated in the callus and become fixed.

Favorable operating facilities for repair

also must obtain to justify this operation, i.e., the primary repair cannot be undertaken in an emergency room equipped to deal only with minor lacerations, etc. Good help, proper instruments and sutures and a suitable anesthetist must be available. If satisfactory operating conditions do not obtain, regardless of where the patient is, the surgeon cannot be criticized for refraining from primary repair. Here also it is to be remembered that secondary repair under more favorable circumstances is possible three or four weeks later if the wound can be closed primarily and if healing without reaction follows.

It was hoped by the local introduction of the sulfonamide drugs to permit more extensive early repairs and to extend the time limits within which such repair is safe. Rather it has seemed to me that the critical study of wound healing which has followed the local application of sulfonamides served to focus the surgeon's attention on this important phase of surgery and to emphasize the importance of primary wound healing in wound care.

The careful survey of wound care supervised by Meleney has shown that the sulfonamides have not reduced local infections and whatever beneficial effects there may be following sulfonamide therapy are due to the general and not the local action of the drug. Experiments conducted by Dr. Harvey S. Allen and myself on the effect of local sulfonamides on tendon healing have shown a severe exudative reaction at the site of implantation and have demonstrated a significant delay in tendon healing. The U. S. Army after an extensive trial in the local use of these drugs issued a directive advising against its use. Emphasis in local care of wounds has swung almost entirely away from the use of any local agents.

Penicillin has been little used as a local agent in this country. Its use intramuscularly or intravenously has undoubtedly lessened spreading infections and permitted an extensive program of secondary closures of war wounds. However, its use does not allow disregard of good surgery, but rather emphasizes the need for careful technic and wound care. Certainly no one would advocate nerve and tendon repair in a questionably contaminated or old wound simply because one had penicillin at his disposal. It seems possible that penicillin by reducing spreading infections following initial surgery may permit earlier secondary repair.

It has seemed to me that the advent of chemotherapy and antibiotic therapy has altered very little our initial care of open wounds. They have enlarged the scope of secondary surgery in that local wound infections have been kept under control and prevented from spreading, and the stimulus

to a study of wound healing has had as concomitant an improvement in surgical technic. No one has claimed that they are a substitute for good surgery or that well established principles can be disregarded. Certainly in our judgment of the immediate injury we cannot yet afford to overstep the limits that have been established in nerve and tendon repair.

Secondary repair of nerve and tendon damages should be undertaken as soon as the condition of the wound permits. There must be no infection present. In wounds which have healed per primum, it may be assumed that there was no infection. Such wounds may often be reopened for secondary repair within three to four weeks after they have been sustained, providing the other prerequisites are met. If infection has been present it is necessary to wait six to 12 months after the process has subsided, depending upon the severity of the infection.

The induration must be gone from the wound, otherwise the isolation of nerves and tendons is very difficult, healing will be interfered with and latent infections may flare up.

The joints must be movable, otherwise the repair of tendons which move these joints will be fruitless. The covering tissues of the hand must be supple and the skin normal with a good layer of subcutaneous fat to overlie the area of proposed repair. If dense scar or atrophic skin overlies the operation site it will require removal and replacement by a pedunculated flap before a nerve and tendon operation can be done.

In instances therefore of deficient covering tissues, stiff joints, etc., time will be required to remedy these defects before secondary repair can be undertaken. Much can be accomplished in the way of physical therapy by the patient himself, by soaking the hand in warm soapy water once or twice daily and gently massaging and moving stiff joints for a period of 15 to 20 minutes. While waiting for appropriate time for repair of divided nerves the muscles paralyzed by these nerves must be kept relaxed by proper splinting to prevent irreparable damage to them by their unopposed antagonists.

Secondary tendon repair may consist of tendon suture or may entail the use of tendon grafts. In most instances it is possible to predict ahead of time whether or not a graft will be required. The source of these grafts may be occasionally the sublimis tendons, in cases where the profundus tendons only are repaired. The palmaris longus tendon is occasionally available. Most often, however, parts of the extensor digitorum longus of the toes will be needed and it is possible to remove four long segments from each foot. In removing these grafts from the foot great care must be taken to preserve the thin layer of areolar tissue (paratenon) which immediately surrounds the tendons since this serves as a gliding mechanism for the newly grafted tendon. It has never seemed logical to surround tendons with artificial membranes or other foreign matter in hopes of preserving or permitting motion. Our observations on the use of amniotic membrane and tantalum foil have been confined to attempt to repair the damage occasioned by their use. Dense adhesions and excessive fibrosis, caused by these substances have just the opposite effect to that for which they were used.

Incisions for secondary repair must take into account the scars of the original injury and previous operation. The surgeon follows the general principles laid down for enlarging incisions noted earlier. Some judgment must be exercised in making these incisions since it may happen that if the scar is disregarded and raised in the flap it may be so poorly vascularized as to break down. Also a narrow strip of skin between the scar and an operative incision may become gangrenous. As a rule all or part of the original scar is excised and enlarging incision made along appropriate lines to gain adequate exposure.

Tendon wounds in the wrist or palm in which there has been no infection or loss of substance are frequently amenable to suture. Where there has been loss of tendon, however, or in old cases where great contraction of the muscle has occurred, it is usually necessary to graft tendon segments into the defect. Where the injury involves the fingers with the digital sheaths a graft is always indicated. The profundus alone is repaired since it is impossible to obtain free gliding of two grafted tendons, within the narrow sheath. In order to avoid a suture line within the sheath attachment of tendon to the distal phalanx may be accomplished by bringing the Y-shaped tendon graft about the base of the distal phalanx and suturing the stump of the profundus into the crotch of the Y, as recommended by Koch.

Unless secondary operation is performed very early the fibrous sheaths will be found to be collapsed and unusable, or destroyed and in these cases transverse ligaments will require to be fashioned from bits of tendon to hold the newly grafted tendon in place and prevent bowstring deformity.

Following tendon repair absolute immobilization is maintained for a period of approximately three weeks, after which some active motion is permitted with the appropriate parts protected from over-stretching by means of a splint or check rein. At the end of four or five weeks the patient is fitted with a removable splint which permits free motion but protects the part against the extreme pull of the antagonists or against sudden forceful movements. As soon as the removable splint has been applied the patient is instructed to soak the hand once or twice every day and to exercise it carefully, avoiding over-stretching. Physical therapy may be instituted three or four weeks after operation although many patients will perform their own quite successfully after a little instruction.

Nerve repair poses several problems. First, of course, is that of the accurate diagnosis, nature of and extent of nerve damage. It is not necessary to go into the details of diagnosis of peripheral nerve lesions. There are a few simple pathognomonic signs by which lesions of the nerves involving the hand may be confidently recognized. The typical wrist drop of radial nerve damage is never missed; and the restricted area of sensory loss on the dorsum of the hand between the first and second metacarpals is just as pathognomonic. Division of the ulnar nerve produces the typical wasting of the interosseus muscles, the extension deformity of the metacarpophalangeal joints of the third, fourth and fifth fingers. Inability to abduct and adduct the fingers is easily demonstrated. Median nerve lesion besides the extensive sensory loss is revealed by the loss of the intrinsic motions of the thumb (rotation) and the wasting of the thenar eminence. While it is occasionally difficult to be certain that regeneration is taking place after a supposed nerve suture, it has been our experience that in case of doubt it is wise to explore, and invariably it is found that the damage has not been repaired.

Secondary nerve repair must also be done in a field of soft tissues as in the case of tendons, but the problem of obtaining end to end suture is not always so easily solved since the use of nerve grafts has not yet been shown to be as universally applicable as the tendon graft. The nerves must be first isolated in the normal positions above and below the site of injury and followed to the scar. It is usually necessary to free the proximal and distal nerve ends for quite a distance above and below the site of damage so as to permit suture without tension. Extra length of the ulnar nerve may be obtained by transferring the nerve forward from its position back of the medial epicondyle. Positional changes in the neighboring joints, e.g., flexion of elbow and wrist will often produce enough relaxation to permit suture without tension. I have never been able to bring myself to bone shortening operations. However, there occurs the case in which no maneuvers suffice, and it is here that the nerve graft holds the only hope of a solution. In contrast to a few favorable reports of nerve grafting, notably by Bunnell, most neurosurgeons are quite sceptical of its value in the human despite the favorable results in animal experimentation. Recently, however, Davis and Perret have reported four carefully studied cases in which there is undoubted evidence of nerve regeneration. A point they make is that regeneration requires a much longer time than we have realized and that those who have reported unfavorably· upon the procedure may not have waited a long enough time. That nerve regeneration requires a long time is well realized, and that it may require a much longer time following nerve graft comes hardly as a surprise. Certain it is that those who have been following nerve repair cases over a period of years recognize a slow but steady improvement taking place after the first evidence of regeneration. Slow improvement may be detected, year after year over a period of four or five years.

RESUME

Repair of nerve and tendon damage to the hand may be accomplished at the initial operation if conditions permit, or as a secondary procedure three to five weeks after primary healing of a wound in which primary repair was not initially advisable. In case of doubt either as to the condition of the wound or the technical facilities it is advisable to refrain from nerve and tendon repair.

Present Status of Immunization Procedures[*]

JOHN F. HACKLER, M.D., M.P.H.

*Professor of Preventive Medicine and
Public Health
University of Oklahoma
School of Medicine*

OKLAHOMA CITY, OKLAHOMA

The value of active immunization against Diphtheria, Pertussis, Smallpox, Tetanus, and Typhoid Fever can no longer be questioned. These immunizing agents are effective in prevention of their respective disease when properly administered, allowing for a suitable length of time for development of antibodies. Only one of these—Pertussis—falls short of being almost one-hundred per cent effective, but there is ample justification for its widespread use. While complete protection may not be attained in all susceptible children, the disease is modified to the extent that loss of life is unlikely to occur and other complications are reduced materially.

DIPHTHERIA

Although diphtheria immunization has been known to be effective for many years, application of the procedure has lagged. It is known that immunization of only 60 per cent of preschool children will prevent general outbreaks of the disease, yet throughout the United States few areas are known to have reached that percentage. In Oklahoma during the past 5 years we have had an average of 396 cases with 50.4 deaths per year. In fact, Oklahoma, 1940-42, ranked third in the United States in deaths from diphtheria under 10 years of age with a rate of 13.5 per 100,000 children of that age. For the

*Delivered before the Section on Public Health, Oklahoma State Medical Association Annual Meeting, May 2, 1946.

country as a whole, the rate was 5.3.[1]

As shown in Figure 1, during the late war years we lost ground in Oklahoma in our fight against this disease, due in part perhaps, to loss of medical men to the armed forces, particularly younger men, and to depletion of health department staffs. In 1944 there was a definite upswing in an otherwise steadily declining death rate. This rise was maintained through 1945.

FIGURE I
Deaths from Diphtheria per 100,000 population by years, 1936-45, - Oklahoma.

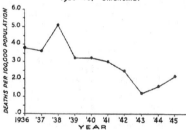

Alum precipitated diphtheria toxoid is the product of choice for immunizing children against this disease and requires at least two doses given at intervals of one month. Only slightly less effective is three doses of fluid toxoid at monthly intervals. One of these procedures should be carried out during the latter half of the first year of life. A booster dose should be given about five years later, just previous to or at the time of school entrance, always in case of a local epidemic, and, in view of the recent increase in diphtheria cases in the "teen" ages, an additional booster at 10 to 12 years of age seems indicated. Satisfactory booster response occurs in 75 per cent of previously immunized children in five days and 97 per cent in 10 days.[2]

PERTUSSIS

Great progress has been made in the control of Pertussis during the past ten years. Improved products have been introduced and controlled studies reported[3] which now place this immunization along with those for smallpox and diphtheria in importance. Eighty to 85 per cent complete protection is now obtainable in comparison with an escape rate of 10 to 15 per cent in the non-immunized. Whooping Cough has for years been a leading cause of death among the common childhood communicable diseases. It heads the list in Oklahoma where it has caused an average of 70.8 deaths per year for the past five years (1940-44), as indicated in Fgure II.

FIGURE II

Average Number of Deaths per Year from Common Acute Infectious Diseases -- Oklahoma, 1940-44.

Disease:

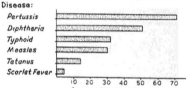

Average Number of Deaths per Year

Since children have not been thought to develop antibodies satisfactorily until the latter half of the first year of life, this immunization has generally been reserved until that period. However, when one studies the data regarding serious complications and particularly, deaths, from whooping cough, one finds that two-thirds of the damage has already been done. Protecting antibodies are not usually carried over from the mother against this disease in sufficient quantity for protection as is the case with most communicable diseases. Immunization of pregnant mothers, with the hope of sufficient placental transfer of antibodies for protection of the young baby has been tried now for some time with encouraging results.[4] As yet however, no conclusive epidemiological studies have been reported which indicate this method may be relied upon. The danger of reaction in the mother must be kept in mind.[5]

Table I indicates that in 1944 in Oklahoma 65.9 per cent of the 41 deaths from Pertussis were under one year of age, 88 per cent under three years, and 97.6 per cent under five years. This is the more startling when compared with diphtheria where only 9.1 per cent of deaths were under one year and 66.7 per cent under five years of age. Of the deaths during the first year, the majority were under six months of age.

TABLE I.

Number and Accumulative Percentage of Deaths by Age from Whooping Cough, Diphtheria and Measles in Oklahoma, 1944....

Age in years	Whooping Cough		Diphtheria		Measles	
	Number	Accum.%	Number	Accum.%	Number	Accum.%
Under 1	27	65.9	3	9.1	13	38.2
1	6	80.5	3	18.2	9	64.8
2	3	88.0	9	45.4	4	76.5
3	3	95.0	5	60.7	–	–
4	1	97.6	2	66.7	1	79.4
5-9	–		9	94.0	4	91.2
10 and over	1	100.0	2	100.0	3	100.0
Total	41		33		34	

Recent studies by Sako, et.al.,[6] and Sauer[7] indicate that young infants do respond by antibody production sufficiently to prevent deaths. This may however be of shorter duration than when given later, and for that reason a booster dose should be given at one year of age. To further protect the individual child and to extend immunity well into the school age so that it will not be brought home to younger children another booster at three years would be helpful. It probably should not be given after six years of age.[8] Whooping Cough immunization should be started early, preferably before two months of age, with a total dosage of at least 90 billion organisms. Sauer has demonstrated effective results with a total of 30 billion organisms using alum precipitated vaccine.[8]

Combined Alum Precipitated Diphtheria Toxoid and Pertussis Vaccine gives quite satisfactory results for both diphtheria and pertussis immunization, however, the importance of giving the pertussis vaccine early in life, in my opinion, outweighs the advantage to be gained by combined procedures at a later date.

TETANUS

If one wishes to combine immunization procedures, the logical combination is tetanus toxoid along with diphtheria toxoid. Delay of both these procedures until the latter half of the first year of life will not likely result in an undue exposure risk to either disease. Both products are toxoids and may be given as fluid (plain) toxoid, or as alum precipitated toxoid. Booster or stimulating doses should be given at least every five years, for both diseases.

While the number of cases from tetanus is not so great, there were in Oklahoma 14.8 deaths per year during the five year period 1940-44. Army and Navy experience has proved beyond doubt that toxoid may be relied upon when given sufficiently long before injury for immunity to develop, and when stimulated by a booster injection at the time of an injury which might result in infection. There is some evidence even that infection acts as a stimulating agent in the previously immunized. Dr. Edward L. Pratt of the Department of Pediatrics, Harvard Medical School, reports[9] a study of cases in the Infants and Childrens Hospital in Boston from 1924 to 1944. His report indicates that 80 per cent of the cases could not have been prevented by reliance upon passive immunity (antitoxin) because they followed injuries which were so slight that a physician was not consulted or were of such a minor nature or under such conditions that one would not usually expect tetanus to develop.

Active immunity as produced by toxoid will eliminate the necessity of sensitizing many pesons to passive agents (antitoxins) containing animal sera. Antitoxin may be required on several occasions, or some may need serum treatment for other diseases. The possibility of severe or unpleasant reactions following such repeated injections is disturbing, to say the least.

If tetanus toxoid is used alone it probably is not necessary to give it before two years of age. The alum precipitated toxoid is preferable in young children. Fluid toxoid should probably be used in persons over 12 years of age, to avoid painful local reactions which occur in increasing numbers as age advances.

SMALLPOX

Even more neglected at present is smallpox vaccination. This has been a mild disease in the United States in recent years. We have had no deaths in Oklahoma during the past five years (1940-44), but have had an average of 57.4 reported cases per year. Recent appearance of the disease in virulent form on our west coast should serve as a reminder that this can be a serious disease and a high level of immunity should be maintained.

Only the multiple pressure method of vaccination can be recommended and this should be applied at three to five months of age, repeated at intervals of five to seven years, and at any time in case of a local epidemic. Serious complications such as encephalitis have not been reported following vaccination in the first year of life, to my knowledge. Some type of reaction should follow each vaccination—either immune reaction, accelerated reaction, or the typical "primary take". If neither of these occurs, the chances are than the vaccine was not potent. This vaccine must be kept in the freezing unit of the refrigerator, to retain its potency.

SCARLET FEVER

Active immunization against Scarlet Fever is of value in selected groups and under certain circumstances, but in recent years and with present medication, the disease is not of sufficient severity to justify widespread use, particularly in view of the prevailing opinion that it protects only against the rash (or erythrogenic toxin) and not against the invasive characteristics of the organism itself.

TYPHOID FEVER

Typhoid Vaccine is so well accepted that it is necessary only to state that it may and should be given when and where indicated. It is seldom necessary under two years of age in urban areas.

MEASLES

Since measles and its complications are of considerable public health importance, mention should be made of available facilities for prevention and modification of this disease. Oklahoma still has a death experience from measles averaging 30 per year (1940-44), 76.5 per cent of which are under three years of age, as shown in Table I. If this disease can be postponed until after three years of age, many lives will be saved and complications will be reduced to a minimum.

Active immunization is not as yet successful but in recent years it has been found that passive protection can be transmitted by the use of convalescent serum, or by immune globulins. The globulin products are more concentrated and at present Human Immune Serum Globulin (gamma globulin)[10] is the product of choice, and is rapidly replacing Placental Globulin. Given within the first five or six days after exposure, in suitable dosage (usually 2 c.c. under three years of age), measles will be prevented. If given after that time but before the onset of symptoms, the disease will be modified and complications will be rare. For older children, modification is to be desired rather than prevention (unless the child is debilitated by other illness), for he will then develop a permanent immunity.

Human Immune Serum Globulin is distributed free to all local physicians by The American Red Cross through the state and local health departments. It is prepared as a by-product from blood donated to the American Red Cross for use by the armed forces as blood plasma during the recent war period. It is also now prepared and distributed through the usual commercial biologic firms.

As a general rule in giving immunizations

it should be remembered that lengthening the interval between injections within reason is to be preferred to shorter intervals. Particularly is this true with alum precipitated products which are in general preferable to plain products in that they give a more complete and longer lasting immunity. For example, pertussis immunization is more effective at three to four week intervals than at one to two week intervals. Even two to three month intervals are satisfactory for some alum precipitated products. As a rule intervals of one month are optimal from the standpoint of immunity production, and in public health clinics more immunizations are completed when given at one month than at longer intervals.

A period of two to three months is required for development of active immunity, which reaches its height usually within that period following the last injection of the series, then gradually declines over a period of months or years, but can be quickly restimulated to effective protective levels within five to 10 days by a single additional injection of the immunizing agent. Usually one-half the final dose of the original series is sufficient for this "booster" effect.

No attempt has been made to discuss other immunizations such as for Rocky Mountain Spotted Fever, Plague, Typhus Fever, Yellow Fever, etc., all of which are quite effective under circumstances demanding exposure to those diseases.

SUMMARY

In summary, I would suggest the following schedule of immunizations, in view of the public health importance of the diseases, and with due regard to adequate protection of the individual.

1. Pertussis Vaccine at one, two and four months of age.
2. Smallpox Vaccination at three or five months of age (at least between three and 12 months).
3. Diphtheria and Tetanus Toxoid (combined) during the last half of the first year, preferably beginning at the ninth month.
4. Booster Pertussis Vaccine at one year and three years.
5. Human Immune Serum Globulin following exposure to measles. Preventive—under three years. Modifying—three and over.
6. Booster Smallpox, Diphtheria and Tetanus at fifth year or at school entrance, always during a local epidemic, or following injury in the case of tetanus.
7. Booster Smallpox, Diphtheria and Tetanus Toxoid at 10 to 12 years of age.

BIBLIOGRAPHY
1. Metropolitan Statistical Bulletin; August, 1945.
2. Vladimir K. Volk, Wm. E. Bunney, and John T. Tripp, American Journal of Public Health, Volume No. 33, page 475; 1943.
3. J. A. Garvin, Ohio State Medical Journal, Volume No. 41, page 229; 1945.
4. Pearl Kendrick, Mary Thompson and Grace Eldering, American Journal of Diseases of Children, Volume No. 70, page 25; 1945.
5. Report of the Committee on Therapeutic Procedures for Acute Infectious Diseases and Biologicals of the American Academy of Pediatrics, Revised March, 1945.
6. W. Sako, W. L. Treuting, D. B. Witt and S. J. Nichamin, Journal of the American Medical Association, Volume No. 127, page 379; 1945.
7. Louis W. Sauer, Proceedings of Institute of Medicine of Chicago, Volume No. 13; 1945.
8. Louis W. Sauer, W. H. Tucker and Eva Markley, Journal of the American Medical Association, Volume No. 125, page 949; 1944.
9. Edward L. Pratt, Journal of the American Medical Association, Volume No. 129, page 1243; 1945.
10. Morris Greenberg, Samuel Fant, David D. Rutstein, Journal of the American Medical Association, Volume No. 126, page 944; 1944.

Small Town Practice*

CARL BAILEY, M.D.
STROUD, OKLAHOMA

Mr. Chairman and Gentlemen:

I do not apologize for the unscientific text of this paper because I feel it is opportune.

Several papers have been written about the country doctor—many referable to the horse and buggy era. Time has advanced and the country practice has been replaced by small city practice with outlying country trade. This is due to better roads and faster means of transportation, a decrease in the number of contagious and infectious diseases such as smallpox, typhoid and malaria, and the centralization of trade areas.

People in the country need good medical care as well as people in the larger cities, but lack of proper hospital facilities for which the recent graduate is trained and the desire of the recent graduate to centralize and specialize, the small towns are often found wanting. Not that I here criticize those who specialize, but far too many "so called" specialists are modified general practitioners. The country practitioner needs all the higher education he can get and should specialize in general practice, for his work is varied and at times, taxes the best qualified.

The small towns and communities need good, young doctors now. The doctor should be young because the work is hard, and because his variety of opportunities is unlimit-

*Delivered before the Section on General Medicine, Oklahoma State Medical Association, Annual Meeting, May 3, 1946.

ed. He should be good because his knowledge of medicine and human nature will be taxed to the utmost. He is needed now because many towns, even counties are without good medical care and in far too many communities his place is being taken or has been taken by the unskilled, or cultists. This should and can be changed.

The responsibility to supply all small towns and communities with doctors does not rest entirely with the medical profession. Some of the responsibility must lie with the community itself. The community should and must be civic minded enough to cooperate and see that its obligations are met. It should make itself into a desirable location by furnishing or seeing that modern, adequate, facilities can be supplied with the personnel required to give the young doctor and his colleagues the desire to locate and furnish the people adequate medical attention.

By adequate medical attention, I mean the fundamentals, at least, of good medicine. It would naturally be impossible for a very small community to expect to be supplied with on the spot over-all medical attention, but it could supply the location whereby the specialists from the larger areas could be called in and do their work without fear and trembling, at the sugestion and recommendation of their local doctor.

I do not believe the lifetime of any one individual is sufficient to supply a community with a garage for human beings, namely, a hospital, carry on his work as a physician, and do both adequately. If and when the doctor dies, the hospital is disposed of along with his personal effects, then the next doctor has to start all over again. I believe the hospital could and should be taken over by the community itself, as something lasting and permanent.

There should, of course, be someone to lay the groundwork or foundation. This responsibility lies within the medical profession itself. Let it encourage the towns to supply adequate workshops, itself supplying the personnel, and the direction and guidance of the workshops.

In a small community, the doctor's business is everyone's business. This, fortunately, does not apply to the doctor only, and it is not entirely a disadvantage. One does not always have to see the patient to know how he is getting along, nor to wonder long whether he is still satisfied with the doctor's services. It also makes it more essential for the doctor to follow the golden rule and the Oath of Hippocrates.

If one is unfortunate enough not to have a colleague with whom one can entrust one's patients, this is a distinct disadvantage, because one does not feel free to have enough leisure hours, vacation time, or time for post graduate study. This, of course, can be remedied by having a colleague, or colleagues. Partnership or group practice can apply equally well to the small community as to the city.

Since the need is great, a doctor cannot help but make a living, and regardless of our politics, an adequate living, the education of our children, and security in our old age are the aims in life for most of us. It is my understanding that they are still not putting pockets in shrouds. If wealth is the doctor's only consideration, it would have been much better if he had entered some other business or profession. The net income between the average city physician, and the average small town physician does not vary appreciably chiefly because the country doctor's expenses are less. There are exceptions both ways but considering everything—the question of remuneration averages up rather closely.

Another advantage in small town practice, is the fact that we naturally live nearer to Mother Earth. I don't mean to get sentimental, but, gentlemen, it does something for a man's perspective to be constantly within five minutes of God's great outdoors and amid the handiwork of His firmament.

One of our poets has said, "The world is too much with us late and soon and in getting and spending we lay waste our powers"— well, there's something about an early morning ride down a lonely country road on a mission of mercy that does something for a man's mind and heart. We have a little more opportunity to reflect and think and make the most of our resources within.

Then too, the people themselves get you and hold you. Very close friendships are made both within and without the profession. "From the cradle to the grave" *really* applies to small town practice.

In conclusion I think we'll all agree that our profession at its best must be based on service—and the ability to bring out the best that is in us individually. In many ways we are better able to do this in an environment that lends itself to adequate remuneration, time for reflection, close friendships, and most of all, the satisfaction of meeting the most vital need facing the medical profession today, that of "bringing well-trained, well-rounded medical attention to rural communities". On this basis, I appeal to the young doctor to consider a noble calling—a doctor flying his best colors—in a small town amid the people of the soil.

Although it is humiliating to confess, yet I do confess, that cleanliness and order are not matters of instinct; they are matters of education, and like most great things, mathematics and classics, you must cultivate a taste for them. *Disraeli.*

Book Reveiws

CLINICAL ELECTROCARDIOGRAPHY. By American Authors. Edited by David Scherf, M.D., F.A.C.P., Associated Professor of Medicine, New York Medical College, Flower and Fifth Avenue Hospitals, and Linn J. Boyd, M.D., F.A.C.P., Professor of Medicine, New York Medical College, Flower and Fifth Avenue Hospitals. Second edition. Price, $8.00: J. B. Lippincott Company, Publishers, Philadelphia, January 22, 1946.

This edition has been completely revised and rewritten. The authors begin the book with a simple and clear explanation of the principles of the electrocardiogram; a discussion of the principles of the apparatus and the production of the various complexes of the electrocardiogram as produced by the action of the heart. The physiology of the heart's action is well correlated with the electrocardiogram. This places the entire matter on a sound basis for a clear understanding of the abnormal electrocardiogram. The basic principles have been over simplified for a definite purpose and although there are many theories which have been clearly worked out and are now acceptable, the electro-physieal principles involved are very complex. Many of these theories and principles have not been explained in detail and a more simple and logical basis has been discussed on which to base beginning interest and information regarding the subject.

It is particularly well written for the beginner who is interested in this phase of cardiology. Both the old and the new nomenclature are considered so that one gains a thorough understanding between the two theories. The various alterations of the individual complexes making up an electrocardiogram are discussed in detail both as to changes which fall within normal limits and those changes which have a pathological significance. These changes are well illustrated by electrocardiograms throughout the book.

The effects of extra cardiac factor in producing an abnormal electrocardiogram is clearly shown and illustrated. Such extra cardiac factors as the endocrine glands and avitaminosis are particularly well covered. Abnormal records resulting from cardiac factors such as coronary thrombosis or myocardial infarction, acute pericarditis, cardiac injury and trauma are well illustrated and discussed with adequate correlation between the clinical problems and the interpretation of the electrogardiograms which is taken up with full consideration in the chest leads. An explanation of the arrhythmias includes a pathological physiology of the origin of the arrhythmias, the clinical aspects and the relationship of one arrhythmia to another.

Part four is given over to selective problems and interpretations with differential diagnosis. The book is recommended to all interested in this field and especially to those just becoming interested in this field. F. Redding Hood, M.D.

BRONCHIAL ASTHMA. Leon Unger, B.S., M.D., F.A.C.P., Assistant Professor, Department of Medicine, Northwestern University School of Medicine. Charles C. Thomas, Springfield, Illinois. $9.00. 1945.

This book, divided into three parts, namely the Clinical, the Laboratory and the Scientific, compiles detailed information on the sources of allergens, elimination diets, and a discussion of the various drugstore remedies of the treatment of Asthma, and is a valuable addition to the library of an internist as well as the allergist.

The clinical section takes up in detail the history, etiology, pathology and symptomatology as well as the different diagnosis and treatment of bronchial asthma. The continuity of thought in this section makes the reading interesting as well as instructive and yet includes scientific data necessary to sustain the point. These chapters are sthorough and comprehensive and are supplemented with an excellent bibliography.

The chapter on treatment is of great value to the individual practitioner, including as it does all forms of therapy.

The laboratory section contains information as to the preparation of extracts and the technic of pollen counts and shows that much time and effort was devoted to make this chapter as practical as possible.

The illustrations and charts provided in this book are excellent and they indicate that the publisher did an excellent job in printing.

On the whole this comprehensive study of asthma is a scientific yet practical treatise of great value to all individuals in the field of medicine.—James R. Huggins, M.D.

Obituaries

T. J. Jackson, M.D.
1874-1946

Funeral services were held Thursday, May 2, for Dr. T. J. Jackson, Ardmore, who died May 1 in his home following a critical illness of two weeks duration. Dr. Jackson was graduated from Atlanta College of Physicians and Surgeons in 1905 and has practiced medicine in Ardmore for 25 years.

He was a member of the Carter County Medical Society, the Kiwanis Club and the Masons. Dr. Jackson is survived by his wife, Daisy, a brother and two sisters.

C. L. Sullivan, M.D.
1880-1946

On January 27, 1946, Dr. C. L. Sullivan, Elmore City, died unexpectedly of a heart ailment.

Dr. Sullivan received his medical degree in 1905 from the Barnes Medical College in St. Louis. He moved to Elmore City in 1906 and has practiced medicine there for the past 40 years. He helped organize the First State Bank of Elmore City of which he was a director and a vice-president. He was a member of the Scottish Rite Temple of Guthrie, the First Baptist Church of Elmore City, the County Medical Society, the Oklahoma State Medical Association and the American Medical Association.

Dr. Sullivan is survived by his wife, one daughter, three sons, one brother and two sisters.

Medical School Notes

Word has been received that 1st Lt. David U. Geigerman, MC, 2819 Welborn Street, Dallas, Texas, graduated from the Army Air Forces School of Aviation Medicine, Randolph Field, Texas, on the 8th of February, 1946. Under the guidance of its Commandant, Brig. Gen. Eugene G. Reinartz, the School of Aviation Medicine specializes in training physicians and surgeons in a special branch of medical knowledge, practially unknown during World War I, but which now aids in safeguarding the lives of Army pilots and Air Force personnel. The intensive course Lt. Geigerman has just completed is one prerequisite for attaining the wings of a "Flight Surgeon" in the Medical Corps, U. S. Army Air Forces. Dr. Geigerman received his degree of Doctor of Medicine from the Oklahoma University School of Medicine in 1944.

The base hospital at Will Rogers Fie'd is under consideration by the Veterans Administration for a Veterans General Hospital. At the request of the Veterans Administration a Dean's Committee has been set up at the Medical School to cooperate with the Veterans Administration in working out plans for staffing such an institution. Conferences have been held, and it is thought that such an arrangement will be made although there has been no official announcement by the Veterans Administration.

)

Clinical Pathological Conference

University of Oklahoma School of Medicine
Presented by the Departments of Pathology and Orthopedics
DON H. O'DONOGHUE, M.D.—BELA HALPERT, M.D.

OKLAHOMA CITY, OKLAHOMA

DR. HALPERT: The patient whose story we are considering this morning died of a fairly common disease but one which does not commonly result in death. Early in the course of the disease, this condition was somewhat of a diagnostic problem. By the time the diagnosis became readily apparent, the patient was moribund. Dr. O'Donoghue will present the clinical aspect of the case.

PROTOCOL

Patient: J. H., White Female, age 13; admitted July 24, 1945; died July 26, 1945.

Chief Complaint: Inability to swallow or drink water, difficulty in speech.

Present Illness: On the morning of July 20, 1945, the patient suddenly became nauseated and vomited; vomiting persisted until 4:00 P. M. of that day. There were no associated aches, pains, nor was there headache. Her physician gave her some calomel. She had a temperature of 101° F. On July 21, 1945 fluids were regurgitated through the nose whenever she attempted to drink and she was unable to swallow or to talk plainly. Her physician thought that she was developing a retropharyngeal abscess, and sulfonamides were prescribed. Other physicians were called in consultation and on July 24, 1945 a spinal fluid examination was done. This was suggestive of poliomyelitis and she was referred to this hospital on that date.

Past and Family History: Noncontributory.

Physical Examination: On admission she was an adolescent girl, rather large for her age, complaining only of inability to swallow or speak. Respiratory movements were shallow, irregular, and thoracic in character.

Laboratory Findings: On admission the urine was amber, cloudy and acid, with a specific gravity of 1.032; there was a trace of albumin, no glucose. Numerous red blood cells and white blood cells (the latter in

clumps) were found microscopically. The findings suggested menstrual urine. The hemoglobin was 14.5 Gm., the red blood cell count was 4,950,000 and there were 6,200 white blood cells and 76 per cent neutrophils (18 per cent stab and 58 per cent segmented forms), 22 per cent lymphocytes and 1 per cent eosinophils and 1 per cent monocytes.

Clinical Course: The use of a suction apparatus was necessary to clear mucus from the throat at frequent intervals. Feeding was by stomach tube which was left in place. At 12:30 a.m. on July 26, 1945, a slight twitching of the submental region was noticed; this became marked by 2:00 a.m. The patient became irrational. At 2:15 a.m. there was irregularity of respiration which approached apnea. Manual artificial respiration was given until the patient could be placed in the respirator and continuous oxygen administered. Synchronization of respiration with the machine was poor and she died at 5:00 a.m.

CLINICAL DIAGNOSIS

DR. O'DONOGHUE: We have an unusual opportunity to learn something this morning because the death rate in poliomyelitis is very low, consistently under 5 per cent, and even when a death does occur in one of these children, it is usually very difficult to obtain permission for post mortem examination. To start off with then, we can say that this particular case is atypical—the typical case does not die. Regarding the diagnosis of such a case as this, it should be emphasized that paralysis is by no means necessarily an early symptom of poliomyelitis. As a matter of fact the non-paralytic group will make up the majority of hospital cases. In 1935, we had over 350 patients at Children's Hospital and approximately 60 per cent did not exhibit paralysis. This group is often classified as the abortive type, that is; they do not, in the early stage of their disease, exhibit paralysis.

Many of these are not diagnosed at all; others, who we might say are in the pre-paralytic state, may be diagnosed later when paralysis does occur. Many of these cases do not present symptoms which point directly to the causative disease; perhaps they will have only a gastric upset and vague muscle soreness. It is often difficult to examine the spinal fluid in such instances with what appears to be so little indication for this procedure and yet, many times, spinal fluid changes have been diagnostic when no positive symtpoms were noted. So-called spinal poliomyelitis affects principally the spinal cord, more especially the lumbar region so that the lower limbs are most often affected. The bulbar type is fortunately less common because it is harder to diagnose and the mortality with this type is much higher. That is because the brain stem is involved principally—an involvement that may lead to paralysis of the respiratory mechanism and paralysis of the palate and throat muscles. I am not going to read this protocol in its entirety but I will select from it certain pertinent facts for our consideration. First, the time of year (July) is a very common time for poliomyelitis. This year by July 1st we had more cases here than we usually have by the last of July. The reason I mention this is because it is during an epidemic that cases are most likely to be suspected. Inability to drink water was a chief complaint and this is certainly very signifiant to a person familiar with polio— it immediately suggests bulbar poliomyelitis. Nausea and vomiting were complaints. They are included in that indefinite group of symptoms previously mentioned. They are common complaints of children and could indicate almost anything. The history presented to you was taken after the patient was sent in here and was taken with the idea that this might be a case of poliomyelitis. The day following her initial symptoms, the patient regurgitated water through her nose and was unable to talk. This should certainly lead one to suspect paralysis of the palate and throat and thus some lesion in the nervous system. A retropharyngeal abscess might be considered. I do not believe, however, that if you carefully examined such a patient you would be apt to confuse a retrapharyngeal abscess with paralysis. She was initially treated for a retroperitoneal abscess but not for any great length of time for she was admitted as a case of poliomyelitis to this hospital three days later. Would treatment have done any good if it had been instituted earlier? In this particular case I doubt it. I think the message we have to interpret in this history is one that you find in many histories; careful inquiry and examination usually give the information necessary to make a diagnosis but through improper analysis, the diagnosis may be unduly delayed or missed altogether. The fact that she could not swallow or talk well was very important. The physical examination was pretty sketchy. Although she was a large adolescent girl, she was not breathing with her diaphram, but with her chest. The lungs should have been examined and also the heart and abdomen. We think that we might have obtained considerable important information about the patient had these examinations been done. Otherwise there is no particular information added that you can't get from the history. The laboratory findings, to me, did not mean a great deal. There was no spinal puncture done here.

The patient was not acutely ill on admission but she did die rather suddenly. She was put in bed with instructions to disturb her only when necessary. Suction was necessary to clear mucus from the throat. Such accumulation of mucus is very common in children when they have a paralysis of the palate and is extremely annoying and psychologically bad because it induces a feeling of panic. For these reasons, and to prevent serious interference with respiration, it is extremely important to keep mucus out of the throat. She was fed by stomach tube. I saw her the evening of the day on which she was admitted at which time involvement of the peripheral type was certainly minimal and there was questionable, if any, muscle spasm. We have carefully studied the effects of peripheral involvement much more of late and consider always two types of involvement. First there is the flaccid paralysis illustrated by foot-drop, but in addition there is often hyperirritability and spasm. Often the muscle is tight and resists stretching. You may have both effects in many muscles. To consider for a moment the respiratory difficulty, there are at least two or three causes for respiratory failure of this type:

1. A flaccid paralysis of certain of the muscles of respiration
2. A spastic paralysis of these muscles
3. Paralysis of the glottis.

The diaphragm is usually not affected so much as are the intercostal muscles. Hot packs are excellent for certain type of "tight" muscles. If the muscle is completely flaccid there is nothing in the world that you can do for it. On the other hand, the muscles in spasm can be treated by rest and heat and careful stretching. The "tight" cases are the only ones in which we get any function restored. If one finds a tight expanded chest there should be application of hot packs of some sort. A number of very hot blanket pads changed frequetly will be of great help. This patient did not present the picture of spastic chest muscles. One can tell this by careful examination of the chest to see whether there is any attempt at expansion—whether or not there is any pulling-in of the intercostal spaces with breathing. Sister Kinney has said that the respirator should not be used. She was right in so far as the spastic type of chest is concerned, but it is certainly of great value in those with flaccid paralysis of the respiratory muscles. This patient was very apprehensive and there is a question whether or not she should have been put in the respirator before she was. I did not think she was acutely ill when I saw her, in spite of her difficulty in breathing and swallowing. She was put into the respirator but her respiratory efforts were never well synchronized with the action of the machine. She was never cyanotic. I wonder if she died of a respiratory failure or if she died of cardiac failure. This of course cannot definitely be determined from our clinical data. Perhaps Dr. Halpert can give us some information on this. I have given little time to a discussion of the treatment of polio. Such a discussion can more appropriately be left until some time when we consider a case of the spinal type.

CLINICAL DISCUSSION

DR. HALPERT: I would like to ask if you recall whether the child preferred to lie on one side or the other?

DR. O'DONOGHUE: I do not recall this, but she was lying on the right side when I examined her.

QUESTION: What about the use of prostigmine in patients with spastic muscles?

DR. O'DONOGHUE: Prostigmine may relieve spasm and may be given to a patient with a "tight" chest.

QUESTION: What form of sedation would be most appropriate for use in a case such as this?

DR. O'DONOGHUE: We do not use very much sedation. With rest and heat they do not require sedatives.

QUESTION: It is true that there is no successful treatment in the bulbar type of poliomyelitis?

DR. O'DONOGHUE: There is no specific treatment for polio and the only treatment we have ever found is symptomatic.

ANATOMIC DISCUSSION

DR. HALPERT: There are a number of problems in conection with this disease—poliomyelitis. It is now fairly certain that it is produced by a virus. The portal of entry and exact manner of spread is not quite clear however. The most recent idea is that spread occurs from person to person. Spread by insects has been demonstrated; however, the stage when polio is most infectious is approximately three days prior to the onset of symptoms and for a period of approximately three days thereafter. The period of incubation lasts on an average of about 12 days.

As to the lesions resulting from this disease, it should first be emphasized that the organism of poliomyelitis is very highly selective for nervous tissue, i.e., it is a neurotrophic virus. In fact, histopathologic changes are confined to the nervous system except for certain changes in muscle which occur presumably as a result of this nervous involvement. The course by which spread of the virus takes place within the body is not known. It used to be thought that spread occurred from the nasal passages along the olfactory nerves and although this does occur in the case of monkeys, it apparently is not the major route of anatomic spread in human beings. It is possible that we may have to revise our concept of this disease altogether. A group who studied the disease in New York State found that during an entire year there were definitely cases of polio although not a single instance of paralytic manifestation occurred. It is possible that some of the cases of so-called "flu" which are going around now may be poliomyelitis in an abortive form. As Dr. O'Donaghue has stated, there are two major types of poliomyelitis, the spinal and the bulbar type. We were particularly concerned in this case to learn just where the lesions were and their character. There were no significant changes other than those in the central nervous system. The findings in this instance suggest that the important effects of the disease were principally respiratory. This patient died of anoxemia. The most striking findings were in the lungs; both lungs; particularly the left, were collapsed and almost airless. The left weighed 200 Gm. which is normal, but the right appeared partially solidified, dark red, jelly-like and on the cut surfaces presented a granular appearance. This lung weighed three times that of the left lung. It is possible that the patient developed pneumonia on the right side because she preferred to lie on this side and the influence of gravity led to stasis, edema and hypostatic pneumonia. Upon microscopic examination we found that much of this consolidation and increase in weight was the result of hemorrhage so that we should probably consider, in addition to pneumonia, an additive effect produced by the respirator. Necropsy findings, excluding the central nervous system, were otherwise essentially negative. In removing the brain is presented a gray-red hue similar to that often seen in patients dying of malaria. It weighed about 200 Gm. more than normal. There were no hemorrhages or areas of softening recognizable grossly. Microscopically, the picture was quite characteristic of acute poliomyelitis. Histopathologic changes fell into three major categories: 1) hyperemia with some interstitial hemorrhage, 2) perivascular and interstitial infiltration of lymphocytes, plasma cells and a few polymorphonuclear granulocytes, and 3) degenerative changes in the nerve cells proper. Such findings readily explain those symptoms which suggest encephalitis as well as those specific neurologic findings which relate to focal involvement of nerve cells.

Although particularly in the spinal type, there is a preferential involvement of the anterior horns, the microscopic changes are usually wide-spread. Cases of the frank spinal type usually show at least slight changes in the brain and those with bulbar polio usually show, microscopically considerable spinal involvement.

Classified Advertisements

FOR SALE: Small Clinic now conducted by a general practitioner and an E. E. N. & T. Specialists both of whom wish to retire, either or both will sell. The office building housing the Clinic is one story, air conditioned, well located and practically new. The Clinic is thoroughly established and doing a well paying practice and physicians are badly needed in this community. Correspondence and investigation solicited. Write Box C, Journal, Oklahoma State Medical Association, 210 Plaza Court, Oklahoma City, Oklahoma.

FOR SALE: Chainomatic Balance, Christian Becker; Nelson's Loose Leaf Medicine. Mrs. Ralph E. Myers, 1122 N. E. 13th, Oklahoma City, Oklahoma.

FOR SALE: Retiring because of failing health. Am offering Urological and G. U. instruments and office equipment including Cystoscope, Urethroscope, Catheters, Sounds, Microscope, in fact all instruments and equipment found in active office at a sacrifice. Location optional. Box B, c/o Journal, Oklahoma State Medical Association, 210 Plaza Court, Oklahoma City, Oklahoma.

FOR SALE: New Barnstead Still, capacity 1 gal./hr. $50.00. Biolite Infrared Lamp, $25.00. Telephone 2-4333, Oklahoma City.

WANTED: Physicians for health officer positions in county and district health departments in Oklahoma. Salary range according to public health training and experience $4800 to $6600 plus travel expense. Beginning salary with no previous training experience $4200 to $4800 plus travel expense. Address Commissioner of Health, Oklahoma State Department of Health, Oklahoma City 5, Oklahoma.

FOR SALE: Excellent General Practice, income $12,000; College town 3000; established 20 years; nice 3 room office; x-ray and office equipment original cost $4400. Cash price $2500; agriculture. N. E. Ruhl, M.D., Weatherford, Oklahoma.

FOR SALE: 1 each Keleket No. 4036 type KXP combination X-Ray, complete. For information, please contact the Oklahoma Medical Center, P. O. Box 1191, Oklahoma City, Oklahoma.

FOR SALE: Brown-Buerge Convertible Cystoscope, 24 fr. with concave and convex sheaths, examining and convertible telescopes and two No. 6 fr. catheters. In walnut case. Used one time; perfect condition. $190.00. Marvin Elkins, M.D., Muskogee, Oklahoma.

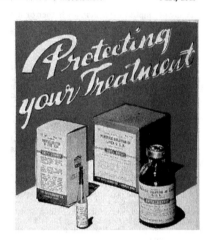

UNCERTAIN SUCCESS in the treatment of pernicious anemia is due to many unpredictable factors.

One element of certainty is added to your treatment when the Solution of Liver prescribed never varies from rigid standards.

Purified Solution of Liver, Smith-Dorsey, is unfailingly uniform in purity and potency. It has earned and maintained the confidence of thousands of physicians.

Purified Solution of Liver, Smith-Dorsey, will help to protect your treatment—to assure you of good results where the medication is the controlling factor.

PURIFIED SOLUTION OF *Liver*

Supplied in the following dosage forms: 1 cc. ampoules and 10 cc. and 30 cc. ampoule vials, each containing 10 U.S.P. Injectable Units per cc.

THE SMITH-DORSEY COMPANY
LINCOLN • NEBRASKA
Manufacturers of Pharmaceuticals to the Medical Profession Since 1908

Special Article

DR. JOHN VANMORE ATHEY

Bartlesville, Oklahoma

The friendly blackjacks and the rustling cottonwoods of the Osage Country welcomed Dr. John Vanmore Athey when in March, 1908 he left his practice in Ohio for the undeveloped new State of Oklahoma. He was born in West Virginia, studied medicine and practiced in Ohio from 1899 until 1908.

With his charming wife Dr. Athey located in Bartlesville, then a mere village, with a hopeful future in the oil industry. He became a member of the Washington County Medical Society in May, 1908, served as its president in 1914 and again in 1945.

He was secretary of the Northeast Oklahoma Medical Society from 1913 to 1916; was secretary of the Washington-Nowata County Medical Society from 1925 to 1944, twenty years of notable achievement in that organization. The Association of Secretaries of Medical Societies was organized during this term.

Serving as medical officer overseas during World War I, he emerged with the rank of captain. His outstanding contribution to the profession in Oklahoma has come through his service as councilor of the sixth district of the Oklahoma State Medical Association, starting in 1942, which position he held until 1946 at which time he requested that his name not be resubmitted.

His wise counsel has been greatly appreciated by his district, and by other officers of the State Association. Dr. Athey may be said to be young in thought, and word and deed, which, with the experience of accumulated years, make him a valuable councilor.

No greater compliment can be paid a man in any profession than to have his services highly considered by his colleagues. As Robert Browning is the poet's poet, so Dr. Athey is the doctor's doctor. Dr. "Van" has given many hours of service to the families of doctors and is always happy to serve in this capacity.

Having helped make Oklahoma medical history, Dr. Athey has seen the Association grow from an ineffectual group to an influential, scientifically potent organization. He can truly say, with Anaeas, "All of this I saw, and part of it I was."

THE PRESIDENT'S PAGE

Many have said the meeting just concluded was among the best if not the best our Association has ever had. The programs were so arranged that all could attend the sections giving them that which was of most interest to the individual.

The guest speakers were leaders in their field and were enthusiastically and attentively received as was evidenced by the attendance at the round table luncheons, sections and by the questions asked of them.

The technical exhibits were good and the exhibitors were well pleased with the attendance. Your officers are grateful to you for having visited the exhibits.

The program outlined and agreed upon by the House of Delegates for the next year is one that will call for the cooperation of the entire membership. This can be made a year of accomplishments with your help. We must go forward, we cannot remain stationary.

President.

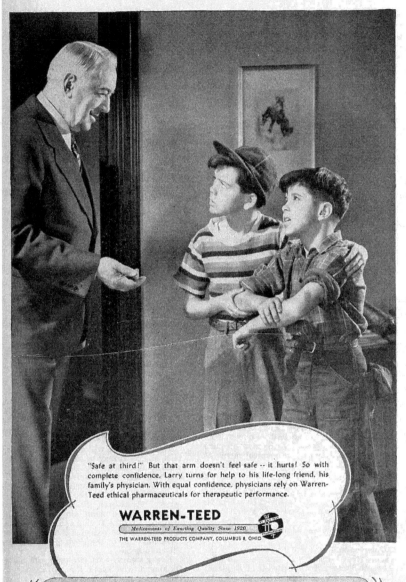

"Safe at third!" But that arm doesn't feel safe -- it hurts! So with complete confidence, Larry turns for help to his life-long friend, his family's physician. With equal confidence, physicians rely on Warren-Teed ethical pharmaceuticals for therapeutic performance.

WARREN-TEED

Medicaments of Exacting Quality Since 1920

THE WARREN-TEED PRODUCTS COMPANY, COLUMBUS 8, OHIO

Warren-Teed Ethical Pharmaceuticals: capsules, elixirs, ointments, sterilized solutions, syrups, tablets. Write for literature.

The JOURNAL Of The
OKLAHOMA STATE MEDICAL ASSOCIATION

EDITORIAL BOARD
L. J. MOORMAN, Oklahoma City, Editor-in-Chief
E. EUGENE RICE, Shawnee
BEN H. NICHOLSON, Oklahoma City
MR. DICK GRAHAM, Oklahoma City, Business Manager
JANE FIRRELL TUCKER, Editorial Assistant

CONTRIBUTIONS: Articles accepted by this Journal for publication including those read at the annual meetings of the State Association are the sole property of this Journal.

The Editorial Department is not responsible for the opinions expressed in the original articles of contributors.

Manuscripts may be withdrawn by authors for publication elsewhere only upon the approval of the Editorial Board.

MANUSCRIPTS: Manuscripts should be typewritten, double-spaced, on white paper 8½ x 11 inches. The original copy, not the carbon copy, should be submitted.

Footnotes, bibliographies and legends for cuts should be typed on separate sheets in double space. Bibliography listing should follow this order: Name of author, title of article, name of periodical with volume, page and date of publication.

Manuscripts are accepted subject to the usual editorial revisions and with the understanding that they have not been published elsewhere.

NEWS: Local news of interest to the medical profession, changes of address, births, deaths and weddings will be gratefully received.

ADVERTISING: Advertising of articles, drugs or compounds unapproved by the Council on Pharmacy of the A.M.A. will not be accepted. Advertising rates will be supplied on application.

It is suggested that members of the State Association patronize our advertisers in preference to others.

SUBSCRIPTIONS: Failure to receive The Journal should call for immediate notification.

REPRINTS: Reprints of original articles will be supplied at actual cost provided request for them is attached to manuscripts or made in sufficient time before publication. Checks for reprints should be made payable to Industrial Printing Company, Oklahoma City.

Address all communications to THE JOURNAL OF THE OKLAHOMA STATE MEDICAL ASSOCIATION, 210 Plaza Court, Oklahoma City 3

OFFICIAL PUBLICATION OF THE OKLAHOMA STATE MEDICAL ASSOCIATION
Copyrighted June, 1946

EDITORIALS

AWAY TO THE A.M.A. VIA THE SANTA FE

Doctor, this is your one chance for a temporary Eutopia. Nobody would want a lasting one, but once in a life time every doctor should mix pleasure with medicine. For generations people have gone west for adventure, and people have gone west for gold, but for the first time since Lewis and Clarke doctors are invited to go west on a lark. This victory vacation provides 18 days of pure fun, interrupted only by a medical picnic at the Golden Gate. If the medical wennies ruffle your gastronomic complacency the restorative juices will be renewed by the roses of Portland, the snow capped brow of Mt. Hood, and the Scenic Columbia River Drive filling you with wonder and insidiously slipping you into the soft mists of beautiful Multonoma Falls where bobbing water ousels bekon you to Heaven.

Then on and on for days of charm in the Pacific Northwest, including an all day cruise to Victoria for a little bit of England. Fascinating drives through sylvan forests, seaside and sunken gardens and then back to the Empress Hotel in time for tea. Cruising back through the light of the setting sun soothes the soul for a peaceful night in the beautiful city of Seattle. This to be followed by one of the most scenic one day trips to be had anywhere in the world; this one day motor trip to Mt. Rainier National Park is something to be remembered a life time. It fills the soul with an abiding appreciation of all things beautiful in the realm of nature. Truly it leads to paradise valley where wild flowers encircled by perpetual snow, literally obscure the good earth.

Time and space will not permit further details. Briefly it may be said that the traveler returns to Seattle for sight seeing in this beautiful city, to the University of Washington with its unrivaled scenic beauty and then the long trek over the northern Pacific, across Washington, Idaho and Montana, through rugged mountains and ravishing vistas, across the Divide and down the eastern slope to the famed Yellow Stone for a three day tour of the Park. Then to Kansas City and home.

Every weary, worn doctor in the State of Oklahoma who hears the nostalgic call of the Atcheson, Topeka and Santa Fe should drop his practice and say goodbye, I am on my way to the A.M.A. and a couple of weeks for genuine play.

THE STATE MEETING

For weeks before the State Medical Association met in Oklahoma City, the State offices were buzzing with activity and every desk and table was stacked with programs, badges and other material for the State Meeting. It was impossible for the Editor to get even a courteous nod and he went about thinking if the Journal does come out it will be only by the grace of God. But like doodle bugs working under a pile of sand the members of the staff came up with the situation well in hand.

Our hats are off to the members of this efficient staff for the part they played in building a fine program and for all mechanical arrangements and at the same time keeping the Journal on schedule. It was a great meeting furnishing an outlet for local medical thought and bringing much of the best in medical progress from other states. It is doubtful if the combined practical and scientific values exhibited at this meeting have been matched by any previous annual meeting. The out of state guests marveled at the quality of papers presented by local doctors and the guest speakers brought to the local profession a wealth of scientific material.

As a result this meeting established a high mark which will stand as a challenge for all future state meetings.

CLOSER CO-OPERATION BETWEEN THE PHYSICIAN AND THE DENTIST

Much has been said and written about this subject, and conditions are much better today than in the past but there is still much to be desired.

It is discouraging for a physician to send a patient to his dentist for a check-up of possible infection in the oral cavity, and have the patient report back that the dentist, after looking in the mouth and without x-ray or other tests, has pronounced that no infection is present.

It is also discouraging for a conscientious dentist to have a physician, after looking in a patient's mouth, give instructions to have this or that tooth or all extracted. Both of these happen, but not so often as in the past.

We believe the average physician feels that the dentist does not give enough consideration to the diagnosis of conditions in the mouth that could affect the patient's general health. Possibly there is some truth in this assumption because anyone practicing a speciality is likely to become so engrossed in his particular field that he could very easily overlook the more general conditions.

Some physicians and a few dentists go so far as to recommend that Dentistry be made a true speciality of medicine by requiring dentist to have an M.D. degree. There are not enough dentists now, and if four more years were required to prepare a dentist for practice, it would further cut down on the number. This would necessitate a subprofession or someone with less training to work under the Physician Dentist to do much of the work now done by the dentist. We do not believe that this would be good for either the dental profession or the public.

We believe that dentists should be taught more about medicine and we also believe the physician should be taught more about dentistry. This should be done in our respective schools for those studying medicine or dentistry. Much could be done along this line by having physicians on dental society programs and dentists on medical society programs.

But we believe the greatest good could be done if the physician and dentist would consult one another more about their mutual patients.—J. B. Ratliff, D.D.S.

THE DOCTOR, THE HOG AND OH POWER ALMIGHTY

On Friday morning a doctor called the O.P.A. to request the privilege of killing a hog. The hog was raised on the doctor's place, the meat would be used for the sustinence of his patients in his own Institution located on his own farm where the hog resided. Unfortunately the doctor does not live on the place with the hog, but he does spend three days a week there looking after the Institution, attending his patients and directing the work on the farm.

When he called the P.O.A. the doctor was passed from one secretary to another, through the heads or representatives of four departments and finally on Saturday morning the fourth department head or representative admitted that the request had some merit but a decision could not be handed down without the opinion of O.P.A.'s legal representative. After some difficulty the legal adviser was located.

He courteously listened to the doctor's story and patiently mulled over the facts while the hog made continued inroads on the dwindling corn supply. After asking many questions and blue printing several possibilities none of which could quite meet the O.P.A. specifications, he was told that the man who took care of the farm and dairy lived on the place. When asked if the hog could be killed in the farmer's name, he pondered the pros and cons and finally it was suggested that the doctor might sell the hog to the farmer who could kill it and sell it back to its rightful owner. The implications were that in this way the O.P.A. would not be embarrassed, the government would not be cheated and the patients would have meat if they were willing to wait for it.

The Saturday noon hour was approaching and the legal representative happened not to be talking from his own office, consequently his printed rules, regulations and directives were not available and the doctor was requested to please call again on Monday. So, the O.P.A.'s legal adviser who was going off the job at noon Saturday to rest until 9:00 A.M. on Monday pleasantly dismissed the doctor who had spent a day and a half pursuing the request and who expected to spend the weekend caring for the sick. But before letting him go the doctor insisted on knowing what difference it would make to Uncle Sam and the hog if he didn't actually live on the place. Also whether or not there would be a government blank to fill out in case he should ultimately secure permission. With the blank hanging over him, and the uncertainty of Monday's negotiations with further delays the doctor decided the fine Poland China hog would have to go to packing town, mix with the common herd and be knocked in the head by a stranger instead of having a private killing. As it now stands the Institution will have to take its quota of fresh pork at O.P.A. prices and the patients will have to take pot luck from the general herd.

According to our lamented Will Rogers, the government always gave more thought and attention to pigs than people. Considering this advantage on the hog's side, and the threatened bureaucratic control of the people and their doctors, the above experience is disconcerting. If the pig-physician relationship can be so disturbed with such serious delays what can we expect re the patient-physician relationship under similar control. If a doctor cannot kill his own hog to save corn and supply meat for his patients, how can he hope to prevent disease, cure the sick and save his patients from disaster under such rules and regulations with weekends off.

SOON OPPORTUNITY WILL BE KNOCKING AT YOUR DOOR

Medical historians have an abiding interest in what doctors are made of, what they live by, and how they die. Many who have pioneered in the building of this great commonwealth are still living. Some have been financially successful, others have lived well, but accumulated little while some have eked out a wonderful existence in the service of humanity, sending up enough good material for a mansion in the sky.

The Alumni Association of the University of Oklahoma School of Medicine is planning a campaign to raise funds for a research institute. When the first gun is fired for this campaign the members of the medical profession should be in line and get off with a good start. Truly this will be a great opportunity for all good doctors who have reaped a material reward from practice or investments.

Opportunity is good enough to knock, but not inclined to wait. Life is short and wealth is troublesome. Sooner or later it must be left behind. Heirs are not always both worthy and wise. The doctor who has been capable and conservative in the accumulation of wealth should employ common sense and sound judgement in its distribution. Even though heirs are worthy and wise they will not need much and they will want less. They will understand that you can't take it with you and will appreciate your desire to place your wealth where it will work for the benefit of humanity.

Certainly the doctors of Oklahoma will not let pass this opportunity to place Oklahoma permanently on the medical map.

When Dr. Ratcliff, one of the recipients of the gold headed cane, died he willed his Yorkshire estate to the Master and fellows of University College forever. This gift to Oxford University provided for the foundation of two traveling fellowships. It made available five thousand pounds for the enlargement of the building of University College where he himself had been educated. It provided forty thousand pounds for the building of a library in Oxford and five hundred pounds yearly forever toward mending the diet of St. Barthalomew's Hospital. Having made provisions for certain individuals he gave to his executors in trust all his estates to be applied to such charitable purposes as they in their discretion should think best, but no part thereof to their own use or benefit.

Out of these bequests came the Ratcliff Library which is perhaps the most beautiful building at Oxford University. In addition that classical city boasts of two other edifices which bear the name of the same munificent benefactor. Nearly three hundred years have elapsed since Dr. Ratcliff's money went to work for Oxford University. It would be impossible to estimate the benefit accrued to humanity.

Our own William Osler participated in Ratcliff's beneficence. If stark materialism and mechanistic developments do not put an end to civilization, students throughout the world shall continue to profit through Ratcliff's bequest.

If you are rich in this world's goods make provision for the future by wise distribution. If you are poor, remember the widow's mite may become mighty.

Death if the liberator of him whom freedom cannot release, the physician of him whom medicine cannot cure, and the comforter of him whom time cannot console.—*Colton: Lacon.*

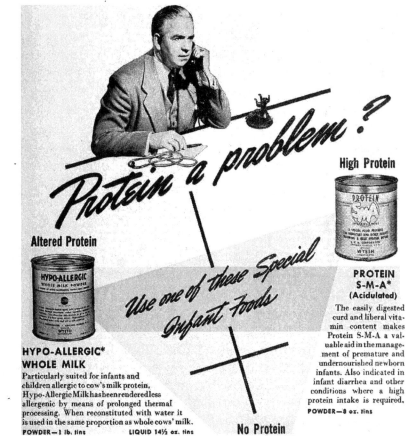

Protein a problem?

Use one of these Special Infant Foods

Altered Protein

High Protein

**PROTEIN
S-M-A***
(Acidulated)

The easily digested curd and liberal vitamin content makes Protein S-M-A a valuable aid in the management of premature and undernourished newborn infants. Also indicated in infant diarrhea and other conditions where a high protein intake is required.
POWDER—8 oz. tins

HYPO-ALLERGIC*
WHOLE MILK
Particularly suited for infants and children allergic to cow's milk protein, Hypo-Allergic Milk has been rendered less allergenic by means of prolonged thermal processing. When reconstituted with water it is used in the same proportion as whole cows' milk.
POWDER—1 lb. tins   LIQUID 14½ oz. tins

No Protein

ALERDEX*
Protein-free Maltose and Dextrins
An all-around milk modifier especially useful in the hypo-allergenic milk diet of the infant sensitive to proteins, Alerdex is prepared from noncereal starch by a special procedure to eliminate every trace of protein.
POWDER—16 oz. tins

S. M. A. DIVISION   *REG. U. S. PAT. OFF.

WYETH INCORPORATED   PHILADELPHIA 3, PA.

53RD ANNUAL MEETING ATTRACTS LARGE REGISTRATION

735 Register

The first post war meeting of the Association was an outstanding success both from the standpoint of scientific medicine and the adoption of a progressive public education program.

Outstanding accomplishments of the House of Delegates were the unanimous approval of the Report of the Publicity Committee which recommended the adoption of an advertising program through the lay press for the purpose of educating the public concerning the advancement in the medical science and medico-economic fields, also the endorsement of a medical care program for veterans, patterned after plans now in operation in Kansas, Michigan, California and many other states.

House of Delegates Votes Special Assessment and Raise in Dues

In keeping with its action to give the public a graphic picture of medicine's place in the every day life of Mr. and Mrs. America through the medium of advertising, the House of Delegates unanimously voted to assess each member twenty-five dollars, the special assessment to be placed in a special fund for advertising purposes. County societies will have this program presented to them in its entirety in the immediate future.

The need for an expansion of the executive office to take care of the increasing activities of the Association was apparent from the report of the Council and the delegates were united in their desire to have all programs of the Association handled in an adequate manner. In order that the programs might be increased in scope the dues of the Association were raised to twenty-two dollars for 1947, an increase of ten dollars. This increase will allow for the employment of an Assistant Executive Secretary which will permit the present Secretary to maintain closer contact with the County Societies and the members by being in a position to attend County, District and Councilor District Meetings.

Allied Professional Committee

The Report of the Council to the House of Delegates which will be carried in the official transcript of the meeting, appearing in this and subsequent issues of the Journal, submitted the following additional recommendations to the House of Delegates: The establishment of a uniform fee schedule for all governmental agencies; the establishment of a committee on rural health to work with farm organizations; the establishment of local committees to advise cities and counties in the construction of hospitals; endorsement of the activities of the Alumni Association of the Oklahoma School of Medicine in promoting a three million dollar research institution; and reorganization of the standing committees of the Association.

Dr. Kuyrkendall, the newly installed president, announced to the House of Delegates that this entire program would be brought to the membership through the Councilor District meetings as soon as possible in order that every member of the Association might have minute details of the program of the Association for the coming year.

NEW OFFICERS AND COUNCILORS ASSUME OFFICE

Paul Champlin, M.D., Enid, President-Elect

Dr. L. C Kuyrkendall, McAlester, was installed as President of the Association by the out-going President, Dr. V. C. Tisdal, Elk City, at the Annual Dinner Dance on the closing day of the Meeting, May 3. He had previously served the Association as Councilor of the Ninth District from 1936 to 1945, when he resigned to assume the duties of the President-Elect. Dr. Kuyrkendall brings to the Presidency of the Association many years of experience in both scientific and economic medical problems and he is still practicing medicine in McAlester, specializing in Opthamology.

Dr. Paul Champlin of Enid was elected to the office of President-Elect to serve in 1947-1948. He is a graduate of Washington University School of Medicine and is a practicing physician in Enid, Oklahoma. Dr. Champlin is the first President to be elected from Enid since 1922 at which time Dr. George A. Boyles served in this capacity.

Dr. Roy Emanuel, Chickasha, newly elected Vice-President, succeeds Dr. Ralph McGill of Tulsa; Dr. Alfred R. Suggs, Ada, Vice-Speaker of the House, succeeds Dr. H. K. Speed, Sayre. Dr. George Garrison, Oklahoma City, was re-elected to serve a succeeding term of two years as Speaker of the House of Delegates.

Dr. James Stevenson who completed his first term as delegate to the American Medical Association was unanimously elected to succeed himself, and Dr. Finis Ewing of Muskogee was unanimously elected his alternate.

New Councilors Elected for Districts No. 2, 3, 4 and 6

The election of Councilors found it necessary to elect a successor to fill the unexpired terms of Dr. Tom Lowry, Oklahoma City, and Dr. J. Wm. Finch, Hobart. Dr. Lowry's vacancy was created by his death and Dr. Finch's by resignation. Dr. Gordon Livingston, Cordell, was elected to complete the term of Dr. Finch and Dr. Carroll Pounders, Oklahoma City, was elected to complete the term of Dr. Lowry. Dr. Pounders was appointed by the Council to fill this position upon Dr. Lowry's death.

Councilors for Districts No. 3 and 6 completed their terms of office and Dr. C. E. Northcutt, Ponca City, was elected to succeed himself in District No. 3. Dr. Ralph McGill, Tulsa, was elected to the office of Councilor for District No. 6, succeeding Dr. John V. Athey, Bartlesville, who requested that the House of Delegates not consider his name for re-election.

SPECIAL TRAIN TO A.M.A. RECEIVING ENTHUSIASTIC APPROVAL

As the Journal goes to press, 100 Oklahoma physicians, their wives and families have already made reservations to go to the American Medical Association meeting in San Francisco July 1-5 and enjoy a post convention trip to the Pacific Northwest.

The Association has extended invitations to other states to participate in the tour and reservations have already been received from Kansas, Texas, South Dakota,

WILLIAM E. EASTLAND, M.D.
F. A. C. R.

RADIUM AND X-RAY THERAPY
DERMATOLOGY

405 Medical Arts Bldg.

Oklahoma City, Oklahoma   Phone 3-1446

Iowa, Mississippi, Indiana and New York.

Each member of the Association has received a direct mail itinerary of the trip and it is urged that all those who may be considering going to San Francisco on the Special Train make their decision as early as possible in order that they may in so far as possible have the accommodations they desire.

The post convention trip to the Pacific Northwest, including stopovers at Portland, Seattle, Victoria, British Columbia, with side trips to Mt. Rainier and the Columbia River Drive; and a three-day tour of Yellow Stone National Park, make this trip almost a must for anyone going to San Francisco.

Complete information can be obtained by writing the Executive Office, 210 Plaza Court, Oklahoma City, or contacting Mr. Harry E. Kornbaum of the Rainbow Travel Service, First National Bank Bldg., Oklahoma City, who will personally conduct the tour.

PRESS RELEASE FROM U. S. PUBLIC HEALTH SERVICE RE: PENICILLIN

Proportion of Element K in supplies of penicillin has not been great enough to reduce seriously the value of the drug in the treatment of syphilis or other diseases. Medical Director J. R. Heller, Jr., Chief of the Venereal Disease Division, U. S. Public Health Service, stated that, ''There is no occasion for alarm on the part of physicians who have used penicillin or of patients who have been treated with it. Penicillin as currently available and employed constitutes the best and safest method of treatment yet devised.''

Commercially prepared penicillin contains not one but several penicillins, known as G, X, F and K. The syphilis study section of the National Institute of Health in the U. S. Public Health Service reports that penicillin K is relatively less valuable than the other penicillins in the treatment of syphilis and certain other diseases because it is rapidly destroyed in the body. Industry has already taken steps to reduce the K content of commercial penicillin and will apply further scientific information as soon as it becomes available. The relative effectiveness of G, X, and F has not yet been determined.

Penicillin has remained a complicated scientific problem since Medical Director John F. Mahoney of the Public Health Service first demonstrated three years ago the curative value of the drug in syphilis therapy at the Venereal Disease Research Laboratory in Stapleton, New York. Subsequently, the Office of Scientific Research and Development sponsored cooperative studies with leading universities and other clinics throughout the country in an effort to determine the effects of drugs upon disease and the relative values of different methods of treatment. Since January 1, 1946, the Public Health Service has assumed complete responsibility for these studies in forty clinics.

NEUROLOGICAL HOSPITAL

Twenty-Seventh and The Paseo
Kansas City, Missouri

Modern Hospitalization of Nervous and Mental Illnesses, Alcoholism and Drug Addiction.

THE ROBINSON CLINIC

G. WILSE ROBINSON, M.D.
G. WILSE ROBINSON, Jr., M.D.

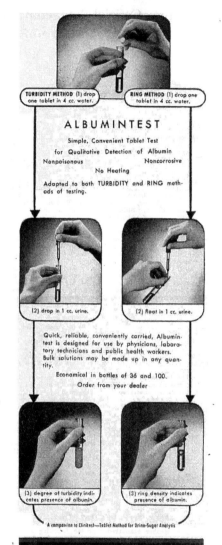

TURBIDITY METHOD (1) drop one tablet in 4 cc. water.   RING METHOD (1) drop one tablet in 4 cc. water.

ALBUMINTEST

Simple, Convenient Tablet Test
for Qualitative Detection of Albumin

Nonpoisonous   Noncorrosive

No Heating

Adapted to both TURBIDITY and RING methods of testing.

(2) drop in 1 cc. urine.   (2) float in 1 cc. urine.

Quick, reliable, conveniently carried, Albumintest is designed for use by physicians, laboratory technicians and public health workers. Bulk solutions may be made up in any quantity.

Economical in bottles of 36 and 100.

Order from your dealer

(3) degree of turbidity indicates presence of albumin.   (3) ring density indicates presence of albumin.

A companion to Clinitest—Tablet Method for Urine-Sugar Analysis

AMES COMPANY, Inc., Elkhart, Indiana

Official Proceedings of House of Delegates
Oklahoma State Medical Association
April 30, 1946

MINUTES OF THE FIRST SESSION
Tuesday, April 30, 1946

The first session of the House of Delegates was called to order in the Skirvin Tower Hotel by the Speaker of the House, Dr. George Garrison.

The Chairman of the Credentials Committee, Dr. McLain Rogers, stated a quorum was present.

It was *moved* by Dr. C. R. Rountree, *seconded* by Dr. James Stevenson, that the minutes of the last meeting be accepted as published. The motion *carried*.

Following the adoption of the above motion, the Speaker appointed the following Reference Committees: *Resolutions Committee*: Drs. E. H. Shuller, McAlester, Chairman; P. J. Devanney, Sayre; C. R. Rountree, Oklahoma City; F. C. Lattimore, Kingfisher; S. A. Lang, Nowata; J. O. Hood, Norman. *Advisory Committee to Resolutions Committee*: Drs. John C. Perry, Tulsa; Julian Feild, Enid; Claude Chambers, Seminole. *Tellers of Elections*: Drs. Phil Risser, Blackwell; Ned Burleson, Prague; Haskell Smith, Stillwater. *Sergeant-at-Arms*: Drs. Charles O'Leary, Oklahoma City; W. F. Lewis, Lawton; L. R. Kirby, Cherokee; E. Eugene Rice, Shawnee.

At this point the Speaker welcomed Mr. Pete Weaver, Stillwater, representative of the State Pharmaceutical Association and Dr. F. J. Reichmann, representative of the State Dental Society, and asked them to say a few words to the House of Delegates.

Mr. Weaver extended the best wishes of the Pharmaceutical Association for a good meeting. Te then commended the medical profession on the past legislation and urged the fight against socialized medicine. It was his opinion that the pharmacists, nurses and other allied professions should band together and join the fight.

Dr. Reichmann then extended the greetings and good wishes of the Dental Society. He stated that the dental profession was proud of what the medical profession was doing and pledged their support in the future.

Dr. Garrison stated that the next item on the agenda was the Annual Report of the Council but that it would deferred until the Report from the A.M.A. Delegates had been given and the Report of the Committees had been given.

The Report of the A.M.A. Delegates was requested and the floor given to Dr. James Stevenson of Tulsa.

Dr. Stevenson explained that the work of the A.M.A. House of Delegates is carried on by referring special topics to reference committees. The voluntary health insurance was referred in order to ascertain what was necessary. The people do not demand compulsory health insurance but want some form of health insurance. Among the fourteen points of the A.M.A. Program, voluntary health insurance is endorsed. A very interesting and enlightening program is anticipated at the meeting this summer in San Francisco.

Dr. C. R. Rountree, Oklahoma City, A.M.A. Delegate was granted the floor. After giving a brief resume of President Truman's Health Program, he outlined in detail the National Health Program of the American Medical Association.

Following the above reports, it was *moved* by Dr. F. W. Boadway, Ardmore, *seconded* by Dr. Ellis Lamb, Clinton, and *carried* that the report of the A.M.A. Delegates be accepted.

The Speaker announced that the following District Councilor Reports had been published and asked the pleasure of the House: Districts No. 1, No. 3, No. 5, No. 6, No. 7, No. 8 and No. 9. On *motion* by Dr. L. S. Willour, McAlester, *seconded* by Dr. James Stevenson, Tulsa, the reports were *accepted*.

---

*This report, appearing in this and subsequent issues, has been cut due to lack of space. The official transcript is in the office of the Oklahoma State Medical Association.

Those Councilor District Reports that had not been published were then in order. District No. 2 Report was called for and, due to the absence of Dr. Wm. Finch, Councilor from District No. 2, no report was given.

Dr. Carroll M. Pounders, Councilor for District No. 4 was then called upon to give his report. Dr. Pounders explained that he had been elected to serve the term left vacant by the passing of Dr. Tom Lowry, former Councilor, and having been in office for only a few weeks, had no report to make.

Dr. John A. Haynie, Councilor for District No. 10 was then called upon and gave the following report:

Report of Councilor District No. 10

To the President and House of Delegates
Oklahoma State Medical Association:

The Tenth Councilor District, composed of Atoka, Coal, Choctaw, Bryan, Johnson, Marshall, McCurtain and Pushmataha Counties, held three Councilor District Meetings during the year, two of the meetings were held for physicians and one for the public and student body of Southeastern State College.

In planning the meetings it was deemed best to hold two Councilor District Meetings, one for the western part of the district and one for the eastern part in order to accomodate the greatest number due to impairment of roads in this part of the State and physicians being overworked. Accordingly, the first meeting was held in Durant on the evening of June 26, 1945 at the White House Cafe and Banquet Room, at which time a most excellent dinner was served consisting of fried chicken, fried and baked fish, fried squirrel and squirrel dumplings, with other accessories. This elaborate and most excellent meal was served to the visitors and all others in attendance complimentary by Dr. W. K. Haynie of Durant, Oklahoma. A large group of physicians attended and everything was most cordial and the finest hospitality prevailed. The meeting was full of interest from beginning to end, the program being furnished by the State Medical Association, consisting of Dr. V. C. Tisdal, president; the late Dr. Tom Lowry; Dr. C. R. Rountree; Dr. L. C. Kuyrkendall; Dr. Joseph Kelso; Dr. A. S. Risser; Dr. E. M. Smith; Dr. Richard M. Burke; Dr. J. T. Bell; Mr. Paul Fessler, Executive Secretary and his assistant Mrs. Jane Tucker and Mr. N. D. Helland. Also present by invitation was Honorable William Parrish, Durant, Representative from Bryan County.

On June 27, 1945, at the assembly hour from 10:00 A.M. to 11:00 A.M. at Southeastern State College at Durant, a meeting was held for the public and student body at which time Dr. Tisdal, the late Dr. Tom Lowry, Dr. Joseph Kelso, Dr. O. R. Rountree and Dr. A. S. Risser addressed the meeting on public health matters of vital importance, including the subject of cancer, great stress being placed on its early recognition, insidious onset and its baneful and pernicious effects. Much interest was manifested by the large and attentive audience.

On the evening of June 27, 1945, the other District Councilor Meeting was held at Hugo, convening in the First Methodist Church where, after a fine meal was served, the entire program was carried out and staffed by the same personnel as at the Durant meeting the evening before, the same outline and the same subject matters being presented. This also was a fine meeting and was largely attended, practically every physician in Choctaw, McCurtain and Pushmataha Counties was present. Also present by invitation and taking part in the meeting were Honorable Bayless Irby, State Senator and Honorable Hal Welch, State Representative.

All the counties have been contacted and most of them visited by the Councilor. However, much of our endeavors have been restricted by the exigencies of War and its aftermath, by excessive rains, lack of bridges

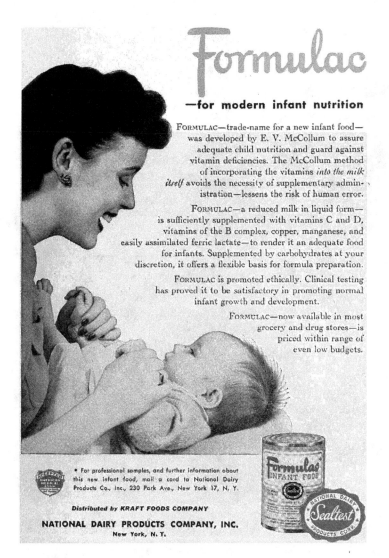

Formulac

—for modern infant nutrition

FORMULAC—trade-name for a new infant food— was developed by E. V. McCollum to assure adequate child nutrition and guard against vitamin deficiencies. The McCollum method of incorporating the vitamins *into the milk itself* avoids the necessity of supplementary administration—lessens the risk of human error.

FORMULAC—a reduced milk in liquid form— is sufficiently supplemented with vitamins C and D, vitamins of the B complex, copper, manganese, and easily assimilated ferric lactate—to render it an adequate food for infants. Supplemented by carbohydrates at your discretion, it offers a flexible basis for formula preparation.

FORMULAC is promoted ethically. Clinical testing has proved it to be satisfactory in promoting normal infant growth and development.

FORMULAC—now available in most grocery and drug stores—is priced within range of even low budgets.

• For professional samples, and further information about this new infant food, mail a card to National Dairy Products Co., Inc., 230 Park Ave., New York 17, N. Y.

Distributed by KRAFT FOODS COMPANY

NATIONAL DAIRY PRODUCTS COMPANY, INC.
New York, N. Y.

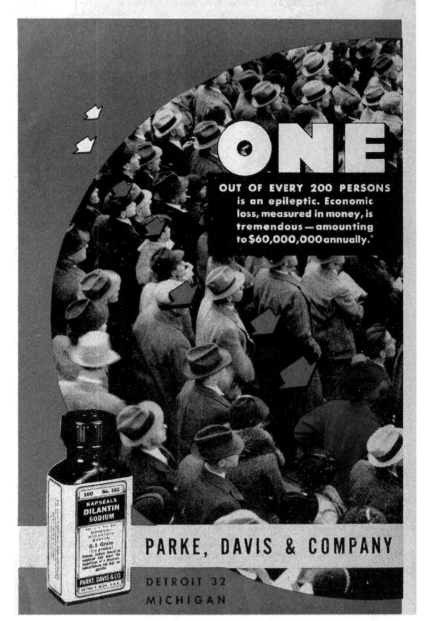

ONE OUT OF EVERY 200 PERSONS is an epileptic. Economic loss, measured in money, is tremendous — amounting to $60,000,000 annually.

PARKE, DAVIS & COMPANY

DETROIT 32
MICHIGAN

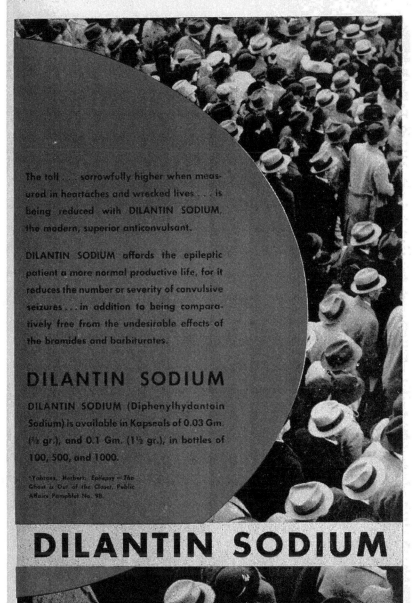

The toll . . . sorrowfully higher when measured in heartaches and wrecked lives . . . is
being reduced with DILANTIN SODIUM,
the modern, superior anticonvulsant.

DILANTIN SODIUM affords the epileptic
patient a more normal productive life, for it
reduces the number or severity of convulsive
seizures . . . in addition to being comparatively free from the undesirable effects of
the bromides and barbiturates.

DILANTIN SODIUM

DILANTIN SODIUM (Diphenylhydantoin
Sodium) is available in Kapseals of 0.03 Gm.
(½ gr.), and 0.1 Gm. (1½ gr.), in bottles of
100, 500, and 1000.

Yahraes, Herbert, Epilepsy — The
Ghost is Out of the Closet, Public
Affairs Pamphlet No. 98.

DILANTIN SODIUM

and poor roads in this part of the State. Yet, with all these handicaps we believe progress has been made. An effort has been made to combine some of the smaller counties which have only a few physicians, and Johnson County, which has not held a meeting for years, has already combined with Bryan County, one or two others are in the formative state of combining.

Since our report a year ago monumental events of great historical importance and world wide significance have transpired, which have affected the thinking and actions of all peoples. Both at home and in the Service striking stories and thrilling episodes of heroic efforts and deeds of valor by medical men inspired by patriotism, love of country and duty to humanity, have brightened the pages of history and have added prestige and enriched tradition to the medical profession. This, rightly, should be the time of great rejoicing and of benevolent adjustment, for the greatest of all wars of history has been fought and won for freedom and following this has been created the United Nations Organization to safeguard the peace of the world which we all hope and pray will meet every emergency for world peace. Just now, howver, there are chaotic and discordant notes and rumblings in some parts of the world and even in our own country we have social, economic and industrial unrest.

John A. Haynie, M.D.
Councilor, District No. 10

It was then *moved* by Dr. Finis Ewing, Muskogee, *seconded* by Dr. James Stevenson, Tulsa, that the Councilor District Reports be *accepted* as published and presented.

At this time, the Speaker of the House stated the next order of business would be the Report of the Standing Committees. He asked the pleasure of the House regarding the Reports of the Medical Education and Hospital Committee which had been published. On *motion* by Dr. James Stevenson, Tulsa, *seconded* by Dr. Earl Woodson, Poteau, the report was *approved*.

Reports were called for from the Annual Sessions Committee, the Scientific Work Committee and the Judicial and Professional Relations Committee. No reports were given from these Committees.

Dr. Garrison then called for the Report of the Public Policy Committee and the following report was read:

Report of the Public Policy Committee

Your Public Policy Committee desires to point out that there has probably been no time in the history of this country when the medical profession has had so many responsibilities for leadership placed upon its shoulders.

Sub-committees of our national Congress are today considering proposed legislation this country would receive medical care. The Public Policy Committee does not feel that it is necessary to speak in detail on the intents and purposes of the Wagner-Murray-Dingell Bill, the Pepper Bill, and other health measures, other than to point out that the medical profession must accept its responsibility in advising the public as to just what these measures would mean in their everyday life. Your Committee further feels that it is of primary importance that the public should know that the Wagner-Murray-Dingell Bill is in reality a compulsory tax and that the type of medical care the individual would receive need not be given first consideration. Your Public Policy Committee likewise feels that medicine must pursue its explorations into the medico-economic fields that will tend to continue to preserve free enterprise and the patient-physician relationship that has made America the most healthy country in the world.

The above objectives will only be obtained by the individual physicians interesting themselves in the selection of the individuals who will act as their elected representatives at both the local state and national levels.

The coming year is an election year. It is imperative that the profession individually and collectively weigh the merits of every person who submits his name to the voters to be elected to a place of trust. Your Committee will in the weeks to come submit to the membership an analysis of all candidates seeking public office in order that you may individually use your best judgement in exercising your prerogative as a citizen.

Have a Coke

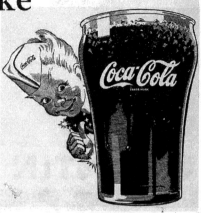

When you laugh, the world laughs with you, as they say—and when you enjoy *the pause that refreshes* with ice-cold Coca-Cola, your friends enjoy it with you, too. Everybody enjoys the friendly hospitality that goes with the invitation *Have a Coke*. Those three words mean *Friend, you belong —I'm glad to be with you*. Good company is better company over a Coca-Cola.

In order that this report may not be too long your Committee submits the following recommendations:

1. That this House of Delegates again go on record opposing the concepts of not only the Wagner-Murray-Dingell Bill, but all other legislation which develops this theory of thinking.

2. That this House of Delegates reaffirm its previous position with reference to sponsoring and endorsing Blue Cross Hospitalization Insurance and the Oklahoma Physicians' Service. There is little doubt that these two organizations have materially met the needs and requests of the general public for a method of budgeting for catastrophic illness and their general health.

Your Public Policy Committee recognizes that the recommendation made by the Council to combine this Committee with the Committee on Publicity is fundamentally sound and concurs in the recommendation. While this Committee has not been in a position to make the detailed study of the advertising campaign recommended by the Publicity Committee and approved by the Council, it, nevertheless, whole-heartedly supports the recommendation. The Committee further would like to point out that in its opinion few physicians recognize the extent to which the field of public relations has become a part of the practice of medicine. Certainly the medical profession must recognize that the most important ally it can have is the general public and that this ally can only be brought into the fight by knowing the principles for which the profession stands and is fighting. The Committee urges that the recommendation of the Council with reference to the educational advertising campaign be adopted.

Your Public Policy Committee does not have at this time any recommendations for a legislative program in the next session of the legislature, other than that program that was adopted for the last session of the legislature.

Dr. Tisdal, President of the Association, appointed during his term of office a special committee composed of Drs. Tom Lowry, Chairman, Howard Hopps, and W. Floyd Keller, to study and promote public interest in a Medical Examiners Bill.

Your Public Policy Committee believes that a Medical Examiners Bill should be introduced into the legislature and every effort made to secure its passage. Your Committee further recommends that this House of Delegates instruct this Committee to continue its efforts to work in behalf of the State Board of Public Health, the State Health Department and the University of Oklahoma School of Medicine. The gains in these fields accomplished in the last legislature must not be lost. Your Committee likewise feels that the assistance given to this program by all members of the legislature who supported it should be recognized and that Senator Louis Ritzhaupt and Representative O. W. Starr should be commended for their support in these matters.

The attention of all Delegates and Alternates and Officers attending this meeting is called to the announcement which was handed to you when you registered, which announces a change in the program wherein there will be representatives from the National Physicians Committee and the American Medical Association appearing on the Friday afternoon program for a report on the hearings now being held in Congress on the Wagner-Murray-Dingell Bill. It is this Committee's opinion that every delegate and alternate must attend this meeting in order that he may be in a position to make an up to-the-minute report to his Society and allied professional organizations. This Committee would also recommend that each delegate and alternate have all other physicians from his county attend this meeting. In closing this report, as Chairman of the Public Policy Committee, I would like to say that I personally endorse the recommendation to enlarge this Committee. It is imperative that all sections of the State be represented and that a thorough dissemination of the public policy problems facing the American people today be placed before the medical profession in order that they in turn may intelligently discuss all aspects of politics that would in any any affect the health of the American people.

Respectfully submitted
McLain Rogers, M.D., Chairman
Finis W. Ewing, M.D.
J. D. Osborn, M.D.,
Louis Ritzhaupt, M.D.
O. W. Starr, M.D.

On *motion* by Dr. James Stevenson, Tulsa, *seconded* by Dr. C. R. Rountree, Oklahoma City, the Report of the Public Policy Committee with its recommendations was *accepted.*

The Speaker then called for the Report of the Necrology Committee. The following Report and Resolution were presented:

Report of the Committee on Necrology
Resolution

That those members who have paid the supreme sacrifice in either civilian or military service may be accorded the honor due them, the Committee on Necrology submits the following resolutions for adoption by the House of Delegates:

WHEREAS, Since the 1944 report made by the Committee on Necrology of the Association, the Grim Reaper has gather 50 of our members.

THEREFORE, BE IT RESOLVED, That the House of Delegates of the Oklahoma State Medical Association give due recognition to the demise of the said 50 fellow members and to the honor we hold for them as well as our deep regret at the parting, and instruct the Secretary to inscribe their names upon the records of the Association as follows:

Name	Born	Died	Residence
Hutchison, Austin	1875	April, 1945	Bixby
*Scott, Frank Waldo	1887	April, 1945	Muskogee
Croston, G. C.	1877	May, 1945	Sapulpa
Weaver, Edward S.	1881	May, 1945	Cordell
*Goad, S. L.	1867	June, 1945	Marlow
Little, Daniel E.	1878	June, 1945	Eufaula
White, Arthur W.	1877	June, 1945	Okla. City
Bonham, James M.	1870	July, 1945	Hobart
Lipe, Everett N.	1878	July, 1945	Fairfax
Powell, Wm. H.	1872	July, 1945	Sulphur
Barker, Nim Lou	1885	Aug., 1945	Broken Bow
*Vickers, Chas. P.	1873	Aug., 1945	Okla. City
*Fuller, Wm. Banks	1897	Aug., 1945	Okla. City
Pemberton, Richard K.	1871	Sept., 1945	McAlester
*Vaughn, Benj. F.	1864	Sept., 1945	Bethany
*Dossey, Wm. J.	1869	Sept., 1945	Cyril
Drasbach, Harry V.	1867	Sept., 1945	Okla. City
*Bramblett, James C.	1877	Sept., 1945	Amber
Stough, Daniel F., Sr.	1875	Sept., 1945	Geary
*Nafus, Charles Allen	1871	Oct., 1945	Ft. Gibson
McKellar, Malcolm	1885	Oct., 1945	Tulsa
*Deberry, Lemnel S.	1866	Oct., 1945	Idabel
Cain, Philip L.	1860	Nov., 1945	Albany
Birnbaum, William	1905	Nov., 1945	Tulsa
Gardner, Powell B.	1889	Nov., 1945	Guthrie
*Hahn, Charles J.	1857	Nov., 1945	Sand Springs
*Lowther, Robert D.	1868	Dec., 1945	Norman
*Jones, Edward D.	1882	Dec., 1945	Nowata
Preston, J. R.	1876	Dec., 1945	Weleetka
Henry, J. W.	1888	Dec., 1945	Cheyenne
*Hilsmeyer, P. E.	1864	Dec., 1945	Amber
*Baugh, J. H.	1873	Dec., 1945	Meeker
Lowry, Tom	1891	Dec., 1945	Okla.City

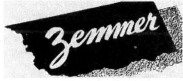

PRESCRIBE OR DISPENSE
ZEMMER PHARMACEUTICALS
A complete line of laboratory controlled ethical pharmaceuticals.   OK 6-46
Chemists to the Medical Profession for 44 years.
THE ZEMMER COMPANY • Oakland Station • Pittsburgh 13, Pa.

*Nickell, Benjamin F.	1862	Dec., 1945	Davenport
Davenport, Albert L.	1872	Dec., 1945	Holdenville
*Bates, Samuel R.	1872	Jan., 1946	Wagoner
Floyd, William E.	1880	Jan., 1946	Holdenville
Fullenwider, C. M.	1878	Jan., 1946	Muskogee
Smith, Charles E.	1873	Jan., 1946	Okla. City
Sullivan, C. L.	1878	Jan., 1946	Albany
*Whisenant, J. W.	1869	Jan., 1946	Duncan
*Sellers, Robert L.	1865	Feb., 1946	Westville
*Driver, Charles M.	1869	Feb., 1946	Mounds
Preston, Charles R.	1881	Mar., 1946	Snyder
Adams, John W.	1878	Mar., 1946	Chandler
Collins, Benjamin F.	1878	Mar., 1946	Claremore
*Slover, George W.	1878	Mar., 1946	Sulphur
Myers, Pirl B.	1874	Mar., 1946	El Reno

*Not members of Association

On *motion* by Dr. Finis Ewing, Muskogee, *seconded* by Dr. J. G. Edwards, Okmulgee, the Report of the Committee on Neerology was *accepted*.

Upon completion of this report it was *moved* by Dr. Louis Ritzhaupt, Guthrie, that the House of Delegates approve a form resolution to be prepared and sent to the immediate families of the deceased from now on. The motion was *seconded* by Dr. R. Q. Goodwin and *carried*.

The Speaker then called for the Report of the Postgraduate Committee. The following report was given:

Report of the Committee on Postgraduate Medical Teaching

The Committee on Postgraduate Medical Teaching submits the following report to the House of Delegates:

Dr. Patrick P. T. Wu of Rochester, Minnesota, was employed by the Postgraduate Committee on June 1, 1945, to complete the course in Surgical Diagnosis which had been discontinued October 1, 1944.

Doctor Wu has completed three circuits including the centers of: Bristow-Sapulpa, Stillwater-Cushing, Pawhuska, Ponca City, Guthrie, Wewoka, Shawnee, Pauls Valley, Norman, Chickasha, Lawton, Altus, Frederick, Duncan and Ardmore. Total registrations for the three circuits numbered 315 with an average attendance of 87 per cent (which is the highest percentage of, attendance of any previous course.) Physicians in the armed forces or who have returned from World War II have been urged to attend the lectures. These doctors are admitted without paying the regular fee of $9.00 and are entitled to all the privileges of the course. Certificates of attendance have been issued to those whose attendance averaged 70 per cent or more and a manual on Surgical Diagnosis has been given to each physician enrolled. During these three circuits Doctor Wu has held 324 private consultations with physicians. In addition to his regular lectures he has given 19 lay lectures in 16 different communities with an approximate attendance of 1,670.

The course is now in progress in the centers of Watonga, Woodward, Guymon, Alva and Enid with a registration of 92 physicians. The attendance is excellent.

Plans are now being made for the next postgraduate course which will succeed almost immediately the present course in Surgical Diagnosis. It is the opinion of the majority of the physicians that the next postgraduate teaching should be in gynecology or psychiatry.

Receipts from February 1, 1944 to April 1, 1946 have amounted to $30,545.00. Total disbursements for this period were $23,701.93, leaving a balance of $6,843.07 to complete the course.

The Commonwealth Fund of New York has. during the past eight years, contributed $86,160.00 to this program in Oklahoma. Your Committee desires to point out that all activities of The Commonwealth Fund are designed to assist in the promulgation of medical education and not for propitiation. Your Committee feels that it is not particularly to the credit of the profession in Oklahoma to find it necessary to secure financial assistance from the East to continue such a worthy and worthwhile program. Your Committee will, therefore, attempt to make the postgraduate courses self sustaining in the future.

It is contemplated that the Oklahoma State Health Department and the State Medical Association will continue to appropriate money for this program until the time arrives when these courses may possibly become entirely self sustaining.

Therefore, be it recommended that the fee for the course to the individual physician be raised to $15.00 in order that additional contributions from The Commonwealth Fund will not be necessary.

Since the resignation of Mr. L. W. Kibler, December 1, who had been a full-time employee of the Postgraduate Committee for many years, Mr. Dick Graham, the Executive Secretary of the State Association, has carried on the work formerly done by Mr. Kibler. The Committee is delighted to report that this new plan is definitely successful in that Mr. Graham carries out the duties expeditiously and to the entire satisfaction of everyone concerned. Mr. Graham not only has made numerous contacts with the physicians in the various teaching areas but the expenses of carrying on the course have already been definitely reduced. This change in no way has detracted from the efficiency of the course management and is a long step forward in making the Postgraduate Committee work self supporting.

The Committee desires to thank The Commonwealth Fund of New York, the Oklahoma State Health Department, the United States Public Health, and the Oklahoma State Medical Association for their financial assistance and further recommends that the House of Delegates, by resolution, express its appreciation to these contributing agencies.

Respectfully submitted,
Gregory E. Stanbro, M.D., Chairman
On *motion* by Dr. Finis Ewing, Muskogee, *seconded*

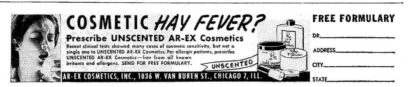

COSMETIC *HAY FEVER?*

Prescribe UNSCENTED AR-EX Cosmetics

Recent clinical tests showed many cases of cosmetic sensitivity, but not a single one to UNSCENTED AR-EX Cosmetics. For allergic patients, prescribe UNSCENTED AR-EX Cosmetics—free from all known irritants and allergens. SEND FOR FREE FORMULARY.

UNSCENTED

AR-EX COSMETICS, INC., 1036 W. VAN BUREN ST., CHICAGO 7, ILL.

FREE FORMULARY

DR._____
ADDRESS_____
CITY_____
STATE_____

J. E. HANGER, Inc.

ARTIFICIAL LIMBS, BRACES, AND CRUTCHES

Phone: 2-8500   612 N. Hudson

L. T. Lewis, Mgr.   BRANCHES AND AGENCIES IN PRINCIPAL CITIES   Oklahoma City 3, Okla.

AUTHORITATIVE clinical investigators place strong emphasis on the importance of the barrier in conception control.

In a recent comprehensive report,[1] physicians indicated an overwhelming preference for the diaphragm and jelly method (93% of 36,955 new cases).

In keeping with these expressed opinions we continue to suggest that for the optimum in protection the physician prescribe the combined use of occlusive diaphragm and spermatocidal jelly.

You assure your patient a product of highest quality when you specify *Ramses*

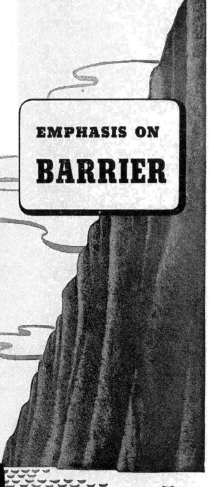

EMPHASIS ON
BARRIER

Competent observers report:

"Jellies and creams used without mechanical devices yield relatively high protection, but studies have not proven them fully dependable to block the external os, or to invalidate all sperm."[2]

"When no type of occlusive pessary can be fitted, or when the woman refuses to use one, the only other reliable method is the use of the condom. With proper technic and instruction this method is highly reliable but has many disadvantages which the diaphragm method overcomes."[3]

1. Clinic Reports: Planned Parenthood Services in the United States. Human Fertility 10: 25 (Mar.) 1945.
2. Dickinson, R.L.: Techniques of Conception Control. Baltimore, Williams and Wilkins Co., 1942.
3. Warner, M.P.: I.A.M.A. 115: 279 (July 27) 1940.

gynecological division

JULIUS SCHMID, INC.

423 West 55 Street • New York 19, N. Y.   QUALITY FIRST SINCE 1883

by Dr. R. Q. Goodwin, Oklahoma City, the Report of the Postgraduate Committee with its recommendation to raise the fee to $15.00 was *approved.*

The Report of the Committee on Study and Control of Tuberculosis had been published in the April issue of the Journal and the Speaker called the attention of the House to the recommendations in this report.

On *motion* by Dr. L. Chester McHenry, Oklahoma City, *seconded* by Dr. C. R. Rountree, Oklahoma City, the Report of the Committee on the Study and Control of Tuberculosis with its recommendations was *approved.*

The Speaker then called for the Report of the Committee on the Study and Control of Venereal Disease. The following report was given:

Report of the Committee on the Study and Control of Venereal Disease

The committee wishes to call attention to the report in the November, 1945 issue of the State Journal.

It seems wise in the presence of the newer drugs to consider improvements in the methods of venereal prophylaxis. At best it seems that drugs of caustic nature have been too frequently employed. Attention should be given to some of the newer mild antiseptics, which do not stain the clothing and are effective bactericidal agents.

Attention is called to a suggestion which Dr. C. B. Taylor made, that the short period of treatment for gonorrhea may delay the symptoms or mask the presence of an associated syphilitic condition. This should be considered. Perhaps it would be wiser to give an adequate amount of penicillin to cover the early treatment of syphilis when treating a case of gonorrhea.

Attention should be given to the correction of poor urethral or prostatic drainage in clearing gonorrhea or non-specific urethritis.

Respectfully submitted,
Robert H. Akin, M.D., Chairman

On *motion* by Dr. Ned Burleson, Prague, *seconded* by Dr. F. P. Baker, Talihina, the Report with its recommendations was *approved.*

The Speaker then called for, in turn, reports from the following Committees: Conservation of Vision and Hearing; Crippled Children; Industrial and Traumatic Surgery; Medical Economics; Advisory to Womans Auxiliary; Library; Maternity and Infancy; Advisory to Public Welfare; Military Affairs; Post-War Planning; Public Health. There were no reports given.

At this time the Chair declared a five minute recess.

At the end of the five minute recess, Mr. Dick Graham was granted the floor. Mr. Graham stated that no memorial or resolution shall be issued in the name of the Oklahoma State Medical Association until it has been approved by the House of Delegates. He asked that the House of Delegates consider the presenting of memorial certificates to Dr. W. W. Rucks, Sr., Dr. C. R. Rountree and Dr. Henry H. Turner for their service in connection with the Procurement and Assignment Service.

Dr. Louis Ritzhaupt, "It is fitting that the three men who served in this capacity be presented a memorial certificate. I *so move.*" This motion was *seconded* by Dr. Carroll Pounders, Oklahoma City and *carried.*

The Speaker then asked that Mr. Dick Graham read the Annual Report of the Council.

Annual Report of the Council

In submitting this report to the House of Delegates, the Council feels that it is necessary to stress the fact that the last twelve month's activity of the Association has, of necessity, digressed from the initial program recommended by President Tisdal and endorsed by the House of Delegates.

The Council believes that it is only fitting and proper that this House of Delegates take cognizance of the fact that this is the first post-war meeting of the Association. There is, today, in this House of Delegates, many physicians who served their country honorably and gloriously. These same physicians have returned to this state to again take up the practice of medicine and it is the

C. A. GALLAGHER, M. D.

CURT VON WEDEL, M. D.
(Consultant)

PLASTIC and RECONSTRUCTION SURGERY

610 N. W. Ninth Street

Oklahoma City, Oklahoma

Office 2-3108

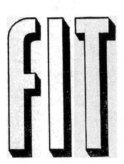

THE unique CAMP system of controlled adjustment incorporated in many specialized models graded to the various types of body build gives Camp Anatomical Supports the endless number of fitting combinations called for by the endless variations in the human figure. Full benefit of this precision design is assured for the individual patient's well-being and comfort because Camp Scientific Supports are precision fitted by experts ethically trained at Camp instructional courses in prescription accuracy.

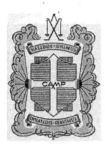

Camp Anatomical Supports ethically distributed under the inspiration of this hallmark have met the exacting test of the profession for four decades. Prescribed and recommended in many types for prenatal, postnatal, postoperative, pendulous abdomen, visceroptosis, nephroptosis, hernia, orthopedic and other conditions.

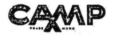

ANATOMICAL SUPPORTS

S. H. CAMP & COMPANY
Jackson, Michigan

*World's Largest Manufacturers
of Scientific Supports*

Offices in NEW YORK • CHICAGO
WINDSOR, ONT. • LONDON, ENG.

If you do not have a copy of our "Reference Book for Physicians and Surgeons", copy will be sent upon request.

solemn obligation of every physician, irrespective of his practice or location, to recognize the terrific sacrifice that has been made by these men and to do everything in his power to assist in helping those who have returned to re-establish themselves. Words are not sufficient and the most adequate manner of expressing sincerity of our esteem for the sacrifice that they have made can best be done by the referring of patients. The Council welcomes home these men and trusts that they will enter wholeheartedly into the affairs of the profession.

During the past year the medical profession has found that its thoughts and abilities, of necessity, must be directed into the fields of economic and political thinking of our country. What had initially been planned as a program for 1945-46, namely a progressive, over-all educational program, utilizing four points, i. e., public education; postgraduate education; post-war planning; a closer fostering of our county societies, has not been accomplished in the manner originally conceived, namely, a militent effort to place before the people individually and collectively an educational program comprising all of the problems that affect their health whether or not they were political, economic or scientific.

The Council desires to pay particular tribute to the Oklahoma County Medical Society for initially instigating a public educational advertising campaign through the lay press. In addition, the Council desires to offer this same commendation to all other County Societies and allied organizations who have followed the same program. There can be little doubt that unless the public is educated to its responsibilities in protecting itself from outside forces that would regiment it, there is little that the medical profession can do as its sole guardian.

While the above paragraphs may substantiate some of the greatest threats and problems to be checked by medicine, the Council is fully cognizant of the fact that other activities of the Association must be continued.

The following reports and recommendations from the Council reflect what the Council believes to be the major activities of the scientific, economic and public policy questions to be sponsored by the profession not particularly for the year to come, but as a long range program.

Finances

The finances of the Association are in satisfactory condition for its present *activities*. The auditor's report for our fiscal year ending December 31, 1945 has been published in the Journal. Total assets excluding bonds on December 31, 1945 amounted to $7,248.37. Income from dues on April 1, 1946 was up $2,048.00 over the same period in 1945 and in the main, represents members who have returned from military service.

Income from Journal advertising for 1946 will approximate that of 1945 inasmuch as the 1946 advertising schedules represent war time contracts let in 1945. It is anticipated that 1947 revenue will drop from the war time level.

The Council recognizes that this body will later in its deliberations consider the advisability of placing a special assessment on the membership for the purpose of putting in operation a statewide educational program through the newspapers and radio, but feels, nevertheless, compelled to advise the House of Delegates that it is its responsibility to determine the scope of the Association's activities and the manner in which they will be financed.

The Council is not recommending salary increases for any of the employees but it is necessary to point out that the facilities of the Executive Office have had to be enlarged in order to take care of the increasing demands on the office in such programs as the Oklahoma Physicians' Service, Medical Care for Veterans, Public Policy work, Mal Practice and Health and Accident Insurance Programs, etc.

For the reasons that have been enumerated and with the belief that the membership desires to have the Association continue its progressiveness, the Council recommends that there be a raise in the dues for 1947. The Council would prefer that a motion for a raise in dues come from the floor of the House and for this reason does not specifically recommend any raise other than to observe that in its opinion the raise should be $10.00.

The Council is refraining from presenting a budget to the House of Delegates until such time as the amount of dues has been established.

Membership

The membership of the Association as of April 15, 1946 was as follows: 1393 active members of which 120 are still serving in the Armed Forces and have paid no dues, 30 honorary and six associate members.

The total number of paid memberships recorded as of April 15 was 1237 which is an increase of 173 over the same date of the previous year.

The Council in its deliberations believes that there have developed certain major issues that bear the careful consideration of the House of Delegates. The Council herewith presents these issues and its observations and in some instances specific recommendations.

Educational Program with Newspaper and Radio Advertising

Each delegate and alternate has received advance information on this suggested program. The Council feels that the profession must accept its responsibility in educating the public on matters of health. The Oklahoma County Medical Society and other societies have seen the excellent results that came from the series of ads carried in the Daily Oklahoman. The Council in authorizing the Chairman of the Publicity Committee to contact an advertising firm, felt that it should acquaint itself with what the modus operandi would be and what might be expected in the way of results. Two programs were advanced by the agency which have been reported to you for your study. The Council feels this method of approach is the only feasible one to follow and that the program should be financed by a special assessment against each member. While more pertinent details will be brought out in discussions from the floor, the Council would like to point out that each newspaper in the state would be utilized and that all ads appearing in the separate counties would be to the credit of the local county society. The Council also believes that the House should understand that this program would not be a negative one. That the ads would be prepared under Council direction and be progressive in nature. The ads would follow the trends in medicine and diseases, warning the public against abuses and false claims as well as pointing out unsound and unfounded economics and political schemes. The Council requests that each Delegate give careful consideration to this proposal. The public is looking to this profession for leadership. The Council, therefore recommends that a special assessment of $25.00 be made on each member.

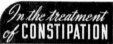

you will find a useful adjunct in

YOUNG'S RECTAL DILATORS

Constipation, nervousness and other conditions caused by tight sphincter muscles are often alleviated. Set of 4, both adult and children's sizes. Sold on physician's prescription only—not advertised to the laity. At ethical drug stores or your surgical supply house. Write for brochure.

F. E. YOUNG & COMPANY . . . . 424 EAST 75TH STREET, CHICAGO 19, ILLINOIS

Medical Care Program for Veterans

No doubt many of the Delegates have followed the development of state plans in Kansas, Michigan, California and many other states and are acquainted with their interests and purposes. President Tisdal has appointed a special committee to study a plan for Oklahoma and this Committee headed by Dr. John Burton of Oklahoma City will report to the House of Delegates at a later time. The Council has already considered the report of this committee and recommends to the House of Delegates that it give approval to the committee's recommendations.

Fee Schedules

From literally time immemorable the problems of fee schedules have been with the medical profession but it has not been but within recent years that governmental agencies have, by their entrance into the medical care field, brought about a need for a consolidation of the thinking in this field. Your Council is well aware that today the physician is faced with performing his work under a schedule of fees for insurance companies, state insurance fund, vocational rehabilitation and public welfare commission, etc. It is the Council's recommendation that the Association take steps to work out a fee schedule that will apply to professional care rendered for all governmental agencies irrespective of whether they are local, state or federal. It is believed by the Council that the fee schedule established for Veterans Administration work could well become the schedule for all agencies.

Rural Health

During World War II the public in general and the medical profession in particular realized that the necessity for physicians to enter the armed forces would place a great burden upon all physicians remaining at home and especially rural physicians and rural populations and it is to the credit of both that the crisis was met with such fortitude and understanding. Today, however, with the great majority of physicians returned from the war there remains a serious problem in the rural areas on matters of health. It is obvious to the profession

CREDIT SERVICE

330 American National Building

Oklahoma City, Oklahoma

(Operators of Medical-Dental Credit Bureau)

We offer a dignified and effective collection service for doctors and hospitals located anywhere in the State. Write for information.

28 YEARS
Experience In Credit and Collection Work

Robt. R. Sesline, Owner and Manager

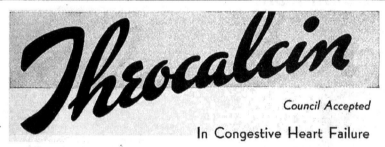

Council Accepted

In Congestive Heart Failure

For the reduction of edema, to diminish dyspnoea and to strengthen heart action, prescribe Theocalcin, beginning with 2 or 3 tablets t. i. d., with meals. After relief is obtained, the comfort of the patient may be continued with smaller doses. Well tolerated.

Theocalcin, brand of theobromine-calcium salicylate, Trade Mark reg. U. S. Pat. Off.

Available in 7½ grain tablets and in powder form.

Bilhuber-Knoll Corp. Orange, N. J.

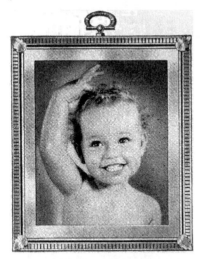

DOCTOR, MEET THE DARICRAFT BABY

Perhaps you are "meeting" the Daricraft Baby every day in your own practice. If not, may we call to your attention the following significant points of interest about Vitamin D increased Daricraft:

1. Produced from inspected herds; 2. Clarified; 3. Homogenized; 4. Sterilized; 5. Specially Processed; 6. Easily Digested; 7. High in Food Value; 8. Improved Flavor; 9. Uniform; 10. Dependable Source of Supply.

Producers Creamery Co.
Springfield, Mo.

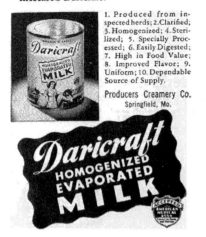

Daricraft
HOMOGENIZED
EVAPORATED
MILK

that all the blame for this condition should not be placed on the doorstep of medicine. Local communities themselves have failed to meet their own responsibilities in providing physical facilities for attracting physicians to their area. The Hill-Burton Bill will no doubt assist in alleviating this condition but in the interim the profession should not lose sight of its responsibilities. The Council recommends that a special committee be appointed to work with farm groups and other interested agencies to attempt to work out a temporary solution to many acute and critical rural problems.

Construction of Hospitals

Construction of hospitals in communities in need of such facilities is receiving, as has been stated, a great impetus from the Hill-Burton Bill (Senate Bill 191) now being considered by the House of Representatives after passage by the Senate. This Association has along with the American Medical Association and like organizations endorsed and supported the Bill. Your Council feels that it must point out to this House of Delegates that the medical profession has a great responsibility to the individual cities considering such construction. The local county medical societies must take the initiative in such programs as it will be discovered that very unsavory conditions can develop with reference to the cults. It is recommended that every society appoint a committee on the construction of health facilities and immediately communicate the makeup of the committee to all civic groups as well as city and county officials in order that they may know of the cooperative attitude of the profession. Your Council also feels that careful consideration should be given to the need for hospital construction. On the present impetus there are perhaps many areas that are becoming too enthusiastic and will regret at a future day their venture. The profession must guide and council in these matters. Your Council likewise feels that the State Board of Public Health should immediately complete and release the results of its hospital survey in order that communities may know of their relative positions and be allowed to make their appeals if there seems to be an injustice.

Medical Research

The recent action of the Alumni of the School of Medicine of the University of Oklahoma has the full support of the Council. This project which is envisioned to be a three million dollar research institute without political interference calls for the complete support of every physician. The Council has heard rumors of lack of interest in this project because of its location in Oklahoma City and the Council feels that such observations are without factual foundation. No great medical center would ever have been established had there not been a unification of facilities. Certainly this research should be connected with the Medical School. It is ironical that the benefits which would accrue to the state as a whole would seem to mean that its location in Oklahoma City should not have state support. The Council would look with favor on any resolution that would come from the floor of this House that would in any way bring about the creation of an endowment fund from physicians only for this worthy project. Every physician should know that any contribution he might give would be deductible from his income tax and that the money could be given for no more worthy ideal.

State Board of Health

The State Board of Health which was created by the last legislature, and in turn supported by the Association, has made many strides in perfecting its organization. While the Council realizes that revolutionary changes were not contemplated or in order, nevertheless feels that it must go on record as recommending to the Board of Health and the State Health Department that their actions become more positive and progressive and that upon its shoulders rests a responsibility to the people that transcends all other considerations. The Council again recommends the full support of the Association be placed at the disposal of the State Board of Health.

Reorganization of Association's Committees

During recent years it has become increasingly obvious to the Council that the method of studying problems placed before the profession in the fields of economics,

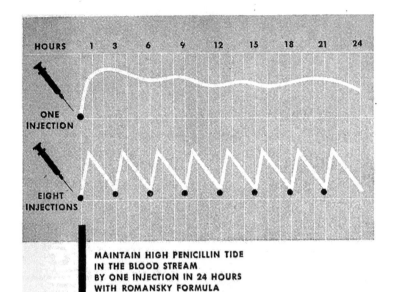

MAINTAIN HIGH PENICILLIN TIDE
IN THE BLOOD STREAM
BY ONE INJECTION IN 24 HOURS
WITH ROMANSKY FORMULA
. . . OFFERED BY BRISTOL LABORATORIES

Office or home treatment now becomes practicable through administration of Penicillin in Oil and Wax as developed by Captain M. J.
Romansky (M.C.) at the Walter Reed General Hospital, Washington,
D. C. With this preparation it is possible to hold a penicillin therapeutic blood level by one injection in 24 hours, thus replacing the
previous use of 8 injections of penicillin in saline over 24 hours.

There is usually less discomfort to the patient, and hence better
cooperation. Also, by eliminating repeated injections the cost of
treatment to the patient is lowered. and there is an appreciable saving
in physicians' and nurses' time. This can be readily attained by the
single injection of 1 cc. of 300,000 units in the oil-beeswax medium—
known as Romansky formula, Bristol.

Bristol Laboratories now offer the Romansky formula with calcium
penicillin. Due to special processing, the Bristol preparation is especially easy to inject. Write for new literature.

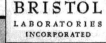

BRISTOL
LABORATORIES   SYRACUSE 1, NEW YORK
INCORPORATED

public policy and scientific medicine have, of necessity, called for the creation of special committees inasmuch as the By-Laws of the Association only provides for the following Standing Committees with a staggered membership: Annual Session; Credentials; Judicial and Professional Relations; Medical Education and Hospitals; Publicity; Public Policy; Scientific Work; while in turn the Association has seventeen Special Committees with little if any reports to make from one year to the next.

Your Council has studied the advisability of reforming the Standing Committees to include many of those that are now carried as Special Committees and tin turn to consolidate some of these. As an example, it has not proven feasible to attempt to maintain both a public policy Committee and a Publicity Committee and it is the belief of the Council that these two Committees should be placed on one, holding the name of the Committee on Public Policy and Publicity. Your Council also feels that the number of members on Standing Committees should be increased to six, with two members retiring each year and the President empowered to vote in place of a tie.

In order that this matter may be brought before the House of Delegates for discussion, the Council recommends that the By-Laws be amended in the following respect: *Chapter IX, Section 1;* amended to read in the sixth line "Public Policy and Publicity" and that the word "Publicity" in line 8 be stricken. *Chapter IX, Section 1;* be amended by adding following line nine, the following lines consecutively, "Medical Economics" "Study and Control of Infectious Diseases" "Conservation of Health". *Chapter IX;* be further amended by striking Section 8 and including the wording of this Section in Section 6. *Chapter IX;* be further amended by renumbering Section 9 as Section 8; Section 10 as Section 9 and adding the following: Section 10—Committee on Medical Economics; Section 11—Committee on Study and Control of Infectious Diseases; Section 12—Committee on Conservation of Health. *Chapter IX, Section 2;* be amended to substitute in line 5 the word "six" for the word "three" and in line nine the word "two" for the word "one".

Your Council feels that if these amendments are adopted it will be possible to decrease the number of Special Committees and at the same time develop a more comprehensive field of work for the Standing Committees which, in turn, will mean a greater activity on the part of the Standing Committees.

Annual Session

During the years immediately preceding the war and as evidenced by this meeting, it has become extremely difficult to hold the Annual Session in any of the hotels in the state. This difficulty is occasioned by the fact that to pay the expense of eleven or more guest speakers, print programs, etc., it is necessary to promote an attractive meeting from the standpoint of the exhibitors. It might be of interest to the House of Delegates to know that the exhibitors that are attending this meeting have paid to the Association, $2,880.00 which, in turn, will pay for the entire expense of the meeting. In turn the Scientific Work Committee must provide meeting space for nine different section meetings. The Council has considered the report from the Scientific Work Committee and concurs, recommending to the House of Delegates that this report and amendment to the By-Laws be adopted.

Public Policy

Your Council is refraining from recommending specific proposals on matters of Public Policy. The Council has received the report of the Public Policy Committee and endorses this report in its entirety.

Postgraduate Medical Teaching

The Council would point out to the House of Delegates that the Postgraduate Teaching Program has maintained its excellent standard. The Council feels that the House of Delegates should know that during the past eight years the Commonwealth Fund has contributed $86,160.00 to this Program and that in line with the report that will be made by the Postgraduate Committee, the profession should take steps to make this program financially independent from outside sources.

Medical Education

The Council recognizes that the Oklahoma University School of Medicine has a very important bearing on the

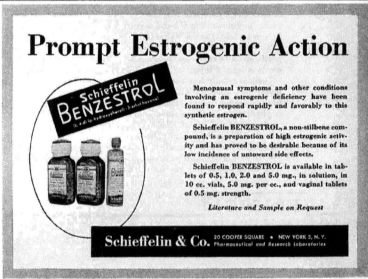

Prompt Estrogenic Action

Schieffelin BENZESTROL
α, 4-di(p-hydroxyphenyl) -3-ethylhexane)

Menopausal symptoms and other conditions involving an estrogenic deficiency have been found to respond rapidly and favorably to this synthetic estrogen.

Schieffelin BENZESTROL, a non-stilbene compound, is a preparation of high estrogenic activity and has proved to be desirable because of its low incidence of untoward side effects.

Schieffelin BENZESTROL is available in tablets of 0.5, 1.0, 2.0 and 5.0 mg., in solution, in 10 cc. vials, 5.0 mg. per cc., and vaginal tablets of 0.5 mg. strength.

Literature and Sample on Request

Schieffelin & Co. 20 COOPER SQUARE • NEW YORK 3, N. Y.
Pharmaceutical and Research Laboratories

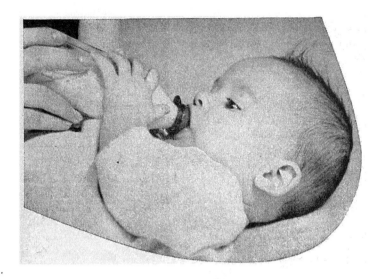

Silencer for midnight phones

When pediatricians prescribe 'Dexin' brand High Dextrin Carbohydrate for their infant patients, the physicians are no longer wakened so frequently by frantic late-night phone calls. Because of the high dextrin content, 'Dexin' feedings tend to (1) diminish intestinal fermentation and the resultant colic and diarrhea and (2) promote the formation of soft, flocculent, easily digested curds.

'Dexin' babies sleep more soundly, physicians' phones jangle less, and the doctor himself obtains more undisturbed sleep. Not unpalatably sweet, 'Dexin' is readily soluble in hot or cold milk or other bland fluids. 'Dexin' does make a difference.

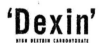

'Dexin'
HIGH DEXTRIN CARBOHYDRATE

Composition—Dextrins 75% • Maltose 24% • Mineral Ash 0.25% • Moisture 0.75% • Available Carbohydrate 99% • 115 calories per ounce • 6 level packed tablespoonfuls equal 1 ounce • Containers of twelve ounces and three pounds • Accepted by the Council on Foods and Nutrition, American Medical Association.
'Dexin' Reg. Trademark

Literature on request

BURROUGHS WELLCOME & CO. (U.S.A.) INC., 9 & 11 East 41st St., New York 17, N. Y practice of medicine in Oklahoma and the type of physicians who will carry on the profession in this state and for this reason believes that the Association should interest itself in the school's welfare.

The Council feels that the Oklahoma University School of Medicine, with its additional appropriation from the last legislature and the building program of the Alumni, is in a position to increase its stature not only in Oklahoma but in the great Southwest. The Council recognizes that the Medical School has been seriously handicapped by the loss of its Dean, Dr. Tom Lowry, and appreciates the sacrifice that the present Acting Dean, Dr. Wann Langston, is making in maintaining the integrity of the School.

It is the opinion of the Council that the University of Oklahoma School of Medicine must have, at the earliest possible moment, a full time Dean who can grow with the School and become a forceful leader in medical education. The Council recognizes that Dean Langston does not desire to remain as Dean and for this reason wishes it definitely understood that no statements with reference to the School should reflect upon him. As a matter of fact, the Council desires to pay him all homage. It is recommended that the Resolutions Committee draw up suitable resolutions for transmission to Dr. George Cross, President of the University of Oklahoma and to the Board of Regents, urging the securing of a full-time Dean at the earliest possible date.

Your Council realizes that this report has only touched upon a few of the high points of the policies of the Association and its business transactions but, nevertheless, feels that from this report can come many constructive advancements in the conduct of the Association's affairs. The Council further feels that it should point out that it is the responsibility of each delegate to consider all proposals submitted to the House of Delegates not in the light of how it will affect the Delegate individually, but more particularly what his vote on the proposal will mean to his profession, the public and the physicians who will enter the profession in the years to come.

Every Delegate should remember that this is a changing world, that today's problems are not met with antiquated practices of the past and that every physician, though he or she be yet unborn, should have from this present profession sound, proven and demonstrated advancements irrespective of the fields in which they fall, be they economic, political or scientific.

After the reading of the Council Report the Speaker stated, "It would seem more feasible to break this report down. As was stated earlier, we will take out of this report two specific recommendations which will come from Special Committees: first, the recommendation having to do with the education program and the recommendation of the special assessment; second, to take out of the report the recommendation concerning the medical care program for veterans. These two will be covered by special committee reports. If there is no objection the Chair will entertain a motion to the effect that these two recommendations in the Council Report be removed from the Report to be considered under the special committee reports." On *motion* by Dr. McLain Rogers, Clinton, *seconded* by Dr. Finis Ewing, Muskogee, this suggestion was *aproved*.

Dr. Garrison continued: "As your Chairman sees it there remains eight specific recommendations to the House of Delegates and it is his opinion that the best disposition of this report is to present these recommendations for your consideration one by one and then give you an opportunity to vote on each one."

It was *moved* by Dr. J. S. Fulton, Atoka, *seconded* by Dr. W. A. Howard, Chelsea, that a raise in dues for 1947 be approved. The motion *carried*.

On *motion* by Dr. F. W. Boadway, Ardmore, *seconded* by Dr. H. A. Higgins, Ardmore, the Council's recommendation in regard to the fee schedule was accepted and *approved*.

On *motion* by Dr. Finis Ewing, Muskogee, *seconded* by Dr. James Stevenson, Tulsa, the Council's recom-

mendation that a special committee be appointed to work with farm groups as outlined was accepted and *approved*.

On *motion* by Dr. McLain Rogers, Clinton, *seconded* by Dr. Earl Woodson, Poteau, the Council's recommendations regarding these committees on construction of health facilities was *approved*.

On *motion* by Dr. E. H. Shuller, McAlester, *seconded* by Dr. Ned Burleson, Prague, this recommendation of the Council regarding the creation of an endowment fund from physicians, was *approved*.

The Council went on record as recommending to the Board of Health and the State Health Department that their actions become more positive and progressive and that upon its shoulders rests a responsibility to the people that transcends all other considerations. The Council again recommended the full support of the Association to be placed at the disposal of the State Board of Health.

On *motion* by Dr. Louis Ritzhaupt, Guthrie, *seconded* by Dr. Robert Akin, Oklahoma City, the first part of this recommendation was *not approved*.

On *motion* by Dr. Finis Ewing, Muskogee, *seconded* by Dr. Ned Burlson, Prague, this recommendation regarding Standing Committees was *approved*.

On *motion* by Dr. Louis Ritzhaupt, Guthrie, *seconded* by Dr. Phil Risser, Blackwell, a commendation to Dr. Cross and the Board of Regents was *approved*.

Dr. Garrison: "We have presented and passed all recommendations of the Council with the exception of the two specifically left for the special committees. I will entertain a motion as to the acceptance of the Council Report.

On *motion* by Dr. McLain Rogers, Clinton, *seconded* by Dr. Finis Ewing, Muskogee, the Council Report was *accepted*.

Bureau Calls the Turn

The following incident points up the current campaign of the American Cancer Society to educate the public to the danger of cancer and the importance of prompt examination by qualified physicians and responsible clinics.

A western Oklahoma man recently inquired about a cancer clinic in a nearby city which claimed to be able to "cure" this dread disease. Later the inquirer reported back that the Better Business Bureau had "called the turn" on this concern.

The inquirer's brother, stricken with cancer and grasping at straws, was already on his way to the clinic was made. The report of the Better Business Bureau indicated that concerns of this type wrought their "cures" on superficial cancers or non-malignant growths or infections which would respond successfully to treatment by any physician or surgeon, but that when analysis showed actual cancer the clinic would decline the case because "the disease was in too advanced a stage to respond to treatment". This is exactly what happened, the inquirer reported.

There is no scientific evidence as yet to show that any diet, salve, serum or combination of drugs will cure cancer. Taken in time cancer may be cured by competent surgery and sometimes by the use of radium and X-ray but even these methods may not be adequate to save the victim who has wasted precious time trying to cure a cancer with worthless remedies.

Dr. Sam Binkley Locates on West Coast

Word has been received in the Executive Office that Dr. J. Samuel Binkley, formerly of New York City is now associated with the Los Angeles Tumor Institute. He will be remembered as having conducted a short course in cancer education here in this State in 1941. Dr. Binkley served in the Medical Corps of the Navy and was discharged from the service in January, 1946.

Many readers judge of the power of a book by the shock it gives their feelings. *Longfellow*.

Description is always a bore, both to the describer and to the describee. *Disraeli*.

OFFICERS OF COUNTY SOCIETIES, 1946

★

COUNTY	PRESIDENT	SECRETARY	MEETING TIME
Alfalfa	W. G. Dunnington, Cherokee	L. T. Lancaster, Cherokee	Last Tues. each Second Month
Atoka-Coal	J. B. Clark, Coalgate	J. S. Fulton, Atoka	
Beckham	P. J. DeVanney, Sayre	J. E. Levick, Elk City	Second Tuesday
Blaine	W. F. Bohlman, Watonga	Virginia Curtain, Watonga	Third Thursday
Bryan	W. K. Haynie, Durant	Jonah Nichols, Durant	Second Tuesday
Caddo	Preston E. Wright, Anadarko	Edward T. Cook, Jr., Anadarko	
Canadian	G. L. Goodman, Yukon	W. P. Lawton, El Reno	Subject to call
Carter	J. Hobson Veazey, Ardmore	H. A. Higgins, Ardmore	Second Tuesday
Cherokee	P. H. Medearis, Tahlequah	R. K. McIntosh, Jr., Tahlequah	First Tuesday
Choctaw	Floyd L. Waters, Hugo	O. R. Gregg, Hugo	
Cleveland	James O. Hood, Norman	Phil Haddock, Norman	Thursday nights
Comanche	Wm. Cole, Lawton	E. P. Hathaway, Lawton	
Cotton	G. W. Baker, Walters	Mollie Scism, Walters	Third Friday
Craig	Lloyd H. McPike, Vinita	J. M. McMillan, Vinita	
Creek	W. P. Longmire, Sapulpa	Philip Joseph, Sapulpa	Second Tuesday
Custer	Ross Deputy, Clinton	A. W. Paulson, Cordell	Third Thursday
Garfield	Bruce Hinson, Enid	John R. Walker, Enid	Fourth Thursday
Garvin	M. E. Robberson, Jr., Wynnewood	John R. Callaway, Pauls Valley	Wednesday before Third Thursday
Grady	Roy Emanuel, Chickasha	Rebecca H. Mason, Chickasha	Third Thursday
Grant	I. V. Hardy, Medford	F. P. Robinson, Pond Creek	
Greer	J. B. Lansden, Granite	J. B. Hollis, Mangum	
Harmon	W. G. Husband, Hollis	R. H. Lynch, Hollis	First Wednesday
Haskell	Wm. S. Carson, Keotah	N. K. Williams, McCurtain	
Hughes	Victor W. Pryor, Holdenville	L. A. S. Johnson, Holdenville	First Friday
Jackson	E. W. Mabry, Altus	J. P. Irby, Altus	Last Monday
Jefferson	F. M. Edwards, Ringling	J. A. Dillard, Waurika	Second Monday
Kay	L. G. Neal, Ponca City	J. C. Wagner, Ponca City	Second Thursday
Kingfisher	John W. Pendleton, Kingfisher	H. Violet Sturgeon, Hennessey	
Kiowa	Wm. Bernell, Hobart	J. Wm. Finch, Hobart	
LeFlore	S. D. Bevill, Poteau	Rush L. Wright, Poteau	
Lincoln	J. S. Rollins, Prague	Ned Burleson, Prague	First Wednesday
Logan	James Petty, Guthrie	J. E. Souter, Guthrie	Last Tuesday
Marshall			
Mayes	L. C. White, Adair	V. D. Herrington, Pryor	
McClain	S. C. Davis, Blanchard	W. C. McCurdy, Purcell	
McCurtain	J. T. Moreland, Idabel	R. H. Sherrill, Broken bow	Fourth Tuesday
McIntosh	F. R. First, Checotah	W. A. Tolleson, Eufaula	First Thursday
Muskogee-Sequoyah			
Wagoner	R. N. Holcombe, Muskogee	William N. Weaver, Muskogee	First Tuesday
Noble	A. M. Evans, Perry	Jesse W. Driver, Perry	
Okfuskee	W. P. Jenkins, Okemah	M. L. Whitney, Okemah	Second Monday
Oklahoma	W. F. Keller, Okla. City	John H. Lamb, Okla. City	Fourth Tuesday
Okmulgee	F. S. Watson, Okmulgee	C. E. Smith, Henryetta	Second Monday
Osage	Paul H. Hemphill, Pawhuska	Vincent Mazzarella, Hominy	Third Monday
Ottawa	C. F. Walker, Grove	W. Jackson Sayles, Miami	Second Thursday
Pawnee	H. B. Spalding, Ralston	R. L. Browning, Pawnee	
Payne	F. Keith Oehlschlager, Yale	C. W. Moore, Stillwater	Third Thursday
Pittsburg	Millard L. Henry, McAlester	Edward D. Greenberger, McAlester	Third Friday
Pontotoc-Murray	John Morey, Ada	R. H. Mayes, Ada	First Wednesday
Pottawatomie	F. P. Newlin, Shawnee	Clinton Gallaher, Shawnee	First and Third Saturday
Pushmataha	John S. Lawson, Clayton	B. M. Huckabay, Antler	
Rogers	W. A. Howard, Chelsea	P. S. Anderson, Claremore	Third Wednesday
Seminole	Clifton Felts, Seminole	Mack I. Shanholz, Seminole	Third Wednesday
Stephens	Everett King, Duncan	Fred L. Patterson, Duncan	
Texas	Daniel S. Lee, Guymon	E. L. Buford, Guymon	
Tillman	H. A. Calvert, Frederick	O. G. Bacon, Frederick	
Tulsa	John C. Perry, Tulsa	John E. McDonald, Tulsa	Second and Fourth Monday
Washington-Nowata	Ralph W. Rucker, Bartlesville	L. B. Word, Bartlesville	Second Wednesday
Washita	L. G. Livingston, Cordell	Roy W. Anderson, Clinton	
Woods	John F. Simon, Alva	O. E. Templin, Alva	Last Tuesday Odd Months
Woodward	T. C. Leachman, Woodward	C. W. Tedrowe, Woodward	Second Thursday

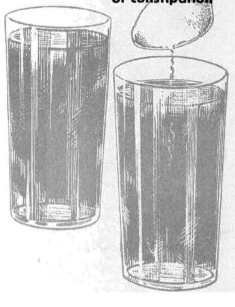

The "SMOOTHAGE" regimen in the treatment of constipation

A rounded teaspoonful of Metamucil stirred into a glass of water, milk or fruit juice, three times a day, provides the soft, mucilaginous bulk which is desirable for natural elimination. Metamucil contains no roughage, no oils, no chemical irritants.

Metamucil is the highly purified, nonirritating extract of the seed of the psyllium, Plantago ovata (50%), combined with anhydrous dextrose (50%). It mixes readily with liquids, is palatable, easy to take.

Supplied in 1-lb., 8-oz. and 4-oz. containers.

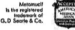

Metamucil is the registered trademark of G.D Searle & Co.

ACCEPTED AMERICAN MEDICAL ASSN.

SEARLE
RESEARCH IN THE SERVICE OF MEDICINE

THE JOURNAL
of the
OKLAHOMA STATE MEDICAL ASSOCIATION

| VOLUME XXXIX | OKLAHOMA CITY, OKLAHOMA, JULY, 1946 | NUMBER 7 |

Rheumatic Myocarditis *

ROBERT H. BAYLEY, M.D.

Oklahoma University School of Medicine

OKLAHOMA CITY, OKLAHOMA

Rheumatic heart disease is a major cause of death, second only to tuberculosis, between the ages of fifteen and twenty-five years. With the exception of the few of these patients who die of a fulminating acute rheumatic carditis, death occurs from chronic cardiac invalidism. We should, therefore, be greatly interested in the factor which leads to chronic rheumatic cardiac invalidism. This factor is active rheumatic myocarditis. We hear so much about rheumatic mitral stenosis, rheumatic aortic insufficiency, and rheumatic pericarditis that I am sure undue emphasis is placed upon these factors. These factors are unimportant in the production of cardiac invalidism. For example, it is not uncommon to encounter high-grade chronic rheumatic valve disease in perfectly healthy individuals in their fourth, fifth, or even sixth decade. Other diseases such as subacute bacterial endocarditis, pneumonia, hypertension, and arteriosclerosis are required to cause death in these people, their chronic rheumatic valve disease does not. Moreover, active or healed rheumatic pericarditis is of almost no clinical importance in the production of cardiac invalidism. Pick's disease or constrictive pericarditis is not caused by the rheumatic disease process.

Active rheumatic myocarditis presents a great problem in both the diagnostic and therapeutic fields. However, it is diagnosable and treatable in the vast majority of instances. Consequently, the high mortality rate from rheumatic cardiac invalidism is unjustified. Let us examine, first, the diagnostic and, second, the therapeutic problem.

DIAGNOSIS

There are two natural subdivisions of the diagnostic problem presented by rheumatic

myocarditis. In one group are the patients with extracardiac manifestations of active rheumatic disease. In the other group are patients without these extracardiac manifestations. In the first group we are duty-bound to make the diagnosis of rheumatic myocarditis by inference in any and all subjects which present the extracardiac manifestations of active rheumatic disease. The situation here is analogous to the diagnosis by inference of minimal or subliminal active pulmonary tuberculosis in the patient who has developed an acute pleurisy with effusion. Let us carry the analogy further. If the rheumatic myocarditis and the minimal pulmonary lesion are not thus diagnosed, attention and treatment will be directed primarily at the extracardiac rheumatic lesions and at the pleural effusion. In each instance the effort is ninety per cent misdirected, for both of the latter phenomena heal without event in spite of treatment if not because of it. The patient is fortunate who develops edema with his acute nephritis, pleural effusion with his minimal or subliminal pulmonary tuberculosis, and sore red joints with his rheumatic myocarditis, for these will enable a diagnosis by inference and the opportunity for treatment will thus occur. In this connection it should be remembered, however, the rheumatic fever is the single most common cause of unexplained fever. Hence, fever alone is not always a helpful extracardiac manifestation. The diagnostic importance of additional extracardiac manifestations, muscle and joint pains, nodules, and chorea, is self-evident.

Of particular importance are the cardiac manifestations of rheumatic myocarditis. Unfortunately, from the diagnostic standpoint, the cardiac manifestations are those

*Presented at the Annual Meeting, Oklahoma State Medical Association, Friday, May 3, 1946.

of myocarditis in general. There is not a single etiologically specific clinical cardiac sign of rheumatic myocarditis. Moreover, since the specific extracardiac manifestations are absent in the *majority* of instances, particularly in warmer climates, the magnitude of the diagnostic problem becomes evident.

First of all, a diagnosis of myocarditis in general and one of rheumatic etiology in particular will only be possible for those who maintain a high index of suspicion. The evidence must be searched for in most instances. Fortunately, the causes of myocarditis other than rheumatic disease, particularly in subjects under thirty years of age, are few indeed. The imbalance of this ratio enables one to entertain a rheumatic etiology in all instances of myocarditis under thirty years, unless the etiology can be definitely proved otherwise. A few of these subjects will have *lupus erythematosis disseminatus* which is to be suspected if bright red skin lesions are present or if the urine shows red cells, casts, and albumen. A few patients in this group will have *periarteritis nodosa* which should be seriously considered if there is a history of allergy or a high eosinophil count. A muscle biopsy may settle the question. A few of the women will have *post-partal myocarditis*. This lesion develops within eight weeks of delivery. A few patients in this group will have *beri-beri heart*. These patients cure rapidly with thiamine chloride and have little or no slowing of their circulation time at the outset. The occasional subject with *myxedema heart*, but without edema, might give difficulty. Ordinarily the associated sinus bradycardia is quite characteristic, and a low B.M.R. should settle the question. Finally, a few patients of the group will have so-called *isolated myocarditis*. Here the rapidly fatal course with treatment for rheumatic myocarditis may arouse the suspicion that one is dealing with a so-called isolated myocarditis.

The subject with myocarditis presents some if not all of the following signs and symptoms. They have been listed in approximate order of their diagnostic importance.

1. Cardiac enlargement.
2. Certain electrocardiagraphic changes.
3. Transient pericardial friction rub.
4. Diminished pulse pressure.
5. Sinus tachycardia and gallop sound.
6. Dyspnea on exertion without orthopnea.
7. Elevated venous pressure.
8. Palpitation and precordial pain not necessarily associated with exertion.
9. Rapid sedimentation rate.

Because of their importance, certain of these items require further comment. Cardiac enlargement is the single most valuable diagnostic sign, particularly when it is ob-

served to be progressive or regressive. The six-foot roentgenogram is the only reliable method of detecting and following cardiac enlargement. The severity of active rheumatic myocarditis is directly proportional to the amount of cardiac enlargement. The enlargement is due to hypertrophy as well as dilation, and both are produced by the effects on the myocardium of the rheumatic inflammatory process. The enlargement is not primarily dependent upon the endocardial or the pericardial lesions. The rheumatic inflammatory process attacks chiefly the walls of the left ventricle and the interventricular septum and hypertrophy is most striking in these regions. Moreover, both dilatation and hypertrophy due to rheumatic myocarditis are reversible, or subject to regression, under proper management. As cardiac invalidism and death are approached by the rheumatic patient, cardiac enlargement invariably becomes marked. Progressive cardiac enlargement without any other manifestations of rheumatic disease is presumptive evidence of the active rheumatic state and demands proper treatment. In this connection, I have recently observed the case of a teen-aged boy whose cardiac enlargement progressed from normal to marked within a year. The heart weighed fourteen hundred grams, or nine times its proper value. The endocardial and pericardial lesions were negligible. In general, the cardiac hypertrophy appears to depend upon two factors, the presence of an active inflammatory rheumatic process and excessive heart work, either one of which, when acting alone, is essentially ineffective.[1] Another important feature of the hypertrophy is that, to a limited extent at least, the hypertrophy is regressive in the continued absence of operation of both factors which produce it.

The electrocardiographic changes of rheumatic myocarditis are often of considerable diagnostic aid. It has been repeatedly emphasized that transient prolongation of the P-R interval, which indicates a partial atrio-ventricular heart block, appears in ninety or ninety five per cent of electrocardiograms recorded daily from subjects throughout the active attack. More recently, the routine recording of multiple unipolar chest leads from these subjects has disclosed additional information of diagnostic and therapeutic value.[2] Repeated electrocardiograms constitute one of the more important laboratory procedures with which to follow the course of rheumatic myocarditis. Electrocardiographic changes which indicate activity may outlast all other laboratory evidence of activity.

The transient precordial friction rub in the rheumatic subject is to be regarded as evidence of underlying active rheumatic myocarditis, a part of the so-called pancarditis of this disease. Its diagnostic usefulness is limited by the rarity with which it is detected. Its absence is of no diagnostic use. Its presence in a subject suspected of having myocarditis should certainly suggest a rheumatic etiology. *Lupus erythematosis disseminata* and *periarteritis nodosa* may also produce friction rub.

In adults, disproportionally small pulse pressure (20 mm. Hg. or less in a subject whose heart rate is under 110 per minute) should command attention. In younger subjects, the pulse pressure value is lower, and the rate value is higher normally, and allowance must be made. A small pulse pressure is related to the more severe grades of myocardial damage and is not etiologically specific. In addition to factors which cause myocarditis, the low pulse pressure is observed routinely in acute myocardial infarction. The latter is of rare occurrence, however, in subjects under twenty-five years of age and is observed only occasionally in subjects between the ages of twenty-four and thirty years. If pulsus alternans or electrical alternans is present, the myocardial damage is usually severe.

Sinus tachycardia and gallop sound, particularly when the former is out of proportion to the fever, should direct attention to the myocardium. The extra sound which contributes to the gallop is diastolic in time but does not create the gallop sound in rates under one hundred per minute. These signs are not etiologically specific.

Dyspnea on exertion is important in connection with this discussion because of the frequency with which it may justly serve to call our attention to the myocardium. Orthopnea also ocurs in connection with rheumatic myocarditis. However, it makes its appearance only in the terminal stages of the disease. When other physical findings of myocarditis indicate clearly a precarious state, the patient is usually able to rest in the supine position without shortness of breath. The elements of so-called congestive heart failure appear only as terminal events in the vast majority of instances of myocarditis. In many instances sudden death intercedes before congestive heart failure can terminate the illness.

As in the case of tuberculosis, the sedimentation rate has proved to be one of the valuable laboratory aids with which to follow the course of the rheumatic disease process. The increased rate is not etiologically specific for rheumatic disease, but the normal sedimentation rate very strongly suggests that active rheumatic disease in general, and active rheumatic myocarditis in particular, are not present.

Diastolic murmurs which are diagnostic of chronic rheumatic valve disease frequently vanish when the myocarditis is active and reappear later when activity subsides. Therefore, their diagnostic usefulness is limited at the time when it would be most useful.

THERAPY

It is now known that streptococcic sore throat is somehow followed within three weeks by active rheumatic disease in susceptible subjects. Preventive treatment has become important, for it is now known that the prophylactic use of sulfonamide is decidedly successful in preventing streptococcic sore throat. The adult dose of sulfadiazine is 1 gm., two or three times daily, throughout the fall and winter seasons when streptococcic sore throat is common. Smaller doses are required for children. Tonsillectomy has not proved to be of preventive or curative value. The operation with adenoidectomy should be done when the local status of these tissues warrants. Moreover, when any surgical procedure is undertaken on subjects who are known to have or have had rheumatic disease, the prophylactic use of sulfonamide or penicillin should always be employed. The danger here is not from rheumatic carditis but an induced transient bacteremia which may lead to subacute bacterial endocarditis.

It is apparent that good nursing care, for the purpose of obtaining a minimal work demand on the heart, outranks all other therapeutic measures which are used in treating active rheumatic disease. The use of sodium salyicate has been thought to be important primarily because of the symptomatic relief which it affords. However, some of the more recent studies[a] suggest that when it is employed in large doses with equally large doses of sodium bicarbonate, it may have some curative value. I am sure that doses which afford symptomatic relief afford rest and thereby lessen the work demand on the myocardium, and in this manner help in the prevention of ultimate cardiac invalidism. There is a recent tendency, on the part of some physicians, to get the patient "up and about" who is suffering from active rheumatic disease. If, in a given case, this procedure lessens, rather than increases, the work demand on the heart, it is justified, otherwise it is to be forcefully condemned. The articles which recommend the "up and about" treatment have been very incomplete from the standpoint of long-time followup. The situation reminds one of the "up and about" treatment of tuberculous pleurisy with effusion which was supposed to commence as soon as the evidence of active pleuritis is over. Most of the subjects treated on this plan found their way into tuberculosis sanitoria with advanced pulmonary disease before a subsequent five-year period had ended. It is my present conviction that a routine "up and about" treatment for active rheumatic disease will lead to unnecessary cardiac invalidism by the time young adult life is reached. I urge, therefore, that this recommendation not be accepted except in those instances where it clearly decreases the work demand on the myocardium. A sharply curtailed work demand for the myocardium throughout the stages of active myocarditis is the keynote

of prevention of chronic rheumatic cardiac invalidism.

BIBLIOGRAPHY

1. H. B. Taussig and M. Goldenberg: Roentgenologie Studies of Size of Heart in Childhood; Three Different Types of Teleroentgenographic Changes Which Occur in Acute Rheumatic Fever, American Heart Journal, Volume No. 21, page 440; April, 1941.
2. S. R. First and R. H. Bayley: Electrocardiographic Studies in Rheumatic Heart Disease with Reference to Interpretation of Multiple Unipolar Percordial Leads. (Unpublished).
3. A. F. Cobrun: Salicylate Therapy in Rheumatic Fever, Rational Technique; Bulletin of Johns Hopkins Hospital, Volume No. 73, pp. 435-464; December, 1943.

Endocrine Complaints in the Eye, Ear, Nose and Throat Area*

E. H. COACHMAN, M.D.

MUSKOGEE, OKLAHOMA

Eye complaints arising from an endocrine basis form the most numerous, as well as the most easily detected group, of the Eye, Ear, Nose and Throat area. The subjective symptoms are not so varied but that the repetition of these complaints should suggest to the oculist and otolaryngologist that they have a common origin, and can be relieved by a common procedure.

SYMPTOMS

Headache, arising from use of the eyes, is the most constant symptom especially from reading, sewing, picture shows, riding on the train or in cars. Accompanying these they may have skipping of lines, or figures, inability to draw or determine when a line is level, trouble threading a needle even with their ordinary glasses worn, photophobia with lacrimation, stinging and burning of the lid margins, periodic spasm of the lids, inability to read more than 20 to 30 minutes without tiring and associated inability to concentrate. Where they have used their eyes the night before such as with card playing or night driving, the headache is present on awakening.

The location of the headache is usually in one of three places in this frequency: (1) unilaterally, above, in, or behind one eye; (2) medially, between and behind the two eyes; (3) unilaterally again, but in the occiput area, and descending down the neck between or into the scapula area. Many patients have dizziness and even nausea accompanying these headaches which frequently misleads to the diagnosis of migraine headaches, Menieres syndrome, and worst of all "sinus trouble".

*Presented at the Annual Meeting, Oklahoma State Medical Association, Wednesday, May 1, 1946.

General complaints like paraesthesias of the hands and feet are felt by the patient, especially a "going to sleep" of the ring and little fingers which are supplied by the ulnar nerve. Accompanying this they have a stiffness of the arms and legs, especially after sitting or lying down for 20 or 30 minutes. For this reason many of them are regular attendants with the massaging cults. Massage gives but temporary relief, so they persist in further search. It is odd that they should be diagnosed by an eye examination but since extraocular muscles are quite small their departure from normal can be detected rather early.

Fatigue is another general symptom almost as constantly complained of as headaches, and is described by the patient as being "easily tired", "having to slow down", "can't do a day's work" and "as tired on arising in the mornings as when retiring". Nothing ever relieves their tired, worn-out feeling so they trudge along from one day to the other "just getting by". They are therefore irritable, "lose their tempers easily", and become anti-social, which makes them try to pass the time by reading, only to find they cannot concentrate, and if they force themselves to do so their headaches and ocular complaints start afresh. So they change glasses one pair after the other, with no relief, and finally come in with an "up against it" feeling and none too kindly disposed towards still another "change in glasses". This skepticism is easily dispelled if the oculist will turn and enumerate the patient's symptoms and show thereby he has a grasp of the situation.

Dizziness and lacrimation are equal in rate of occurrence. The lacrimation is especially noticed in bright lights or sunshine, so squinting and colored glasses are commonly resorted to, in an attempt to lessen the photophobic symptoms. Never have I examined such a wearer of colored glasses but that the latent vertical phoria was found, for it is this latent phoria which gives rise to the eye complaints.

Often the dizziness is felt spontaneously, but is more apt to be noticed when changing positions, as in stooping or arising from bed or turning suddenly. It is transient, yet annoying, and gives a feeling of helplessness, which increases with its repetition. It is because of this feature that the Menieres syndrome is injected, since occasionally these patients fall and bruise themselves noticeably, but are immediately able to regain their equilibrium and continue. Such incidents worry them and lessen their confidence so that they live a plagued existence.

Transient scotomata are not uncommon, and are detected by the patients themselves, when they notice that several words in a sentence, or portions of familiar objects, are missing in one or both eyes. These are projected as dark spots and may scintillate, but are more apt to persist for a period and disappear spontaneously, then repeat the course all over again, in no rhythmic fashion.

School children having a visual acuity of 20/20 in both eyes or better, will often be poor readers, unable to concentrate, and consequently do not understand what they read due to their latent vertical phoria. The reason they do not comprehend the meaning of what they read is simply because the higher eye will read across the page, then the lower eye will take over when a new line is started, thus skipping a line or so and losing the meaning expressed. Bookkeepers "jumble" their columns of figures for the same reason, and find it necessary to use a ruler to stay on the right line. Carpenters and painters have difficulty making a straight line, while aviators experience the same trouble in making a landing from lack of stereoscopic vision, when the two eyes fail to focus in the same horizontal plane.

SIGNS

It is also characteristic of this group when 35 to 45 years of age that they look so healthy, with their added "middle age spread", that they receive little consideration when their complaints do not befit their appearances. This added weight is of itself a sign of the onset of latent vertical phoria, and it must be unearthed by occluding the eye, since less than 10 per cent of the cases will show perceptible amounts of vertical phoria without patching the weaker eye a couple of days. Many of the premenopause and climacteric headaches are due to this

imbalance of the extraocular muscles in the two eyes. It is this same condition which spells satisfaction or dissatisfaction with their bifocal glasses, for if the two eyes are not aligned upon the same horizontal plane when the visual acuity of each is improved with lenses, their headaches are more increased, and their eye strain enhanced until they prefer going back to their old lenses, with which they saw less well in order to avoid the strain of the stimulated weaker eye trying to maintain binocular vision.

When the vertical prism is incorporated into the correcting lenses, they not only see better with less effort, but lose their anxiety over the change, and are more dependent upon their new glasses than ever before, simply because without the prism to hold the eyes to the same horizontal plane, they revert to their old imbalance and all its symptoms. You will find few of these patients going without their glasses, since the comfort they furnish overcomes all the objections. Your change from single lenses to bifocals is thus relieved, since the closer the work, the more dependent the patient becomes upon the vertical prism to maintain alignment of the two eyes.

Another enjoyable feature to the inclusion of vertical prisms is the certainty with which you may predict which patient will require them. This is done by finding a subnormal temperature, low blood pressure and low pulse rate; e. g., 98° temperature, 110/60 blood pressure, 60 pulse, in an individual of 35 to 45 years of age. Accompanying these findings there is usually found pitting along the lower inner third of the tibia, puffing of the eye lids, and a suggestion of bloating, or fullness to the face. This oedema is generalized but best detected in these locations. There is a noticeable thinning of the outer third of the eye brow, or even the entire brow. The hair of the scalp may be scant, or bald, and the skin itself seems to be devoid of its oily filament, leaving it dry and leathery in appearance. Otomycosis is a frequent accompaniment, since the wax secretion is lessened, the skin is subsequently unable to ward off infection when moisture from head bathing, etc., is left undried in the ears.

I have yet to see an otosclerosis case not have a latent vertical phoria, which adds strength to the contention it is endocrinal in origin, and they too, as a rule have the subtemperature, low blood pressure and slow pulse, and persistent oedema. The same is true of drug idiosyncrasies, especially to sulfa, aspirin, and atropine, for they will be found to have all these findings, plus the latent vertical phoria. These same cases tolerate infections poorly, by having more pain, distress, and prostration than patients with apparently the equivalent condition but with different constitutional tolerance. People of low stature are more frequently found in this group, than the medium and tall, also blondes (especially red heads) are more numerous than brunettes. Gentiles, Jews, Negroes and Indians seem to be equally represented, and people of all ages from all parts of the United States are affected since the local influx at Camp Gruber furnished ample material for determining this point.

Men and women are equally represented but the condition is prone to run in family groups, predominating when one or more parent is involved and not found at all in other families. Therefore when a parent is found carrying a latent vertical phoria generally fifty per cent or more of their children will have the same trouble. If both parents are sufferers the percentage and certainty is increased while with neither parent having the condition it is rare to find their children possessing a latent vertical phoria. These details, plus an alertness in taking their history will lead the oculist to suspect the latent character of vertical phoria in many previously undiagnosed cases.

Once having suspected the phoria how can it be proven? The visual acuity is taken without glasses for each eye, and the eye having the lower acuity is patched for at least 48 hours, at which time it will show the amount of drop in focus, producing the headache and eye symptoms of which the patient complains. Almost as surely as you have two eyes with different visual acuities, you have a latent vertical phoria! And as surely as you have a visual acuity of 20/20 of one eye and a 20/15 of the other you likewise are dealing with a latent vertical phoria, giving rise to greater symptoms, than if the visual acuity of the two eyes differed more widely, simply because the eyes put forth a greater effort to maintain binocular vision where the visual stimuli are nearer equal than where they are not. Most oculists make the mistake of brushing these off as "needing no glasses". Glasses are for more purposes than correcting hyperopia, myopia, and astigmatism, although you would never suspect it, by the frequency with which oculists overlook the correction of latent vertical phoria.

Even the few cases that show a vertical phoria on the initial examination will consistently have a greater phoria following the two day occlusion of the weaker eye. Seventy five per cent of those not showing any vertical deviation when first examined will show a latent vertical phoria following 48 hour patching. This shows the necessity of occluding the eye, otherwise it is missed.

In those rare cases, where the patient is unable to decide which eye has the greater acuity, especially where they have 20/15 in both eyes and still the symptoms are those of latent vertical phoria, the procedure is to patch one eye at a time, each for two days, and make recordings of the vertical deviations, and the eye occluded which gives the greater deviation finding is taken as the weaker eye and the full prismatic correction prescribed. Often this is the only correction needed, since the spherical and cylindrical errors are found too small to adequately explain the severity of the complaint.

A gauze patch of half an inch thickness which prevents the lids opening, thus occluding the eye for approximately 48 hours, is held firmly with adhesive and worn continuously, otherwise the test is not satisfactory, since the eye must be rested as much as possible to allow it to settle to its natural level. When the patch is removed the eyes are kept closed tightly until ten diopters prism base in are placed before each eye, (for diplopia) along with whatever spherical or cylindrical correction (which previously has been determined) and a vertical Maddox rod before the left eye. The eyes are then opened and the head held in its natural erect position, rather than a faulty position, which of itself could introduce a vertical error, but constant care will prevent this happening.

A round green light is projected upon the screen and the patient sees a horizontal green streak through the vertical Maddox rod before the left eye and the green dot before the right. A rotary prism is placed before the right eye base up or down, and the patient asked to state when the green line is level with the center of the green dot. The number of prisms base up or down to level these two objects is the amount of latent vertical phoria, for distance, and by placing an additional fifteen diopters of prism base in and repeating the process (adding bifocal correction if a presbyope) the amount for near is quickly secured at 13 to 16 inches, and the full amount incorporated into the patient's new lenses.

They are cautioned not to be alarmed if they have diplopia for five, ten, or fifteen minutes, when they first place their glasses on in the morning, since this period of time is necessary for the eyes to come to the same horizontal plane when the correction is placed before the eyes. Upon removing the correction at night the eyes again become imbalanced, but this is noticed only for a few moments. Even this on and off phenomenon is not noticed by the patient after a couple of weeks, and by that time they are so wedded to their glasses nothing matters. Patients wearing vertical prisms have more difficulty getting along without their correction than the same patient where the prisms are not included. In fact, without the prisms they continue to have eye strain and soon give up their continuous use, since the increased visual acuity of the two eyes only increases the effort of the two eyes to work together, which they cannot continuously do without the vertical correction incorporated, therefore they prefer seeing less well, to keeping the headaches and eye symptoms. Once the vertical element is taken into consideration, the situation is reversed and you have a patient relieved when the visual acuity is increased instead of punished, and they become more and more dependent upon their glasses, thus wearing them without being urged since eye comfort was their original reason for consulting you.

Now there is nothing new about latent vertical phoria, since it has been discussed pro and con since Von Graefe's time. Marlow found it present in 84 per cent of 700 cases and for the last five years my routine has been to patch every eye case in order to determine the amount of latent vertical phoria. My technique has not been as elaborate as Marlow's since he occluded the *dominant* eye for one to two weeks and took measurements in more than the vertical plane, to study the deviations of the two eyes. My search was for something quickly secured, practical, and symptom relieving, which the patient would tolerate. This procedure has trebbled my refractions and dwindled the complaints from patients to a new low, and it will do the same for you.

After reading considerable literature on occlusion[1] [2] [3] [4] [6] [7] [8] [10] [11] [12] [13] tests, vertical[14] phorias, unlevel[4] orbits causing heterophoria, and determining how consistently[5] these cases had low temperature, slow pulse and low blood pressure, low B.M.R.'s, ankle pitting, with negative (urinalyses, heart examinations and blood wassermans,) together with absence of infections, then seeing Howard's[8] description of the role of hypothroidism in ophthalmology, I felt the subnormal findings and latent vertical phoria had a common origin. The gynecologist removing ovaries and ovarian cysts, helped to show that ovarian dysfunction also played a part in latent vertical phoria causing headaches and eye strain, and not until the latent vertical phoria and pelvic pathology were both corrected, was the patient permanently benefitted. The same has been noticed with diabetics, hypoglycemias, hyper and hypothyroidism, and of course at the menopause it is most frequent of any age span, thus clinically proving the connection between endocrine dyscrasia and latent vertical phoria, which is the only link in the chain of evidence, original with me. The significance is simply that there is a dyscrasia within the endocrine chain, and is not specific as to any one gland or its rate of activity. It is purely general in character, indicating, I feel, a loss of muscle tone, which

gives rise to the patient's complaints.

Since most of these cases are hypothyroids, thyroid (grains 1 to 5 after meals) is prescribed until the pulse rate is normal, continuing it for months or years, which relieves them of their generalized symptoms of fatigue, insomnia, dizziness, muscle cramps and paraesthesias, lack of concentration, and general inertia. Only in children is there a chance to correct the latent vertical phoria by combining endocrine therapy and corrective lenses, and only rarely then, since most of them get to feeling better and consider continuous medication unnecessary. In those who cooperate the least, the phoria usually has progressed the most, when their eyes are again examined, so there seems to be a definite connection between the endocrine function and the eye muscles. Since vitamin therapy has become well established, a maintainance dose, especially of B complex, is given to take care of the increased matabolism induced by the thyroid therapy, which I feel are the vitamins' chief contribution. No dieting is permitted, so that these patients do not vary materially in weight during the course of the thyroid therapy.

Much information can be gathered by a study of the variations in the three findings, viz. temperature, blood pressure and pulse, e.g. with the temperature 98°, the blood pressure 120/70, and pulse 95 in a 50-year-old male, nicotine is probably the cause of the rapid pulse, and he is advised to eliminate it and return in three to four weeks, when it will often be 60 or 65, thus showing the true picture which accompanies these latent vertical phoria cases. Nicotine, caffeine and alcohol are the stimulants most frequently causing increased pulse rates such as illustrated, and for that reason their removal is obtained before beginning thyroid therapy, so as not to complicate the pulse rate, which is checked at semi-monthly or monthly intervals.

Where a rise in temperature, plus a fast pulse, is encountered the cause of the fever usually eliminates the rapid pulse. But where stimulants and fever are missing and a fast pulse is present with a low blood pressure, we often find allergy, or some endocrine pelvic pathology, and refer them for that purpose. It will amuse you to witness the curiosity of your fellow M.D.'s wanting to know how you suspected these conditions from examining the eyes! The practice of medicine in any branch is eternally interesting if we but keep hunting for puzzles to solve. It was puzzling to me why so many patients had increased eye strain by increasing their visual acuity, so I set out to find the reason.

Patients who come with a complaint of "sinus trouble", and show nothing abnormal in the nose and throat, and whose transillumination and X-ray of sinuses are normal we always check for temperature, blood pressure, pulse, and look for oedema about the eyes and ankle, then note the thinning eye brow, and if confirmed the eyes are refracted, vertical phoria tests done, and then the weaker eye is patched for two days. The patch is removed and the eyes kept closed until the ten diopters prisms are before each eye for maintainance of diplopia, before the eyes are opened. The patient's correction is placed before each eye, the Maddox rod vertically before the left eye, while the prism to measure the amount of vertical phoria is before the right eye. The full amount of vertical prism is incorporated into the prescribed lenses, and the patient placed on thyroid and daily maintenance dose of vitamins (especially vitamin B complex) and the "sinus trouble" ceases to give the patient further trouble.

In so called vasomotor rhinitis, where a great deal of clear mucoid discharge is present, especially post nasally, and all allergic history and search net us nothing, we usually record the subnormal temperature, blood pressure and pulse, then test for latent vertical phoria, and if found, the case will respond to the same thyroid, and vitamin therapy, without any further manipulation. Where allergy leaves off and endocrine dyscrasias begin their manifestations is impossible to determine, but clinically if allergy is suspected and not found, treat for the endocrine trouble and results will usually be forth coming. We need to keep endocrine malfunctions in mind, just as a few years back we had to be trained to be on guard for allergies, and soon we will relieve a great deal of distress which we are now failing to do.

It is hard for us to overcome the errors of our medical school teachings, where we were admonished against thyroid medication, as though a toxic goitre was the inevitable result. This is a gross misrepresentation, for I have given 2 and 3 grains to patients daily for months with high blood pressure to study its effects, and instead of raising the blood pressure it always lowers it ten to thirty points, even though the pulse rate may advance five to ten per minute.

On the background of low temperature, low blood pressure, and slow pulse, with orbital and ankle odema, thyroid therapy has been given to literally hundreds of cases, months on end, and not a single toxic goitre, or perceptible injury of any kind has resulted. I myself have taken thyroid daily (2 to 4 grains) for nearly four years and intend doing so the rest of my life, since I had all the findings of a latent vertical phoria, an

ambulatory B.M.R. of only minus 6, and looked too healthy to get much medical attention, yet, got to the point where it was a task for me to do an ordinary day's work, so I went to work on the thyroid, vitamins, and vertical prisms and have never dared turn loose!

Patients complaining of "tightness" and a "smothering sensation" in the throat, or of excessive post nasal drippage, especially where they have "to clear" their throats before starting to talk, will usually show all the positive signs of an endocrine dyscrasia, and will respond almost without exception to thyroid and maintenance vitamin therapy. Nothing can be found on examining these cases, so the history is the lead, and where in doubt, take the temperature, blood pressure, not the orbital oedema, and outer third of the eye brow, and pit the ankle along the lower inner third of the tibia, then refract and occlude the weaker eye and you will be surprised how often the syndrome comes to light, and you with it!

The ear may be the only complaint the patient mentions, and the examination usually shows a few flakes of desquamating skin in the outer external canal, or nothing abnormal is found, even on audiometer reading, yet the trouble is an aggravating roaring, noises of various types, itching, and a tightness which runs down the neck perpendicularly from the canal, or along the course of the eustachian tube into the throat. Again if we work the case up the associated low findings in temperature, blood pressure, pulse, orbital and ankle oedema, latent vertical phoria are all present and mean the same thing as if the same patient had complained of the eye, nose or throat area instead of the ear.

Patients having unaccounted for swelling about the face, especially when the lids are swollen on arising, will often produce this syndrome and respond to the same treatment, since in hypothyroidism there is a water retention, which gives rise to the persistant oedema, long before myxoedema appears. Thyroid therapy increases the urinary output and relieves the pitting, along with its other benefits.

CONCLUSIONS

Endocrine dyscrasias are frequently undiagnosed due to failure to correlate the history, with subnormal temperature, low blood pressure, slow pulse, generalized oedema, (especially about the orbits and ankles) and to search for a latent vertical phoria.

Latent vertical phoria is easily demonstrated by sufficient monocular occlusion and inclusion of the *full amount* of prism gives relief to the ocular complaint.

Latent vertical phoria is a constant associate of endocrine dyscrasia, usually hypo-thyroidism, but may be found along with hypo or hyper function of other glands in the endocrine chain. Therefore it is a general and not a specific indicator of endocrine dysfunction.

Latent vertical phoria can be easily demonstrated in children as well as adults, suffering from endocrine dyscrasia, and is an early sign, guiding the ophthalmologist to the diagnosis oftentimes before the internist can arrive at one.

BIBLIOGRAPHY

1. S. V. Abraham, Department of Ophthmology, University of Chicago: Bell's Phenomenon and the Fallacy of the Occlusion Test; American Journal of Ophthalmology, page 656; 1931.

2. H. Barkan: The Occlusion Test for Latent Hyperphoria and Its Clinical Results; XIII Concilium Ophthalmologicum Amsterdam; September, 1929.

3. Carl Beisbarth: Hyperphoria and the Prolonged Occlusion Test; American Journal of Ophthalmology, page 103; 1932.

4. A. L. Brown: The Role of Unlevel Orbits in Heterophoria; American Journal of Ophthalmology, Volume No. 12, page 815; 1929.

5. E. H. Coachman: The Association of Latent Vertical Phoria with Endocrine Dycrasia; Oklahoma State Medical Journal; August, 1945.

6. G. E. De'Schweinitz: Discussion of Paper by L. F. Appleman - A Method of Uncovering Latent Hyperphoria; Archives of Ophthmology, Volume No. 3, page 651, 1930.

7. Duane and C Berens, Jr.: Ophthalmic Literature, Volume No 17, page 53; 1921.

8. E. Fuchs: Subjective Symphmatology of Ocular Disorders; American Journal of Ophthalmology, pp 13, 113-117; February, 1930.

9. Harvey J. Howard: The Relationship of Hypothroidism to Ophthalmology; Read before State Medical Association, Oklahoma City; 1938.

10. W. L. Hughes: Prolonged Occlusion Test; Archives of Ophthalmology, Volume No. 11, pp. 229-236; February, 1934.

11. F W. Marlow: The Technique of the Prolonged Occlusion Test; American Journal of Ophthalmology, Volume No. 15, page 320; 1932.

12. R. O'Connor: Diagnosis of Vertical Deviation of the Eyes; British Journal of Ophthalmology, Volume No. 8, page 449; 1924.

13. K. L. Roper and R. E. Bannon, Dartmouth Eye Institute: Diagnostic Value of Monocular Occlusion; Archives of Ophthmology, page 316, April, 1944.

14. C. Worth: Worth's Squint, page 435; Edited by F B Chavasse, Edition No. 7, Phil. P. Blakiston, Sons & Co.; 1939.

Surgery in the Treatment of the Stomach and Duodenum[*]

C. C. FULTON, M.D.

OKLAHOMA CITY, OKLAHOMA

A few years ago a discussion of the treatment of inflammatory diseases of the stomach and duodenum would have been largely devoted to the relative merits of medical management and surgery. However, today I believe that most physicians will agree that the treatment of peptic ulcer belongs in the hands of the internist, who should be especially interested in gastroenterology. At the same time I believe that it is equally well established that there are a number of patients whose ulcers fail to respond to conservative measures or develop serious complications, and that these patients require surgery for the relief of their distress.

No recent outstanding new facts have been established as a cause of peptic ulcer. The concept that was taught when I was in medical school still prevails, namely that peptic ulcer is a disease in which spasm and increased secretion of hydrochloric acid play an important role, and that both spasm and hyperchlorhydria are associated with local irritation or with neurogenic stimuli, which may be purely central in origin, or which may be on a circulatory or infectious basis. In other words, this means that certain people have an ulcer diathesis and that in these individuals, fatigue, nervous tension, infection, disturbances in circulatory integrity,

*Presented at the Annual Meeting, Oklahoma State Medical Association, Friday, May 3, 1946.

as well as too severe digestive burdens, are precipitating factors; and it also follows that in such individuals, ulcers may heal and later recur at the same or new sites.

The diagnosis of peptic ulcer does not strictly fall within the province of this paper, however, there are a few remarks that I believe should be made. The history obtained from ulcer patients is most frequently that of the typical, clearly defined, upper abdominal distress, occurring at a definite time after meals and relieved by food or neutralizing medication. Sometimes, however, intercurrent diseases of the colon or gallbladder may so confuse the picture that it is difficult to make a definite diagnosis of either condition. Absence of ulcer symptoms in patients with hemorrhagic ulcer is another diagonstic problem, especially if the hemorrhage is the first one and if there is no definite X-ray defect. The diagnosis often rests between hemorrhage from esophageal varices with possible liver cirrhosis and hemorrhage from peptic ulcer. There may be no X-ray evidence of abnormality of the esophagus, stomach or duodenum. It is often true, however, that in these cases, careful questioning will reveal a previous half forgotten ulcer history. Also in many cases an X-ray defect will often be seen later at a site where, at the first examination, no ulcer was seen. It is a safe rule to regard all typical ulcer hemorrhage as

having been caused by a gastroduodenal lesion, even in the absence of history or X-ray
findings, unless typical findings of liver cirrhosis or blood dyscrasia are found. Too, I
believe it well to frequently remind ourselves
that all gastric ulcers are not accompanied
by hyperchlorhydria. In only about twenty-
five per cent of gastric ulcers, will increased
acid be found, while a duodenal ulcer will
rarely be found unaccompanied by increased
acidity. In gastric ulcer, the finding of no
acid has long been considered to be suggestive of malignancy. This may still be true, but
by no means is it a decisive diagnostic factor,
since benign ulcer with achlorhydria and malignant lesions with acid, are both found,
quite frequently.

The problem of differentiation between
gastric ulcer and carcinoma has been and
continues to be a vital one. In most instances
a trial of good medical management should
be instituted. However, certain accomplishments must be demonstrated. The lesion
must promptly disappear by roentgenological
examination; the patient must be free of
symptoms and occult blood must disappear
from the stools. If these conditions have been
maintained for a year, as shown by periodic
examinations during this year, then we can
consider that the medical management of
this gastric ulcer has been successful. The
responsibility for repeated examinations
every two months during this year must be
assumed by the physician, as we are all
familiar with the case histories, which recite
the fact that upon first examination no evidence of malignancy was found, but upon
whom a subsjquent operation revealed an
inoperative malignant lesion. When the
above criteria have not been fulfilled, the
lesion may be properly considered to be an
unhealable ulcer in an area notoriously susceptible to malignancy.

Based upon the experiences of the internist and surgeon, familiar with this field of
medicine, definite indications for surgical
intervention are recognized. In general, ulcers which are intractable to medical management, whether known to be malignant or
not; ulcers with a tendency to repeated serious hemorrhages, or ulcers which produce
obstruction due to repeated episodes of inflammation, all require surgery. Obviously,
acute perforation of a peptic ulcer demands
immediate surgical intervention. Sometimes
the economic status of peptic ulcer patients
prohibit the necessary regulation and maintenance of the prescribed medical treatment.
In these cases, a sub-total gastric resection
may be the expedient method of treatment.
The cooperative study of the internist and
surgeon is of the greatest importance in the
selection of these cases for surgery. Especially is this so in gastric lesions where it is
difficult to distinguish between a benign and

a malignant ulcer. All lesions of the stomach
should be considered malignant until proven
otherwise, as only in this manner will malignancy be diagnosed early enough to permit operation at the most favorable time.
The necessity for an adequate sub-total resection of the stomach for most of the intractable or complicated ulcer cases is obvious.

Dr. Lahey has made the statement that he
has never seen a benign lesion of the greater
curviture of the stomach, although they have
been reported. He believes these patients
should be immediately subjected to a high
sub-total gastrectomy.

Prepyloric gastric ulcers are extremely
dangerous but not necessarily malignant, and
they may with safety, be given the above
mentioned trial of medical management. In
a situation where a prepyloric spasm persists, which on roentgenologic examination,
a cancer cannot be ruled out, surgical exploration is justified, after explaining to the
patient that negative findings may be determined at operation. Even though the exploration is negative, this is far better than
allowing an early malignant lesion to become
inoperable. If a gastric ulcer responds satisfactorily to medical management, that is, it
closes and then reopens, the patient should
immediately be subjected to a high sub-total
gastrectomy.

Duodenal ulcer still is much more common
than gastric ulcer. Marshall reported that of
8,380 patients with peptic ulcer which were
seen at the Lahey Clinic up to January 1,
1944, 6.4 per cent were gastric ulcers and
93.6 per cent were duodenal ulcers. Further,
he stated that 19.3 per cent of the gastric
ulcer cases required surgical intervention,
whereas only 6.2 per cent of the duodenal
cases required surgery for the relief of symptoms.

The management of duodenal ulcer is
pretty well standardized. For perforation,
only the simple closure of the perforation
must be done. No involved or extensive surgical procedure is permissible. At this time
the main mission of the surgeon is to save
the patient's life and nothing else. Intractable pain, after good medical management,
involves either the acceptance of the pain
or a surgical procedure.

There are two distinct types of pyloric obstructions. First, there is the cicatrical pyloric obstruction which is caused by the con-
tracting scar of a healed ulcer, unaccompanied by ulcer symptoms. Since this obstruction
is entirely mechanical, a simple gastroenterostomy is the operation of choice.

The second type of pyloric obstruction is
one associated with a chronic or subacutely
active duodenal ulcer. The obstruction is
caused by the scarring due to repeated ulcer

activity as well as edema and pylorospasm due to the active ulcer. It is difficult to foretell which of this latter group will have to be submitted to surgery. A trial at medical management is usually made.

With the exception of acute perforation, hemorrhage in spite of adequate medical management, is the most common and most definite indication for surgical intervention. Sub-total gastrectomy is the procedure of choice. Hemorrhage in the presence of good medical management indicates that the ulcer is continuing to spread and erode. Further, this ulcer is very probably on the posterior wall and may be penetrating into the pancreas, and is therefore difficult to close and to keep closed under medical management.

Some ulcers bleed once or twice and then the patient recovers without further complications. Other ulcers bleed repeatedly and profusely. In this latter type, something must be done if the patient's life is to be saved. If surgery is to be utilized, it should be offered during the early part of the bleeding, as otherwise the mortality is extremely high, even in spite of repeated whole blood transfusions. It is very difficult to decide when to offer surgery in some of these situations.

In most peptic ulcers that are to be subjected to surgery, when possible, a period of time in bed on an ulcer diet and alkaline therapy is most helpful to the surgeon. This reduces the inflammatory exudate about the ulcer and may convert a potentially difficult technical procedure, into a relatively simple one. Signs of acute inflammation should have subsided before surgery is done. Also in the face of a markedly dilated stomach from obstruction, at the pylorsis or in the duodenum, sufficient time should be taken to decompress the stomach and allow return of normal tone to the muscular wall, before surgery is attempted.

If surgery is elected for a peptic ulcer that is chronically or subacutely active, an operation should be done that will lower the gastric acidity to the greatest extent. We know that the removal of three-fourths to four-fifths of the stomach will lower the remaining gastric acidity to ten degrees or lower. Therefore, sub-total resection is the procedure of choice unless it is considered that the patient's condition would not permit such a formitable procedure. In such cases the less desirable operation of anterior gastroenterostomy must be done.

A chronic penetrating callous ulcer of the first part of the duodenum can usually be removed without difficulty or risk. One involving the second part of the duodenum may be difficult, because of its encroachment on, or involvement of, the common duct by the inflammatory exudate. The relationship of the ulcer and the common duct must be es-

tablished before resection is undertaken. The duodenum must be mobilized and in some instances, the common duct is opened and a catheter passed through to the ampulla of vater before it can be determined whether enough duodenum will be left, after resection of the ulcer area, for satisfactory, safe closure of the duodenum.

Jejunal ulcers are complications of surgery. That is, they are most often seen following gastroenterostomies or sub-total gastrectomies. They follow gastroenterostomy in 15 per cent or more of the cases and in two or three per cent of the sub-total gastrectomies. Contrary to previous opinions these jejunal ulcers should be given a trial of medical management, unless the ulcer is lying close to the transverse colon. It has become well established that all ulcer patients must assume that they will have to remain on some sort of dietary restrictions for the rest of their lives, whether they have been treated successfully by medical management or surgery. A patient who has had a sub-total gastrectomy must not lose sight of the fact that he has the so-called ulcer diathesis and that he must not abuse the remaining, apparently normally functioning portion of his stomach.

A more serious complication of surgical intervention is the gastrojejuocolic fistula. This occurs when the gastrojejunal ulcer lies close to, and becomes adherent to, the transverse colon and then ruptures into the colon. Immediate surgery is indicated for this complication. The diagnosis of this condition can usually be made from the passage of undigested food in the feces, as it is passed directly from the stomach into the transverse colon; by diarrhoea and by the unusual and extreme emaciation associated with this fistula. In addition the lesion can usually be demonstrated by a barium enema, roentgenogram.

There are several reasons for the occurrence of this distressing complication. The finsterer resection by exclusion operation is not a satisfactory operation for the reason that gastrojejunocolic fistula frequently occurs following this procedure. This operation as you know, has been advocated in those cases where the duodenal ulcer has so involved the common duct that the ulcer cannot be removed without running great risk of damaging the common or pancreatic ducts, or that the duodenum has become so shortened by scar tissue contraction that the duodenal stump cannot be safely turned in. Finsterer has advocated leaving the duodenal ulcer along with a small part of the pyloris and doing a sub-total gastrectomy. I believe that it has been well established that if any part of the pyloric gastric mucosa is allowed to remain, a jejunal ulcer is very likely to occur. This procedure may have to be done in some cases, if one does not wish to accept the greater risk of transplanting the common and pancreatic ducts into the distal loop of the jejunum after gastrectomy. If the Finsterer exclusion procedure is done, then the abdomen must again be invaded within a short time, after induration and edema has decreased around the duodenal ulcer, at which time the ulcer and all of the remaining pyloric mucosa must be resected.

A common cause for the formation of this colic fistula is the placing of the anastamosis of the gastroenterostomy through the mesentary of the transverse colon. This is a so-called posterior procedure. When this is done, the anastomosis is lying quite close to the transverse colon. Because these complications do occur it seems far better to make the anastomosis anterior to the colon. The percentage of occurrence of gastrojejunocolic ulcer is less and also if one does occur, it is far easier to do another resection, or any other surgical procedure, if the anastomosis is anterior to the transverse colon. Lahey has devised a two stage procedure for the treatment of gastrojejunocolic fistula. In the first stage the terminal ileum is implanted into the descending colon. In the second stage the ascending and transverse colon are removed along with a high sub-total gastrectomy. In his hands this has been followed by a lower mortality than with any other procedure.

Tumors of the stomach are most commonly malignant, but occasional benign neoplasms are found. Marshall reported a series of 464 patients upon whom operation was done at the Lahey Clinic during a five year period ending in 1943, all having a tumor involving the stomach. Ninety-eight per cent of these patients had a malignant tumor. Having in mind this high percentage of malignancy, it is of interest to note that in only 53 per cent was it possible to resect the tumor. In other words, almost half of the patients who presented themselves for surgery had malignant lesions too far advanced for successful extirpation. Yet a review of the symptoms in the unresectable cases, disclosed that the majority had gastrointestinal distress over a long period of time. It is not unreasonable to assume that earlier diagnosis might have made resection possible.

In view of the frequency of gastric carcinoma, we must remember that, it is a distinct possibility in any patient, middle aged or older, who has persistant gastric distress. Therefore any person with persistant gastro-intestinal distress, unrelieved by a trial of diet and conservative therapeutic measures, should have a thorough gastro-intestinal investigation, which should include gastric analysis, roentgenologic and if possible gastroscopic examinations. Furthermore, if malignancy cannot be ruled out, these examinations should be repeated within two month's time. In the event a definite decision can still not be made, a laparotomy is justifiable and indicated.

The mortality in sub-total gastrectomy when done by experienced surgeons is around three per cent. In a group of 530 consecutive sub-total gastric resections to July 1, 1945 in the Lahey Clinic for gastric, duodenal and jejunal ulcer, there were eight deaths, a mortality of 1.5 per cent. This low mortality rate can of course be attained only by those interested and experienced in this type of surgery. Good assistance and good anesthesia, preferably continuous high spinal, promoting as it does complete, prolonged relaxation at all stages of the operation, are necessary. Further, good post-operative care is essential, being alert for complications, especially atelectasis which so frequently follows high abdominal operative procedures and the equally speedy treatment of these complications. Bronchioscopic clearing of the bronchus both immediately after surgery, while still in the operating room, and later if the bronchus becomes obstructed, is necessary to prevent this complication from raising the mortality rate for the operative procedure.

There should be developed here, as in other teaching centers, greater cooperative effort between the internist and surgeon in the study of these problems so that better care shall be made available to the gastric patient, who is not immediately relieved of his trouble. It is surprising how few cases for gastric surgery appear on local hospital operating room schedules. We are either not recognizing these surgical indications or the patients are going elsewhere for more thorough and complete medical or surgical treatment. I am sure that we have sufficiently conscientious and well trained medical talent to properly care for these complicated gastric problems, that, statistically we know are occurring every day.

DISCUSSION

MINARD F. JACOBS, M.D.

OKLAHOMA CITY, OKLAHOMA

It is both an honor and a pleasure for an internist interested in gastroenterology to have the opportunity to discuss a surgical paper. It certainly shows the increasing acceptance by the surgeon of the close cooperation necessary if the best interests of the patient are to be served. Dr. Fulton's paper is one of the best it has been my pleasure to hear and he is to be commended for his wide grasp of the situation bringing out clearly the presently accepted indications for surgery, the type of surgery best suited and the reasons, with which I fully agree.

The preoperative and some phases of the postoperative care of the patient I believe are best handled by the gastroenterologist primarily. I do not believe I am presumptious when I state that probably the biggest single factor responsible for the marked reduction in the mortality in gastric surgery in the past twenty years has been the preoperative preparation of the patient.

In consideration of the patient with pyloric obstruction there are several conditions to be watched and treated if necessary. The patient will obviously be dehydrated and because of the vomiting is frequently in alkalosis. The latter is best determined by obtaining a carbon dioxide combining power of the plasma, a blood chloride and blood urea. If alkalosis is present there will be an increased CO_2 combining power, decreased chlorides and increased urea. This condition can usually be readily overcome by adequate amounts of intravenous sodium chloride in a physiological concentration. One should give 0.5 gm. Na Cl per kilo body weight for every 100 mg. per cent the blood chlorides must be raised. As to the amount of fluid itself one gives an amount equal to that vomited, lost by tube suction plus the normal requirement of 1000 cc. of normal salt. If you wish to use another gauge give enough fluids to obtain a urine output of 800-1000 cc. daily. Glucose may be added for its caloric value. Patients operated upon while in a state of alkalosis frequently die. The stomach of the patient must be lavaged twice daily and the amount of retention should be recorded so as to evaluate the progress of the condition and to help in determining the amount of parenteral fluids necessary. Proper lavage really requires a trained person. As Dr. Fulton mentioned decompression is important to allow the return of muscular tone. I recall seeing one patient several years ago in whom this consideration apparently had been neglected. The stomach was markedly dilated and atonic and the surgeon consequently was unable to tell just where to place the gastroenterostomy opening so that unfortunately it was made too high and as a result could not function properly. Frequently whole blood or plasma is indicated as many of these patients have a low blood protein due to their inability to absorb food. It is here that intravenous amino-acids are of value. They have the disadvantage, however, of running through even an 18 guage needle slowly and consequently the time required to give adequate amounts becomes very fatiguing to the patient. Don't forget that adequate glucose must always be given when giving amino-acids so they will not be used by the body to meet its caloric requirements. Roughly it takes about twice the amount of glucose in grams as amino-acids. As an average the preoperative care of this type of case requires from seven to ten days.

The preoperative care of the hemorrhaging ulcer case requires usually only adequate transfusions of whole blood and plasma as the patient should not be operated upon in shock or on the verge of shock. The blood count should be restored to a safe level as well as the blood volume and protein. Here again amino-acids have been found to be of value. The patients who require immediate surgery as mentioned by Dr. Fulton are generally those in the older or arteriosclerotic age group whose vessels cannot contract. The mortality rate in these is especially high. In general, I think it is agreed by both the surgeons and the internists that hemorrhaging ulcers are best treated medically during the stage of active bleeding, surgery being postponed until the bleeding has ceased and the patient's general condition improved.

May I re-emphasize one very immortant point mentioned by Dr. Fulton that regardless of surgery these patients must adhere to some degree of medical regime the rest of their lives. Too often the surgeon on dismissal of the patient neglects to tell the patient this and instruct him or see that he is instructed properly by the internist. I believe that at least some of the so-called failures of surgical management are due entirely to this.

Regarding the immediate postoperative care of these patients the internist's chief function is to advise properly regarding the diet and its graduations, to watch for complications in the chest, heart and kidney so that appropriate treatment may be promptly instituted. Here too the fluid, and electrolyte balance must be watched as the operated patient loses water by sweating and loss of blood. Vomiting, too, causes a loss of fluids and continuous syphonage loses fluid. These last two may mean 4000-5000 cc. water lost a day and it must be replaced. Generally 2000-3000 cc. of fluid is adequate the first two postoperative days and after that 1000 cc. normal saline.

I should like to ask Dr. Fulton why he states than an anterior gastroenterostomy instead of the orthodox posterior procedure should be done when a resection is not feasible.

DR. FULTON: In answer to Dr. Jacobs' question, I would first like to say that it is technically easier and quicker to perform.

Secondly, if gastrojejunal ulcer develops and further surgery is indicated, it is technically easier to resect the involved parts of the stomach and jejunum, and to do whatever surgical procedure is indicated at the time.

Third, there is less tendency to have the major complications of a gastrojejunocolic fistula occur.

Fourth, the experiences of the large groups who have used this procedure extensively, show just as good functional results as when the posterior gastroenterostomy is done.

BIBLIOGRAPHY

1. Samuel F. Marshall: Surgical Management of Chronic Peptic Ulcer; Surgical Clinics of North America; June, 1944.

2. F. H. Lahey: Inflammatory Lesions of the Stomach and Duodenum; Journal of American Medical Association, Volume No. 27, pp. 1030-1036; April 21, 1945.

3. Sara M. Jordan: The Problems of Peptic Ulcer; Surgical Clinics of North America; June, 1941.

4. Samuel F. Marshall and B. L. Aronoff: Tumors of the Stomach; Surgical Clinics of North America; June, 1944.

5. C. G. Morlock: Journal-Lancet, Volume No. 65, pp. 8-12; January, 1945.

6. Samuel F. Marshall: Ulcer Resulting from Inadequate Gastric Reaction; Lahey Clinic Bulletin; October, 1945.

Clinical Pathological Conference

University of Oklahoma School of Medicine

Presented by the Departments of Pathology and Medicine

H. THOMPSON AVEY, M.D.—HOWARD C. HOPPS, M.D.

OKLAHOMA CITY, OKLAHOMA

DR. HOPPS: You have all had an opportunity to study the protocol of this case and have doubtlessly arrived at the proper diagnosis. At the present time there is little effective therapy for the disease leukemia. We must continue our study of such cases, however, if we are ever to arrive at a complete understanding of this condition. Dr. Avey will present and analyze the clinical aspects of this case.

PROTOCOL

Patient: E. S., white female, age 57; admitted January 1, 1945; died January 4, 1945.

Chief Complaint: Weakness and loss of weight.

Present Illness: The patient became ill in February, 1944, at which time she complained of intermittent "gas pains", abdominal distress with pain, dyspnea, anorexia, weakness and headaches. These symptoms persisted and progressed and she became bedridden in August, 1944. In September she noticed a "swelling" in her neck. In October she complained of an infection in her throat with some bleeding of the gums and soreness of the mouth. During this time she lost approximately 50 pounds. Generalized enlargement of all lymph nodes had been noticed for several months.

Past and Family History: Not obtainable.

Physical Examination: On admission the patient was very weak and was unable to give a history. The information was obtained from a doctor's letter and from her husband. Her temperature was 99.6° F., pulse rate 105, and respiration 16. The patient was pale

and seemed acutely ill. There were a few bleeding points in the mouth. There was generalized lymphadenopathy and matted firm nodes were particularly prominent in both cervical regions, more marked on the right. The nodes were not tender. Examination of the chest was essentially negative except for a soft blowing systolic murmur at the apex. Cardiac rhythm was regular. The heart was not enlarged. Blood pressure was 142/92. Palpation of the abdomen was difficult because of poor cooperation by the patient and generalized abdominal tenderness. The liver was markedly enlarged as was the spleen. The skin was pale and numerous petechial hemorrhages were present. Rumpel-Leede test was positive.

Laboratory Data: Hemoglobin measured 4 Gm. per cent. There were 1,250,000 red blood cells and 28,000 blood cells/cu.mm.: with lymphoblasts 13 per cent, prolymphocytes 46 per cent, lymphocytes 32 per cent neutrophils 9 per cent (juveniles 3 per cent and stabs 3 per cent); platelets 52,500; occasional normoblasts were seen. The peroxidase stain was negative.

Clinical Course: The patient became progressively weaker and lapsed into a semicomatose state the day after admission. She died the following night, January 4, 1945, at 4:45 a.m.

CLINICAL DIAGNOSIS

DR. AVEY: It is rather obvious that this case falls into the category of lymphoblastoma so that we shall keep this fact in mind as we analyze the clinical history and formulate a differential diagnosis.

First to consider the patient's age. She was 57 and this itself is of significance. For instance, acute leukemia usually occurs before the age of 25; chronic myelogenous leukemia is more common between the ages of 30 and 50; chronic lymphatic leukemia occurs principally from 45 to 54; and lymphosarcoma is perhaps most common between the ages of 25 and 55. On the basis of probability then, our patient, according to her age, would be most likely to have either chronic lymphatic leukemia or lymphosarcoma. The chief complaints of weakness and loss of weight do not help us a great deal because these are present in a great variety of conditions. They are quite compatible with leukemia however. As far as the patient knows, she was ill until about February of 1944. She was brought into this hospital January 1, 1945, so that her illness was of approximately eleven months duration. At the time of onset the patient complained of intermittent gas pains and abdominal distress. She suffered also a certain amount of dyspnea, anorexia, loss of strength and headaches. Again, none of these complaints are very specific. In a woman of this age and with this duration of illness, however, some type of malignant neoplasm should certainly be considered in the differential diagnosis. As to the abdominal complaints, in the event that this is one of the lymphoblastomas, these could well be due to pressure of enlarged lymph nodes on some of the abdominal viscera. Dyspnea might also be due to pressure from nodes or could be the result of some "metastatic" lesion in the lungs. On the other hand, it might be simply a manifestation of profound anemia. Headaches could be a manifestation of general toxemia from any of a considerable variety of conditions. As this case illustrates, it is important to realize that leukemia, early in its course, may give symptoms which are all of a general nature and which may be compatible with cardiac disease, renal disease, malignant neoplasms of many types, etc.

We have more or less a gap in the patient's history from February through August although she was apparently getting worse, and finally became so sick that she had to go to bed. According to the relative's story, she noticed a swelling in her neck sometime in September. Additional information from the local physician indicates that in October, she had a severe throat infection and a middle ear infection, following which there developed swelling underneath the ears in the "parotid" region. This was diagnosed as "parotitis". At about this time generalized lymphadenopathy first became evident and the patient began to notice bleeding from the gums and soreness of the mouth. This bleeding is quite significant. A variety of causes are possible including hypovitaminosis C, pyorrhea alveolaris, thrombocytopenic purpura, etc. Actually, bleeding from the gums is a common complaint of patients with leukemia. During this time in which the patient was gradually getting worse, she lost weight, a total of 50 pounds, and her lymph nodes continued to enlarge. Her local physician states that between October and the time she came to the hospital she had two severe acute attacks of "asthma", which again brings up the question as to whether or not there might have been enlarged lymph nodes pressing on the tracheobronchial tree. Her physician stated that she had not had any fever for at least four weeks prior to admission at University Hospital, and this information is of great value in helping to eliminate a good many inflammatory conditions such as tuberculosis, mycotic infection of the lungs, chronic bronchitis, etc. The lack of productive cough would be additional evidence against such an inflammatory process in the lungs.

One of the most prominent physical findings was generalized lymphadenopathy. A description of these nodes is quite important; they are described as being matted, firm and non-tender. The term "matted" is rather significant because it suggests tuberculous lymphadenitis or lymphosarcoma. The fact that they were non-tender pretty well eliminates a non-specific inflammatory basis. Lymphadenopathy was most marked in the cervical region, especially on the right side.

Examination of the chest didn't reveal a great deal in so far as the lung fields were concerned. There was, however, a soft blowing systolic murmur at the cardiac apex. The patient exhibited marked pallor and we have every reason to suspect a profound anemia so that we must consider that this may have been a so-called hemic murmur. Until we confirm our impression of anemia by referring to the laboratory data, we must keep in mind the possibility of an organic cardiac lesion however. The fact that the cardiac rhythm was regular is one further point against cardiac disease per se. The blood pressure was 140/92 which isn't unusual for an adult 57 years old. It might have been higher prior to the patient's illness however.

Palpation of the abdomen didn't reveal a great deal and that is unfortunate because we would like to know whether there were any nodular masses. The examiner was able to determine that the liver was markedly enlarged however and he observed splenomegaly also. We see the largest spleens in cases of chronic myelogenous leukemia, although there may be marked splenic enlargement in chronic lymphatic leukemia also. Patients with acute leukemia usually die before there is time for marked splenomegaly. The duration of the patient's history, approximately one year, pretty well excludes a diagnosis of acute leukemia.

Bleeding points were observed on the patient's gums and further evidence of increased capillary fragility was afforded by a positive Rumpel-Leede test. As you know, patients with leukemia often exhibit a hemorrhagic diathesis. In acute leukemia, occasionally death is the direct result of extensive capillary bleeding. A more detailed description of the skin might have afforded important information. It sometimes happens that in chronic lymphatic leukemia the skin is invaded by leukemic cells and that such areas of cellular infiltration can be seen and palpated. Occasionally such patients are primarily concerned with their dermal lesions and consult first a dermatologist who may make the diagnosis of leukemia entirely on the basis of characteristic skin manifestations.

In considering the laboratory data, we had already received helpful information from the local physician, a report that on the 28th day of December, the patient had a hemoglobin of 50 per cent, red blood count of 1,500,000 and a white count of about 96,000. A differential count was not supplied. In referring to the protocol you see that the patient's anemia had become even more marked. The finding of normocytes is characteristic of myelophthisic anemia and indicates that the bone marrow was trying its best to correct the anemia. The leukocytes had dropped somewhat (28,000) and there was 13 per cent lymphoblasts, 46 per cent prolymphocytes and 32 per cent lymphocytes. There were only a small number of neutrophils, 9 per cent. The negative peroxidase stain was confirmatory evidence that the abnormal cells were of the lymphocytic series. From this then, we have ample laboratory confirmation for our diagnosis of lymphatic leukemia.

What about prognosis in cases of this type? In the acute forms of leukemia, duration is usually but a few months, although some survive for as long as six months. This particular case survived for almost a year so that it corresponds to chronic lymphatic leukemia. This particular patient was unfortunate in that persons occasionally live for many years with chronic lymphatic leukemia. The average length of life with either chronic lymphatic or myelogenous leukemia is 3½ years. X-ray therapy seems to be of little value in acute forms of leukemia, more often it is actually harmful. Irradiation may provide considerable symptomatic relief and may prolong life for months or years in chronic forms of this disease. The hemoglobin is a pretty good prognostic guide. If the hemoglobin is less than 7.5 grams and it does not rise after X-ray therapy, death usually

occurs within a few weeks or a few months. When this patient entered the hospital her hemoglobin was only 4 grams and she was entirely too sick to consider X-ray therapy.

CLINICAL DISCUSSION

QUESTION: Why do patients with leukemia usually have a marked anemia?

DR. AVEY: The pathologic findings in this case should answer the question. It is probable that the anemia here was on the basis of extensive invasion of the bone marrow by leukemic cells with resultant mechanical displacement of those elements which normally manufacture erythrocytes.

ANATOMIC DIAGNOSIS

DR. HOPPS: Dr. Avey's clinical impression of lymphatic leukemia was confirmed by our pathologic findings. It remains for us, however, to explain the various signs and symptoms which this patient presented and to correlate altered function with altered form.

To consider first the anemia, it was of a myelophthisic type as is usual in any sort of leukemia. Approximately 90 per cent of the marrow elements comprised abnormal cells of the lymphocytic series. There was, therefore, inadequate space remaining for that amount of erythropoietic marrow necessary to maintain a normal red blood count. An effect of this anemia was seen in the marked fatty change of both heart and liver. The cardiac murmur described must have been of hemic origin since there was no valvular defect, nor was the heart markedly dilated. There was evidence of abnormal bleeding in internal organs as well as that which was clinically evident. There were petechial hemorrhages in the mucosa of the intestinal tract, pelvis of the kidney and urinary bladder, underlying the peritoneum and pleura and in the lung. These were relatively recent and it is unlikely that the patient's bleeding contributed materially to her anemia.

The abdominal symptoms of which this patient complained are often observed in patients with chronic leukemia. They are usually, as in this case, due to multiple areas of infarction of the spleen with involvement of the capsule and adhesions to neighboring viscera. You will say that the spleen has no pain fibers in the usual sense of the word and that is true. It is important to remember, however, that peritoneal membranes do give rise to considerable pain when they are stretched. In this case there were seven fairly recent infarcts with fibrinous adhesions over these areas. In addition, there were older infarcts and older areas of fibrous adhesions. It is difficult for us to evaluate just what masses were palpated upon abdominal examination and misinterpreted as liver and spleen. Actually both of the organs lay well above the costal margins and were pretty well fixed at that level by the adhesions which I have just described. This illustrates the degree of splenic enlargement which may be necessary before the spleen actually becomes palpable. In this case the spleen was enlarged approximately four times (460 grams) and its lower pole was still 3 cm. above the costal margin.

Symptoms related to the chest were, as Dr. Avey postulated, also related to the leukemia. Tracheobronchial lymph nodes were enlarged up to four or five times the normal size and were compressing and displacing slightly the major air passages. There was an old, solitary, calcified, subpleural tubercle near the apex of the right lung and old fibrous adhesions over the lateral aspect of the upper lobe. Otherwise, save for slight recent hemorrhage, there was little change.

Most pathologists consider leukemia to be a malignant neoplasm and, if we consider it so, we find that there were extensive "metastases" in this case. Lymph nodes throughout the entire body were markedly involved as was also the spleen and bone marrow. In addition, there was a spectacular infiltration of the kidneys by leukemic cells to the extent that their weight was almost doubled (225 grams). This must have interfered with renal function to some extent and calls to mind the rare case in which renal failure is a prominent manifestation of leukemia. The porta hepatis was rather extensively involved and there was obstruction of occasional bile ducts, but yet the major portion of liver was not markedly altered. The leukemic infiltrates or "metastases", if you prefer, were all composed of cells essentially similar to those abnormal lymphogenous forms observed in the peripheral blood because, after all, those cells are just as neoplastic as the ones which become localized in various tissues.

QUESTION: What was the cause of death in this case?

DR. HOPPS: In any case of cancer, that is a hard thing to put your finger on because these patients have so many organs and tissues which are considerably altered. In this case, speaking of the immediate cause of death, we would have to consider anemia with its associated degenerative changes in the heart, the leukemic involvement of the kidneys and liver, malnutrition (reinforced by an increased metabolism) and perhaps some toxic metabolic process. That is about as far as we can go. This patient did not have any significant degree of bronchopneumonia and we have observed that, peculiarly enough, people with marked anemia rarely develop terminal bronchopneumonia. I know of no reason for this—as a matter of fact this phenomenon is not generally appreciated. It is interesting too that in this patient there was all the more reason for pneumonia in that people with leukemia are quite predisposed to infection. The cells in the peripheral blood are immature and the function of these cells varies directly with the degree of immaturity so that, although a patient may have a blood count of 100,000 or even 1,000,000, he may have inadequate leukocytic *function.*

QUESTION: Could the increased metabolic rate usually shown by these patients possibly be due to leukemic invasion of the vital centers in the brain?

DR. HOPPS: I don't think that this is the complete explanation. Twenty per cent of patients with leukemia develop neurological symptoms sometime in the course of their disease so that you can see the possibility for such a basis. Many of these patients develop fever, some intermittent, others constant, with elevation over a period of months. This, I think, is to be correlated with the increased metabolism. I believe that the increased metabolism is more directly related to the marked over-production of leukocytes and some metabolic by-product of these neoplastic cells which act as a stimulus.

MID-WEST SURGICAL SUPPLY
CO., INC.
Kaufman Building
Wichita 2, Kansas

FRED R. COZART
2437 N. W. 36th Terrace
Phone 8-2561   Oklahoma City, Okla.

NEUROLOGICAL
HOSPITAL
Twenty-Seventh and The Paseo
Kansas City, Missouri

Modern Hospitalization of Nervous and Mental Illnesses, Alcoholism and Drug Addiction.

THE ROBINSON CLINIC
G. WILSE ROBINSON, M.D.
G. WILSE ROBINSON, Jr., M.D.

Special Article

Cleveland County Honors Dr. D. W. Griffin

At an annual dinner meeting on April 26 the Cleveland County Medical Society, assisted by the Ladies' Auxiliary, paid tribute to Dr. and Mrs. David Wilson Griffin. This meeting in the beautiful Woodruff Room at the Student Union, University of Oklahoma was very impressive. After a program of inspiring music and a season of delightful reminiscing by Dr. D. O. Howell, an avowed country doctor by choice, the meeting was devoted to Dr. Griffin.

It was pointed out that Dr. Griffin had traveled all the way from a log cabin environment in Lenoir, North Carolina, where he was born in 1873, to the high position he now holds in the Central Oklahoma State Hospital at Norman. During his 47 years tenure in this position Dr. Griffin has built a great institution with ever expanding possibilities. Through the evolution of this great institution Dr. Griffin has not only served the state of Oklahoma, but he has set an example for other states in the middle west. One of the most notable achievements in Dr. Griffin's career as head of this institution has been the training of young men in this field of endeavor. He has imparted to them not only the scientific knowledge of psychiatry, but the elements of his own sterling personality.

It is remarkable that through all the political upheavals in the State of Oklahoma Dr. Griffin has held this administrative position for 47 years and that during this time there has never been a successful attack upon his administration policies. There has been no serious criticism, no charge of inefficiency, no lack of integrity, no question of judgment and no doubt of the wisdom employed.

It was pointed out that Mr. Churchill's speeches, appearing in two great volumes, were printed without alteration; no change was deemed necessary. Even political expediency made no demands; no living person could improve upon what Churchill had said. As this notable meeting closed it was stated that likewise Dr. Griffin's life might be presented without alteration to stand as an example for others in his profession. With loud acclaim his moral, social and economic services to the great commonwealth of Oklahoma and to the Nation were heralded. With modest means the ruddy faced recipient of these encomiums arose in the midst of great applause and after a few words of grateful acknowledgement he resumed his seat, obviously unchanged by the world's plaudits and ready to go on about his professional business.

The following facts are taken from the biographical sketch "Oklahoma's Premier Medical Institutional Executive" printed in the Cleveland County Medical Society Program:

"Longest tenure of any Oklahoma Institutional Head—47 years. Born in one-room log cabin, October 28, 1873, near Lenoir, North Carolina—fourth in a family of 13 children. Descended from poor but humble, honest and ambitious parentage. Attended the post-Civil War schools two or three months in the year. Finished the equivalent of a high school course in Amherst Academy and Barnes Academy, North Carolina. Attended Rutherford College, North Carolina, one year in preparation for a medical career. Entered University College of Medicine, Richmond, Virginia, September, 1895, and was graduated M. D., May 13, 1899.

"Licensed by Board of Medical Examiners, North Carolina. Opened Practice, home rural community, North Carolina, 1899. Tendered Superintendency of Territorial Sanitarium, (Central State Hospital) Norman, Oklahoma. Offered $50.00 per month and board, with raise to $75.00 per month in six months, if mutual. Accepted. Was raised to $100.00 per month before six months, and has remained since. Professor of Psychiatry, 1915, School of Medicine, University of Oklahoma, Professor Emeritus now, Author, and Counsellor in laws pertaining to care and treatment of the mentally ill of the State. Elected to 'Oklahoma Hall of Fame', November 17, 1935."

The JOURNAL Of The
OKLAHOMA STATE MEDICAL ASSOCIATION

EDITORIAL BOARD

L. J. MOORMAN, Oklahoma City, Editor-in-Chief

E. EUGENE RICE, Shawnee   BEN H. NICHOLSON, Oklahoma City

MR. DICK GRAHAM, Oklahoma City, Business Manager

JANE FIRRELL TUCKER, Editorial Assistant

CONTRIBUTIONS: Articles accepted by this Journal for publication including those read at the annual meetings of the State Association are the sole property of this Journal.

The Editorial Department is not responsible for the opinions expressed in the original articles of contributors.

Manuscripts may be withdrawn by authors for publication elsewhere only upon the approval of the Editorial Board.

MANUSCRIPTS: Manuscripts should be typewritten, double-spaced, on white paper 8½ x 11 inches. The original copy, not the carbon copy, should be submitted.

Footnotes, bibliographies and legends for cuts should be typed on separate sheets in double space. Bibliography listing should follow this order: Name of author, title of article, name of periodical with volume, page and date of publication.

Manuscripts are accepted subject to the usual editorial revisions and with the understanding that they have not been published elsewhere.

NEWS: Local news of interest to the medical profession, changes of address, births, deaths and weddings will be gratefully received.

ADVERTISING: Advertising of articles, drugs or compounds unapproved by the Council on Pharmacy of the A.M.A. will not be accepted. Advertising rates will be supplied on application.

It is suggested that members of the State Association patronize our advertisers in preference to others.

SUBSCRIPTIONS: Failure to receive The Journal should call for immediate notification.

REPRINTS: Reprints of original articles will be supplied at actual cost provided request for them is attached to manuscripts or made in sufficient time before publication. Checks for reprints should be made payable to Industrial Printing Company, Oklahoma City.

Address all communications to THE JOURNAL OF THE OKLAHOMA STATE MEDICAL ASSOCIATION, 210 Plaza Court, Oklahoma City 3

OFFICIAL PUBLICATION OF THE OKLAHOMA STATE MEDICAL ASSOCIATION

Copyrighted July, 1946

EDITORIALS

THE TONGUES OF THINGS

Always it is interesting to contemplate with what eloquence and accuracy objects of historic interest may portray the past and impliment the pattern for the future.

In the field of medicine we may say that from the mute voice of pre-historic hunchbacks beneath desert sands on through the code of Hammurabi, the Asklepion of Cos, the bust of Hippocrates, the Acropolis at Pergamos, the tongues of medicine as a free enterprise eloquently proclaim its progress in behalf of human kind. Its evolutionary response to human needs under changing conditions has been in keeping with nature's demands, in so far as human ingenuity, directed along scientific channels, is able to interpret natural phenomena. Medicine's traditions indicate that its natural course should not be interrupted by designing politicians who have no knowledge of its fundamental principles.

The above title was suggested by Catherine Drinker Bowen, the author of A Yankee of Olympus, now avidly gathering information for a volume on John Adams.[1] A reading of her article in the May Atlantic with her account of a visit to the heirloom sale in New York, of the belongings of two ladies living in the environs of Boston, bearing names in which figures the words Adams and Quincy, is most stimulating. As we contemplate the present plight of our country and the lives of two great contemporaries, Jefferson and Adams, friends and rivals dying on the same day, this discussion by Catherine Drinker Bowen takes on a significant aspect and furthers the consummation of our theme.

"The bowl sat on a pedestal in the middle of the auction gallery. There was no glass over it, no lock or key. Big and round and fragile and cobalt blue, with the shield on one side. 'Diameter 14 inches,' the catalogue said. 'Script initial J (for Jefferson), surmounted by a helm, and having a banderole with motto *Rebellion to Tyrants is Obedience to God.*' Lowestoft pitcher *en suite.* Both bowl and pitcher are understood in the family to have been given by Thomas Jefferson to President John Adams."

This Journal in an effort to represent the consensus of opinion for the medical profession of Oklahoma has been so militant in its rebellion toward tyranny, the Editor finds much comfort in this motto, *Rebellion to Tyrants is Obedience to God.*

In the light of what is happening to our people and our profession the members of the State Medical Association would do well to study the lives of the two great contemporaries mentioned above. John Adams, not knowing that Jefferson was dying, employed his last breath to say with comforting assurance, "Thomas Jefferson still survives". Though at that moment Thomas Jefferson was passing it is reported that he once said of Adams, "As disinterested as the being who made him".

What we need today in Washington is a courageous representation, a few statesmen with puritan fortitude, as disinterested as the God who made them. No doubt this famous bowl in the hands of a trusted messenger traveled the hard way from Monticello to Quincy, Massachusetts, and no doubt the motto was mutually acceptable and mutually adhered to.

To our legislators we propose a toast from this bowl, *"Rebellion to Tyrants is Obedience to God"*. It would be interesting to observe the countenances of Wagner, Murray and Dingell when confronted with such a toast. Tyranny, sugar coated, is worse than tyranny in the raw.

1. John Adams His Bowl by Catherine Drinker Bowen, the Atlantic, May, 1946.

THE GLORY OF MEDICINE

The glory of medicine in Oklahoma finds expression through the bright halo of scientific accomplishment, through the ambitious stride of young doctors keeping abreast of those advancing. Lest we forget, our ambitious youth in the field of medicine should be reminded that the effulgence of this halo is drawn largely from the sacrificial life of the country doctor whose pioneering spirit more than a half a century ago poured the foundation upon which they stand.

Though the stimulating environment of the country doctor is a thing of the past, and his horse and buggy hardships are folded among our treasured souvenirs. we should never lose the spirit which enabled him to surmount all difficulties and made him responsive to human needs, regardless of financial, moral, cultural or religious rating.

These pioneerinig doctors were not Gods from Olympus, but they were endowed with certain etherial attributes which set them apart. They were much more concerned with patient welfare than about worldly goods. Business appointments and material interests immediately lost caste in the face of charity calls. Often the poor took precedence of the well-to-do. The larger life came through response to duty, not in search of booty. Physical fortitude was sustained by a strange spiritual urge which must never be forgotten.

Young man, herein lies your challenge. Shall we keep that halo bright? The last paragraph of Maimonides' Prayer may help:

"May there never rise in me the notion that I know enough, but give me strength and leisure and zeal to enlarge my knowledge. Our work is great, and the mind of man presses forward forever. Thou hast chosen me in Thy grace, to watch over the life and death of Thy creature. I am about to fulfill my duties. Guide me in this immense work so that it may be of avail."

HOW IS YOUR HEALTH AND ACCIDENT PROGRAM, DOCTOR?

Looking to the future in insurance should bə a part of every doctor's economic program. Most of us realize early in life that we should have a definite life insurance program, both for our protection and the protection of our families during our years of productivity and for the purpose of building up an estate when, in late years, we are unable to carry on at all, or are hampered by partial disability of one kind or another. Since doctors are regarded as poor investors of the money they make through their professional efforts many adhere to the idea that investments in life insurance is the wisest and safest. Others of us are so busy in the practice of medicine and are so concerned over our professional success that we are inclined to neglect our personal affairs. The insurance agent often has to force us to buy the protection we need.

Other types of insurance should also be given proper consideration. We must be protected against lawsuits to which we are constantly endangered, regardless of the sincerity of our efforts and the conservative practice of medicine. The State Medical Association has established a group of policies of this type of insurance with an excellent company which gives us the best protection.

As we are able to extend our personal protection with insurance we should be concerned with the loss which results from accidents or illness. This loss of time not only involves an outlay of cash money, but the current expenses of our offices and homes go on just the same.

Members of the medical profession in Oklahoma have the privilege of joining their own particular county group in the Blue Cross to obtain hospitalization insurance at a most reasonable price and with a broader coverage than commercial companies will give. Yet it is most surprising that only a small percentage of our doctors have taken advantage of this privilege. When hospitalization for themselves and families is necessary they can only regret their careless neglect and procrastination. It would be a very simple matter to send a check to the secretary of the county society to take part in the next group participation. On renewal dates the doctor would then be reminded.

The insurance committee, in selecting a policy on health and accident insurance for members of the State Society has purposely avoided inclusion of hospitalization, so that the doctor could get a much better coverage price.

With his health and accident disability the doctor should already be participating in the Blue Cross, and the two kinds of policies will give him an unequaled protection for such misfortunes. Our policy gives world wide coverage and pays sickness disability for as much as five years in any one accident.

If this policy is accepted on the first call of the company's representative no proof of insurability is required, but if at some later date the doctor wishes this insurance this proof is required. This makes it possible for every practicing physician up to the age of 70 years to participate. Should an accident result in immediate death, or, even in death after a period of disability up to six months, the family receives, in addition to what has been given for his disability, the principal sum which may be $1000.00 to $5000.00. Yes such help is duely appreciated, and when the test has been made the beneficiary is indeed thankful that enough foresight was exercised to secure such protection. Health and accident insurance in anyone's economic program is good business.—Victor K. Allen, M.D.

OKLAHOMA HOSPITALS

The Journal of the Oklahoma State Medical Association welcomes "Oklahoma Hospitals" in the field of medical service. Volume No. 1, Issue 2, June, 1946, is now in circulation. The Oklahoma State Hospital Association and the Editorial staff are to be congratulated upon the character of this new publication. Judging from the present showing, this Journal has a bright future.

The leading article in this issue should be worth 10 years' subscription to any hospital. It appears under the caption "What's Cookin'". The appeal is universal. Sooner or later all people who enter hospitals are interested in food. Even those who go to the operating room to be opened with prayer are soon ready to be filled with food; provided it is good. It behooves the hospital to ask "What's cookin'?" Good luck "Oklahoma Hospitals".

MEDICAL RESEARCH

At Atlantic City a few weeks ago while waves of the Atlantic rolled upon the sands of this relatively new country, nearly a thousand of the best doctors in the world were assembled in the ballroom of a great hotel. Far removed from the marts of trade, untouched by the evils of an exigent world and uninterested in political or material expediency, these men were pursuing medical science for the sake of mankind. The members of the Association of American Physicians were in the second day of their intensive annual meeting. Scientific presentations were temporarily interrupted. Three illustrious physicians stood on the rostrum, Warfield T. Longcope, Oswald T. Avery and Rufus I. Cole. All three were marked by the march of time, but shining through their aging faces was an intellectual glow undimmed by their years.

The President of the Association, Dr. Longcope, announced that Dr. Avery was to be awarded the George M. Cober medal for outstanding medical research. The presentation was to be made by his friend and long-time associate, Rufus I. Cole, in medical research.

It is unfortunate that this inspiring event could not have been witnessed by every young doctor in the land. Oklahoma is a vigorous young state, richly endowed. As it goes forward agriculturely and industrily it must not lag intellectually. In the latter field science must take its place.

The Alumni Association of the University School of Medicine is planning a research institute. Naturally the consummation of this plan will bring trained research workers. But in the State of Oklahoma there must be young men with latent abilities and a love of humanity which potentially transcends all obstacles. The wealth of Oklahoma must recognize the worth of such young men and lay the fire for genius in the service of humanity. This proposed research institute should represent a broad vision and an unlimited scope, in the field of scientific investigation in order that these young men may suffer no annulling limitations. In science there is no place for selfish interests.

May every young man who reads this story ponder the possibilities in pure scientific research and at least may one or two join the crusade against the awful tyranny of the unknown.

Classified Advertisements

FOR SALE: Hospital equipment, including 1 Keleket No. 4036, type KXP combination X-Ray complete. Contact Oklahoma Medical Center, P. O. Box 1191, Oklahoma City, Oklahoma.

FOR SALE: Practice in county seat town of approximately 2,500, situated between two oil fields, one recently discovered. Physician desires to retire. Will sell practice and office equipment including X-Ray. Office space available. Write Box J, Oklahoma State Medical Association Journal, 210 Plaza Court, Oklahoma City, Oklahoma.

FOR SALE: Retiring because of failing health. Am offering Urological and G. U. instruments and office equipment including Cystoscope, Urethroscope, Catheters, Sounds, Microscope, in fact all instruments and equipment found in active office at a sacrifice. Location optional. Box B, c/o Journal, Oklahoma State Medical Association, 210 Plaza Court, Oklahoma City, Oklahoma.

THE PRESIDENT'S PAGE

The educational program of the Association is shaping up nicely and will soon be in such form as to be started. This is the program authorized by the House of Delegates and it will be carried out as they directed.

The committee appointed to draft and put before the members of the Association the G. I. treatment program is awaiting confirmation of the program by the Veterans Administration. It is possible this may happen before this is published.

The committee are to be commended for the work they have done on this plan, and it is hoped all will enter actively on the plan if and when it is confirmed.

Each committee chairman is urged to familiarize himself with the duties of his committee and as early as possible enter upon their duties as each committee is important and has its particular place in our organization.

President.

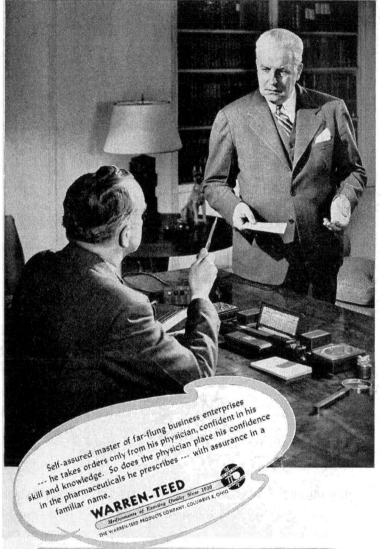

Self-assured master of far-flung business enterprises --- he takes orders only from his physician, confident in his skill and knowledge. So does the physician place his confidence in the pharmaceuticals he prescribes --- with assurance in a familiar name.

WARREN-TEED

Medicaments of Exacting Quality Since 1920

THE WARREN-TEED PRODUCTS COMPANY, COLUMBUS 8, OHIO

Warren-Teed Ethical Pharmaceuticals: capsules, elixirs, ointments, sterilized solutions, syrups, tablets. Write for literature.

VETERANS, HERE'S HOW YOU CAN OBTAIN SURPLUS PROPERTY.

It is requested that the attached communication from the State Post War Planning Commission concerning *Surplus Property* be read at your County Medical Meeting or its contents made known to members of your society who are veterans of World War II.

Eligible veterans who reside in counties other than as hereinafter stated should address inquiries to:

Mr. H. W. McGinness, Chief Examiner
Veterans Certification Unit,
War Assets Administration
324 Key Building
Oklahoma City, Oklahoma

Those who reside in Kay, Noble, Payne, Pawnee, Osage, Washington, Nowata, Craig, Ottawa, Delware, Mayes, Rogers, Tulsa, Creek, Okmulgee, Wagoner, Cherokee, Adair, Sequoyah, Muskogee, Okfuskee, McIntosh, Haskell, LeFlore, Latimer, Pittsburg, Hughes, Seminole, should write to:

Mr. Raymond Ferguson, Chief Examiner
Veterans Certification Unit
War Assets Administration
512 Petroleum Building
Tulsa, Oklahoma.

Those who reside in McCurtain, Pushmataha, Choctaw, Atoka, Bryan, Coal, Johnston, Marshall, should write to:

Mr. William Jasper, Chief Examiner
Veterans Certification Unit
War Assets Administration
5th Floor, Mercantile Bank Building
Dallas, Texas

The following letter was received by the Executive Secretary from the State Post War Planning Commission:

"For the information of World War II veterans who are members of the Oklahoma State Medical Association, we are providing you with the following information regarding veterans preference in the purchase of surplus property.

"An amendment was signed by the President May 3rd which placed the veteran in a much more advantageous position in regard to the preference granted him under the Surplus Property Act of 1944. That amendment authorized the War Assets Administrator to set aside certain items found to be in demand by veterans, such items to be held for sale to veterans only.

"The following medical, surgical and dental apparatus and equipment are at this date included on the Administrator's Set Aside List:

Major Operating Tables	Dental Units
Operating Lamps	Dental Chairs
Field X-Ray Units	Dental Cabinets
Diathermy Machines	

"As yet the above list are the only articles of medical and surgical equipment which have been so set aside but the list is subject to change from time to time by action of the Administrator.

"Other types of equipment not on the Set Aside List may from time to time be available as surplus and will be sold to veterans on a priority, second only to purchases of Federal Agencies, for their own use.

"For the veteran to purchase any surplus property, either that on the Set Aside List or otherwise, it is necessary that he make application to the Veterans Certification Unit of War Assets Administration at the appropriate office as indicated by the enclosed map of the State of Oklahoma. That application is filed on SWPC Form 66 which must be accompanied by a photostatic copy of the applicant's discharge.

"Veterans who have received the above certification will be notified when the articles for which they have been certified are available at which time they will have an opportunity for inspection and purchase if they desire. Certificate holders will be notified in the chronological order in which their certificates have been issued. Each certificate holder will be notified of three such sales after which his certificate will become inactive if he has not purchased the articles on which he has been notified.

"Under the law as it now stands, it is impossible for War Assets Administration to see small items individually since the expense of such transactions would make it impossible for them to operate on an economical basis.

"If any member of the Oklahoma State Medical Association feels that he is not being given the proper consideration in his attempts to purchase surplus property through War Assets Administration, we would appreciate information in regard to the particular case in order that we may take the necessary steps for correction of any irregularities."

U. S. PUBLIC HEALTH SERVICE ESTABLISHES FELLOWSHIPS

An announcement has been received that the National Foundation for Infantile Paralysis has established a grant to be utilized by the Committee on Training of public health personnel of the U. S. Public Health Service for 125 Fellowships to train physicians and sanitary engineers in public health work.

The Fellowships provide a year's graduate training in a school of public health or sanitary engineering. They are available either during the academic year beginning in the fall of 1946 or fall of 1947 and are open to men and women who are citizens of the United States.

The purpose of the Fellowships is to aid in the recruitment of trained health officers, directors of special medical services, and public health engineers to help fill some of the 900 vacancies in public health medical positions and 300 vacancies for public health engineers, existing in State and local health departments over the country. The Fellowships are reserved for newcomers to the public health field, and are not open to employees in State and local health departments, for whom Federal Grants-in-Aid are already available to the States.

Applicants for Fellowships may secure further details by writing to the Surgeon General, U. S. Public Health Service, Attention: Public Health Training, 19th and Constitution Avenue, N. W., Washington, D. C., Owing to the anticipated heavy enrollment in graduate schools, completed applications for training in the fall term of 1946 should be filed promptly. The awards committee will act on applications on the following dates: June 15, July 1, July 15 and August 1.

OFFICIAL PROCEEDINGS OF HOUSE OF DELEGATES, OKLAHOMA STATE MEDICAL ASSOCIATION

(Conclusion)

The Speaker then called for the Report of the Publicity Committee. Dr. John Burton, Chairman was granted the floor and read the following report:

Report of the Publicity Committee

The Publicity Committee endeavoring to carry out President Tisdal's program of public education relative to medicine, learned at the onset that to be heard effectively one must have the public's wholehearted respect. Secondly, it was quite evident that there were many forces working adversely in this regard. Some were outright in their attacks, others more subtle, in that they attempted to minimize or depreciate the position of the doctor in the life of the community.

An intensive study was made as to the best way to combat these forces. Advice and counsel were obtained from the American Medical Association, the National Physicians Committee, and from other State societies which were carrying on like programs. It was well agreed that any effort made should be of a high type, presented with force and dignity, and one with an appeal for all levels of society. Acting upon these premises, the problem was presented to a national advertising and public relations agency—the Erwin-Wassey Advertising Agency of Oklahoma City.

Several meetings with varied discussions were held. Out of these were crystallized the following: 1. That a definite program of public relations should be inaugurated. 2. That this program should embody public education, advertising and better public opinion. The advertisements would be prepared under the direction of the Council and would be progressive in nature. They would follow modern trends in medicine, warning the public against abuses and false claims. They would also point out the weakness of political and economic ideas being advanced against the medical profession. The copy would all be of a positive type and not negative.

3. Radio publicity was discussed but it was thought that it was too expensive at this time.

4. The Agency has recommended that the Association utilize each newspaper in the State on the basis of a 40 inch ad each month. This is a quarter of a page. This size ad being considered large enough to accomplish the purpose, yet small enough to avoid waste. The cost of this program is $25,027.20.

In considering the number of the public that would be contacted through the newspapers, it is important to point out that the total paid subscriptions of newspapers in Oklahoma is 639,247 and based upon 3.5 persons per family, this makes a reading public of 2,237,364. This program obviously would be a most advantageous one for the Association to promote.

5. The Constitution and By-Laws provide three means of raising funds for the activities of the Association, namely; raising dues; special assessment; voluntary contributions. It is felt that the most equitable way to meet this expense would be by an assessment.

6. The Committee, in considering this over-all project, would recommend if favorably voted upon by the House Veterans Administration to make available to veterans examinations and medical care through private physicians and recommends to the Council that at the earliest possible date the Council put this plan into operation in Oklahoma.

Respectfully submitted,
John F. Burton, M.D., Chairman
Ben Ward, M.D.
Everett King, M.D.,

After the reading of the report the following motion was made: On motion by Dr. Louis Ritzhaupt, Guthrie, seconded by Dr. Ned Burleson, Prague, the report and recommendations were approved.

At this time, the Speaker called for presentation of amendments to the Constitution and By-Laws from the floor. Mr. Graham was recognized and presented several amendments to the By-Laws which would be necessary in revising the set up of Standing Committees. (These amendments appear in the Council Report). The Speaker stated that final consideration would be given to the amendments to the By-Laws the following morning.

Th Chair then called for the invitation for the next Annual Meeting. A letter was read by the Tulsa Delegation.

On motion by Dr. R. Q. Goodwin, Oklahoma City, seconded by Dr. F. W. Boadway, Ardmore, the invitation was accepted.

The Speaker stated that the next order of business to be considered would be the election of Honorary Members to the Association. The name of Dr. A. C. Lucas of Castle, Oklahoma, had been submitted to the office of the Association for election. On motion by Dr. James Stevenson, Tulsa, seconded by Dr. J. G. Edwards, Okmulgee, Dr. Lucas was elected to Honorary Membership.

The Speaker then stated that there were no applications for Associate Membership.

Dr. Garrison then stated that it was his duty as Speaker of the House to set a definite time for the election of officers. He stated that the time would be 10:30 P.M., April 30, 1946, at the second session of the House.

At this time Dr. Garrison declared the meeting adjourned to reassemble at 9:00 P.M. in Parlor A of the Skirvin Tower Hotel.

MINUTES OF THE SECOND SESSION

The second session was called to order by Dr. Garrison, at 9:00 P.M.

The Credentials Committee announced a quorum present and upon motion the report was accepted.

The Chairman stated that the House had passed a motion at the previous session awarding memorial certificates to Dr. W. W. Rucks, Sr., Dr. Henry H. Turner and Dr. C. R. Rountree, all of whom had served as State Chairman for the Procurement and Assignment Service.

Dr. V. C. Tisdal, President, was granted the floor and made the following remarks: "On behalf of the Oklahoma State Medical Association I present these certificates to you in recognition of the work that you have done in service to your country and to the Association in the recent emergency. We commend the great service that you have rendered the profession."

The three memorial certificates were presented to Dr. Rucks, Dr. Turner and Dr. Rountree. Speaking for all three Dr. Rucks acknowledged with appreciation the receipt of the certificates.

The Speaker then informed the House that a letter had been received from the United States Department of Agriculture with the urgent request that it be presented to the House of Delegates of the Oklahoma State Medical Association. He read the letter.

WILLIAM E. EASTLAND, M.D.
F. A. C. R.

RADIUM AND X-RAY THERAPY

DERMATOLOGY

405 Medical Arts Bldg.

Oklahoma City, Oklahoma   Phone 3-1446

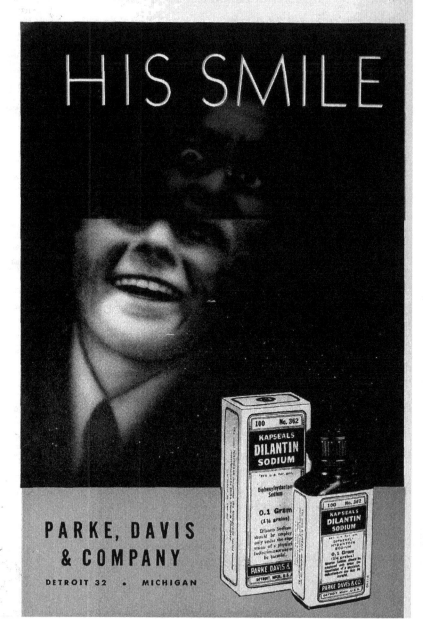

BETRAYS
THE SHADOW
ON HIS MIND

Behind the smile of the epileptic may be the feeling of insecurity and the dread of his next seizure. DILANTIN SODIUM favorably influences such epileptic psychologic factors and is effective in controlling convulsions. This superior anticonvulsant...relatively free from sedative, hypnotic or depressant action...provides complete control of seizures in a substantial percentage of cases. In others it lengthens the interval and diminishes effects of the seizures.

Available in Kapseals of 0.03 Gm. (½ gr.) and 0.1 Gm. (1½ gr.).

DILANTIN SODIUM
(DIPHENYLHYDANTOIN SODIUM)

After the reading of the letter the following motion was made: On *motion* by Dr. R. Q. Goodwin, Oklahoma City, *seconded* by Dr. Lee Emenhiser, Oklahoma City, the House of Delegates went on record as being 100 per cent behind the Famine Emergency Campaign. The motion *carried.*

Mr. Dick Graham was next called upon to present to the House of Delegates the plan for the reorganization of the County Societies. Mr. Graham gave the report, indicating the proposed changes on the map.

After the report a limited discussion followed. Mr. Graham assured the House that the map and suggestions as to grouping were not the final set up—that this would be entirely up to the individual counties and Districts. On *motion* by Dr. C. H. Cooke, Perry, *amended* by Dr. A. R. Sugg, Ada, *seconded* by Dr. Ellis Lamb, Clinton and carried, the plan was *adopted* as outlined providing that the individual county and the Councilor Districts agree to the changes. The motion *carried.*

The Chairman then called for final disposition of the Publicity Report and suggestions made by Dr. John F. Burton, Chairman of the Committee. On *motion* by Dr. James Stevenson, Tulsa, *seconded* by Dr. C. R. Rountree, Oklahoma City, the report was *approved.*

The Speaker then recognized Dr. P. J. Devanney, Sayre, who *moved* that $25.00 be assessed each member of the Association this year to pay for the plan as, outlined. The motion was *seconded* by Dr. F. C. Lattimore, Tulsa and *carried* after the discussion.

Election of Officers

The Speaker then stated that the next item of business was the election of officers. A ten minute recess was declared for the purpose of the members of the various Districts to get together.

The first officer to be elected was the President-Elect. Nominations were as follows: Dr. Paul Champlin, Enid was nominated by Dr. John Burton, Oklahoma City; Dr. Clinton Gallaher, Shawnee was nominated by Dr. Sam McKeel of Ada; Dr. George Garrison, Oklahoma City

was nominated by Dr. W. T. Andreskowski of Ryan. Dr. Garrison asked that his name not be considered.

On *motion* by Dr. C. H. Cooke, Perry, *seconded* by Dr. E. H. Shuller, McAlester and *carried,* the nominations ceased.

While the Tellers were counting ballots for the election of President-Elect, the floor was granted to Dr. L. C. Kuyrkendall, McAlester, who said, "You have adopted a plan here tonight that I promise within the next four months, will be carried to every County Society in the state so that each member will know what we plan to do."

The results of the balloting showed Dr. Paul Champlin of Enid to be the President-Elect. On *motion* by Dr. Sam McKeel, *seconded* by Dr. C. R. Rountree, the election was declared *unanimous.*

Dr. Champlin was called to the stand and said, "I have just a few words. This is an honor you have bestowed upon me that no doctor could refuse. On the other hand it is a job for which I feel ill-equipped. I have been rather a consistent attendant of medical meetings since entering the profession and I don't believe that I ever attended a medical meeting that I did not get something out of. It is a most important thing for all of you to attend all meetings regularly. I was very much interested in the reorganization of the county societies and districts that was proposed as I feel that the closer and the more doctors you can get to attend, more work will be accomplished. As I have said, I feel totally ill-equipped for this job that you have given me but I assure you that I will do my very best for the medical profession of the state and for medical education and research. Thanks very much—I am humiliated with the honor that you have so kindly bestowed upon me."

Following the election of President-Elect, nominations were in order for Vice-President. The following nominations were received: Dr. Phil Risser, Blackwell nominated Dr. Roy Emanuel of Chickasha; Dr. H. K. Speed, Sayre nominated Dr. J. B. Hollis, Mangum; Dr. E. H. Shuller,

FOR CLIMACTERIC CONTROL

- *Dosage to Meet the Patient's Needs*
- *Proven Clinical Potency*
- *Marked Tolerance*
- *Economy*

Possessing these desirable qualities, Schieffelin BENZESTROL meets the requirements of the most critical physician for the estrogenic control of the instabilities of the climacteric.

A non-stilbene compound, this synthetic estrogen tides the patient over the period of adjustment involved in hormonal regression with a high degree of safety and satisfaction.

Schieffelin BENZESTROL Tablets—0.5, 1.0, 2.0 and 5.0 mg. —50's—100's—1000's.

Literature and Sample on Request

Schieffelin BENZESTROL Solution—5.0 mg. per cc.—10 cc. vials.
Schieffelin BENZESTROL Vaginal Tablets—0.5 mg.—100's.

Schieffelin & Co.　　20 COOPER SQUARE　•　NEW YORK 3, N. Y.
Pharmaceutical and Research Laboratories

McAlester nominated Dr. J. T. Phelps, El Reno. On *motion* by Dr. A. R. Sugg, *seconded* by Dr. Ralph McGill, the nominations *ceased*.

After two ballotings the election of Dr. Roy Emanuel of Chickasha was announced.

The Speaker then stated that the election of Councilors of Districts No. 2, No. 3, No. 4 and No. 6 were in order. Regarding the election of a Councilor for District No. 2, the Speaker announced that a resignation had been received from Dr. Wm. Finch of Hobart, present Councilor, which had been duly accepted by the Council. Regarding the election of the Councilor for District No. 6, the Speaker stated that a letter had been received from Dr. J. V. Athey, present Councilor whose term expires, stating that he did not wish to be considered for re-election.

The Speaker called for nominations for Councilor for District No. 2. Dr. V. C. Tisdal was recognized and nominated Dr. Gordon Livingston, Cordell. There being no other nominations, on *motion* by Dr. L. Chester McHenry, *seconded* by Dr. E. H. Shuller, the election of Dr. Gordon Livingston was declared *unanimous*, Dr. Livingston being elected to finish the term of Dr. Finch.

Dr. Garrison then called for nominations for Councilor of District No. 3. Dr. Julian Feild was recognized and nominated Dr. C. E. Northcutt for re-election. There being no other nominations, on *motion* by Dr. Julian Feild, *seconded* by Dr. C. H. Cooke, Dr. Northcutt's election was declared *unanimous*.

Nominations were now in order for Councilor of District No. 4. Dr. R. Q. Goodwin was recognized and nominated Dr. Carroll Pounders who had been serving as Councilor to fill the unexpired term of Dr. Tom Lowry. There being no other nominations, on *motion* of Dr. R. Q. Goodwin, *seconded* by Dr. E. H. Shuller, Dr. Pounders was *unanimously elected* to fill the unexpired term of Dr. Tom Lowry.

The Speaker then called for nominations for Councilor of District No. 6. Dr. W. A. Howard, Chelsea was recognized and nominated Dr. Ralph McGill of Tulsa. There being no other nominations, on *motion* by Dr. J. V. Athey, *seconded* by Dr. W. F. Keller, Dr. McGill was *unanimously* elected.

Dr. Howard was again recognized and said, "I would like to say a word on behalf of our District for the man who has served as Councilor for our District. We want the House of Delegates to know that we hold in high esteem and respect our former Councilor, Dr. J. V. Athey."

The Speaker then announced that the next office to be filled with that of Speaker of the House. He asked that Dr. H. K. Speed, Vice-Speaker, take this nomination. Dr. Speed recognized Dr. W. S. Larrabee, Tulsa, who nominated Dr. George Garrison for re-election. The nomination was *seconded* by Dr. C. R. Rountree. There being no other nominations, upon *motion* by Dr. E. H. Shuller, *seconded* by Dr. W. A. Howard, Dr. Garrison's

RADIUM

(Including Radium Applicators)

FOR ALL MEDICAL PURPOSES

Est. 1919

Quincy X-Ray and Radium Laboratories
(Owned and directed by a Physician-Radiologist)

HAROLD SWANBERG, B.S., M.D., Director

W.C.U. Bldg.   Quincy, Illinois

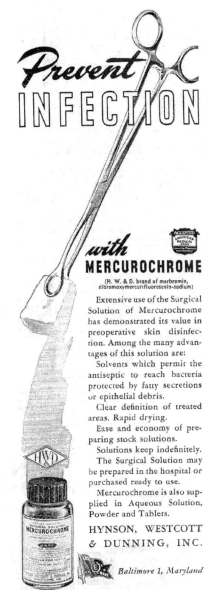

Prevent INFECTION

with MERCUROCHROME

(H. W. & D. brand of merbromin, dibromoxymercurifluorescein-sodium)

Extensive use of the Surgical Solution of Mercurochrome has demonstrated its value in preoperative skin disinfection. Among the many advantages of this solution are:

Solvents which permit the antiseptic to reach bacteria protected by fatty secretions or epithelial debris.

Clear definition of treated areas. Rapid drying.

Ease and economy of preparing stock solutions.

Solutions keep indefinitely.

The Surgical Solution may be prepared in the hospital or purchased ready to use.

Mercurochrome is also supplied in Aqueous Solution, Powder and Tablets.

HYNSON, WESTCOTT & DUNNING, INC.

Baltimore 1, Maryland

election was *unanimous.*

Dr. Garrison again took the Chair and called for nominations for Vice-Speaker of the House. Dr. Louis Ritzhaupt was recognized and nominated by Dr. A. R. Sugg of Ada. There being no other nominations, upon *motion* by Dr. R. Q. Goodwin, *seconded* by Dr. John Perry, Dr. Sugg was *unanimously* elected.

Next in order was the nomination of Delegate to the A.M.A. Dr. John Burton was recognized and nominated Dr. James Stevenson for re-election. There being no other nominations, upon *motion* by Dr. C. R. Rountree, *seconded* by Dr. John Burton, Dr. Stevenson was *unanimously* elected.

The next office to be filled was that of Alternate Delegate. Dr. McLain Rogers was recognized and nominated Dr. Finis Ewing for re-election. There being no other nomination, upon *motion* by Dr. Sam McKeel, *seconded* by Dr. W. S. Larrabee, the election of Dr. Ewing was *unanimous.*

At this point in the agenda, Dr. Garrison read the Official Call of the American Medical Association to Delegates for the Annual Meeting of the American Medical Association in San Francisco, July 1 through July 5. Upon *motion* by Dr. McLain Rogers, *seconded* by Dr. John Burton, the Call was *accepted.*

Dr. V. C. Tisdal was recognized: "We need an Allied Professions Committee in order to carry to all interested groups the present medical economic problems. We need the united support and cooperation of all of these groups and for that reason we ask that we form such a committee. I *move* that we form an Allied Professions Committee." The motion was *seconded* by Dr. James Sterenson and *carried.*

The next item of business was the consideration of the dues for 1947. Dr. Garrison called for discussion.

After lengthy discussion regarding the exact amount of the raise in dues, it was decided that the raise should be approved and no amount indicated. The *motion* by Dr. C. R. Rountree, Oklahoma City, *seconded* by Dr. R. Q. Goodwin, Oklahoma City, that the dues for 1947 be raised, *carried.*

It was suggested by the Chairman and approved by the House that the House of Delegates should meet on the morning of May 1 at 9 A.M. to consider the amount of dues and to be advised of the budget. A Council meeting was called for 8:30 A.M. for the purpose of drawing up a budget for presentation to the House of Delegates.

The next item called for by the Speaker was the report of the Resolutions Committee. Dr. E. H. Shuller, Chairman, was recognized and read the following Resolutions on:

Council on Medical Services and Public Relations:

On *motion* by Dr. McLain Rogers, Clinton, *seconded* by Dr. Finis Ewing, Muskogee, the resolution was *adopted.*

George F. Lull: On *motion* by Dr. J. V. Athey, Bartlesville, *seconded* by Dr. McLain Rogers, Clinton, the resolution was *adopted.*

Olin West: On *motion* by Dr. James Stevenson, Tulsa, *seconded* by Dr. C. R. Rountree, Oklahoma City, the resolution was *adopted.*

Dean of the Medical School: On *motion* by Dr. Louis Ritzhaupt, Guthrie, *seconded* by Dr. J. V. Athey, Bartlesville, the resolution was *adopted.*

The Commonwealth Fund: On *motion* by Dr. O. C. Newman, Shattuck, *seconded* by Dr. J. G. Edwards, Okmulgee, the resolution was *adopted.*

Postgraduate Instruction: Upon *motion* by Dr. James Stevenson, Tulsa, *seconded* by Dr. R. Q. Goodwin, Oklahoma City, the resolution, as amended, was *adopted.*

Crippled Children: On *motion* by Dr. C. R. Rountree, Oklahoma City, *seconded* by Dr. James Stevenson, Tulsa, this resolution is to be held for investigation by the Council.

Pontotoc County Medical Society: On *motion* by Dr. O. C. Newman, Shattuck, *seconded* by Dr. A. R. Sugg, Ada, the resolution was *adopted.*

The next order of business was the final disposal of the Amendments to the By-Laws. In this connection Dr. Garrison read the following letter which had been referred to the Resolutions Committee in order asked the pleasure of the House as the letter would call for an amendment to the Constitution at the next Annual Meeting.

"For some time I have thought about an idea which I feel would be for the improvement and the betterment of the State Medical Association. I am writing this letter to ask you to bring this before the Council of the State Medical Association for their consideration.

"Under the present rules, the governing body of the State Association is the Council, composed of one man elected from each of the ten councilor districts with the State officers also as members.

"It occurs to me that if alternate councilor members were elected at the time of election of the councilors, it would afford definite assurance that the districts would always be represented at the Council meetings. Likewise, it would afford a means of training men in the working and functioning of the State Medical Association so that their talents could be used at a later date."

On *motion* by Dr. Ned Burleson, Prague, *seconded* by Dr. H. A. Higgins, Ardmore, this suggestion was *approved.*

Amendments to By-Laws
(See Report of Council)

J. E. HANGER, Inc.

ARTIFICIAL LIMBS, BRACES, AND CRUTCHES

Phone: 2-8500　　　　　　　　　　　　　　　　　　　　　612 N. Hudson

L. T. Lewis, Mgr.　　　BRANCHES AND AGENCIES IN PRINCIPAL CITIES　Oklahoma City 3, Okla.

Prescribe or Dispense

ZEMMER　　**Zemmer Pharmaceuticals**
A complete line of laboratory controlled
ethical pharmaceuticals.　　OK 7-46
Chemists to the Medical Profession for 44 years.

The Zemmer Company　　Oakland Station
Pittsburgh 13, Pa.

Effective Against
CHIGGERS
(RED BUGS)

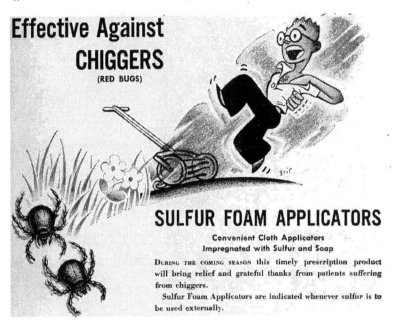

SULFUR FOAM APPLICATORS

Convenient Cloth Applicators
Impregnated with Sulfur and Soap

DURING THE COMING SEASON this timely prescription product will bring relief and grateful thanks from patients suffering from chiggers.

Sulfur Foam Applicators are indicated whenever sulfur is to be used externally.

They have the advantage of ...
- ... even dispersal of fine sulfur particles
- ... convenience—they are easy to use
- ... elegance—no grease, mess or stain
- ... safety, minimizing the possibility of sulfur dermatitis

Complete directions with each package

TREATMENT

PROPHYLAXIS

SULFUR FOAM APPLICATORS

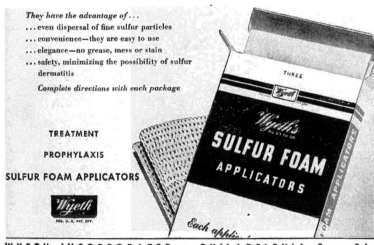

WYETH INCORPORATED • PHILADELPHIA 3 • PA.

On *motion* by Dr. W. S. Larrabee, Tulsa, *seconded* by Dr. Lee Emenhiser, Oklahoma City, the amendments were *adopted* as presented.

The Speaker declared the meeting adjourned until 9 A.M., May 1.

THIRD SESSION

The third and final session of the House of Delegates convened at 9:00 A.M., May 1.

After the call to order by the Speaker of the House, the Credentials Committee stated that a quorum was present.

Mr. Dick Graham was given the floor and read the budget for the year 1947. After the reading of the budget there was discussion from the floor concerning the proposed raise in dues and the budget as presented.

On *motion* by Dr. J. S. Fulton, Atoka, *seconded* by Dr. C. R. Rountree, Oklahoma City and *carried*, the dues for 1947 were increased in the amount of $10.00.

On *motion* by Dr. L. S. Willour, *seconded* by Dr. James Stevenson, Tulsa, the budget was *approved* as presented.

On *motion* by Dr. C. E. Northcutt, Ponca City, *seconded* by Dr. J. G. Edwards, Okmulgee and *carried*, it was requested that a budget be prepared in advance of the next Annual Meeting.

At this time Dr. Louis Ritzhaupt was granted the floor and stated that he thought a delegation from the House of Delegates should call upon Roy Turner, candidate for Governor. Mr. Dick Graham stated that he felt this was an excellent idea and that within the next three days, each candidate for Governor who had established offices should be called upon by the same delegation. The following motion was made. On *motion* by Dr. C. R. Rountree, Oklahoma City, *seconded* by Dr. McLain Rogers, Clinton and *carried* it was requested that a member from each Councilor District be appointed for this purpose.

The Chair appointed the following: Dr. O. C. Newman, District 1; Dr. McLain Rogers, District 2; Dr. C. E. Northcutt, District 3; Dr. Louis Ritzhaupt, District 4; Dr. F. W. Boadway, District 5; Dr. Ralph McGill, District 6; Dr. Ned Burleson, District 7; Dr. Finis Ewing, District 8; Dr. Earl Woodson, District 9; Dr. John Haynie, District 10.

Dr. C. R. Rountree was next recognized and said, "It is with pride that I rise at this time to make the following motion: I *move* that this House of Delegates express its appreciation to Dr. V. C. Tisdal, President, for the great amount of work and energy he has put into his presidency. The motion was *seconded* by Dr. R. Q. Goodwin, Oklahoma City and *carried*.

At this time the Chair declared the meeting adjourned.

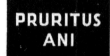

PRURITUS ANI

YOUNG'S RECTAL DILATORS

The itching of pruritus ani may often be relieved by dilatation, especially when caused by a tight or spastic sphincter muscle which prevents bulky or dry stool from being expelled regularly and smoothly.

have been found very effective in breaking the impulse of rectal muscle to keep itself locked. Sold only by prescription. Obtainable at your surgical supply house; available for patients at ethical drug stores. In sets of 4 graduated sizes, adult, $4.75, children's set $4.50. Write for Brochure.

F. E. YOUNG & COMPANY, 424 E. 75th St., Chicago 19, Ollinois

Have a Coke

When you laugh, the world laughs with you, as they say—and when you enjoy *the pause that refreshes* with ice-cold Coca-Cola, your friends enjoy it with you, too. Everybody enjoys the friendly hospitality that goes with the invitation *Have a Coke*. Those three words mean *Friend, you belong —I'm glad to be with you.* Good company is better company over a Coca-Cola.

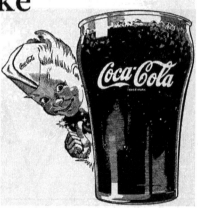

Medical Abstracts

SCIATIC PAIN: ITS RELATION TO PAIN IN THE BACK AND SPINAL DEFORMITY; E. N. Wardle. The Medical Press and Circular. Volume L, pp. 197-201; 1945.

The author states that, of 120 consecutive cases in which the patient complained of pain in the leg, eighty-one were found to have neuralgia only, and 39, a true neuritis. Many patients with true sciatic neuralgia will admit having had attacks of intermittent back pain. Examination reveals regidity of the lumbar spine, and painful limitation of movement in all directions. Twenty-nine cases of this type of osteo-arthritis were treated by simple immobilization of the spine in a plaster jacket for approximately four weeks. There was one failure.

Eighty cases of sciatic scoliosis, which was characterized by severe pain, list of the whole body to one side, strong spasm of one erector spina, and wasing of the whole quadriceps muscle, where treated by the application of a head-suspension plaster jacket. There were eleven failures. In some cases, laminectomy and removal of a herniated disc were indicated, and six operations were done. Four patients returned to work, one had good recovery after removal of a meningioma, and one died.

Treatment of thirty-seven cases of sciatic pain associated with congenital lumbar abnormalities were successful in twenty cases, unsuccessful in seventeen. Fifteen cases of injury to the erector spinae and lumbar aponeurosis were helped by injection of two or three cubic centimeters of a one per cent novocaine solution into the painful area, and by manipulation.—E.D.M., M.D.

INCREASE IN RESISTANCE OF TUBERCLE BACILLI TO STREPTOMYCIN: A PRELIMINARY REPORT. Guy P. Youmans, M.D., Ph.D., Elizabeth H. Williston, M.D., Department of Bacteriology, Northwestern University Medical School, William H. Feldman, D.V.M., M.S., Division of Experimental Surgery and Pathology, Mayo Foundation and H. Corwin Hinshaw, M.D., Ph.D., Division of Medicine.

Since various bacteria apparently may rapidly acquire a resistence to streptomycin, experiments were carried out to determine if the resistance of tubercle bacilli would increase on continual exposure to this drug. Two procedures were employed.

1. Tubercle bacilli were cultured from twelve tuberculous patients, both before and after treatment with streptomycin, and their sensitivity to the drug compared. This revealed that in eight of the twelve patients, the terbercle bacilli showed marked increase in resistance to streptomycin, up to 500 to 1,000 fold after treatment.

2. Tubercle bacilli were exposed in vitro, the concentrations of streptomycin which inhibited but did not completely prevent growth. The strains of mycobacterium terberculosis, one of human and one of avian type, showed an increase in resistance more than 1,000 fold.

(Complete results will subsequently be published in greater detail.)—H.J., M.D.

PULMONARY EMBOLISM IN FRACTURES OF THE HIP: COLLES' FRACTURE, J. Warren White. Southern Medi-Harry Golodner, Louis J. Morse and Alfred Angrist. Surgery, Volume 18, pp. 418-423; 1945.

Heart disease and bronchopneumonia have been thought to be the most common cause of death, following fractures of the hip. Pulmonary embolism has not been considered so often as this article would indicate that it should be. Of 304 patients who were treated for intertrochanteric or intracapsular fractures of the neck of the femur, there were eighty-six deaths. Twenty-five autopsies were performed, and the causes of death in these patients were as follows: Pulmonary embolism in nine, bronchopneumonia in seven, artheriosclerotic heart in four, and miscellaneous causes of death, including sepsis, in five.

This study would indicate that pulmonary embolism from venous thrombosis in the veins of the lower extremities is the most frequent cause of death in cases of fracture of the hip. From their observations, the authors conclude also that this complication is less frequent in

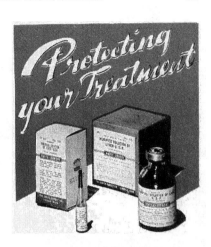

UNCERTAIN SUCCESS in the treatment of pernicious anemia is due to many unpredictable factors.

One element of certainty is added to your treatment when the Solution of Liver prescribed never varies from rigid standards.

Purified Solution of Liver, Smith-Dorsey, is unfailingly uniform in purity and potency. It has earned and maintained the confidence of thousands of physicians.

Purified Solution of Liver, Smith-Dorsey, will help to protect your treatment—to assure you of good results where the medication is the controlling factor.

PURIFIED SOLUTION OF *Liver*

Supplied in the following dosage forms: 1 cc. ampoules and 10 cc. and 30 cc. ampoule vials, each containing 10 U.S.P. Injectable Units per cc.

THE SMITH-DORSEY COMPANY
LINCOLN • NEBRASKA
Manufacturers of Pharmaceuticals to the Medical Profession Since 1908

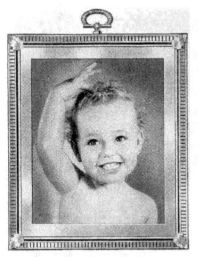

DOCTOR, MEET THE DARICRAFT BABY

Perhaps you are "meeting" the Daricraft Baby every day in your own practice. If not, may we call to your attention the following significant points of interest about Vitamin D increased Daricraft:

1. Produced from inspected herds; 2. Clarified; 3. Homogenized; 4. Sterilized; 5. Specially Processed; 6. Easily Digested; 7. High in Food Value; 8. Improved Flavor; 9. Uniform; 10. Dependable Source of Supply.

Producers Creamery Co.
Springfield, Mo.

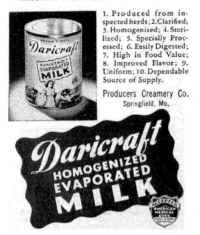

patients who become ambulatory early. They have suggested prophylactic bilateral ligation of the superficial femoral vein, combined with lumbar sympathetic block, for the prevention of pulmonary embolism in fractures of the hip of patients who cannot be made ambulatory early.—E.D.M., M.D.

ANNOUNCEMENT

The Rocky Mountain Radiological Society is resuming its mid-summer Radiological Conference, which is to be held in Denver, Colorado, August 8-10, 1946. The program committee is arranging an excellent program. The guest speakers are: Dr. John Camp; Dr. William E. Costolow: Dr. Ross Golden, and Dr. Dabney Kerr.

All physicians interested in radiology are urged to attend this conference. The radiologist should plan his vacation to come to Colorado and participate in this excellent program.

Reveal not to a friend every secret that you possess, for how can you tell but what he may some time or other become your enemy? *Saadi: The Gulistan.*

Money and time are the heaviest burdens of life, and the unhappiest of all mortals are those who have more of either than they know how to use. *Johnson: The Idler.*

Book Reviews

THE CARE OF THE AGED. Malford W. Thewlis, M.D., Attending Specialist, General Medicine; Attending Physician, South County Hospital, Wakefield, R. I.; Director, Thewlis Clinic. Fifth Edition, 65 Illustrations, Six Collaborators, 500 pages. C. V. Mosby, St. Louis.

The care of the aged (geriatrics), gracefully or physiologically growing old (senescence), pathologically growing old (senility), the study of the aged (geratology) and government by the aged (gerontocracy). Thus has sprung up a new specialty in medicine. "It is estimated that about 45 per cent of the diagnoses in old age are incorrect as shown by necropsies.' In old age anatomic structures, relations and functions are altered. Therefore pathologic processes affect alterations differently and disease is modified in character, symptoms and signs.'' Since problems of the aged are separate and distinct from the problems of maturity and pediatries, a firm footing is established for the development of the above specialty.

This book on geatries is just off the press. A very creditable magazine on geriatries made its bow in January, 1946. Insurance actuaries figure the average expectancy now is 65 years. If Bogomolets antireticular cytotoxic serum lives up to its claim, the life expectancy will be 150 years.

This is a well written and well edited book by the author and six collaborators. It is the fifth edition which shows its worth. The texts are much altered in this edition and the book consists of eight parts. Prevention of geriatrics is stressed, stress and longevity, as well as other recent accomplishments in medicine. It is dedicated to the memory of I. L. Nasher, M.D., the father of modern geriatrics. The late LeRoy Peters, M.D., wrote the chapter on tuberculosis. It does not pretend to be a general medical text book, but deals with the involutional changes and the diseases most occurring in chronological later life, as well as premature involutional changes. This book should be in the hands of all physicians, as the care of the aged is becoming more and more a medical, political and social, as well as an economic problem, and the profession should be alerted on this ever changing phase of medicine.—Lea A. Rieley, M.D.

Doubting Thomas...

and Richard...

and William...

and James...

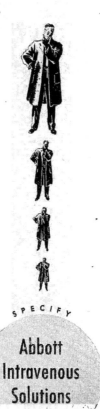

Yes, they are all "Doubting Thomases," these Abbott control technicians, when it comes to testing Abbott Intravenous Solutions. They insist upon rigid tests and searching examinations throughout *each step* of manufacture to insure utmost purity and sterility. Starting with the selection of raw materials in the stockroom, their exacting control on each lot is not relaxed until after it is packed and ready for shipment. In the interim, they make sterility and pyrogen tests, with special pharmacological and biological tests when needed; pH determinations; tests for dissolved chemical impurities; light-inspections of each finished container for color, clarity and freedom from foreign particles. If any of these tests should indicate that the lot is not up to standard, the entire lot would be destroyed. As a final precaution, each cap is vacuum-tested to insure an airtight fit. These tests and controls are your assurance that you can use Abbott Intravenous Solutions in bulk containers with fullest confidence. ABBOTT LABORATORIES, North Chicago, Illinois.

SPECIFY

Abbott Intravenous Solutions

In Bulk Containers

INDUSTRY TUBERCULOSIS SILICOSIS AND COM-PENSATION. A Symposium, prepared by the Committee on Tuberculosis in Industry of the National Tuberculosis Association and American Trudeau Society. Leroy U. Cardner, M.D., Editor. National Tuberculosis Association, New York, N. Y. $2.00, 1945.

In the light of present day medicine in relation to industry the knowledge in this small condensed volume is indispensable even for the general practitioner. It is not safe for the average doctor to think he can leave all these questions in the hands of specialists in industrial medicine.

In the preface Dr. Kendall Emerson makes this significant statement: "The new symposium is intended to give useful information on tuberculosis, pneumoconioses with particular reference to silicosis and workmen's compensation, not only to those who specialize in industrial medicine, but also to those generally interested in a subject that lately has commanded much attention."

The interesting story in this valuable compendium is highlighted by the table of contents:

Part I—Tuberculosis

1. Tuberculosis and Industry, W. P. Shepard, M.D.
2. Conquest of Tuberculosis in Industry, Herman E. Hilleboe, M.D., and David M. Could, M.D.
3. The Attitude of Industry Toward X-Ray Examinations of the Chest, C. D. Selby, M.D.

4. Control of Tuberculosis in an Industrial Group, Ada Chree Reid, M.D.

Part II—Pneumoconioses

5. Review of Silicosis for the Industrial Hygienist and Medical Practitioner, L. E. Hamlin, M.D.
6. The Respiratory Hazards of Electric Arc Welding, O. A. Sander, M.D.
7. Elements of Diagnosis and Prognosis in Pneumoconiosis, Leroy U. Gardner, M.D.
8. Management of the Silicotic Patient, Paul J. Bamberger, M.D.
9. Aluminum Therapy in the Prevention and Treatment of Silicosis, A. J. Lanza, M.D.

Part III—Compensation

10. Medical Aspects of Compensation for Partial Disability from Silicosis, George W. Wright, M.D.
11. Occupational Diseases—The Physician and the Law, Leopold Brahdy, M.D.
12. Occupational Disease Liabilities—Financial and Humanitarian, B. E. Kuechle.

It will be easy for the doctor to realize the importance of this book if he will read Leopold Brahdy's article dealing with the physician and the law and remember that "The law answers no medical questions." Particularly note-worthy are the articles by Hamlin, Sander, Gardner and Wright.—Lewis J. Moorman, M.D.

DIAGNOSTIC CLINIC OF INTERNAL MEDICINE AND ALLERGY

Phiilp M. McNeill, M. D., F. A. C. P.

General Diagnosis

CONSULTATION BY APPOINTMENT

Special Attention to Cardiac, Pulmonary and Allergic Diseases

Electrocardiograph, X-Ray, Laboratory
and Complete Allergic Surveys Available.

1107 Medical Arts Bldg.
Oklahoma City, Okla.

Phone 2-0277

COSMETIC *HAY FEVER?*

Prescribe UNSCENTED AR-EX Cosmetics

Recent clinical tests showed many cases of cosmetic sensitivity, but not a single one to UNSCENTED AR-EX Cosmetics. For allergic patients, prescribe UNSCENTED AR-EX Cosmetics—free from all known irritants and allergens. SEND FOR FREE FORMULARY.

UNSCENTED

AR-EX COSMETICS, INC., 1036 W. VAN BUREN ST., CHICAGO 7, ILL.

FREE FORMULARY

DR.
ADDRESS
CITY
STATE

THE JOURNAL
of the
OKLAHOMA STATE MEDICAL ASSOCIATION

VOLUME XXXIX	OKLAHOMA CITY, OKLAHOMA, AUGUST, 1946	NUMBER 8

Acute Otitis Media; Its Management By the General Practitioner and Pediatrician *

J. D. SINGLETON, M.D.

DALLAS, TEXAS

Acute Otitis media is, primarily, a disease of infancy and early childhood, but it occurs not infrequently in older children and adults. In the management of this condition the objective is to eradicate the infection, guard against recurrences, and if possible, prevent such complications as acute surgical mastoiditis, chronic atorrhea and mastoiditis with impaired hearing, lateral sinus thrombosis, meningitis and brain abscess.

A practical knowledge of the anatomy of the middle ear and its adnexa, and an understanding of the pathological processes that occur in the presence of infection combined with a knowledge of the susceptibility of the infecting organism to specific chemotherapeutic agents will aid greatly in the choice and application of the measures necessary to obtain the above mentioned objective.

ANATOMY

In the infant the eustachean tube is relatively shorter, broader and more patulous than in the adult. The bony external auditory canal is undeveloped and the annulus is incomplete in its upper segement. The drum membrane is set at a more obtuse angle. The mastoid process is not developed. The cortex is thin, and porous over the antrum. Pneumatization is confined to the antrum with possibly a few surrounding small cells. The bony middle ear cavity and the ossicles are well developed and approximately adult in size. The mucosa is thick and embryonal in character; in the attic and antrum it is redundant, lying in folds.[1 2]

Normally development in the middle ear and mastoid is rapid and by the end of the fifth or sixth year full adult development has

occurred;[3] at this stage the mucous membrane has resorbed, become thin and closely adherent to the underlying bone; occasionally resorption is delayed predisposing to infection, chronicity and complications. The mastoid is well developed, and pneumatization is complete. At this point I wish to call attention to the fact that the mastoid is composed of two distinct parts, the squama and the petrosa; the two parts are often separated by a dense septum known as Korner's septum.[4] Infection often enters and is confined to the deeper petrosal cells with little or no involvement of the superficial squamosal cells. Sellers[3] has demonstrated in some original work that a section made through the posterior half of the attic shows it to be shaped like an inverted truncated cone, wide above and narrow below. If the tympanic membrane is intact, the cavities of the attic and tympanum are separated by a constriction giving roughly the shape of an hour glass. In this region are the ossicles with their ligaments, the tendon of the tensor tympani muscle, the folds delimiting Prussac's space, and the chorda tympani nerve, all tending to further block the constricted space separating the posterior portion of the attic from the tympanum. Above the ossicles, extending from the antrum to the eustachean tube, lies a free space with its long axis in a direction from postero lateral to antero-infero-medial which Sellers has designated the antro-tubal drainage way. This drainage way is of prime importance in the presence of infection because of the ease with which it becomes blocked in the region of the ossicles by swelling and exudate thus damming pus in the posterior portion of the attic and forcing it back into the antrum and mastoid.

*Delivered before the General Session, Oklahoma State Medical Association Annual Meeting, May 1, 1946.

PATHOLOGY

Acute infections of the middle ear may be classed as follows:

1. Catarrhal
2. Serous or purulent
3. Hemorrhagic or thrombotic

In acute catarrhal otitis media the infection is usually mild, but it varies with the age of the patient and the virulence of the infecting organism. It occurs most often in infants and young children, because of the ease with which infection ascends the short open eustachen tube. The child may be fretful and may cry with pain. It runs little or no fever. Examination of the drum membrane shows slight redness with little or no bulging. These patients usually recover without drainage either by paracentesis or spontaneous rupture. If the infection is severe and drainage through the tube fails to occur, or is insufficient and paracentesis is too long delayed, exudation, ulceration, and necrosis occur. The disease then progresses to become a purulent otitis media.

In older children and adults the disease is less frequent. The course is similar to that seen in infancy, and resolution usually occurs without rupture or paracentesis; in these patients fluid, usually serous but some times mucoid, may collect and remain in the middle ear; such a condition produces a feeling of fullness with marked impairment of the hearing in the affected ear; there may be slight congestion of the drum membrane with some loss of luster but there is no bulging.

In acute serous or purulent otitis media the pathology is more severe. In this type of disease the infection invades the deeper layers of the mucous membrane and reaches the middle ear by spreading along the intercellular spaces and the lympatics. Once in the middle ear the infection spreads to involve the mucosa of the attic and often invades the mucosa of the mastoid antrum and other mastoid cells as evidenced by the post-auricular swelling, redness, and tenderness over the antral area, and tenderness over the mastoid tip. Post auricular edema, even to the extent of displacing the ear downward and forward, is not an uncommon finding in infants and young children during the first few days of an acute otitis media often becoming manifest before drainage occurs from the ear. The severe edema that occurs in the mucosa of the middle ear, especially in those cases where normal resorption of the membrane failed to occur, along with the accumulation of thick fibrinous exudate tend to block off the posterior constricted portion of the attic in the region of the ossicles thus damming pus in the attic and forcing it back into the mastoid antrum and other mastoid cells. Such a condition if improperly treated tends either to become chronic or produce the coalescent surgical mastoiditis described by Kopetzky.[6]

Symptoms and physical findings in patients suffering from this type of infection also vary with the age of the patient and the severity of the infection. In children the temperature ranges from 101 to 105, they usually have severe pain in the ear and there is often tenderness and swelling over the mastoid. The drum membrane is inflamed with moderate to marked bulging, or it may have ruptured spontaneously and be draining a serous, sero-sanguinous or purulent drainage. Adults do not run such high fever and are not so likely to have tenderness and swelling over the mastoid. This type of infection constitutes a great majority of the acute otorrheas that we are called upon to treat; with the proper management, the results in these cases are almost 100 per cent satisfactory.

In the hemorrhagic or thrombotic type of otitis media the infection reaches the middle ear through the smaller blood vessels in the form of a thrombophlebitis. Untreated, the infection rapidly spreads through the middle ear to invade the mastoid. It may involve the larger blood vessels including the lateral sinus giving a lateral sinus thrombosis or septecemia; intracranial complications are not uncommon. Patients suffering from this type of infection are desperately ill, run a high temperature often septic in character, and are not relieved by paracentesis and drainage of the middle ear. The drainage is thin, blood stained, and profuse. Fortunately this type of middle ear disease is rare.

Bacteriology: De Sanctis and Larkin[7] in a bacteriologic study made on 268 cases of otitis media found streptococcus hemolyticus in 29 per cent, staphylococcus aureus in 25 per cent, pneumococcus in 19 per cent, a mixture of streptococcus hemolyticus and staphylococcus aureus and pneumococcus in 2 per cent. Three per cent of the culture were negative.

TREATMENT

In view of the fact that the present day treatment of the more severe acute middle ear infections is largely a combination of chemotherapeutic and surgical measures, I wish to call your attention to three general principles laid down by Williams[8] of the Mayo Clinic. First, he states that the infecting organism should be identified before chemotherapy is started. Second, in mild infections a chemotherapeutic agent capable of producing more frequent and more serious complications in itself should not be given. Third, the drug should be given every opportunity to produce a good effect; the dose should be adequate; it should be given at regular intervals throughout the 24 hours; it should be given over a sufficiently long period of time; and all collections of pus should be drained, and regions of necrotic soft tissue and bone should be removed. Adherence to these principles in the management of acute middle ear disease will give highly satisfactory results.

Acute Catarrhal Otitis Media: In the treatment of acute catarrhal otitis media palliative measures such as ear. drops, nose drops, sedatives and bed rest usually suffice. If pain persists and bulging of the drum membrane increases, paracentesis should be resorted to; the ear canal should be kept clean with small cotton wicks. With these simple measures one can expect recovery in most cases in a few days. In case of failure, measures to be described in the treatment of the more serious suppurative otitis media will have to be resorted to. The catarrhal cases with fluid in the middle ear require inflation of the eustachean tube and usually incision of the drum membrane followed by mass suction; the fluid is not under pressure and will not evacuate itself unless suction is applied; these cases should be referred to an otologist; if neglected they tend to become chronic and may result in permanent impairment of the hearing; often the condition is most stubborn and repeated incisions of the drum membrane may be necessary before recovery occurs; chemotherapy is not indicated in these cases.

Acute Serous or Purulent Otitis Media: In view of the fact that the organisms found in acute otitic infections are predominantly from the groups sensitive to the sulfonamides and to penicillin, and since the disease is the first in a chain of serious complications that may follow upper respiratory infections, it is my belief and practice that bed rest and one of the sulfonamides, usually sulfadiazine, should be given in the early stages of the more severe cases of this disease. The dosage should be adequate and it should be continued for several days after all symptoms have subsided. Such treatment will abort many cases that would otherwise go on to suppuration and complication.

If there is sufficient fluid in the middle ear cavity to produce bulging of the drum membrane at the time of the first examination, it is freely incised at the point of greatest bulging; if practical a culture is taken at this time; a small cotton wick is placed gently against the drum membrane at the site of the incision and left in place for 1 to 2 hours; on removal any blood clot that may

have formed will come away with the cotton; the external canal is kept clean with special cotton wicks. Ear drops and irrigations are not advised at this time. Sulfadiazine in adequate doses is started; an initial dose equal to one-half grain per pound of body weight is given; subsequent doses are such that the patient receives 1 grain per pound of body weight in 24 hours; this dosage is continued until the temperature is approximately normal for 24 hours at which time the dosage may be reduced but the drug is not discontinued. Sedatives are given if needed and one-fourth per cent or one-eighth per cent neosynephrin hydrochloride in normal saline solution is used as a nasal spray or in drops 3 or 4 times daily. Where spontaneous rupture of the drum membrane occurs within a few hours after the onset of earache and fever, the above treatment with the necessary modification is instituted.

With the above treatment the infection usually subsides or shows definite improvement within 24 to 72 hours. However, if the drainage continues and pain and fever persist with or without tenderness over the mastoid, it indicates a blocking of the antrotubal drainage way with damming of pus in the posterior portion of the attic and antrum; this is a critical stage and these patients should be seen by an otologist. The blocking and inadequate drainage that is producing the pain and fever is usually relieved by daily applications of gentle mass suction with a Siegel's type otoscope under direct vision; the amount of pus that can be evacuated by this procedure is often amazing. If an otologist is not available, as is often the case in this section of the country, the sulfonamide should be continued for a few days longer and special attention should be given to keeping the external canal clean and open. At this stage the pus is usually thick, creamy, and often profuse; it is best removed by irrigation with a rubber tipped medicine dropper using sterile normal saline or saturated boric acid solution; following the irrigation the canal is dried with special cotton wicks; these procedures can be safely carried out by a nurse or the mother. However, these patients should be seen at least once every two days, more often if the symptoms warrant, in order to see that the canal is free of all debris as shown by a good view of the drum membrane, and to watch for complications. If the perforation is posterior or superior and marginal, one must suspect mastoiditis; in the presence of definite mastoid infection an ear should not be permitted to drain longer than 6 weeks without resorting to mastoid surgery. If the perforation is central and located anteriorly one must suspect that the drainage is persisting because of an associated infection of the sinuses, tonsils or adenoids; such infections when present should be eradicated if possible. Recovery is often hastened and recurrences prevented by the eradication of naso-pharyngeal disease.

Hemorrhagic or Thrombotic Otitis Media: In the presence of an acute fulminating otitis media with high fever, 104 to 105 or higher, associated with pain in the ear not relieved by drainage, pain and tenderness over the mastoid, and profuse thin blood stained drainage, one should proceed on the assumption that he is dealing with an acute hemorrhagic otitis media. A patient suffering from this type of infection should be immediately hospitalized if possible, and a culture should be taken to determine the type of infecting organism. In dealing with such an infection, I think that both sulfadiazine and penicillin should be started at once. Sulfadiazine should be given in amounts necessary to establish and maintain a blood level of 15 to 20 mg. per 100 cc of blood. The initial dose of penicillin should be 40,000 to 60,000 units followed with 15,000 to 20,000 un. q. 3 h. until the infection is brought under control. These patients should be watched carefully for signs and symptoms of mastoiditis and intracranial complications.

COMMENT

The post auricular edema and swelling that occurs in infants and young children in the early stages of an acute ototis media even to the extent of displacing the auricle downward and forward is not an indication for mastoid surgery; free incision of the drum membrane and the establishment of adequate drainage results in a rapid disappearance of the edema with complete recovery in a short time. However, post auricular edema, associated with redness, pain and tenderness, that appears at an interval of 2 weeks or longer after the onset of acute otitis media in infants or adults must be viewed with grave concern; such a condition almost invariably indicates a surgical mastoiditis; in older children, due to extensive pneumatization of the mastoid, swelling may occur in the zygomatic region above and in front of the auricle.

In performing a paracentesis on infants, one frequently notes that on piercing the drum membrane, the knife does not fall into a cavity but meets resistance; this occurs because of a thickened swollen embryonal type of mucous membrane; in these cases it is often necessary to reopen the ear once or twice daily for several times before free drainage is established and maintained; the above condition is found occasionally in older children and infrequently in adults; such cases are prone to become chronic if neglected or improperly treated.

In the administration of a sulfonamide in the treatment of acute otitis media, the drug should be started early; the dosage should be adequate; it should be continued for several days after al lsymptoms have subsided, and care shquld be exercised to prevent toxic reactions. What seems to be a practice, in scme localities, of prescribing a total of 12 tablets with instructions to stop the drug as soon as the temperature reaches normal or. when the prescribed 12 tablets have been taken cannot be too strongly condemned.

CONCLUSIONS

1. Acute otitis media is the first in a chain of complications that may follow upper respiratory disease.

2. Untreated or improperly treated acute otitis media is often complicated by acute surgical mastoiditis, chronic otitis media and mastoiditis with partial deafness and chronic surgical mastoiditis. Meningitis, brain abscess, lateral sinus thrombosis, septicemia and labyrinthitis are some of the more serious but less frequent complications.

3. In the treatment of this disease, if the organism is identified and the proper chemotherapeutic drug administered in adequate doses for a sufficient period of time; and if free drainage is established and maintained in association with thorough cleansing of the canal, rapid recovery in most cases will occur, thus preserving the hearing and preventing other and more serious complications.

4. All cases of acute otitis media that do not recover satisfactorily, within a reasonable length of time, should be referred to a competent otologist.

BIBLIOGRAPHY

1. George Morrison Coates: Middle Ear and Mastoid Infection in the Infant as a Focus of Systemic Disease; Archives of Pediatrics; May, 1930.

2. George Morrison Coates: Mastoid Infection in the Infant; Annals of Otology, Rhinology and Laryngology, Volume No. 36, pp. 931-924; December, 1927.

3. Oscar V. Batson: Surgical Anatomy of the Temporal Bone; Surgery of the Ear, Kopetzky, page 132; 1938.

4. J. D. Singleton: Pneumatization of the Adult Temporal Bone, the Mastoid Portion; An Anatomic and Clinical Study, The Laryngoscope, Volume No. 54, page 324; July, 1944.

5. Lyle M. Sellers: Clinico-Pathologic Observations of Otitis Media and Paratympanitus; Annals of Otology, Rhinology and Laryngology, Volume No. 46, page 1074; December, 1937.

6. S. J. Kopetzky: Otologic Surgery, page 4; 1929.

7. Adolph G. DeSanctis, Vincent P. Larkin: Otitis Media and Mastoiditis in Children. The American Medical Association Journal, Volume No. 120, page 1087; December 5, 1942.

Low Spinal Anesthesia in Obstetrics*

PHIL RISSER, M.D., BLACKWELL, OKLA.

ROY EMANUEL, M.D., CHICKASHA, OKLA.

We are convinced that spinal anesthesia for labor and delivery is a procedure which should have a foremost place among the many analgesic and anesthetic methods used. We realize that the subject is a controversial one and that a series of 118 cases is not large enough to permit final conclusions. However, we do feel that our cases have been so carefully observed that, by analysis, we can show that this procedure, if used properly, is a step toward making childbirth safer for mother and newborn while at the same time affording the mother more comfort than other methods now used, caudal excepted.

We are reporting a series of 118 consecutive deliveries under spinal anesthesia. We have worked independently and these cases represent approximately one-third of the patients delivered by us over a two year period. The initial breakdown shows 76 primiparous patients, 23 para one and 19 para two or more. Twenty-three delivered spontaneously, 70 were delivered with outlet forceps, 19 with corrective forceps or other manipulative procedure, and 6 by Caesarian section. Three breech presentations occurred in the entire group, and one set of twins. Of the breech presentations, one delivered spontaneously and the other two were extracted.

It is important to explain what appears to be a high percentage of operative deliveries. We routinely use outlet forceps and episiotomy in the delivery of primipara, or in patients of any parity where the perineal tissues are retarding delivery of the head. Spinal anesthesia was chosen in these cases because it is the anesthesia which most facilitates delivery; the operative procedure was in no case made necessary by the use of spinal. We would use spinal in many more cases which deliver spontaneously, except for the fact that we have not yet yearned how early spinal anesthesia can be introduced in multipara, and so are unable to use it because we misjudge the rate of progress in labor. I mention this because the large number of operative deliveries might, by

some, be attributed to the type of anesthetic used.

In contradistinction to outlet forceps, we use the term corrective forceps to designate those cases in which they were used to correct an unfavorable position of the presenting part, or to bring the head down from pelvic planes above the outlet. Here again the anesthetic was chosen for this type of delivery and cannot be considered a causative factor of the abnormality. In deliveries of this kind it is the infant's life which is more greatly jeopardized. It is accepted that the degree of respiratory depression of the baby increases directly in proporation to the length and amount of inhalation anesthesia administered to the mother. We are convinced that spinal anesthesia is the anesthesia of choice in these cases because it does not add to the shock which the baby exhibits as a result of the strenuous delivery. A second reason is the great increase in the ease of these deliveries which follows the complete relaxation obtained.

It should be emphasized here that spinal anesthesia is not to be used for cases requiring version. This is because the regular uterine contractions of labor continue with undiminished tone and so render such maneuvers extremely dangerous, as well as difficult.

For years it has been considered that spinal anesthesia for obstetrics is unsafe because it predisposes to circulatory collapse. This may be the case in the hypertensive patient, but in normal patients it definitely is not true. We think this belief originated in the days when spinal anesthesia was in its infancy and the possibility of shock was great in any case where it was used, regardless of the type of operative work. It was inevitably so, considering the lack of experience and the uncertain drugs used. We know now that the formerly inexplicable sudden death was the result of the anesthetic drug ascending too high in the spinal canal, and not of any supposed change in abdominal pressure.

There were no maternal deaths in the series. Only one patient showed a degree of shock which necessitated active treatment. In this case, it followed a long manipulative

*Delivered before Section on Obstetrics and Gynecology, Oklahoma State Medical Association Annual Meeting, May 1, 1946.

delivery and occurred three hours after the introduction of the anesthesia, and cannot be considered as due to the type of anesthetic. the patient responded promptly to routine measures. Spinal anesthesia, as we use it for obstetrical purposes, is actually far safer than it is for general surgery. The reasons are obvious. Smaller amounts of drug than are used for even the lowest abdominal surgery will give obstetrical anesthesia lasting from 2 to 4 hours. The drug is given in not more than one to one and one-half cc of liquid vehicle, with no barbotage. It is introduced low in the spinal canal — between L 3 and 4 or even between L 4 and 5 — while the patient is in such a position that her hips are lower than her shoulders. The patient's head is kept elevated on a pillow at all times after she is turned on her back. In a few cases these precautions will keep the anesthesia so low that labor pains will be incompletely relieved. Anesthesia will still be found adequate for any type of pelvic delivery and repair, and will last from 2 to 4 hours.

The number of infant deaths, three, is large for 118 deliveries. One was a hydrocephalic monster delivered by section. It's respirations were weak, and resuscitation was not attempted. The second was an infant delivered spontaneously, which looked good immediately following delivery. Respirations and heart-beat became steadily weaker, and in spite of all supportive measures it died. Autopsy revealed both kidneys to be cystic to the extent that it was difficult to find any normal kidney tissue. The third did not survive a long, difficult manipulative delivery. None of these deaths can in any way be attributed to the type of anesthesia.

Of the remaining infants delivered, only two were cyanotic enough to cause the obstetrician to use restorative measures. Both of these responded promptly to the administration of CO_2 and O_2. I think this is significant, in view of the fact that there were 19 difficult deliveries 3 breech presentations, and 6 sections. Excepting the hydrocephalic, not one infant delivered by section needed resuscitation. This speaks more eloquently than anything else of the value of spinal anesthesia as a means of reducing neo-natal mortality. It is pharmacologically impossible for drugs of the cocain series, introduced intra-spinally, to in any way depress the baby. Slowing of the fetal heart can be detected following the induction of spinal anesthesia in the mother. I ascribe no clinical importance to this, in view of the excellent condition of the infants after delivery. Since the factors responsible for variations in fetal heart rate during uterine contractions are

ceiving intravenous Ergotrate showed no tendency to bleed. The greatest amount of blood loss in a single patient was 360 cc, and several bled so little that the drapes were not stained. The old belief which has been often repeated, that spinal anesthesia in delivery was attended by increased bleeding and danger of hemorrhage, is not substantiated by observation.

Blood loss in cases delivered by section could not be measured, so these cases were omitted in calculating averages. We can only say that bleeding was not profuse and shock did not occur in any case of section.

The length of labor in these patients is also a matter of interest. Again we were forced to reduce the number of cases analyzed to 65 because of lack of accurate figures for the remainder. These are not selected cases. The truth is that a sleepy practitioner neglected to record his data on some cases, and so they could not be used. In computing average length of labor we considered the patients only as primiparous or multiparous. No attempt was made to divide the time in labor into first, second ,and third, stages. The average length of labor in the 38 primiparous patients included was 14 hours. The average multiparous labor was 7 hours and 30 minutes, the average being figured on the remaining 28 cases.

so poorly understood, and since the amount of slowing, if detected, is slight, I cannot feel that it indicates any danger to the child. A possible explanation may be that the expansion of the arterial bed in the anesthetized area results in increased oxygenation of the infant's blood and reflex slowing of the heart.

This does not mean that there is an increased tendency to bleeding following delivery. The amount of blood loss was recorded in only 66 of our cases. The average estimated blood loss in this group was slightly less than 100 cc. Most of the patients were given an ampoule of Ergotrate, intravenously, as the anterior shoulder was delivered. While this undoubtedly reduces blood loss during the third stage of labor, we feel that the maintained tone of the uterus is the essential factor that explains why the average blood loss in our patients was less than the average stated in textbooks. Patients not re-

In spite of these figures, it is difficult to answer the question as to whether or not spinal anesthesia administered in the second stage of labor prolongs labor. It is certainly true that some patients with well established, active, and regular contractions wil lap-. parently become less active following the introduction of spinal anesthesia. Contractions continue regularly, but they become less frequent and. of somewhat shorter duration.

However, I cannot recall any patient in active second or late first stage labor at the time of introduction of spinal, in whom the contractions become less frequent than every 4 or 5 minutes. In some cases there will even be some apparent loss of progress—the head will seem higher on rectal examination and the dilatation slightly less. This probably is what has convinced some that labor is prolonged by the use of spinal anesthesia.

Our feeling is that labor has become less violent without becoming less effective. I do not believe that it is necessary for a woman to become the straining, suffering figure that we have so long accepted as an essential step in successful labor. In my opinion the possibility of less violent labor is more than offset by the great relaxation of the cervix and perineum. It is impossible for the woman in labor to grip the sides of the table with her hands, brace all of the muscles of her lower extremities and abdomen, close her glottis, and "bear down," and leave her perineal muscles relaxed. In addition there is the reflex spasm of the perineal muscles as they are forcefully spread and over-stretched by the advancing presenting part. It is these soft tissues that are the only barrier to progress after engagement of the head in the normal pelvis. If they are completely relaxed the extreme voluntary effort of the patient does not need to be added to the power of the uterine contractions to force the presenting part over the perineum.

The patient under spinal anesthesia can still "bear down," though she must be told when she is having a contraction. Furthermore, she is free from pain and fear and cooperative in every possible way. Now, as she strains with her voluntary muscles, her expulsive force is no longer actively opposed by the soft tissues of the birth canal. I have on several occasions seen the cervical dilatation progress from two fingers at the time the spinal was given to complete dilatation in the course of three hard uterine contractions.

An obstetrician using spinal anesthesia very soon comes to disagree with the teaching that voluntary effort on the part of the patient is necessary for progress during the second stage of labor. He disagrees because he repeatedly observes the complete fulfillment of the mechanism in this stage without any use of the voluntary muscles by the patient. Recently one of us had a para one with a breech presentation to deliver. Spinal anesthesia was introduced when dilatation of the cervix was complete. The patient had been given Demerol and hyoscin and almost immediately after the anesthetic took effect,

was asleep. The presenting breech was well above the perineum and it was estimated it would be one or two hours before she could be delivered. Called back less than fifteen minutes later, it was found that while she had continued to sleep, and with no voluntary effort, the patient had precipitated a 7 pound 14 ounce baby — restituting the shoulders and delivering the head without manual aid of any kind and without even a mucosal tear. The placenta was in the vagina and was easily expelled with fundal pressure. The amount of bleeding was so small that the linens were not stained.

The disgraceful mismanagement of this case is being reported because it demonstrates that while labor may become apparently less active after introduction of spinal anesthesia, it will not necessarily be prolonged. The figures on our few cases bear this out. We feel that it is unimportant, for if labor is slightly proloned, the increase in comfort and safety afforded the mother and child will surely be worth a little more of the physician's time.

In cases where spinal anesthesia is only for delivery this question does not arise.

In concluding, we want to make a few points clear so that we will not be misunderstood. We are not proposing that spinal anesthesia in obstetrics is the best solution to the problem of analgesia and anesthesia for childbirth. We do not advocate or encourage its use by all physicians practicing obstetrics.

On the other hand, for us it has yielded good results, and we believe that the study of our cases justifies our use of it and entitles us to doubt the objections commonly raised. In summarizing, we would say that it is a valuable procedure in the hands of any physician experienced in the use of spinal anesthesia who will adhere to a systematic technique, is willing to give all the time necessary to the patient in labor, and who will respect certain definite contra-indications.

Under these limitations, we maintain that it offers a safe, satisfactory and convenient way to deliver obstetrical patients with the greatest freedom from pain, compatible with the greatest possible safety to them and their newborn babies. We urge open minded consideration of the method.

DISCUSSION

ALBERT D. FOSTER, M.D.

OKLAHOMA CITY, OKLAHOMA

There can be little argument over the efficacy of spinal anesthesia in relieving the pain and discomforts of childbirth, and few persons will dispute the statement that the method affords no direct pharmacologic depression of the fetus. Therefore, any discussion of a presentation of a series of obstetrical cases in which spinal anesthesia is employed will be concerned with the relative safety of the method to the mother.

All methods of anesthesia carry a certain definite risk to the patient. In rare instances the risk may be ascribed to an undesirable side-effect of the drug, but the majority of anesthetic difficulties are related to the technique of administration; some are unavoidable, others are distinct technical errors on the part of the anesthetist. Therefore, the safety of any anesthetic method depends mainly upon the ability of the anesthetist. Spinal anesthesia is relatively safe only if it is properly conducted and the patient is constantly attended by one who is versed in the art of resuscitation. It is not a safe method when used by the surgeon as a substitute for the constant attendance of an anesthetist or as an alternate method in the absence of adequate equipment for resuscitative purposes.

The hazards of spinal anesthesia are primarily those of alterations in the circulatory status of the patient. Spinal anesthesia alone without concomitant surgery is an insult to normal circulatory processes. Paralysis of sympathetic nerves with resultant vasodilatation in the anesthetized areas demands a compensatory vasoconstriction in the unanesthetized areas if peripheral circulation and blood pressure are to be maintained. This is the chief objection to spinal anesthesia in major procedures where severe blood loss is anticipated or for patients who are in a state of surgical shock. Not only is a portion of the compensatory vascular bed paralyzed, but that portion which remains intact is already in a state of partial vasoconstrictive activity which has been necessitated by the circulatory changes induced by the spinal anesthetic itself. Thus, it becomes obvious that the level of spinal anesthesia must be kept as low as is consistent with adequate relief from pain, if adverse circulatory effects are to be minimized and if as much of the vascular bed as possible is to be kept in a state where it is capable of compensation for insult such as blood loss and trauma incident to the surgical procedure. A level of sensory anesthesia as high as the tenth thoracic segment (skin anesthesia level at the umbilicus) is adequate to provide relief from pain accompanying uterine contractions. A higher level adds nothing to the comfort of the patient, but merely increases the hazard of circulatory complications. Spinal anesthesia which is sufficiently high to cause paralysis of even the lower intercostal muscles adds to the respiratory embarrassment which the parturient suffers in common with

other patients who have huge abdominal tumors and whose respiratory movements are predominantly thoracic in character because of the abdominal interference with diaphragmatic activity.

"Spinal anesthesia calamities" usually appear with dramatic suddenness and within the first twenty minutes following the injection of the anesthetic drug. In less than five minutes, a patient who appears to be perfectly normal and with adequate circulation may progress to a state of complete collapse in which he is pulseless, without respiration, and appears to be dead — indeed if treatment is not instituted immediately, the latter appearance will become permanent.

Circulatory collapse and respiratory failure constitute the most important complications of spinal anesthesia.

Circulatory collapse is characterized by subnormal blood pressure, pale blanched skin and mucous membranes, anxiety, restlessness, nausea, syncope, and in extreme instances — death. Treatment is usually a simple matter if instituted within one to two minutes of the onset of this complication. 50 mg. of ephedrine administered intravenously will generally correct the situation by enhancing the vasoconstrictive activity in the unanesthetized areas and by increasing cardiac output. The state of circulatory collapse induced by the spinal anesthetic per se should be differentiated from this due to true surgical shock which occurs during the operative procedure, generally following severe loss of blood. In the latter instance, the treatment differs; it should be constituted of measures designed to restore the circulating blood volume — namely, fluid replacement preferably by transfusion of whole blood.

Respiratory failure is the other important complication of spinal anesthesia. This may be due to diaphragmatic paralysis if the anesthetic drug has reached a sufficiently high level to anesthetize the motor components of the third to fifth cervical nerves. This is a rare occurrence — generally the anesthetic drug is sufficiently dilute by the time it ascends to such a level that it anesthetizes only the sensory and autonomic nerve fibers, while the more resistant motor roots remain unaffected. Nonetheless, respiratory failure is not an uncommon complication of spinal anesthesia. In most instances interference with respiratory activity is due to depression of the respiratory center by cerebral anemia resulting from circulatory collapse. The treatment of this state consists of artificial inflation of the lungs with oxygen and the immediate intravenous administration of a "vasopressor" drug — ephedrine, which is generally readily available in any operating room, is satisfactory. None of the newer synthetic vasopressor drugs has been conclusively demonstrated to have any definite superiority over ephedrine. Analeptic drugs such as Coramine and Metrazol should never be used — not that they do harm, but that they do no good, and their administration frequently delays prompt initiation of proper resuscitative measures which are (1) 50 mg. of ephedrine intravenously, and (2) artificial respiration with oxygen *delivered to the lungs through a clear airway.*

If a surgeon elects to induce spinal anesthesia in patients whom he expects to deliver, he may do so with safety only if he is well versed in the art of resuscitation and is willing to remain by the patient's side in constant supervision. Once the operative procedure is to commence, he may then delegate to an assistant the details of observation, including the recording of blood pressure and pulse rate at frequent intervals, and at the first indications of trouble he must be willing to drop everything else to attend to resuscitative measures — temporizing for but a few moments may result in either a serious temporary complication or even fatality.

Providing the technique of spinal anesthesia is satisfactory and a proper level of anesthesia is attained, dangerous complications will be few and far between, i.e., one in several hundred cases; nonetheless, the hazard is real and the penalties so great that every case demands the closest possible attention. Practically all "spinal anesthesia deaths" are avoidable — fatality is generally the result of either negligence or improper or delayed attempts at resuscitation.

The safety of any method of anesthesia depends primarily upon the anesthetist, secondarily upon the method or choice of drug.

The Practical Treatment of Neuroses*

M. P. PROSSER, M.D.

NORMAN, OKLAHOMA

The neurosis is a disordered functioning of the personality, and it must be differentiated from the normal personality, from the psychotic or insane personality, and from the personality distorted by organic disease. The symptoms of the psychoneuroses are generally considered as an alternative for normal conduct; and reality changes are only quantitative in the neuroses, while they are qualitative in the psychoses.

In considering the importance of a psychoneurosis and treatment of a psychoneurotic disorder, one must consider the entire personality of the individual who is suffering the neurosis. The balance between the individual's assets and liabilities must be taken into account. An individual with many personality assets will not appear very neurotic although he may have a degree of neurotic phenomena which would cripple a less capable individual. The question always to be answered in treatment, and repeatedly during treatment, is, "How do the assets and the liabilities of this particular personality now balance?" At this point it should be mentioned that in some instances the neurosis should not be treated but should be left undisturbed, for it may well be functioning as a useful defense to preserve the integrity of the personality from unmodifiable and intolerable environmental forces.

Several types of neuroses are encountered and commonly described, but the classification I shall use is that employed by military services, inasmuch as this classification has been used constantly, and per force, by the single largest group of physicians to use any single classification. This group begins with:

A.   The normal personality with neurotic traits, manifested by transitory emotional disturbances and mildly unprofitable responses to difficult environmental situations. These persons are seen frequently and their disorders should be summarily handled during their early visits to a physician. They may be seen again on other occasions with

*Delivered before the Section on Neurology, Psychiatry and Endocrinology, Oklahoma State Medical Association Annual Meeting, May 2, 1946.

similar disturbances, but they will rarely develop a chronic neurotic pattern of behavior unless encouraged by over treatment or too much sympathy. Poor treatment of this type lends dignity to thei rdisorder and gives the personality an unwarranted secondary gain (in attention, lifting of responsibility, and emotional support) that makes the development of a chronic neurotic pattern an almost normal response.

B. The psychoneurotic personality, warped by emotional conflict or stunted from the maturity of independent thinking and feeling, and developing, in the face of disappointment, one or more of the following distorted reaction patterns:

1. Anxiety — tension states, with or without.
2. Hypochondriasis
3. Hysteria
4. Neurasthenia
5. Obsessive — compulsive disorders
6. Reactive depressions.

B-1 Anxiety states manifest themselves through attacks of fear of disaster, tremors, perspiration, dyspnea and palpitation. This is a normal response to real and impending danger, but in the neurotic personality it frequently results from a trigger-like reaction to some event which threatens the return of repressed memory or wish.

B-2 Hypochondriasis is a defensive conversion in which the anxiety, mentioned above, has been transferred to an organ or organ system, with resultant overconcern for the organ selected. The afflicted personality is otherwise found to be empty and considerable difficulty is encountered in developing a normal affection for other persons. The heart and digestive apparatus are common seats for these hypochondriacal trends.

B-3 Hysteria, resulting from an essential personality conflict which has been solved by the conversion of psychic tension to the production of a physical complaint, is usually manifested by a disturbance of sensation or function. When hysteria is monosymptomatic, such as a hemi-paralysis, or pain in a particular area, it may be very difficult to diagnose.

B-4 Neurasthenia, occurring as a by-product of excessive repression, is manifested by chronic fatigue, introspection, and vague unorganized somatic complaints.

B-5 the obsessive-compulsive disorders, (also termed psychasthenia and the obsessive-ruminative tension states) are manifested by fears, compulsions and rituals; and are associated with mental mechanisms frequently approaching psychotic degree.

B-6 Reactive depressions, resulting from actually depressing circumstances, are mani-fested by exaggerated and prolonged despondency which far exceeds the normal response to the depressing event. This particular disorder actually belongs in the affective or "mood-swing" group, rather than to the true neuroses, and it is frequently seen in those individuals who later develop Manic-Depressive or Involutional psychoses. The treatment of this disorder is based upon the same premise as the treatment of the psychoses named, and such patients must be carefully watched for suicidal efforts.

C. Character neuroses, occurring most commonly in cultured people who are making a satisfactory social adjustment. Usually no symptoms are apparent to an outsider, but the personality has been internally modified through compromising with the neurotic trend. The individual can usually recognize the disorder himself by finding some things very difficult to do, which ordinarily should be easily accomplished. The mode of living is narrowed, and occasionally life becomes intolerable. Hypertension, digestive disturbances, skin conditions, allergies, hyperthyroidism, and other psychosomatic disorders occur in people having character neuroses. Unfortunately, this disorder is most difficult to approach and usually the symptoms prove most unyielding to our present day knowledge of psychoterapy. Here the patient's understanding of the cause and mechanisms involved in the production of the disease does not produce an alleviation of symptoms; and when improvement is achieved, it is usually due to changes in the environment rather than in the personality.

In approaching the treatment of the psychoneurotic personality, we should look for positive rather than negative signs of the neuroses. A lack of evidence of organic disease to explain the patient's complaint is not enough, for we do not know that we, as physicians, understand all organic syndromes, as yet. We cannot be sure how severe or prolonged the pain will be in, for example, a wrenched knee under all circumstances. Then too, the psychoneurotic may be organically ill as well, and this presents an insurmountable problem if exclusion of organic disease is used as the basis for diagnosis.

Therefore, in approaching the diagnosis of our patient we cannot deal with a simple dichotomy of organic or psychoneurotic disease. We have, instead, to differentiate between:

1. Organic illnesses involving primarily structural changes.
2. Functional, but not personality-integrated illness, such as hemic murmurs and fatigue following toxic disease.
3. Psychosomatic diseases, such as angioneurotic edema, gastric ulcers, asth-

ma and rheumatoid arthritis, where both organic and psychic factors co-operate to produce or precipitate clinical syndromes. (The character neuroses).

4. Transitory, easily dispelled neurotic traits occurring in stable personalities under great stress.

5. Personality d i s o r d e r s producing chronic somatic complaints. (the psychoneuroses and psychoses).

6. Hypersuggestibility, or poor verbal reporting by a mentally defective; confusing any clinical picture.

7. More or less conscious exaggeration of organic complaints by a person who has something to gain.

8. Frank malingering.

Treatment of the neuroses is largely dependent upon the development of the art of interviewing the patient. During the interview, positive evidence of the disorder may be accumulated, and subsequent treatment planned accordingly. Neurotic phenomena demanding treatment are:

I. ANXIETY. Anxiety operates in producing psychoneurotic symptoms in a way similar to bacterial action in producing an infectious disease. Anxiety may be recognized in the form of:

a. Free floating anxiety, with fear of impending disaster, dyspnea, palpitation, etc.

b. Anxiety dreams.

c. Excitement, with trembling and hyperidrosis.

d. Apprehension, with anxious expectation, or

e. Reasonless worry.

II. Manifestations of defenses against anxiety. These neurotic symptoms are comparable to the inflammatory process the body employs in combating bacterial infections. These appear as:

a. Character traits; excessive ambition, orderliness, cleanliness, petulancy, parsimony, etc.

b. Hysterical conversions: pain, anesthesia, blindness, paralysis, amnesia, etc.

c. Regression: enuresis, oral activities, alcoholism, and dependency.

d. Compulsions, tics, rituals, hand-washing, etc.

e. Hypochondriasis; diet fads, exercises, enema artists, and patent medicine addicts.

f. Phobias: Aerophobia, hemophobia, claustrophobia, etc.

g. Exaggerated alertness: hypersensitivity to noise and light, car sickness, increased muscle tension,

startle reaction, irritability, restlessness, and self-consciousness.

III. Manifestations of by-products between anxiety and psychic events. These may be compared to pus exuded from an infection. They appear as:

a. Fatigue

b. Backache

c. Headache

d. Moodiness and depression.

With these diagnostic aids well in mind, we can now consider the practical treatment of the neuroses. Treatment is logically divided into prophylactic measures and therapeutic procedures.

Prophylactic measures, or mental hygiene, are particularly important in the adequate care of patients suffering organic diseases, or injuries, or those who are to be subjected to surgical procedures. Such patients are in anxiety producing situations, and are prone to suffer not only pain of their illness, but the anguish provoked by the threat of death, of financial insecurity, or the loss of their emotional security in the household. This anguish provokes psychosomatic visceral responses which may in turn produce even more anxiety and dread. Good mental hygiene consists of orienting the individual not only to the nature of his organic illness, but in explaining to him the mechanisms and meaning of the symptoms of anxiety which he suffers. The man who is to have his gall stones removed may suffer additional and unnecessary dread because of palpitation of emotional origin. He may fear that he also has some heart disease which will take his life during the coming operation. And the man hurt in an industrial accident may develop chronic functional headaches and anorexia of compensable degree unless he is quickly enlightened regarding the relative normalcy of these disorders in a fear producing situation.

In turning to the therapy of the neuroses, it cannot be emphasized too strongly that success is largely dependent upon the art of interviewing the patient. This requires time and patience, and the physician who will understand his patient will allow the patient to speak freely and fully about the problems which concern him. He must impart to the patient, by attitudes and implication, that he is capable of understanding (rather than sympathy). He must imply he is not satisfied with the initial recitation of the patient's symptoms, which usually have been rehearsed on many occasions for family and various physicians.

With this approach perfected, the physician will frequently find that the patient has a fairly good understanding of the situational factors precipitating his disorder, but has hesitated to tie cause and fear together because of fear of being ridiculed, or fear that some organic disease is also present. This latter fear is particularly common because of the emphasis placed upon "watching for early signs of organic disease" during the past few decades.

Frequently the physician finds that the patient can be satisfactorily adjusted and his symptoms relieved in a few interviews, if only he can be assisted in successfuly working out the problems of the immediate precipitating cause. Definite decisions, aggressive behavior, and hard work to attain the desired success are the channels into which the physician must guide this patient. Throughout treatment, useful activity is important, and bed rest or unearned vacations have little value.

It is true that this brief form of treatment does little acquaint the patient with the basic personality disorders which made him susceptible to the development of his neurotic symptoms. But even leaders of the psychoanalytic school are now aware that this knowledge on the part of the patient is not necessary to successful and adequate treatment. Admittedly this brief therapy occupying only a few hours does not prevent future exaserbations of similar disorders, but even the most intensive forms of psychotherapy or shock therapy also fail to attain this goal upon occasion. While the application of this brief therapy is limited, it proves quite adequate in many cases where the symptom complex is of short duration; and especially satisfactory where the symptoms are dramatic in nature (i.e. Hysteria, Anciery-tension states, early Hypochondriasis and Neurasthenia-. One successful plan of brief therapy involves (1) the establishing of the relationship between the symptoms and the precipitating situation; (2) the development of a course of action whereby the patient may (3) the presentation of these two factors to the patient in a logical and acceptable manner, and (4) the forceful suggestion to the patient that "now you no longer need your symptom to defend you, for you have a more successful and more tolerable solution to the disturbing problem at hand". Too, suggestion backed by a good plan of action is far more permanent in its effect than is suggestion alone.

While intensive analysis of the patient's early emotional development is by no means necessary to good therapeutic results; a thorough knowledge of mental mechanisms, basic human motivations, and common emotional patterns are most helpful to the physician. This knowledge permits him many short cuts to the patient's problems. However, these "good guesses" must be employed with utmost caution for a poor guess destroys the patient's confidence in his doctor and strongly mitigates against response to treatment. Likewise, reassurance must be used sparingly and thoughtfully lest the patient feel that his doctor is simply discounting all symptoms.

The more chronic neuroses involving greater social or physical disability require other therapeutic approaches. In neurasthenia a reawakening of social interest and responsibility as a substitute for the regressive trend is quite successful. Philanthropic enterprises in which the patient may work out his own repressions through the lives of those he assists are especially beneficial. Frequently prolonged psychotherapy of a supportive nature is a necessary adjunct in such patients. The obsessive-compulsive states are most resistive to all forms of therapy and not infrequently do not respond, or respond only temporarily to intensive or prolonged psychotherapy, or to shock therapy .

The value of shock therapy in the treatment of the neuroses deserves consideration, both because of the dramatic recoveries frequently obtained, and the organic damage and mental deterioration which occasionally follow in its wake. A review of th ecurrent literature[3][4][5] reveals almost uniformly good results in Reactive Depressions, and uniform attenuation of the depressive features in other neurotic states. Anxiety is usually temporarily relieved, but frequently recurs as the amnesias associated with shock disappear. The conversion hysterias or hypochondriacs respond well at first, but too frequently new symptoms appear and the total results are discouraging. The obsessive compulsive states respond only fairly well, but always require prolonged treatment and relapses are common. Hysterias respond least of all, and frequently are made worse and more anxious. Certainly, if shock therapy is to be used in the neuroses, it should be only an adjunct of active and continuous psychotherapy; and many workers report excellent results with the combination where no results were evident with one alone.[4][6][7]

No discussion of practical treatment would be complete without commenting upon narcoanalysis. The most useful agents are intravenous sodium amytal and sodium pentathol in relief of acute anxiety states and the hysterias. Emotional ventilation can be easily obtained in the hypnotic states which results from their use and the patient is found highly suggestible. Recently nitrous oxide as a hypnotic agent for narco-analytic procedures has been suggested,[9] and its quick recovery period offers definite advantages. Narco-analysis involves constant psychotherapy, as the name implies, and efforts at treatment through sedation alone are usually quite sterile.

Group psychotherapy, a recent development in the practical treatment of the neuroses, received great impetus during the war through its widespread use in the military services. This form of therapy is an admixture of mental hygiene lectures, patriotic or social enthusiasm, group hypnotism, and semi-public self-analyses under the guidance of a physician or leader. Results obtained appear to depend largely on the degree of enthusiasm developed within the group; and the individuals enjoying the greatest improvement were usually those who developed the greatest interest in helping other members of the group to get well. This form of therapy appears to have very limited applications in civilian society, though it can be employed to sustain large groups of mildly unstable individuals, with common interests, at a productive level.[10][11] Alcoholics Anonymous makes practical use of this principle in their activities and group meetings.

In conclusion, there are many practical approaches to the treatment of the neuroses, but all hinge upon the art of interviewing the patient and tactfully persuading him to abandon his neurotic symptoms for more useful channels of behavior and emotional response. Healing usually comes as the patient shares his problem with the understanding physician, and relief with the realization that his early and now meaningless traumatic emotions are transposed to contemporary people and situations. Re-education and adequate orientation are important adjuncts, but the main theme of successful adjustment must be work, useful work, well directed work, and purposeful work.

BIBLIOGRAPHY

1. Frank J. Muehler: Nature of the Neuroses, Army Medical Bulletin, July, 1943.
2. Franz G. Alexander: Indications for Psychonalytic Therapy, Bulletin New York Academy of Medicine; June, 1944.
3. Lother B. Kolinski, et al: Electric Convulsive Therapy of Neuroses, Archives of Neurology and Psychiatry; December, 1944.
4. Elsworth F. Baker: Analysis of Convulsive Therapy, Psychiatric Quarterly; Jan. 1945.
5. Harry Gauss: Treatment of the Neuroses, American Journal Digestive Diseases; August, 1944.
6. John W. Bick, Jr.: Problem of Severe Psychoneurotic, American Journal Psychiatry; September, 1945.
7. Robert B. McElroy: Anxiety Neuroses, American Journal Psychiatry; January, 1945.
8. Roy F. Grinker: Neuropsychiatric Experiences Eighth Air Force; 1945.
9. C. H. Rodgerson: Narco Analysis with Nitrous Oxide. British Medical Journal; June 17, 1944.
10. Sam B. Hadden: Group Psychotherapy, American Journal Psychiatry; July, 1944.
11. Howard R. Rome: Group Psychotherapy, American Journal Psychiatry, January, 1945.

Nasal Fractures[*]

O. ALTON WATSON, M.D.

OKLAHOMA CITY, OKLAHOMA

I have chosen the subject of nasal fracture because I feel that it is a neglected one, and thought it would be instructive to review some of the facts we have known and perhaps partially forgotten; to bring out any new ideas that have been developed and to present a few case histories that emphasize certain fundamental points.

Fracture of the nose has not, at least in our own locality, been managed by one group of physicians. It has been shunted back and forth between the Orthopedist and the Rhinologist, neither taking a special interest in the condition, with the result that many patients have been neglected and others mismanaged. To my mind it matters little which group takes care of these patients provided the patient is in the hands of a physician who is thoroughly familiar with the anatomy and physiology of the nose and who has had sufficient surgical training and experience to repair damage to the soft or supporting structures.

ANATOMY

The nose is a triangular pyramid which projects anteriorly between the orbits. The framework is made up of a bony and cartilaginous portion, covered by skin and lined with thick mucous membrane. The bony portion consists of two nasal bones, supported by the perpendicular plate of the ethmoid and by the frontal processes of the superior maxilla. The cartilaginous part comprises the cartilaginous septum uniting with the upper lateral cartilages; two independent lower lateral cartilages, and several minor

*Delivered before Section on Eye, Ear, Nose and Throat, Oklahoma State Medical Association Annual Meeting, Wednesday, May 1, 1946.

accessory sesamoid cartilages. The arterial supply of the nose is chiefly from the external carotid but the root and bridge of the nose is supplied with branches from the ophthalmic branch of the internal carotid. The sensory nerve supply is from the first and second division of the trigeminal. The only motor nerve is a branch of the facial, which is distributed to the alar muscles. This is of great practical significance if one desires to watch the action of the facial nerve when performing a mastoidectomy. The anesthetist may be directed to watch the ala of the nose. With each inspiration they will be seen to dilate, showing continued function of the facial nerve. This can be observed much more easily than the larger less frequent movement of the muscles of expression, thus giving earlier warning if one is dangerously near the facial nerve.

DIAGNOSIS

A history of injury to the nose, associated with nosebleed, ecchymosis about the eyes, is presumptive evidence of a nasal fracture. Pain is usually not pronounced. Inspection early may reveal a flattening of the nasal bridge or a displacement to one side of the midline. Later swelling may partially obliterate the deformity. Intranasal examination frequently reveals a laceration of the mucous membrane, hemorrhage, or edema. Palpation is of great value and can be performed without great pain if done gently. Often one may grasp the nasal bridge between the thumb and forefinger, gently pull it to right or left and feel a distinct movement between the separated fragments. This is of course positive evidence of fracture. X-ray is of little value in fractures of lateral wall but is very helpful in determining the presence and extent of fracture involving the nasal bridge. I have two slides which illustrate this condition. A lateral view is more informative than an antero-posterior view. Another useful procedure is to hold a straight applicator against the face so that it bisects the forehead and extends downward over the center of the lip, thus revealing whether the nose is in the midline or not.

TREATMENT

I. Recent fractures:

a. Lateral displacements. If the fragments are not locked or impacted it is usually a simple matter to anesthetize the nose both intranasally with Cocaine or Pontocaine and externally with a small amount of Novocaine then with a gauze covered thumb, force the bony fragments back into place. If the fragments are not movable, it is because the nasal bones after fracture have been driven down beneath the projecting edge of the frontal process of the superior maxilla. They can be released by applying Walsham forceps, or a large Kelly protected with rubber

tubing and by gently lifting or rocking the impacted fragments will snap back into place.

b. Depressed nose:

Means a fracture of the nasal bone. The location of the depression may be anywhere from the junction of the nasal bone with the frontal bone down to the lower border of the nasal bone. This type of fracture is demonstrated readily with a lateral x-ray view, or can usually be detected by sliding the forefinger along the bridge of the nose, feeling a depression where the fracture has occurred. The treatment consists of anesthetizing the part and with a heavy elevator or small forcep, pushing the bone back in place. A forefinger should be placed over the nasal bone externally to guide in the replacement. There is frequently a combination of lateral displacement and depression but the same principles of treatment should be applied.

2. Old Nasal Fractures: The diagnosis presents no difficulty, because the swelling is gone and the deformity may be seen at a glance. In addition to the deformity there is usually associated a disturbed physiology, i.e., a difficulty in breathing. I should like to emphasize the fact that reconstruction of a nose with an old unreduced fracture is not usually done for appearance only. Nearly all these patients have a badly deviated septum which requires surgical management and in most cases the combination of straightening the external nose and performing a submucous resection of the septum at the same time gives a better functional result than if either or both procedures are done separtely. An added advantage is that in cases of nasal depression, cartilage from the septum may be utilized to build up the defect. I have some pictures which illustrate a case of this kind.

1. Lateral Fractures:

In brief, the nose must be mobilized by subperiosteal saw incision through the bone, along the nasolabial grooves then the nose moved to its proper position and maintained in place with molded Stent dressing. I will spare you the details of this procedure except to state that the incision is in the lateral vesibule of each nostril. The periosteum is elevated and a right angle Joseph saw is used to cut two-thirds of the way through the bone, then by thumb pressure the bones are fractured laterally. Also necessary in this procedure is the freeing of the skin over the dorsum of the nose and the mobilization of the nasal bones one from the other and from the frontal bone. Naturally a resection or reconstruction of the nasal septum should be done at the same time as it allows easier mobilization of the entire nose.

2. Old Depressed Fractures:

There is no method by which the nasal bones can be raised and maintained in place after complete healing has taken place, so that the operation of choice is to repair the septum by submucous resection and if possible salvage enough cartilage and bone to fill in the defect. Two or three pieces of cartilage may be tied together with catgut to increase the thickness if desired. If there is not enough of this material fresh Costal Cartilage may be used.

Preserved septal cartilage and costal hyaline cartilage may also be used but they are not as satisfactory as fresh cartilage in that it tends to absorb in some cases.

I have a few pictures illustrating six different cases:

1. J.B.T.

·A victim of V. J. day celebration. The hump was present before his accident but one may notice the right convex side and the left concave side of the nasal bridge, due to recent fracture. In the head back position notice the twisted tip. This is a recent case and easily repaired but it is evident that in an old unreduced fracture of this sort, a submucous alone would not give good breathing space. In this case there was some impaction of the concave side so that the nasal bone had to be unlocked or freed before the nose could be pushed to the left. The result was excellent but I was unfortunate in not obtaining a picture as the patient left town in three or four days.

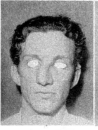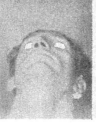

2. C.

This patient was hit with a beer bottle three days before I saw her. Her laceration had been repaired during the first few hours at an emergency room. The picture does not show the depression of the bridge as pronounced as was actually present but it can be seen, as also can the lateral deviation to the right. This patient also had a rather marked high septal deviation as might be expected. Her breathing was much better after replacements of the fragments. The other photograph shows a straight nose after replacement.

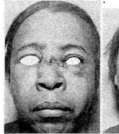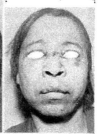

3. C. P.

This is a seventeen year old boy injured while playing football. He was known to have suffered a nasal fracture at the time and another physician reset it. I saw him one week after the accident and there was rather marked lateral deviation to the right and depression of the nasal bridge. X-ray shows a fracture of the nasal bone with drepression and also a fracture along the nasolobial groove. With this information it was not difficult to push the nasal ridge back into place. This was done with gas anesthesia and intranasal packing used to hold the bones in position for a few days.

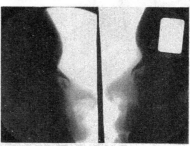

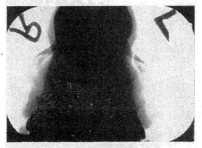

4. D. R.

This is practically the same as in the last case except there was not so much lateral displacement and there was more depression about the middle of the dorsum where the nasal bone may be seen depressed. This was repaired with local anesthesia.

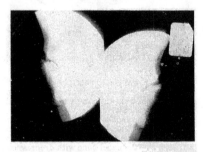

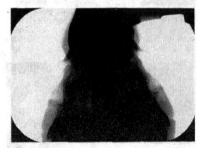

5. M. D. W.

This patient was injured in a car wreck and was treated elsewhere. He had other serious injuries which overshadowed his nasal ones, but a vertical laceration along the right side of the nose was repaired and the nose was "set." He came to me because of difficult breathing and because of the visible deformity. Notice the lateral deviation to the left and the rather marked saddle effect. Also note the twisted tip with the almost complete occlusion of the right nostril due to the dislocation of the cartilaginous septum out of the vomer groove.

This patient was operated under local anesthesia, a submucous resection of the septum with reconstruction of tip was done. Lateral osteotomy with mobilization of the nasal ridge was done. Part of the cartilage removed from the septum was utilized to fill in the saddle defect. One area in the old scar broke down and some serum escaped but healed promptly after a stitch was used to hold the cartilage grafts together was removed. The second group of pictures were taken about three weeks following operation.

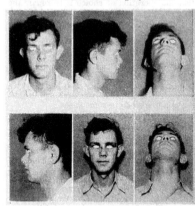

6. F. A. S.

This sixteen year old boy was kicked by a horse three years previously. He and his mother both felt that the deformity was such a distinct handicap. He also had considerable deviation of the septum. Submucous Resection was done and as in the previous case the septal cartilage was used to fill in the defect. There was some infection in the pocket made for the flap and a considerable part of his graft absorbed. Probably it will be necessary to use some Costal cartilage to replace this. I am sorry not to have pictures on this boy as they would show improvement but probably not a desirable result.

The best of a true life is its private part—*A. Bronson Alcott.*

The images of men's wits and knowledges remain in books, exempted from the wrong of time, and capable of perpetual renovation.—*Bacon: Advancement of Learning.*

My books are friends that never fail me. *Carlyle: Letter to his Mother, March 17, 1817.*

Classified Advertisements

FOR SALE: Well equipped 18 bed hospital industrial community. Excellent opportunity for doctor desiring to build practice. Write Box F, Journal, Oklahoma State Medical Association, 210 Plaza Court, Oklahoma City, Oklahoma.

FOR SALE: Hospital, Southwestern Oklahoma County Seat Town. County population 22,817. Only one other hospital and three practicing M.D.'s. Contact R. M. Adams, M.D., 521 N. Boulder Street, Tulsa, Oklahoma.

Clinical Pathological Conference

University of Oklahoma School of Medicine

Presented by the Departments of Pathology and Medicine

ROBERT H. BAYLEY, M.D. AND BELA HALPERT, M.D.

OKLAHOMA CITY, OKLAHOMA

DR. HALPERT: The patient whose story we are presenting today did not appear to present much of a diagnostic problem. It will become apparent, however, that he did not die of the disease from which the clinicians thought that he suffered. The true nature of the disease was not apparent at necropsy either and it was not until we reviewed the microscopic sections that the true cause of death was ascertained. Dr. Bayley will present the clinical aspects of the case.

PROTOCOL

Patient: J. B., Negro male, age 48; admitted October 5, 1945; died October 10, 1945.

Chief Complaints: Chills, weakness and malaise, cough, anorexia, loss of weight.

Present Illness: In July, 1945, the patient began to lose weight. During the last of August, he had a single chill which lasted an hour. This was followed by weakness, anorexia and malaise. On September 24, 1945, he began to have chilly sensations. These occurred at irregular intervals during the succeeding four days and he developed a cough productive of approximately a cupful of foul, yellow, mucopurulent sputum a day. The cough improved in a week's time. Since October 1, 1945 the patient has had dyspnea. He was admitted to University Hospitals on October 5, 1945.

Past and Family History: The patient had the usual childhood diseases. His wife was living and well except for "throat trouble." The patient had six children, living and well. One pregnancy terminated spontaneously at the third month. The patient denied venereal disease. No family history of tuberculosis or diabetes could be elicited. The patient's mother died of cancer.

Physical Examination: The patient was well developed, rather emaciated, and appeared acutely ill. He was semi-comatose and

did not respond to questions. The head and neck were not remarkable. The chest was of the sthenic type. Increased muscle tone was observed over the chest wall bilaterally. Sibilant rales were heard over the right apex and "medium" moist rales over both pulmonic bases. Breath sounds were increased on the right side. The heart was not abnormal. Pulse was 120/min. and regular. The blood pressure was 112/72. The spleen and liver were "questionably palpable." Otherwise the abdomen was negative. Reflexes were physiologic.

Laboratory Data: Admission blood studies revealed 13 grams per cent hgb., 6.42 RBCs/cu.mm. and 12,500 leukocytes/cu.mm. with 84 per cent neutrophiles (4 per cent juveniles and 12 per cent stabs) 15 per cent lymphocytes, and one per cent monocytes. The blood sugar was 96 mg. per cent. The Mazzini test was negative. The sputum contained Gram-positive cocci in chains and questionable lancet-shaped diplococci. No acid-fast organisms were found. On October 9, 1945 the Widal test was negative. Stool cultures revealed no pathogens. Blood cultures were negative. An x-ray of the chest revealed numerous small nodules infiltrating both lung fields.

Clinical Course: On admission, the temperature was 103 degrees F. Throughout the hospital course it was of septic type, varying from 99 degrees to 104 degrees. Respirations increased gradually from 28 to 64. The patient received solutions of glucose intravenously and other supportive therapy. There was slight bleeding from the gums. The patient continued to appear somewhat dehydrated in spite of parenteral fluids. He grew rapidly weaker, became cyanotic and died on October 10, 1945.

CLINICAL DIAGNOSIS

DR. BAYLEY: This 48 year old negro male presented, as his chief complaints, chills, weakness, malaise, cough, anorexia and loss of weight. These are relatively non-specific with two exceptions. The presence of fever strongly suggests an infectious process. On the other hand, "cough" is helpful in localizing the disease to one of two systems, either cardiovascular or respiratory. Our first impression then would be that this patient presents some infectious process, possibly involving the respiratory system. We are told that in July the patient began to lose weight and that in August he had a chill with weakness, malaise and anorexia. This could well be interpreted as the onset of an infectious process which, after a period of relative latency, progressed and resulted in his terminal disease. Later there were chilly sensations and then a cough with expectoration of considerable quantities of purulent sputum. There are not many conditions that will produce such signs or symptoms. *Bronchitis* is pretty well eliminated by the quantity of sputum produced (1 cup per day,. Two things that come to mind in such circumstances are: 1) *bronchiectasis* and 2) *lung abscess*. We know that people with bronchiectasis continue for years with recurrent attacks of pneumonitis which tend to be more severe upon each subsequent attack. I believe that at the time this patient was coughing up a cupful of purulent sputum a day he probably had a lung abscess.

At the time of hospital admission, the situation was somewhat different. It is rather difficult to interpret the chest findings of apical sibilant rales and medium rales over the bases. In bronchiectasis we expect to find medium moist rales, usually in both bases.

Other findings were not significant except in a negative way. We do not know much more about this case after physical examination than we learned from the history. We know that the history is incomplete. Perhaps if the patient had been able to respond to detailed questioning we could have discerned the missing points.

We must consider, I believe, that this patient had a pulmonary infection of some sort which produced death in the course of three months. It is possible that *pneumonia* can present such a picture, complicated by failure to resolve, abscess formation etc. We must consider also that rather loose term, *pneumonitis*, represented by an unusual type of bronchitis and peribronchitis.

Let us refer to the laboratory data for additional help in limiting the differential diagnosis. The hemoglobin was 13 gms. per cent and the red blood count 6.4 million, probably a manifestation of dehydration. With this in mind, the white blood count,

which was proportionately elevated, is not indicative of leukocytosis. Sputum examinations revealed nothing specific. Actually, except for x-ray findings, we have no definite assistance from the laboratory.

CLINICAL DISCUSSION

DR. SHRYOCK: The only films which we have to present are of the chest. There is some haziness over the right lung field and multiple small nodular areas are seen throughout both lung fields. It was our impression that this was probably miliary tuberculosis with right or plural effusion. The possibility of abscesses cannot be excluded however.

QUESTION: What other infection might produce such nodules?

DR. SHRYOCK: *Virus pneumonia* sometimes causes such changes. *Coccidosis* may also give this picture but the nodules are usually not so numerous.

DR. HOPPS: Does the pneumonic form of *plague* ever produce such lesions?

DR. SHRYOCK: I am not familiar with the chest findings in pneumonic plague.

DR. BAYLEY: I am certainly inclined to agree that *tuberculosis* is the most common cause of roentgenographic changes such as we have just seen. This brings up the question as to whether or not this picture is typical of generalized miliary tuberculosis. It is my impression that this picture is more characteristic of hematogenous miliary tuberculosis confined to the lungs. You will note that the left costophrenic angle is free and that the nodules are more dense in the upper lung fields. Roentgenologists have difficulty in differentiating miliary tuberculosis from *silicosis*. Persons with silicosis complain principally of dyspnea and until the disease has reached a late stage there is no cough. Another diagnosis to consider is *actinomycosis*.

DR. HOPPS: As you pointed out there is no leukocytosis. I should think, however, that the "shift to left" indicated by the presence of 4 per cent juveniles and 12 per cent stab cells indicates a reaction of the bone marrow to infection.

DR. HACKLER: Is this picture compatible with tularemia?

DR. BAYLEY: Systemic *tularemia* usually includes a few pulmonic lesions and the picture may simulate tuberculosis; as the patient recovers, however, the pulmonic lesions disappear.

DR. AVEY: Suppose that this man had recently come from a Louisiana sugar mill?

DR. BAYLEY: A by-product of sugar cane called bagasse provides the raw product from which celanese is manufactured. From inhalation of this material the disease bagassosis may result. Patients so affected have a high fever. I have seen one case which simulated miliary tuberculosis. This patient recovered in six months. In the present case we must consider three general categories of disease: neoplasm, bacterial infection and mycotic infection. A diffuse form of *Hodgkin's disease* can produce a ground glass appearance in the lung fields and can give nodular metastases as well. *Lymphosarcoma* may be mentioned in passing, but I do not seriously regard either as a possibility in this case.

ANATOMIC DIAGNOSIS .

DR. HALPERT: At necropsy this patient was markedly emaciated. No significant abnormalities of the skin were noted. The peritoneal cavity was dry, free from adhesions and the liver was not enlarged. There were "pin-point" gray-white nodules scattered over the external and cut surfaces of the liver and the spleen. Otherwise the liver appeared unchanged. The spleen, however, was enlarged about three times and softer than usual. In addition to the pin-point nodules described there were many, three to four millimeters in diameter, which appeared to be fibrocaseous. Other abdominal viscera were not remarkable. The right pleural cavity contained 850 ml. of a murky yellow-brown liquid. The left was similarly involved. Nodules, similar to those seen in the spleen, were scattered on external and cut surfaces of the lungs. These were more numerous in the apex than in the base. There were no larger areas of caseation, nor was there ulceration of bronchi nor cavity formation. Lymph nodes, in the hilus of the lung, were not enlarged and no primary tuberculous complex was evident. This in itself should have aroused our suspicion that this was not tuberculosis. Our provisional gross anatomic diagnosis was miliary tuberculosis with pyothorax. Microscopic study revealed something quite different however. The picture was typical of tularemia. Since Dr. Bayley and I have both resided in New Orleans we should have recognized that these lesions were a manifestation of tularemia. Approximately 212 cases of tularemia have been studied at Charity Hospital, of which 12 died. I performed the necropsy on two of these. The failure to demonstrate acid-fast organisms in the sputum should have focused our attention upon tularemia as a possibility. Histologically, these nodules, at first glance, resemble tubercles, but closer study revealed that the predominant cell was a rather typical macrophage as differentiated

from the epithelioid cell of tuberculosis. There was central necrosis and in those central areas polymorphonuclear leukocytes were often prominent. A few multinucleated giant cells were seen.

This is the first case of tularemia which has been studied at necropsy at this hospital. It is interesting that this disease is almost confined to America although there have been isolated reports from Europe and Russia. The most common form of spread is from rabbit to man. Ticks, flies, etc. may serve as intermediate hosts. The organism was first discovered by McCoy as a result of his studies in California from 1908-1911. The mortality rate is about 4 per cent. The mode of infection in this instance is not quite clear. There was no skin lesion. Perhaps the organisms were ingested with improperly cooked food or contaminated water.

DISCUSSION

DR. HACKLER: In Oklahoma, during the last 6 years, there has been an average of 36 cases of tularemia per year. These cases have been almost limited to the Eastern part of the State. The disease is highly infectious, and nearly all of those persons who have worked extensively with this disease have become infected. Although direct infection from handling diseased rabbits is common, flies also transmit the disease. The organism readily passes through the unbroken skin. Cases have been reported in which the infection resulted from drinking contaminated water.

DR. BAYLEY: In the three cases of fatal tularemia which I have seen at post-mortem, pulmonic nodules were larger and much less frequent and more irregularly distributed. None of these three cases simulated miliary tuberculosis to the extent that this case did.

DR. HOPPS: This is an unusual case of tularemia. Infections with *Pasteurella tularense* fall into four major categories. Approximately 80 per cent are of the ulceroglandular type in which the portal of entry is manifest by an ulcer of the skin and adenopathy of regional lymph nodes. The other 20 per cent comprise the glandular type, the ophthalmic type, and, as this case illustrates, the septic form or "typhoid" type in which superficial lesions are minimal. It is this type which may occasionally, as it did here, closely mimic miliary tuberculosis. This fourth type contributes the majority of deaths from this disease.

The JOURNAL Of The
OKLAHOMA STATE MEDICAL ASSOCIATION

EDITORIAL BOARD
L. J. MOORMAN, Oklahoma City, Editor-in-Chief
E. EUGENE RICE, Shawnee
BEN H. NICHOLSON, Oklahoma City
MR. DICK GRAHAM, Oklahoma City, Business Manager
JANE FIRRELL TUCKER, Editorial Assistant

CONTRIBUTIONS: Articles accepted by this Journal for publication including those read at the annual meetings of the State Association are the sole property of this Journal.

The Editorial Department is not responsible for the opinions expressed in the original articles of contributors.

Manuscripts may be withdrawn by authors for publication elsewhere only upon the approval of the Editorial Board.

MANUSCRIPTS: Manuscripts should be typewritten, double-spaced, on white paper 8½ x 11 inches. The original copy, not the carbon copy, should be submitted.

Footnotes, bibliographies and legends for cuts should be typed on separate sheets in double space. Bibliography listing should follow this order: Name of author, title of article, name of periodical with volume, page and date of publication.

Manuscripts are accepted subject to the usual editorial revisions and with the understanding that they have not been published elsewhere.

NEWS: Local news of interest to the medical profession, changes of address, births, deaths and weddings will be gratefully received.

ADVERTISING: Advertising of articles, drugs or compounds unapproved by the Council on Pharmacy of the A.M.A. will not be accepted. Advertising rates will be supplied on application.

It is suggested that members of the State Association patronize our advertisers in preference to others.

SUBSCRIPTIONS: Failure to receive The Journal should call for immediate notification.

REPRINTS: Reprints of original articles will be supplied at actual cost provided request for them is attached to manuscripts or made in sufficient time before publication. Checks for reprints should be made payable to Industrial Printing Company, Oklahoma City.

Address all communications to THE JOURNAL OF THE OKLAHOMA STATE MEDICAL ASSOCIATION,
210 Plaza Court, Oklahoma City 3

OFFICIAL PUBLICATION OF THE OKLAHOMA STATE MEDICAL ASSOCIATION
Copyrighted August, 1946

EDITORIALS

HEARINGS ON S-1606

Congressional approval of the Wagner-Murray-Dingell Bill S-1606 would be as deadly to people's medicine as 606 was to their syphilis. The socialistically minded predatory politicians who watch the committee hearings on this bill with shifting eyes and dripping chops are resting uneasily in their lairs. As the hearings proceed they see their chances for a deadly raid on the flock rapidly fading. The bleeding public has found wool in their teeth and they must live on what they have dragged down or go hungry.

Good Americans are not willing to give up the last vestige of freedom and submit to coercion; they are not willing to surrender the intangible yet genuine urge for freedom in the choice of a doctor and the safeguarding of their medical secrets; they are not willing to encourage melingering on the part of patients and incompetency on the part of physicians through the approval of federal medicine under the proposed Wagner-Murray-Dingell Bill. Neither are they sufficiently naive to believe that more than a hundred thirty million people can be certified and integrated under the proposed program without additional personnel in the present social security set-up. If this were true as suggested by a member of the committee the people should rise up in righteous wrath against an already existing bureaucracy which at the taxpayers' expense could maintain in idleness a sufficient army of government employees to take care of this anticipated tremendous task. In a democratic country it seems most unfortunate that we must pay taxes to defray the expenses of the interminable Senate Committee hearings on a proposal as undemocratic as the Wagner-Murray-Dingell Bill.

As these hearings proceed before the Committee on Education and Labor ,doctors should strive to educate everyone of their patrons in the meaning of medicine under government control. The record of government care of the sick since World War I presents a sorry story. It would be sad enough if it dealt with livestock and poultry; instead of human beings. Those who doubt the above statements might do well to look into the political care of psychiatric patients occupying hundreds of thousands of beds in the United States and the thousands upon thousands of cases of tuberculosis cared for by the government since World War I.

After having suffered more than twenty years of mismanagement under General Hines, the people of the United States have every reason to be proud of the Veterans Administration under General Bradley with its altered policies and ambitions and its medical department under General Hawley. The people and the medical profession may well be hopeful since the avowed policy is to bring the care of the disabled veterans as nearly as possible in line with civilian medicine by eliminating unnecessary military features, cutting red tape and streamlining paper work. Already the care of disabled veterans is being decidedly facilitated through civilian medical channels. In a straight forward statement before the Senate Committee, General Bradley said, "While the proposals contained in S-1606 would not appear to be designed to impair in any way the hospitalization benefits now administered by the Veterans Administration, I wish to state clearly that in my opinion it is important that nothing be done which will impair it. I also believe that this veterans benefit should continue to be under the exclusive jurisdiction of the Veterans Administration."

After pointing out the fact that the Veterans Administration has more than a hundred hospitals now in existence and that every state in the union except three has veterans hospitals and that hospitals are under construction in these three, he points out the possibility of conflict between care under the Veterans Administration and under the proposed Wagner-Murray-Dingell Bill and the necessity of making exceptions in case the proposed bill becomes a law. In other words veterans already entitled to government medicine and hospitalization should not have to pay the withholding tax for government medicine under the proposed bill. General Bradley and General Hawley have made it clear that V. A. doesn't want the veterans' families because of the difficulty they encounter in their attempt to secure sufficient medical personnel.

If V. A. under its new generous medical plan encounters such difficulties, what may we expect when S-1606 attempts to staff its medical care program under the social security administrator. If good doctors hesitate to accept service under the present high standards of the V. A. medical department and the ethical appeal of General Hawley, how will they react to the contracts offered by the social security administrator under the Wagner-Murray-Dingell Bill? A close perusal of the Senate Committee hearings indicates that some of the proponents of the proposed bill are beginning to be burdened with this question. Will a sufficient number of good doctors be willing to make themselves available for the poor medical care which must inevitably result. If the proposed legislation is passed by congress its implimentation will discover many unexplored problems. The problem of securing a sufficient number of doctors to give so-called adequate medical care may prove to be an insurmountable one. The death of scientific medicine under the government's destructive program would prove to be a costly experience. It is time for every good American to make his protest both audible and legible. Doctors should see that the people are apprised of the danger. They should know how foul it is, how deadly to their freedom and ultimately to their physical welfare. "We hold these truths to be self evident; that all men are created equal, that they are endowed by their creator with certain inalienable rights, that among these are life, liberty and the pursuit of happiness."

The German idiology dominating the Wagner-Murray-Dingell Bill emasculates the Declaration of Independence. Does the spirit of independence still live in our hearts?

IN A NUT SHELL

The war is over. Young doctors returning from service in the Army and Navy are back in the harness, older doctors and those declared physically unfit, or essential, who heroically held the home front are weighted with fatigue. But all are better because of sacrificial service. All readjustments must be amicably and generously negotiated. Medicine in Oklahoma must take on new life and move on to higher ground.

MALPRACTICE INSURANCE

Malpractice insurance is quite old. From stone writings, we find that as far back as the year 2250 B.C., the code Hammurabi, Babylon, imposed an insurer's liability on the Physicians of that day. The code read: "If a physician make a deep incision upon a man with his bronze lancet and cause the man's death, or operates on the eye socket of a man with his bronze lancet and destroys the man's eye, they shall cut off his hand."

This was quite a severe penalty for the doctor of those days, but is just as severe in the courts of today, when a judgment for a large amount of money is obtained against the physician.

Much malpractice litigation arises from the fact that ordinary people expect too much of a doctor, and that the doctor himself fosters these expectations too tenderly. All goes well if the cure is forthcoming. Otherwise there may be a painful contraction of confidence which leads too often to another lawsuit for malpractice.

A doctor who keeps complete records in his office and at the hospital can give a good account of his diagnosis and treatment when he is called before the court in malpractice action. These records should include the mental history, the physical examination, copies of laboratory reports, all instructions and treatment given the patient, a progress record, and any special reports, such as that of a consultant, etc. Especially should be included any failure or refusal of the patient to follow instructions.

It is beyond human possibility for a doctor to remember the history, examination, and treatment of a patient, and yet on the other hand, every detail of treatment, every word spoken, is likely to be well remembered by the patient. This is the view taken by the average jury when there is conflict between the patient's and the doctor's statements of the happenings.

It is unwise to be too secretive. It is advised that the attending physician should in every case inform some responsible person, husband, wife, parent, or guardian, or next of kin, as to the details or essential facts of the case.

A doctor should never be foolish enough to write a letter to the plaintiff's attorney without legal advice.

A surgeon has no legal right to operate on a child without the consent of the latter's parents or guardian, except in very extreme cases.

"In Moss v. Rishworth (Texas)", a tonsillectomy was performed on a boy of eleven. An adult sister had given consent. This was held insufficient. The surgeon was held liable.

Publicity should never be given about any case. A child was born with its heart outside of its body. The family physician took the baby to the hospital for operation. The child died. It was alleged that the hospital permitted a photograph to be made of the child and gave the facts of the case to a newspaper without the permission or knowledge of the parents. After publication the parents sued the hospital and doctor. A judgment was given to the parents.

The consent of both the husband and wife is a prerequisite to the performance of an autopsy on a child. The consent of either the husband or wife must be obtained in the event of an autopsy on one or the other. However, if the husband or wife is survived only by children the consent of all of the children must be obtained. This is true, of course, if the autopsy is not performed, in accordance with law, by the coroner or other authorized person.

A physician employed a diathermy machine in treating his patient. The patient was burned on the neck and shoulder. The doctor told the patient not to worry, that he carried $80,000 insurance to take care of such things. This served as an invitation to be sued. He was!

Failure to give tetanus antitoxin for a "puncture" wound may constitute negligence.

Failure of a physician to treat an infant's eyes with silver nitrate solution at birth, as required by state health regulations, constitutes negligence.

Evidence that a physician administered roentgen treatment to a patient without remaining in the room or within hearing, which treatment resulted in a burn, warrants a finding of negligence, unless satisfactorily explained.

Do not guarantee results, keep good medical records, do not make any statement in regard to malpractice claim, unless you have taken legal advice. Strong defense of malpractice actions is necessary if the incident of these suits is to be reduced. When plaintiffs uniformly fail to obtain favorable judgments, it is obvious that the bringing of such actions will be discouraged.

Remember your policy with the State Medical Association extends to you fee legal advice on malpractice cases. The best attorneys are at your service.—W. M. Eberle.

FROM THE THROAT OF THE CHICKEN—STREPTOMYCIN

Dr. Selman A. Waksman of Rutgers University calls attention to the fact that streptomycin producing organisms namely *streptomyces griseus* was isolated from both the soil and from the throat of the chicken. Dr. Waksman states that in the search for an antibiotic capable of inhibiting or destroying the gram negative bacteria and yet not toxic in its effect, they isolated more than 1000 strains of actinomycetes in the laboratories of the New Jersey Agriculturel Experiment Station. They were searching both against diseases caused by gram negative bacteria and against the so-called acide fast bacteria. The bacillus causing tuberculosis is the classical example of the latter.

The resistance of the tubercle bacillus to all forms of chemotherapy, including penicillin and sulfa-compounds stimulated interest in this project. After many animal tests and continued purification of the crystalline substance, streptomycin is now being employed in the treatment of certain infectious conditions in man. The continued limited supply, because of the difficulties of production and the high cost, has been under careful control and distributed only for experimental purposes, including therapeutic tests in human beings. Its toxicity is now being carefully studied by a group of scientists at the New York City Hospital. This group is working with patients who volunteer to become human guinea pigs. These studies indicate that certain changes in the blood picture and toxic effects upon the kidneys when the drug is employed in the human being are rather disturbing.

At the Mayo Clinic, Dr. Henshaw and his co-workers are carrying out therapeutic tests in the treatment of patients suffering from various forms of tuberculosis. Their experience indicates that the therapeutic influence upon tuberculous conditions is very dramatic and very promising and that the toxic effects are apparently minor. They have employed the purified crystalline form of streptomycin in the treatment of 63-patients suffering from tuberculosis. In practically all cases there has been a reduction in the sensitivity to tuberculin and in many cases of pumonary tuberculosis, serial x-ray films show a remarkable clearing of the lesions. In pulmonary cases, the treatment seems to be most effective in generalized miliary tuberculosis, in hemotogenous, and acute exud…tive pulmonary tuberculosis, and in chronic tuberculosis with acute bronchogenic spread. In no instance has the disease been completely eradicated and it has been noted that even after favorable response relapse or reactivation followed discontinuance of the anti-biotic agent.

The mechanism of action is not known. Neither is the optimum dose well established. There is no definite opinion as to the desirable length of treatment and no well formulated idea as to the interval between doses. It is well known that streptomycin may suppress and even eradicate experimental tuberculosis in guinea pigs, but there is a wide discrepancy between experimental uses and effects in animals and in the human being.

At the Trudeau Sanatorium Laboratory guinea pigs, experimentally inoculated with tubercle bacilli developing gross lesions in the various organs of the body before being treated with streptomycin, manifest a marvelous response to the administration of the drug. The gross lesions in all of the organs,

including the lymph nodes, were reduced to small fibrotic scars and the guinea pigs were in good condition when killed. The controles suffering from lethal disease, showed evidence of widespread gross tuberculous lesions when killed. As reported in experimental tests conducted on human beings the treated guinea pigs showed a reduction in sensitivity to tuberculin.

The medical staff of the Veterans Administration is now interested in forwarding the experimental studies in the human being and for this purpose an experimental station is being established for additional clinical tests in the treatment of tuberculosis. Both the laboratory workers and the clinical investigators in the field are to be commended for their conservative attitude in the face of great therapeutics promise.

No doubt the possible toxic effects will soon be determined and clearly defined, the dose and a uniform schedule for treatment established. While awaiting these decisions and adequate production with diminishing costs, let us thank the lowly chicken pecking in the soil that harbors the fungus which may successfully foil the deadly tubercle bacillus.

EDITORIAL NEWS

The editorial policy of the Journal has not changed, but when the avalanche of scientific material from the program of the recent state meeting swept under our mast-head, space in the Journal became precious. During the past four years there have been times when the members of the Editorial Staff worked hard to fill space, occasionally special articles were provided to take up the slack. Now it is difficult to find space. But the staff is proud of the scientific material available for the columns of the Journal. These columns belong to the doctors of the State and we are glad to return them to their rightful owners. With few exceptions the limited editorial space will be devoted to pertinent current topics of local or general interest, not forgetting that *"rebellion to tyrants is obedience to God."*

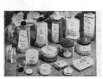

UNSCENTED COSMETICS
FOR THE ALLERGIC PATIENT

AR-EX Cosmetics are the only complete line of unscented cosmetics regularly stocked by pharmacies. To be certain that your perfume sensitive patients do not get scented cosmetics, prescribe AR-EX Unscented Cosmetics. SEND FOR FREE FORMULARY.

AR-EX

FREE FORMULARY

DR
ADDRESS
CITY
STATE

AR-EX COSMETICS, INC.,   1036 W. VAN BUREN ST.,   CHICAGO 7, ILL.

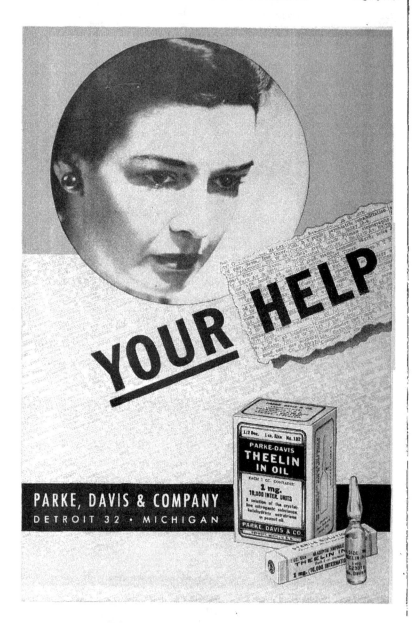

YOUR HELP

PARKE, DAVIS & COMPANY
DETROIT 32 · MICHIGAN

PARKE-DAVIS
THEELIN
IN OIL

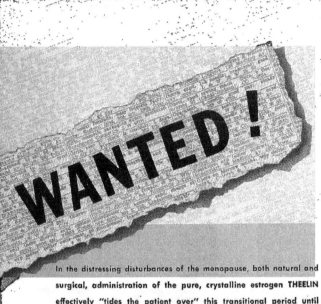

In the distressing disturbances of the menopause, both natural and surgical, administration of the pure, crystalline estrogen THEELIN effectively "tides the patient over" this transitional period until endocrine readjustment occurs. It is also indicated in disorders due to estrogenic deficiency, such as vaginitis, kraurosis and pruritus vulvae.

Theelol Kapseals are available for treatment of the milder menopausal symptoms and for maintenance between injections. Theelin Suppositories, Vaginal, are particularly well adapted for the treatment of gonorrheal vaginitis.

T H E E L I N

Theelin in Oil is available in ampoules of 0.1, 0.2, 0.5 and 1.0 mg., in boxes of 6 and 50. Theelin, Aqueous Suspension, in 2 mg. ampoules, in boxes of 6 and 25. Theelol Kapseals, 0.24 mg., in bottles of 20, 100 and 250. Theelin Suppositories, Vaginal, 0.2 mg., in boxes of 6 and 50.

THE PRESIDENT'S PAGE

It is desirable after the vacation period is over and the different county societies take up their regular meetings that where a merger with an adjoining county will strengthen and improve a county with small membership, that serious consideration be given such merger to the end that all concerned may profit. This does not destroy the identity of any county society. They are still entitled to representation as before in the House of Delegates.

A move has already been started in the 10th Councilor District which, if perfected, will greatly benefit the smaller county societies in this District. It is hoped other districts will as soon as possible do the same.

If your Society is in need of a speaker for any occasion, please remember to call upon your State Office for one or more as speakers are available if you will make your wants known.

President.

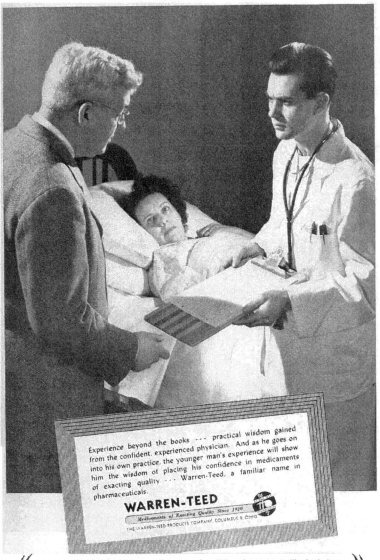

Experience beyond the books · · · practical wisdom gained from the confident, experienced physician. And as he goes on into his own practice, the younger man's experience will show him the wisdom of placing his confidence in medicaments of exacting quality · · · Warren-Teed, a familiar name in pharmaceuticals.

WARREN-TEED

Medicaments of Exacting Quality Since 1926

THE WARREN-TEED PRODUCTS COMPANY, COLUMBUS 8, OHIO

Warren-Teed Ethical Pharmaceuticals: capsules, elixirs, ointments, sterilized solutions syrups, tablets. Write for literature.

69 OKLAHOMA PHYSICIANS ATTEND A. M. A. IN SAN FRANCISCO

Sixty-nine Oklahoma physicians attended the 95th Annual Session of the American Medical Association held in San Francisco July 2, 3, 4, and 5. This representation of Oklahoma physicians is somewhat higher than recent years, no doubt due to the accessibility of the meeting.

California State Medical Association and the San Francisco County Medical Society are to be complimented on handling the meeting in a most expedicious manner. Even California weather was on its best behavior.

Officers Elected

The election of officers was highlighted by the unanimous action of the House of Delegates in selecting Dr. Olin West, past Secretary-General Manager of the A. M. A., as President-Elect. Dr. George F. Lull, having previously been selected by the Board of Trustees for this position, was elected Secretary to continue the work of Dr. West.

Other officers elected were:

Vice-President—Edward L. Bortz, Philadelphia.

Treasurer—Josiah J. Moore, Chicago.

Speaker, House of Delegates—R. W. Fouts, Omaha.

Vice-Speaker, House of Delegates—F. F. Borzell, Philadelphia.

Trustee—Charles W. Roberts, Atlanta, Ga.

Judicial Council—Walter F. Donaldson, Pittsburgh.

Council on Scientific Assembly—Leonard W. Larsen, Bismark, N. D.

Council on Medical Education and Hospitals—Victor Johnson, Chicago.

Council on Medical Service—E. J. McCormick, Toledo, Ohio; Thomas A. McGoldrick, Brooklyn.

House of Delegates to Meet Semi-annually

The House of Delegates, recognizing the need for a closer relationship between the House of Delegates, the Board of Trustees and officers, unanimously approved a recommendation from the Board of Trustees that the House of Delegates meet semi-annually, one meeting to be held during the winter months and the other during the Annual Session.

The Board of Trustees reported that the 1947 Annual Meeting would be held in Atlantic City June 9; the 1948 meeting in St. Louis, Missouri, May 7, the latter date being a month early. Obviously this will mean that state medical associations who have spring meetings will have to set their annual meetings ahead in 1948 in order to comply with the Constitution and By-Laws of the American Medical Association, concerning the certifications of duly elected delegates.

Oklahoma Resolution Favorably Received

A resolution introduced by the Oklahoma delegation urging the establishment of either a bureau or council within the A. M. A. on the History of Medicine was referred to the Committee on Miscellaneous Business. The Oklahoma delegates, Dr. C. R. Rountree, Oklahoma City, and Dr. James Stevenson, Tulsa, appeared before this Committee in support of the resolution and while the Committee did not report the resolution favorably as presented, it did present to the House of Delegates a substitute resolution urging the J. A. M. A. to make available a more comprehensive coverage of medical history, and recommended to both the Council on A. M. A. Medical Education and Hospitals and the Scientific Sections that every effort be made to increase in their respective activities material in the field of medical history.

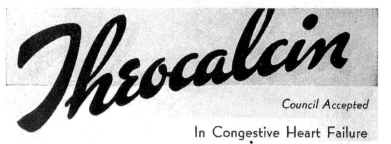

Theocalcin

Council Accepted

In Congestive Heart Failure

For the reduction of edema, to diminish dyspnoea and to strengthen heart action, prescribe Theocalcin, beginning with 2 or 3 tablets t. i. d., with meals. After relief is obtained, the comfort of the patient may be continued with smaller doses. Well tolerated.

Theocalcin, brand of theobromine-calcium salicylate, Trade Mark reg. U. S. Pat. Off.

Available in 7½ grain tablets and in powder form.

Bilhuber-Knoll Corp.   Orange, N. J.

Numerous delegates were extremely complimentary in expressing to the Oklahoma delegation their approval and support of the intent of the original resolution.

Board of Trustees Report Survey of A. M. A.'s Public Relations

Probably the high light of the meeting was the report of the Board of Trustees concerning a survey of the entire structure of the A. M. A. with reference to its activities in the field of public relations. The report which soon became commonly known as the Rich report, getting its name from the author, was most comprehensive in its investigation of the public relations activities of the A. M. A. The complete text of the report was not made available to the individual delegates and this action on the part of the Board of Trustees met some opposition inasmuch as it was felt by some delegates, as indicated by the resolution introduced, that the entire report should have been made available for study and subsequent action.

The outstanding feature of the report was the recommendation that a full time public relations representative be employed to present medicine's program to the American people. The Oklahoma delegation was extremely pleased to see that the recent program adopted by the House of Delegates of the Oklahoma State Medical Association closely parallels the recommendations now being made to the A. M. A.

Dr. Anton J. Carlson Awarded Distinguished Service Medal

The Committee on Distinguished Service Award of the A. M. A. submitted the names of Dr. A. J. Carlson, Chicago, Dr. Torald Sollomann, Cleveland, and Dr. Francis Carter Wood, New York City, for consideration to the House of Delegates for this award, and Dr. Anton J. Carlson was elected on the first ballot. Dr. Carlson's recognition was based upon his many investigations in physiology of the heart and circulation, gastric secretion, the nature of hunger and the glands of internal secretion. He is immediate Past President of the American Association for the Advancement of Science, Past President of the American Physiological Society and the Society for Experimental Biology and Medicine. Dr. Carlson has long been a leader in the fight against quackery and in favor of animal experimentation. He served with the U. S. Army in the first World War and was with the A. E. F. from March to September, 1919. Besides his many contributions to the scientific periodical literature, he is the author of books on Health in Hunger and Disease and Machinery of the Body.

Dr. Carlson was born in Sweden in 1875 and came to this country in 1891. Membership in many scientific societies and many honors have previously come to Dr. Carlson as a result of his eminent scientific and medical contributions.

Oklahoma Delegation Entertains Friends

Following the concluding session of the House of Delegates, Dr. Rountree and Dr. Stevenson entertained informally their many friends among the House of Delegates, Board of Trustees and the officers. This very friendly gesture on the part of Dr. Rountree and Dr. Stevenson was most enthusiastically received by those who attended.

OPS APPROVED BY 27 COUNTIES

Twenty-seven county medical societies have approved Oklahoma Physicians Service officially. They are: Tulsa, Payne, Creek, Washington, Nowata, Murray, Pontotoc, Pottawatomie, Garvin, Oklahoma, Kay, Osage, Okfulkee, Pittsburg, Washita, Kingfisher, Alfalfa, Woods, Muskogee, Sequoyah, Wagoner, Grady, Harper, Dewey, Blaine, Garfield, Woodward.

Approval by a county medical society does not carry any legal or financial responsibilities on the part of the doctor. It merely means that:

1. The doctor will cooperate with the Enrollment Representative in promoting the sale of the Plan to groups of employees in their county.

2. That the doctors will cooperate with the Plan by speaking well of it to the patient and potential groups.

3. That the doctor will not abuse the Plan by charging more for their service than they would normally, but charge the patient as if he were not a member of the Plan.

Book Reviews

THE MODERN ATTACK ON TUBERCULOSIS. Henry D. Chadwick, M.D., Superintendent of Westfield State Sanatorium, 1909-1929; Tuberculosis Controller of the City of Detroit, 1929-1933; Commissioner of Public Health of the Commonwealth of Massachusetts, 1933-1938; Medical Director of Middlesex Tuberculosis Sanatorium, 1938-1941. Alton S. Pope, M.D., Chief, Bureau of Communicable Diseases, Department of Health, Chicago, 1926-1929; Deputy Commissioner of Public Health and Director of the Division of Tuberculosis, Commonwealth of Massachusetts. Revised edition, 184 pages. Commonwealth Fund, New York City. Price $1.00.

The first edition of this valuable hand book was reviewed in the Journal, September, 1942, page 402. The second edition has been revised in an attempt to bring the reader up to date on the ever changing methods of attack. It contains a new section on pathogenesis and predisposing factors.

The authors state that, "New material has been added and various section have been expanded to include: photogluorography and the role of mass x-ray examinations in industry and other population groups, with emphasis on the essential role of an organized follow-up system; the financial aspects of hospitalization; rehabilitation; chemotherapy; immunization; and the Federal case-finding program."—Lewis J. Moorman, M.D.

WILLIAM E. EASTLAND, M.D.
F. A. C. R.

RADIUM AND X-RAY THERAPY
DERMATOLOGY

405 Medical Arts Bldg.

Oklahoma City, Oklahoma   Phone 3-1446

A BIBLIOGRAPHY OF INFANTILE PARALYSIS, 1789-1944. Edited by Morris Fishbein, M.D., Editor, Journal of American Medical Association. Compiled by Ludwig Hektoen, M.D., Chief Editor, Archives of Pathology and Ella M. Salmonsen, Medical Reference Librarian, John Creanar Library, Chicago. Fabrikoid. 672 pages. J. B. Lippincott Company, 1946.

This astonishingly complete bibliography covers the literature on poliomyelitis from 1789 to 1944. It begins with an axcellent abstract of Underwood's description of the disease in 1789. The material is arranged chronologically and has a comprehensive index covering, by numbers, the references and the articles. Suitable explanations and abstracts make the work reveal a heretofore unheard of amount of information in an easily accessible manner. While the bibliography is very complete, abstracts are used only when they bring out new or useful information. As pointed out in the preface, the scientific medical literature of the past few years outside of America and Great Britain has not been easily accessible and future supplements are already planned to remedy this defect.

One need only examine the work briefly to realize that the task of covering the literature so thoroughly over this long period, abstracting the numerous writings, arranging translations, putting it all into chronological order and indexing it was a tremendous undertaking. Furthermore, it will be realized that the whole thing was done by experts and represents a very efficient piece of work.

It is one of the most complete volumes we have seen and is a necessary part of every medical library.—Carroll M. Pounders, M.D.

Gratitude is a nice touch of beauty added last of all to the countenance, giving a classic beauty, an angelic loveliness, to the character.—*Theodore Parker.*

THE
MARY E. POGUE
SCHOOL

For Retarded Children and Epileptic Children

Children are grouped according to type and have their own separate departments. Separate buildings for girls and boys.

Large beautiful grounds. Five school rooms. Teachers are all college trained and have Teachers' Certificates. Occupational Therapy. Speech Corrective Work.

The School is only 26 miles west of Chicago. All west highways out of Chicago pass through or near Wheaton. Referring physicians may continue to supervise care and treatment of children placed in the School. You are invited to visit the School or send for catalogue.

30 Geneva Road, Wheaton, Ill.
Phone: Wheaton 319

Have a Coke

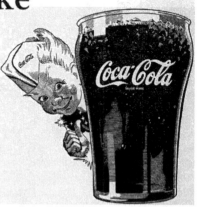

When you laugh, the world laughs with you, as they say——and when you enjoy *the pause that refreshes* with ice-cold Coca-Cola, your friends enjoy it with you, too. Everybody enjoys the friendly hospitality that goes with the invitation *Have a Coke.* Those three words mean *Friend, you belong ——I'm glad to be with you.* Good company is better company over a Coca-Cola.

HIPPOCRATIC WISDOM. William F. Petersen, M.D. First Edition, 268 pages. Charles C. Thomas, Springfield, Illinois. Price $5.00.

The author of this valuable work insists that he has not written a book for Greek scholars, but for medical students and young physicians who must ever seek wider horizons. The reviewer recommends the book for older physicians as well who are mentally alert and young in spirit. It is quite essential for the doctor to distinguish between technical dexterity and medical wisdom. With the help of Hippocrates the author of this little book attempts to show how medical wisdom may evolve from accurate clinical observation and how the union of these two may give rise to the rare gift of intuition — called by Oliver Wendell Holmes, *"Intuitive Sagacity".*

The physician who spurns the wisdom of Hippocrates would do well to remember that even though he may be standing at the top, Hippocrates cuts him under. In medicine nobody can afford to ignore the first scientist, the first anthropologist, the first meteorologist and the first ecologist, all these Hippocrates was. He laid the foundation and left specifications for the super-structure we call modern medicine. If the average physician after returning from the club or his hangout at the drug store would pick up Petersen's *Hippocratic Wisdom* and read a few pages before going to sleep he would find out that the old man of Cos knew more than he and his pals ever dreamed of. He might even lie awake wondering how the Father of Medicine acquired so much knowledge 2400 years ago and his ego might perceptibly shrivel.

Hippocrates said the physician "Must relax what is tense, and make tense what is relaxed. For in this way the diseased part would rest most and this in my opinion constitutes treatment". Again he says "Medicine is, in fact, subtraction and addition; subtraction of what is in excess and addition of what is wanting". The soundness of this principle has not been disturbed by centuries of scientific progress. In the past busy doctors may have been excused for not wading through the Adams translation of Hippocrates in order to glean the diagnostic and therapeutic truisms so characteristic of the Father of Medicine. But with this text available the medical wisdom of Hippocrates stripped of much of the irrelevent verbage should be read by every forward looking doctor in order that he may be humbled and inspired, and in many ways rewarded by the revelations of the masters. Those who have not read Hippocrates should secure this interesting volume and not add another day to the 24 centuries standing between them and Hippocratic Wisdom.—Lewis J. Moorman, M.D.

PREOPERATIVE AND POSTOPERATIVE TREATMENT. Edited by Lt. Col. Robert L. Mason, M. C., A. U. S., Cushing General Hospital, Farmington, Mass.; and Harold A. Zintel, M.D., Harrison Department of Surgical Research, University of Pennsylvania School of Medicine; Assistant Surgeon, Hospital of the University of Pennsylvania. Second Edition. 584 pages, with 157 illustrations. Philadelphia and London: W. B. Saunders Company, 1946. Price $7.00.

This book is not only an excellent present-day review of physiology, bio-chemistry, and pharmacology as applied to surgical diseases, but it is also a practical reference book for the general surgeon.

The second edition has been almost completely re-written due to the great strides that have been made in the care of the surgical patient during the war years.

Most all pre and postoperative complications are adequately covered in detail with stress praced on practical methods of therapy.

The first half of the book includes the diagnosis and care of common complications both general and local, taking up a system at a time. The latter half of the book deals with pre and postoperative care of surgical patients from a regional standpoint. The sections on care of the hyperthyroid and gallbladder patients are especially well covered.

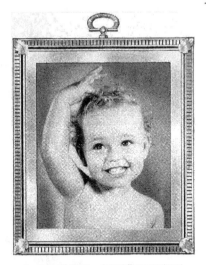

DOCTOR, MEET THE DARICRAFT BABY

Perhaps you are "meeting" the Daricraft Baby every day in your own practice. If not, may we call to your attention the following significant points of interest about Vitamin D increased Daricraft:

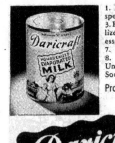

1. Produced from inspected herds; 2. Clarified; 3. Homogenized; 4. Sterilized; 5. Specially Processed; 6. Easily Digested; 7. High in Food Value; 8. Improved Flavor; 9. Uniform; 10. Dependable Source of Supply.

Producers Creamery Co.
Springfield, Mo.

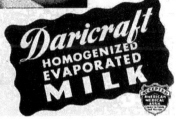

Daricraft HOMOGENIZED EVAPORATED MILK

Every surgeon should have a book of this type within reach at all times. It is a quick reference for almost every type of surgical complication.

It is also recommended for the internist who, after all, will see a majority of poor risk patients being prepared for surgery, and who will see a goodly number of major postoperative complicationss.

It is well organized, well written, and completely up to date.—Everett B. Neff, M.D.

HAY FEVER PLANTS. Roger P. Wodehouse, Ph.D. Chronica Botanica Co., Waltham, Mass. $4.75. 1945. Although there have been other books on hay fever plants and books on allergy containing chapters on hay fever plants, none have contained the clear, concise description that characterizes Dr. Roger P. Wodehouse's book on Hay Fever Plants. An amateur botanist and clinical allergist can identify the plants from the word pictures. The excellent illustrations number seventy-three and are the work of the author. The pictures of the pollen granules are informative.

He states in the preface that he intends "to interpret the botanical facts of hay fever in terms of their clinical significance" and this is the foundation for the untold practical value to allergists and general practitioners. He follows the Latin rules for capitalization.

The most outstanding sources of information found in the book are the regional survey tables of the hay fever plants and their time of pollenization and their significance in that region. These thorough and detailed tables indicate much research and signify even to a reader unacquainted with the reputation of the author that his knowledge of the subject is complete.—Fannie Lou Leney, M.D.

Medical School Notes

Many of the clinical and preclinical staff of the Medical School are attending the Meetings of the American Medical Association in San Francisco. Several of the staff are participating in the scientific program.

Dr. Ben Nicholson, Dr. Robert H. Bayley and Dr. Howard C. Hopps presented papers at the Annual Meeting of the Moton Clinical Society in Tulsa, Oklahoma.

Dr. Robert H. Bayley, Professor of Medicine, recently presented papers on rheumatic heart disease and the treatment of empyema with penicillin, at a combined meeting of County Medical Societies of the Northeastern section of Oklahoma. The meeting was held at the Oklahoma State Hospital at Vinita, Oklahoma.

J. E. HANGER, Inc.

ARTIFICIAL LIMBS, BRACES, AND CRUTCHES

Phone: 2-8500

L. T. Lewis, Mgr.   BRANCHES AND AGENCIES IN PRINCIPAL CITIES   612 N. Hudson   Oklahoma City 3, Okla.

For Estrogen Insufficiency

Schieffelin BENZESTROL
(2, 4 di [p hydroxyphenyl] 3 ethyl hexane)

An important contribution to more effective and more economical estrogen therapy, Schieffelin BENZESTROL offers a dependable means of relieving the distressing symptoms arising from estrogenic hormone deficiency.

Orally potent and unusually well tolerated, this synthetic estrogen is available in forms for three routes of administration: Tablets—orally; Solution—intramuscularly; and Vaginal Tablets—locally.

ORAL	INTRAMUSCULAR	LOCAL
TABLETS: Potencies of 0.5, 1.0, 2.0 and 5.0 mg. Bottles of 50, 100 and 1,000.	SOLUTION: Potency of 5.0 mg. per cc. in 10 cc. Rubber capped multiple dose vials.	VAGINAL TABLETS: Potency of 0.5 mg. Bottles of 100.

Literature and Sample on Request

Schieffelin & Co.   20 COOPER SQUARE • NEW YORK 3, N. Y.
Pharmaceutical and Research Laboratories

CREDIT SERVICE

330 American National Building

Oklahoma City, Oklahoma

(Operators of Medical-Dental Credit Bureau)

We offer a dignified and effective collection service for doctors and hospitals located anywhere in the State. Write for information.

28 YEARS

Experience In Credit and Collection Work

Robt. R. Sesline, Owner and Manager

Dr. Reynold Patzer, Assistant Professor of Surgery, has been granted funds by the Oklahoma Division of the National Cancer Society for an experimental study on the treatment of cancer.

Miss Lilah Heck recently attended the 45th Meeting of the Medical Library Association which was held at the Yale Medical School, New Haven, Connecticut. Enroute she visited numerous medical libraries including the Osler and McGill at Montreal, Boston and Harvard Medical Libraries, the Library of the New York Academy of Medicine and the Army Medical Library in Washington, D. C.

During the next month every physician in the State of Oklahoma and all graduates of the School of Medicine residing in other states, will receive a letter pertaining to life membership in the School of Medicine of the University of Oklahoma Alumni Association. It is particularly important to raise, in the near future, $25,000 in order to begin the campaign for funds required to construct the Aulmni Research Institute.

Medical Abstracts

ORTHOPAEDIC SURGERY FOLLOWING PERIPHERAL-NERVE INJURIES. V. D. Chaklin. Voprosi Neurokhirurgyi, No. 3, 50, 1944.

There are areas of nerve injuries, where all attempts at repair will be useless. There are other areas in which nerve suture gives mediocre results after long convalescence.

In the upper extremity, in the presence of grave injuries to the brachial plexus, the treatment consists in: (1) operative correction through an osteotomized clavicle

THE TABLET METHOD FOR DETECTING URINE-SUGAR

CLINITEST

offers these advantages to physicians, laboratory technician, patient:

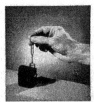

ELIMINATES
Use of flame
Bulky apparatus
Measuring of reagents

PROVIDES
Simplicity
Speed
Convenience of technic
Simply drop one Clinitest Tablet into test tube containing proper amount of diluted urine. Allow time for reaction, compare with color scale.

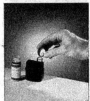

FOR OFFICE USE Clinitest Laboratory Outfit (No. 2108) Includes — Tablets for 180 tests, test tubes, rack, droppers, color scale, instructions. Additional tablets can be purchased as required.

FOR PATIENT USE Clinitest Plastic Pocket-Size Set (No. 2106) Includes — All essentials for testing — in a small, durable, pocket-size case of Tenite plastic.

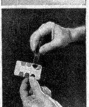

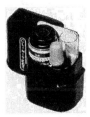

Order from your dealer.
Complete information upon request.

AMES COMPANY, Inc., Elkhart, Ind.

with special attempt to repair the median nerve: (2) support of the extremity with a hinge joint for the elbow; (3) arthrodesis of the shoulder after a period of eight to ten months, followed by immobilization for three months; (4) muscle transplantation for extension, if flexion of the wrist and fingers has been restored. In the presence of total paralysis of all the muscles of the upper extremity, arthrodesis of the shoulder and the elbow with a tenodesis of the wrist is advisable. Radial nerve paralysis may require either transplantation of tendons or a combined suture of the nerve with transplantation of tendons. For median nerve paralysis involving the thenar muscles, one of Bunnell's procedures is recommended.

In the lower extremities, injuries to the femoral nerve involving the quadriceps present difficult problems. Contractures of the knee joint have to be overcome and then transplantation of the biceps performed; or combined transplantations of the tensor fasciae latae and sartorius may be advisable. Among the less desirable corrective measures are arthrodesis and arthroereises of the knee joint.

Injuries to the sciatic nerve require prolonged physiotherapy, the wearing of light braces, and tenodesis of the extensor tendons or posterior arthroereisis of the ankle. Special attention should be given to the often overlooked contracture of the toes.—E.D.D., M.D.

GUNSHOT FRACTURES OF THE SHAFT OF THE HUMERUS.

Gunshot fractures of the shaft of the humerus comprised approximately 3 per cent of all battle casualties among the patients who were admitted to the general hospital from which this study was made. The hanging arm cast was used in treating the majority of these fractures, and bone union was accomplished in almost every instance in which there was no significant bone loss. Ninety-three per cent of the wounds were debrided in forward hospitals. Debridement was performed within the first twelve hours in 69 per cent of all the injured. Sulfanilamide was used locally in every wound, and oral sulfonamides were given to all patients before admission to the hospital.

Most of the patients arrived at the hospital wearing abduction plaster spica casts. In the majority, there was marked disalignment of the fractures, which corrected immediately after the spica was removed and the arm was permitted to drop to the side in a hanging cast. Associated nerve injuries occurred in many of these fractures and were the most frequent cause of permanent disability.E.D.M., M.D.

ANKYLOSIS OF THE TEMPOROMANDIBULAR JOINT: Reed O. Dingman, D.D.S., M.D. American Journal of Orthodontics and Oral Surgery. Volume 32. No. 2. pp. 120-125. February, 1946.

"Chronic ankylosis of the temporomandibular joint is discussed from the standpoint of incidence, etiology, pathology, diagnosis and treatment. Complete excision

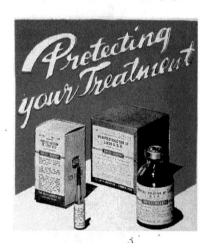

UNCERTAIN SUCCESS in the treatment of pernicious anemia is due to many unpredictable factors.

One element of certainty is added to your treatment when the Solution of Liver prescribed never varies from rigid standards.

Purified Solution of Liver, Smith-Dorsey, is unfailingly uniform in purity and potency. It has earned and maintained the confidence of thousands of physicians.

Purified Solution of Liver, Smith-Dorsey, will help to protect your treatment—to assure you of good results where the medication is the controlling factor.

NEUROLOGICAL HOSPITAL

Twenty-Seventh and The Paseo
Kansas City, Missouri

Modern Hospitalization of Nervous and Mental Illnesses, Alcoholism and Drug Addiction.

THE ROBINSON CLINIC
G. WILSE ROBINSON, M.D.
G. WILSE ROBINSON, Jr., M.D.

PURIFIED SOLUTION OF *Liver*

 ACCEPTED MEDICAL ASSN.

 SMITH-DORSEY

*Supplied in the following dosage forms:
1 cc. ampoules and 10 cc. and 30 cc.
ampoule vials, each containing 10
U.S.P. Injectable Units per cc.*

THE SMITH-DORSEY COMPANY
LINCOLN • NEBRASKA
Manufacturers of Pharmaceuticals to the Medical Profession Since 1908

THE JOURNAL
of the
OKLAHOMA STATE MEDICAL ASSOCIATION

| VOLUME XXXIX | OKLAHOMA CITY, OKLAHOMA, SEPTEMBER, 1946 | NUMBER 9 |

The Diagnosis and Treatment of Pernicious Anemia*

RUSSELL L. HADEN, M.D.

CLEVELAND, OHIO

Pernicious anemia is a true deficiency disease for which specific replacement therapy is available. In idiopathic pernicious amenia the deficiency once present continues throughout the life of the patient. The disease is never "cured". The deficiency responsible for the symptoms is satisfied, however, by complete and continued treatment. A symptomatic deficiency in the specific factor may occur temporarily, as in pregnancy where the need is for a time greater than the supply, or when absorption is interfered with as in sprue or other abnormalitity of the small intestine. Here the deficiency disappears with the relief of the underlying causative disease, although specific therapy is usually helpful.

The seriousness of idiopathic pernicious anemia is best emphasized by the fact that it was always fatal before the introduction of liver treatment by Minot and Murphy in 1926 and is still fatal without specific therapy. While anemia is always present and is usually the early symptom, neurologic involvement occurs almost always in time in untreated cases and usually in patients not completely treated. Subacute combined scler- osis of the spinal cord may lead to a crippling and permanent disability. A disease which is always fatal if untreated and often leads to serious permanent disability if insufficiently treated, merits serious attention.

The first consideration is a correct diagnosis. If it is definitely determined that the patient has idiopathic pernicious anemia, treatment is necessary throughout life. All too often a patient is given liver extract for an anemia which has not been properly studied, and a definite diagnosis of pernicious anemia made. The patient improves but does

*Presented before the General Session, Oklahoma State Medical Association Annual Meeting, May 3, 1946.

not continue treatment because he does not understand that treatment is required permanently. Later a spinal cord lesion develops due to discontinuing therapy; or it may not be realized by the physician that therapy must completely satisfy the deficiency to prevent progress in the neurologic involvement characteristic of the disease. If the anemia is not pernicious anemia, liver extract is seldom needed.

Pernicious anemia is a disease of older people. In 406 cases studied at the Cleveland Clinic only five were less than 30 years of age. In a total number of 558 I have observed the disease began under 20 years of age in only one individual. The disease was first observed over 60 years of age in 41.7 per cent. One patient was 88 years old when first diagnosed. Fifty-two per cent were in the 40 to 60 group.

Three characteristic aspects or phases are observed in pernicious anemia: (1) gastrointestinal, (2) hematologic, and (3) neurologic. The specific factor concerned is formed in the stomach by interaction of a ferment or other substance (intrinsic factor) secreted by the gastric glands on some element of ingested food (extrinsic factor). The substance formed by the interaction of intrinsic and extrinsic factors is absorbed from the gastrointestinal tract. It is necessary for (1) normal gastrointestinal function, (2) the normal growth and development of red blood cells and (3) the normal nutrition of the nervous system. There should be an excess of the specific factor which is stored in the liver after absorption from the small intestine. This represents an overflow after the current needs of the body are satisfied and is stored to supply added demands. The exact structure of the specific factor is unknown. It is possible that this may be folic acid.

No patient with idiopathic pernicious anemia has free hydrochloric acid in the stomach. The achlorhydria seems to precede the anemia and other symptoms of the disease by many years. It probably is congenital in most cases. The mucous membrane of the stomach is atrophic on gastroscopic examination. The papillae of the tongue are atrophic also. A coated tongue in active, untreated pernicious anemia is rarely seen. The surface is almost always clean, giving the tongue a "bald" appearance. The patient ofter complains of a sore tongue. This was a primary complaint in over 10 per cent of our series. Partly as a result of the absence of hydrochloric acid and probably partly as a result of a lack of nutritional factors, diarrhea is common. Many other gastrointestinal symptoms are complained of, such as "indigestion", anorexia, nausea, vomiting, excessive gas formation, and jaundice. As a result of the gastrointestinal disturbances most patients lose weight. With specific therapy the glossitis disappears, the papillae become normal, and the tongue may become coated. Other gastrointestinal symptoms usually clear up. The achlorhydria is permanent.

The blood findings are characteristic. The typical patient has a marked anemia with large red cells filled with hemoglobin (marcocytic and hyperchromic anemia). The mean volume of the erythrocyte is increased, so the volume index is high. Since there is no disturbance in hemoglobin formation, the stroma is filled with hemoglobin. The cells are larger than normal, so the mean cell hemoglobin content is increased and the color index is high. In 558 patients studied for red cell changes all have shown a macrocytosis if untreated. Often the volume index is high when the color index is normal or less than 1. The cell size is by far the best diagnostic indicator of pernicious anemia and is the most important criterion of complete therapy.

The achlorhydria and the macrocytosis of the red cells are the two constant findings in untreated pernicious anemia. An anemic patient with large red cells (increased volume index and mean cell volume) and achlorhydria almost without exception is suffering from pernicious anemia.

The bone marrow reflects the effects of a deficient supply of the erythrocyte-maturing factor. The first change is a slowing of the rate of release of red cells. The cells released are larger than normal since maturation is not complete. This increase in the size of the cell is the first and most sensitive indicator of a deficient supply of the specific factor responsible for pernicious anemia. The immature erythrocytes remain longer and crowd the marrow so the marrow becomes

red due to filling with cells which normally would be delivered into the circulation. As the deficiency progresses, such cells as do reach the blood stream are of many sizes and shapes and some are nucleated. Many cells die in the marrow. The end product of hemoglobin destruction is bilirubin. The increased amount of the bile pigment may exceed the capacity of the liver to excrete it, so definite clinical jaundice may develop. It was once thought that the finding of megaloblasts in the blood film was the best diagnostic criterion of pernicious anemia. The appearance of microcytes, poiklocytes, nucleated red cels and basophilia is a late development of pernicious anemia. The one constant and characteristic early sign is the macrocytosis, and the hematologic diagnosis of pernicious anemia should be based on this finding. The reticulocyte count is low in untreated pernicious anemia. When specific liver therapy is given, the reticulocyte count rapidly rises to a peak since the immature, unfinished red cells are not completed and delivered into the circulation. The height of the reticulocyte rise parallels the hyperplasia and immaturity of the marrow. The redder the marrow the more severe the disease and the higher the reticulocyte count with correct treatment since there are larger numbers of immature cells to be released.

The leukocyte count is seldom above normal in pernicious anemia and often decreased. The leukocytes in the circulation are often larger than normal and usually well lobulated. The hyperplasia of the erythroblastic tissues in the marrow seemingly interferes with the normal growth of granulocytes by crowding out the leukoblastic tissues. The granulocytes remain longer than normal in the marrow so when released show hypersegmentation of the nucleus indicating they are older than the average granular or white cell. The platelets are often decreased, probably for the same reason.

To summarize the blood findings in pernicious anemia: The first change is an increase in volume (macrocytosis) of the red cells into the blood stream. As the disease progresses the anemia becomes more marked, the macrocytosis persists and more immature cells—poikilicytes, megaloblasts, and normoblasts—appear. The reticulocyte count is low. The bone marrow is hyperplastic and red. The leukocyte count is below normal and the white cells in the circulation tend to show increased lobulation. With adequate specific therapy the reticulocyte count rises sharply showing that the erythrocytes are being matured in the marrow. With complete treatment the blood returns to normal and remains so. The one constant abnormality when the disease is active is the macrocytosis of the red cells. It is the earliest variation from normal to appear and the last to disappear and is the best indicator of pernicious anemia from the hematologic standpoint. It is by far the best criterion of the completeness of treatment. All untreated patients in our series of 558 patients with pernicious anemia have had a macrocytic anemia, and often only the macrocytosis. All correctly and completely treated patients show no macrocytosis.

The neurologic lesions are both peripheral and central. There is probably always some degree of neuritis, usually some degeneration of the tracts of the spinal cord, and at times cerebral symptoms due to involvement of the brain. It seems proven that the neurologic lesions are due to a deficiency in the nutrition of the nervous system. It is likely that the same nutritional factor necessary for the maturation of the red cells is required for the nervous system also. It is possible that other substances are involved, but it is known that the deficiency responsible for the neurologic lesions is satisfied by the use of liver and liver substitutes regardless of whether it is dependent on the same factor or some related or independent factor.

The neurologic involvement is manifested by paresthesias of the hands and feet, incoordination or spasticity. The most common finding on examination is a loss of vibratory sense in the lower extremities. Abnormalities in the reflexes and position sense are often present. In 325 patients on whom the vibration sense was tested this was found abnormal (lost or diminished) in 245 or 72.3 per cent. Nearly half (45.8 per cent) of the entire group of 406 patients complained on admission of numbness and tingling in the extremities. Over 10 per cent already had a spinal cord lesion making walking difficult due to incoordination or spasticity. A true psychosis was observed in only one patient.

In treating pernicious anemia the object is to satisfy completely and permanently the deficiency responsible for the disease. Whole liver by mouth, oral stomach extracts, and oral and parenteral liver extracts are available forms of specific treatment. While it is an excellent idea for patients to eat liver as a part of the diet, it is difficult to treat satisfactorily pernicious anemia by eating liver. Stomach extracts can be given by mouth only. Liver extracts given intramuscularly is thirty times as active as the same amount taken by mouth. By far the best method of treatment is the intramuscular of subcutaneous use of a potent liver extract. Some extracts can be given intravenously, but the intravenous method has not advantages over subcutaneous or intramuscular administration. It is probable that a patient is more apt to become sensitive to the extract if given intravenously. There are many different liver extracts on the market varying greatly in strength. There is no exact method for assaying liver extracts. An extract labeled 15 units per c.c. may contain many more. The same manufacturer may offer numerous extracts varying only in potency, which is confusing. I see no point in treating most patients suffering from pernicious anemia with other than a concentrated extract (15 units per c.c.)

Since extracts of different manufacturers may vary, it is wise to select one good extract and use this will all patients. Where the neurologic involvment is serious, some clinicians have thought that a less concentrated extract might contain some substance which is not present in the concentrated extract and which is an aid in relieving the disease of the nervous system. This view is debatable.

Having selected a potent concentrated extract the method of administration must be decided upon. Many different ways have been advised. The whole subject is much colored by personal opinion. I believe strongly that the most satisfactory method is intensive therapy at the beginning of treatment. Certainly in some cases less intensive treatment might be equally as good. There is no way to gauge from the standpoint of the patient the amount of specific factor needed by any individual. The material is not expensive and the results of inadequate treatment are so serious it seems sensible to administer the liver extract in amounts which would cover the needs of all patients. After the initial period of intensive therapy the injections need not be given so often.

The method found uniformly satisfactory is the following schedule:

First two weeks daily injections of 1 c.c. of a potent extract containing 15 units per c.c.

Next three months period twice weekly injections of 1 c.c. of the same extract.

Next three month period weekly injections of 1 c.c. of the same extract.

Remainder of the patient's life monthly injections of 1 c.c. of the same extract.

This plan of treatment has been followed for the past fifteen years. With it the blood is always returned to normal and maintained if the diagnosis is correct. The neurologic lesions never advance and usually improve often to a striking degree; the gastrointestinal symptoms are relieved entirely although the achlorhydria is uninfluenced.

Recent work on folic acid suggests that this substance may be the factor which is responsible for the specific effect of liver and liver substitutes. If this proves to be true the treatment of pernicious anemia will be simplified. Further study is needed, however. It

LIBRARY OF THE
COLLEGE OF PHYSICIANS

is best to do a volume index or other test to determine cell size as even a slight increase in size is a warning that more treatment is needed.

The neurologic signs and symptoms are the hardest to influence and improve much more slowly than the anemia. If progress is not satisfactory, injections should continue to be given at weekly intervals indefinitely. The lack of improvement neurologically may be due to permanent damage to the nerve tract which cannot be altered. So often this damage takes place while the patient is receiving treatment but inadequate treatment. It is remarkable how striking the improvement in a neurologic lesion can be when properly treated. A patient may be completely crippled due to an extensive cord lesion and still regain use of the legs and walk satisfactorily. Seldom is the vibratory sense completely regained—some paresthesia is apt to persist. A neurologic lesion should never develop or progress in an adequately treated patient.

The treatment of any deficiency disease is influenced by certain intercurrent diseases, especially infections. More intensive therapy should be given if such occur.

One troublesome complication of liver therapy is the development of allergic reactions, principally hives, following the injection of liver extract. Most extracts are made from hog liver. Others are made from beef, horse and sheep products. If difficulty is expected, different extracts should be tried. So far I have not seen a patient who could not take some potent extract. Mild reactions may be controlled by giving small doses of adrenalin with the liver extract.

Iron is seldom required unless needed for some reason such as blood loss, apart from the pernicious anemia.

It is doubtful if added vitamins influence the neurologic lesions if liver therapy is given properly and intensively and an adequate diet is eaten. Hydrochloric acid is seldom needed.

SUMMARY

1. Pernicious anemia is a disease characterized by (a) macrocytic anemia with (b) achlorhydria, an atrophy of the papillae of the tongue and other gastrointestinal symptoms and (c) frequent neurologic signs and symptoms manifested by numbness and tingling of the extremities, lost vibratory sense, and disturbances in gait due to combined sclerosis of the spinal cord.

2. In a series of 406 consecutive patients with pernicious anemia: (a) free hydrochloric acid was found in the gastric contents in only one patient, (b) all untreated patients had a macrocytic anemia, (c) the tongue was clean or atrophic in most patients, (d) nearly half complained of pares-

thesias or difficulty in walking, and (e) in three-fourth the vibratory sense was absent.

3. All symptoms and signs except the achlorhydria are due to a lack of some specific substance normally formed by the interaction of a ferment secreted by the stomach on some constituent of the ingested food and stored in the liver.

4. The deficiency in idopathic pernicious anemia is permanent, so treatment is required throughout the life of the patient. The object of treatment is to satisfy completely the need for the lacking substance.

5. A satisfactory method of giving liver extract has been outlined.

6. Folic acid may prove to be the specific factor needed to supply the deficiency.

7. Iron, hydrochloric acid, and other medication is seldom needed. A complete diet should be insisted upon.

8. With adequate therapy (a) the blood returns to normal and remain so, (b) the tongue becomes normal and other gastrointestinal symptoms such as indigestion and diarrhea disappear, (c) the neurologic symptoms improve or even clear completely and (d) the achlorhydria is permanent.

9. In pernicious anemia (a) the seriousness of the disease must be appreciated, (b) the disease must be correctly diagnosed, and (c) treatment must be complete and permanent.

Annual Fall Clinical Conference

The Kansas City Southwest Clinical Society will hold its Annual Conference in the Municipal Auditorium, Kansas City, Missouri, October seventh through tenth this year.

Guest physicians who will take part in the scientific program are E. T. Bell, Minneapolis; Louis A. Buie and John S. Lundy, Rochester; R. B. Cattell, Boston; Warren H. Cole, Paul H. Holinger, Walter L. Palmer, Herbert E. Schmitz, and William Van Hazel, Chicago; Charles A. Doan, Columbus; A. I. Folsom and Tinsley R. Harrison, Dallas; L. H. Garland, San Francisco; Paul B. Magnuson, Washington; G. Glen Spurling, Louisville, and E. H. Watson, Ann Arbor.

A joint meeting with the county medical societies, Monday evening, October 7th, will be a Clinicopathologic Conference. Participants will be E. T. Bell, M.D., (director) and doctors Cattell, Doan, Garland, Harrison, Lundy, Van Hazel and Watson.

There will be daily radio broadcasts, Round Table Luncheons, Scientific and Technical Exhibits.

Special features will include a Stag Dinner with Entertainment, Tuesday evening; Alumni Dinners, Wednesday evening and entertainment for the visiting women.

If you have not received a copy of the Kansas City Medical Journal one will be sent you upon request at the executive office—630 Shukert Bldg., Kansas City 6, Mo.

This is the highest miracle of genius, that things which are not should be as though they were, that the imaginations of one mind should become the personal recollections of another.—*Macaulay.*

God will put up with a great many things in the human heart, but there is one thing that he will not put up with in it — a second place. He who offers God a second place, offers him no place.—*Ruskin.*

A Survey of The Pneumonias*

SAMUEL GOODMAN, M.D., F.A.C.P.

TULSA, OKLAHOMA

I have chosen as the subject of this address "A Survey of the Pneumonias". It concludes a fifteen-year survey of the pneumonias in the Tulsa area, which I began in 1930. The results of previous studies in this series were given in papers[1] [2] [3] read before the Oklahoma State Medical Association in 1936, 1939 and 1942.

Before beginning the discussion I would like to call your attention to the fact that this survey of the pneumonias is a statistical study which required personal interpretation of hospital records. This was necessary since many of the records were incompletely detailed and often lacked some important part of the required data. The reasons for these deficiencies and omissions are more or less well known. To mention only a few of them; the impact of the war on the hospital personnel, the great increase in admissions without adequate facilities to take care of them, and the burden placed upon the civilian physicians, together with important items to be mentioned later, have in no small measure been responsible for inadequacies in some records which could be supplemented only by personal interpretation. Deficiency in hospital records is by no means a local condition. A review of papers published elsewhere shows that during the war years, hospital records were below peacetime standards in many other areas of the country.

With the available data I have selected for analysis those cases which fulfilled the criteria for the diagnosis of pneumonia, omitting all those cases in which incompleteness of records or findings left any doubt as to the correctness of the diagnosis. Secondary and terminal pneumonias incidental to other diseases, such as nephritis, heart failure and infections, and postoperative pneumonias were also excluded from this survey. The above groups comprised 130 of 390 cases of pneumonia admitted to St. John's hospital in the years from 1943 to 1946. The remaining 260 cases of primary pneumonia form the basis of this survey.

The primary pneumonias may be classified into four groups, namely lobar pneumonia,

bronchopneumonia, atypical lobar pneumania and the pneumonias produced by viruses. It should be recalled that typical lobar pneumonia is caused solely by the pneumococcus, whereas the atypical lobar pneumonias are caused by a variety of organisms, such as the staphylococcus, streptococcus, Friedlander and influenza bacillus. The bronchopneumonias due to pneumococci are found almost exclusively in children, while those due to other organisms are found in all age groups. In atypical primary pneumonias caused by a virus the verification of the diagnosis depends upon identification of the virus. Since this is only possible with specialized equipment and is impractical in a General hospital, one must rely on clinical deduction and roentgenological findings for a diagnosis.

In examining the hospital records it became quite evident that exact terminology from an etiological standpoint was frequently ignored. For instance, in relatively few records was the term "pneumococcus pneumonia" used.

TABLE NO. I

Survey of 260 cases of primary pneumonia admitted to St. John's Hospital from January 1, 1943 to January 1, 1946.

Age Groups		Incidence by months		
			Bacterial	Virus
Under one	42	Jan.	48	4
1 to 10	67	Feb.	34	0
11 to 20	15	March	26	2
21 to 30	22	April	13	2
31 to 40	24	May	9	3
41 to 50	28	June	7	2
51 to 60	16	July	6	13
61 to 70	11	Aug.	1	12
71 to 80	9	Sept.	6	11
Over 80	1	Oct.	9	5
Not recorded	23	Nov.	13	2
		Dec.	30	2

Sex		Onset	
Male	140	Sudden	78
Female	117	Gradual	174
Not recorded	3	Not recorded	8

Seasonal incidence: Table one shows clearly that pneumonia does not occur with equal frequency during all seasons of the year. It becomes evident immediately that bacterial pneumonia is by far more frequent during the colder months of the year, while virus pneumonia is more prevalent during the warmer season. Of the 202 cases of bacterial pneumonia in this series, 138 or 70 per cent occured during the months of December, January, February and March, while only

*Delivered before the Section on General Medicine, Oklahoma State Medical Association Annual Meeting, May 3, 1946.

30 per cent were found during the remaining eight months of the year. The seasonal incidence of viral pneumonia shows an interesting reversal of this picture. Of the 58 cases of viral pneumonia in this series, 36 or 65 per cent occurred during the hot months of July, August and September, while only 22 cases or 35 per cent occured during the remaining nine months of the year.

Distribution as to age and sex: While pneumonia may occur at any age, 109 cases or 42 per cent in this series were found in the age group from under one year to ten years. This is in agreement with general statistics on age morbidity. The preponderance of males over females affected is not as evident in this series as has usually been found. There were 140 males and 117 females in this group. In three instances there was no sex specified.

Mode of onset: In 174 or 68 per cent of the cases, an upper respiratory infection preceded the onset of pneumonia. This high incidence is particularly significant. The role of the common cold as a frequent factor in precipitating a pneumonia must not be overlooked. Common colds should be treated energetically rather than lightly, which is so often the case. While it is true that the majority of colds are primarily of viral origin and are uninfluenced by sulfonamides, it seems logical that a persistence of fever or extension into the lower respiratory passages would be an indication for the administration of the sulfonamides. Controlled and extensive studies made by the Army and Navy during the war, repeatedly confirmed this observation.

TABLE NO. II
Site of Lesion

Bacterial		Virus	
Bilateral	71	Bilateral	6
R L L	48	R L L	18
L L L	36	L L L	15
R U L	14	R U L	5
L U L	9	L U L	9
R M L	4	R M L	3
L U L & L L L	3	L U L & L L L	1
Both Bases	5	Both Bases	0
Both upper lobes	2	Both upper lobes	0
Not recorded	18	Not recorded	0

Number of patients x-rayed 177
Number of patients not x-rayed 83

Site of lesion: Table two shows an analysis of 260 cases of pneumonia by localization of the lesion found upon clinical and roentgenological examination. According to Stevens', bilateral lesions occur in almost all cases of bronchopneumonia, while bilateral involvement is found in only about 20 per cent of the cases of lobar pneumonia. The relative frequency of lesions of both lungs in this series, namely 77 cases out of 260, or roughly 30 per cent, can therefore be explained by the fact that a great number of the patients were children under the age of

ten, during which age bronchopneumonia is by far more frequent than the lobar type of pneumonia. Next to bilateral pneumonia the high incidence of involvement of the right lower lobe is noticeable. This is well in accordance with all available statistics and is related to the anatomical structure of the right main bronchus, which is practically a continuation of the trachea. The left lower lobe also shows relatively frequent involvement, which is in accordance with the fact that acute infections of the lung affect predominantly the dependent portions of the organ, while pulmonary tuberculosis shows a predilection for the upper lobes. In this series it will be noted that involvement of the upper lobes is relatively infrequent. It is also interesting to note that, with the exception of bilateral involvement, the incidence of localization in this series follows the same pattern in viral pneumonia as it does in the bacterial type of the disease.

TABLE NO. III

Sputum examination		White Blood Count	
Sputum not examined	171	WBC not done	23
Sputum examined	89	WBC done	231
Type I	6		
Type II	1		
Type III	4	Range of WBC	
Type IV	2	Bacterial 7900-53000	
Type VI	1	Virus 35000-5000	
Type VII	1		
Type VIII	2		
Type XIV	3	Sulfonamide Blood Levels	
Morphol (pneumococci)	42	in 1943 and 1944	
Streptococci	14	Levels done 60
Staphylococci	1	Levels not done 97
Undetermined	12		

Omissions in records are shown again by the number of cases, namely 18, in which a specific site of the lesion had not been recorded in the clinical findings, even though roentgenological reports indicated the presence of pneumonic infiltration. Roentgenological examination is one of the most essential procedures in the diagnosis of pneumonia, although it is noted in this table that 83 or approximately 32 per cent of the cases were not x-rayed. It should be borne in mind that roentgenological evidence of pneumonia is present for hours and even days before typical physical signs can be elicited. It is evident, therefore, that routine roentgenological examination, especially in hospital practice should always be employed.

Further laboratory data are indicated in table three. The fact that of 260 cases there was no sputum examination done in 171, deserves some comment. Since the introduction of the sulfonamides and penicillin in the treatment of infectious diseases there appears to be a tendency on the part of physicians to disregard the necessity of thorough study of each case. Despite the success obtained with the use of the sulfonamides and penicillin, I am convinced that examination of the sputum is of more than academic interest. In this connection it must be recalled that two important organisms, namely the

Friedlander and influenza bacilli are frequent causes of pneumonia.

Neither of these organisms is susceptible to the administration of penicillin. Therefore, it is important that the routine examination of sputums should not be abandoned. The routine use of penicillin without knowledge of the etiology of the disease should be discouraged.

Under the types of organisms is will be noted that in 42 cases there were morphological pneumococci present which would not type. The reason for this is that swelling of pneumococcus capsule frequently does not occur when culfonamides are administered prior to typing.

In 155 cases of pneumonia during 1943 and 1944 the sulfonamides were administered as a specific agent. Given in their order of frequency were: Sulfadiazine, Sulfathiozole and Sulfamerizine. In 1945 when penicillin became available for civilian use, treatment consisted of the use of penicillin alone or penicillin and the sulfonamides in combination. The importance of sulfonamide blood level determination should not be overlooked. It is necessary that safe and therapeutically effective concentrations be obtained in order to assure the most satisfactory results.

Under usual conditions, with adequate levels, one can anticipate a critical fall in temperature within 24 to 72 hours after sulfonamide therapy is begun. Unless blood sulfonamide levels are determined frequently, the efficacy of sulfonamide therapy cannot be properly evaluated since spontaneous recovery often occurs, especially in the pneumococcus pneumonias, as early as the third day of the disease. In this series it is significant that the recovery in fifty patients out of ninety-five, in whom no sulfonamide blood level was done, was retarded beyond the fourth day. A majority of the 58 cases of viral pneumonia was treated with sulfonamides or penicillin. In no instance was there any evidence that the administration of either altered the course of the disease. The ineffectiveness of sulfonamide and penicillin therapy in the viral pneumonias has been amply confirmed by many sources. The average duration of the disease in this series; irrespective of the type of treatment employed, was about 7 days. Up to the present time, none other than symptomatic treatment seems to be indicated in the management of viral pneumonias.

Complications and mortality: In this series of 260 cases all of the deaths occurred in patients who suffered from the bacterial type of pneumonia and none in the pneumonias caused by a virus. There were 21 deaths in all, eight of which occurred within 24 hours after admission to the hospital. The latter were not included in the calculation of the mortality rate as they were in extremely poor condition on admission, and could not have been treated for a sufficient length of time to permit an evaluation of the therapy used.

Therefore in 202 cases of bacterial pneumonia there were 13 deaths a mortality rate of 6.5 per cent, which compares favorably with results obtained elsewhere in the country. It is interesting to note that of the 13 deaths five were above 60 years of age and six were under one year old. Even though the absolute number of deaths is small it conforms to the principle that pneumonias are most dangerous in the very young and the very old. There were only three cases of empyema, an extremely low incidence of this complication, as compared to the period before introduction of the sulfonamides and penicillin.

SUMMARY

A survey of 260 cases of primary pneumonia is presented. This survey includes incidence as to age, sex, season and site of lesion. Laboratory and roentgenological data, treatment, complications and mortality are also evaluated. Of the 260 cases of pneumonia 202 were of bacterial etiology and 58 were of viral origin.

A number of conclusions should be drawn from this study. There was a noticeable lack of accuracy in hospital records during the war years of 1943, 1944 and 1945. In part this was excusable due to factors caused by abnormal condition in these years. On the other hand there was a tendency among physicians to disregard important laboratory procedures in the clinical evaluation of their cases. In this connection, I would like to cite the low percentage of sputum examined, the infrequent use of roentgenological facilities and the lack of obtaining sulfonamide blood levels in instances where the sulfonamides were administered.

It should be clearly understood that the responsibility of the physician does not cease with merely a diagnosis of pneumonia and the administration of rapidly acting drugs. It is still necessary to conduct laboratory tests and roentgenological examinations in order to find the therapy best suited for each form of pneumonia. For example, neither the sulfonamides nor penicillin are effective against the viral type of pneumonia. Much time and effort may be wasted unless all facilities for diagnosis are employed. In addition discomfort to the patient by the administration of penicillin could be avoided if the early diagnosis of viral pneumonia were established. The same holds true in cases of pneumonia caused by the Friedlander and influenza bacillus. It is obvious that the omission of the use of diagnostic facilities, when available, is not consistent with good medical practice. In presenting this survey of the pneumonias I am hopeful that it may stimulate a deeper interest in all phases of investigations pertaining to the disease.

BIBLIOGRAPHY

1. Samuel Goodman: The Recent Outbreak of Lobar Pneumonia in the Tulsa Area. Journal, Oklahoma State Medical Association, 1936.
2. Samuel Goodman: Further Study of Lobar Pneumonia in the Tulsa Area. Journal, Oklahoma State Medical Association, March, 1939.
3. Samuel Goodman: Atypical Pneumonia, Journal, Oklahoma State Medical Association, December, 1942.
4. Stevens: Practice of Medicine.

Myasthenia Gravis*

T. R. TURNER, M.D.

TULSA, OKLAHOMA

While myasthenia gravis is usually considered a rare disease, it is of considerable interest to the practicing physician, not only because of its interesting relationship to muscle physiology, but also because of the rapid advance in methods of treatment during recent years.

For some reason a great many cases of mild and moderately severe myasthenia remain undiagnosed for relatively long periods of time. There are several probable explanations for this. First, many physicians feel that this is such a rare disease that they probably fail to give it due consideration or to search for it sufficiently often. Secondly, the disease is ordinarily chronic with a tendency to remissions and to variations so that the mild case frequently is not seen in the attack. Thirdly, there is a prevailing idea among many that ptosis, diplopia, or facial weakness is always present and in the absence of these obvious signs the possibility is dismissed without further consideration. Finally, the complaint of weakness is so commonly a neurotic one that myasthenia gravis patients are often so labeled.

If the history is carefully taken a great many of these errors will be avoided. History of undue fatigability to the point of true muscular weakness should be sought for. The neurotic will admit, on careful, tactful questioning, that his so-called weakness is really just tiredness, and that by exerting great effort he can always climb the stairs or comb his hair. However, the myasthenic, under the same questioning, will often tell of going up stairs on his all fours, of actually failing to get his arm over his head, of strangling on his food, or of some other incident of true muscle weakness. Further distinguishing characteristics are increasing weakness toward the end of the day, increased weakness eight or ten days before the onset on menses, and variations of severity ranging to frank remissions.

Various groups of muscles may be involved. Thus the symptoms may appear primarily in the eye muscles, the bulbar group of muscles, or the muscles of the trunk and extremities. Various combinations of these may occur.

Examination should include careful tests of individual muscle groups for evidence of weakness, not only those muscles supplied by the cranial nerves, which should be particularly checked, but also the muscles of the trunk and extremities. If definite muscle weakness is found the prostigmin test should be done. It is best to observe carefully for comparison some such objective measures as the length of time the patient can hold the arms extended, his ability to sit up from the recombent position with arms folded on chest, or some similar test against gravity. Usually two or three ampules of prostigmin methylsulfate 1:2000 (to which gr. 1/150 atropine may be added to avoid unpleasant side effects) are given and the time noted. After twenty to thirty minutes the muscle strength is again carefully checked. In the typical case the patient gets dramatic improvement which confirms the diagnosis.

Failing to find definite evidence of muscle weakness on examination of a patient who gives a history suggestive of myasthenia gravis, one of two provocative tests may be chosen to aid in diagnosis. Quinine, having an opposite effect to prostigmin, aggravates

*Delivered before the Section on Neurology, Psychiatry and Endocrinology, Oklahoma State Medical Association Annual Meeting, May 1, 1946.

or produces an attack of muscle weakness. The patient is usually given twenty or thirty grains with instructions to take ten grains at two hour intervals and come to the office two hours after the last dose. He is not told the expected results. Muscle strength is then tested and is compared with that of. the previous day. If weakness is produced, prostigmin is given and the effect again measured.

A second and quicker provocative test is by the use of curare. One tenth the dose commonly recommended for use with electric shock (which is 1 c.c. Intocostrin per 40 pounds body weight) is injected and the effect noted. Normally this will produce little change in muscle strength, but in myasthenia .gravis an attack is precipitated. By way of warning·it should be stated that patients already showing muscle weakness should be given curare with great ca'ution, as fatalities have occurred with this test.

The diagnosis having been established, certain further tests are indicated. Hyperthyroidism occurs with myasthenia gravis sufficiently often that it should be ruled out in every case. Tumor of the thymus occurs rather frequently and special x-ray studies of the chest, including lateral view, are indicated, although the tumor is often difficult to demonstrate and absence of x-ray findings cannot be depended upon to rule it out.

The medical treatment of‿myasthenia, in addition to supportive measures, consists principally of the use of prostigmin, at times in combination with one or more other drugs. The action of prostigmin is thought to be as follows:

Acetylcholine is liberated at the motor end plate by the nerve impulse and is instrumental in producing muscle contraction. Choline esterase is concerned with the destruction of acetylcholine. In myasthenia gravis there appears to be some disturbance in the function of acetylcholine. Prostigmin inhibits the action of choline esterase thus permitting a stronger muscle contraction.

Ordinarily, prostigmin is given orally as prostigmin bromide, which is supplied in 15 mg. tablets. Since the effect wears off in a few hours it must be given five or six times a day so as to produce a smooth response. The dose varies tremendously depending on the 'needs of the patient. Some do well on four or five tablets a day, while others have been known to require up to forty or more. As hypodermic injection is often much more effective than oral administration, severe cases are taught to use a syringe so that they can treat themselves in case of emergency. Atropine may be given if necessary to control such disagreeable side effects as diarrhea and nausea.

After the patient is regulated on the optimum dose 'of prostigmin, certain other drugs may be added, one at a time, so that their value in the individual case can be determined. Of these, ephedrine is usually tried first. It is started in doses of 3/8 grain three times a day, and varied to suit the needs of the patient. It should not be given in the evening because of interference with sleep.

Guanidine hydrochloride is recommended in daily amounts varying from ten to twenty-five mg. per Kg. body weight, divided into three doses. It acts to increase the sensitivity of the muscle to acetylcholine and is an effective supplement to prostigmin in a few cases. Toxic symptoms are mostly gastrointestinal and may be controlled by atropine, but are considered to be an indication to reduce the dose.

Potassium salts in doses of 10 to 12 grams, three times a day, are of value in a few cases.

Glycine in daily doses of 20 to 30 grams was once widely used but has now been largely replaced by other drugs.

X-ray of the thymus region has been used and good results reported in a few cases.

At the present time there is considerable enthusiasm over the treatment of myasthenia by surgical removal of the thymus, particularly where a tumor can be demonstrated. Good results have followed this procedure in a number of cases and some now advocate surgical exploration in all cases, with removal of whatever thymic tissue can be found. The number of patients so treated is rapidly increasing and the true value of the procedure will probably soon be known.

SUMMARY

Myasthenia gravis is a disease of muscle physiology, probably 'related to some hormonal disturbance. With improved understanding of muscle function great strides have been made in the treatment of. this disease in recent years and further advance can be expected in the near future.

BIBLIOGRAPHY

1. C. H. Campbell and J. M. Campbell: The Thymus Gland and Its Relationship to Myasthenia Gravis, Journal of Oklahoma State Medical Association, Volume No. 38, pp. 227-280; 1945.

2. O. T. Clagett and L. M. Eaton: Thymic Tumors in Myasthenia Gravis; Surgical Clinics of North America, Volume No. 23, pp. 1076-1082; 1943.

3. L. M. Eaton: Diagnostic Tests for Myasthenia Gravis with Prostigmin and Quinine; Proceedings of Staff Meeting, Mayo Clinic, Volume No. 18, pp. 230-236; 1943.

4. A. S. Kinot, K. Dodd and S. S. Riven: The Use of Guanidine Hydrochloride in the Treatment of Myasthenia Gravis; Journal of American Medical Association, Volume No. 133, pp. 553-559; 1939.

5. Richard Richter: The Management of Myasthenia Gravis; The Medical Clinics of North America, Volume No. 29, pp. 126-135; 1945.

It is the vain endeavor to make ourselves what we are not that has strewn history with so many broken purposes and lives left in the rough.—*Lowell.*

Clinical Pathological Conference

University of Oklahoma School of Medicine

Presented by the Departments of Pathology and Medicine

REYNOLD PATZER, M.D.—HOWARD C. HOPPS, M.D.

OKLAHOMA CITY, OKLAHOMA

DR. HOPPS: The case for our consideration today presents somewhat of a diagnostic problem. It seems obvious that this man suffered from a malignant neoplasm, but its point of origin was rather obscure. Then too there was some question as to how the neoplasm accounted for the unusual symptoms which this man presented. Dr. Patzer will present the clinical analysis.

PROTOCOL

Patient: N. D., Negro male, age 75; admitted May 31, 1946; died June 8, 1945.

Chief Complaint: Epigastric pain, swelling of the abdomen, and nausea and vomiting.

Present Illness: The patient was apparently well until May 24, 1945 when he first noticed a mass in the epigastrium with severe and sudden pain at the right margin of the umbilicus radiating to the epigastrium. He had had no bowel movement since the onset of this attack. He had had alternate constipation and diarrhea for one year prior to this acute illness. On May 25, 1945 he began to vomit recently eaten food, and the abdomen started to swell. He grew progressively weaker, and was admitted to University Hospital on May 31, 1945.

Past and Family History: Essentially negative.

Physical Examination: This was a well developed, fairly well nourished negro male, apparently acutely ill. His chest was clear to percussion and auscultation. His heart was slightly enlarged to the left; there were no murmurs. The temperature was 100 degrees, pulse rate 120 and respiratory rate 30 per minute. The abdomen was markedly distended and was tympanitic throughout. There was tenderness on deep pressure in the mid-epigastrium. No masses were palpable. Hyperperistalsis was present. His prostate was 2-3 times enlarged, but was not nodular.

Laboratory Data: The urine contained no albumin, 1+ glucose, a few red blood cells and innumerable white blood cells. The hemo-globin was 13 Gm. The red blood cell count was 7,000,000, the white blood cell count was 11,150 with 79 per cent neutrophils. The blood N.P.N. was 40 mg./100 cc. The Mazzini reaction was negative. An x-ray of the abdomen showed many distended loops of small intestine.

Clinical Course: The patient was given intravenous fluids, including blood transfusions, with imporvement, and was operated upon on June 4, 1945. At operation the entire small bowel was very distended. A large neoplastic mass was felt retroperitoneally. A biopsy was taken from a small mesenteric implant. The cause of obstruction was a large metastatic tumer mass 3-4 inches from the ileocecal junction. A catheter was inserted 8 inches proximal to the point of this obstruction. The patient withstood the operation well. The patient did well until the morning of June 8, 1945 when respiration became labored and the patient died suddenly.

CLINICAL DIAGNOSIS

DR. PATZER: From your study of the case history you are aware that this man's chief complaints were epigastric pain, nausea and vomiting. He stated that he felt well until May, 1945 at which time he noticed a mass in the epigastrium with severe and sudden pain. The first symptom that we have to consider then, is pain in the umbilicus radiating to the epigastrium. This directs our attention to the possibility of a lesion in the right lower quadrant and suggests that it is obstructive in nature—perhaps the sequel to a peri-appendiceal abscess. The complaint of alternating constipation and diarrhea is certainly compatible with a partial obstruction of the intestine, especially of the coecum or ascending colon.

Upon extrance to the hospital the patient seemed acutely ill. His abdomen was markedly distended and tympanitic and there was a history of vomiting recently eaten food during the past week. X-rays revealed distended, gas filled loops of bowel.

These various findings confirm our previous impression of intestinal obstruction. The thing that we must try to determine, however, is what kind of obstruction this is and what its etiology is. We wish to know whether or not the patient has much gas in his colon and if he has a fluid level. If the lower small intestine is distended, but not the colon, we know that the obstruction is in the small bowel, above the ileocecal valve. Under such circumstances there is not necessarily a need for immediate surgical intervention. If the obstruction involves the large bowel we should consider the case a surgical emergency. This is because in approximately 10 per cent of these cases the ileocecal valve has more or less of a one-way action. Gas can enter the large bowel from the small intestine, but cannot leave via the ileocecal valve. There results a progressive distention which may ultimately lead to increased permeability and bacterial peritonitis.

From the operative report, we know that the site of obstruction was at the ileocecal junction and that its cause was a malignant neoplasm. We do not know the cause of the patient's death. He was apparently doing well until, suddenly and unexpectedly, he died on the fourth post-operative day. Did the patient have peritonitis? Was there an unbalance of fluid or electrolytes because of improper post-operative management? Was his death related to the primary malignant neoplasm from which he suffered and of which we do not know the origin?

What are the things which may give rise to a mass in the epigastrium? A carcinoma of the stomach may do this, and in addition, there may be metastasis in the intestine which could cause obstruction. The absence of hematemesis or blood in the stools would be somewhat against this. We should also have a history of "digestive difficulty" following certain foods. Another possibility is carcinoma of the pancreas. In this case it would almost certainly be of the body or tail and thus an uncommon type. We can say this because carcinoma of the head of the pancreas almost invariably results in jaundice. Patients with carcinoma of the pancreas often have marked weakness, out of proportion to what might be expected. There is a suggestion that this man had such weakness. There is also, often, very severe pain in the back—this patient did not present such a complaint. From this history I am not sure what this patient had.

CLINICAL DISCUSSION

QUESTION: What do you think was the immediate cause of death?

DR. PATZER: I do not know—I wonder if he didn't have peritonitis. I would consider peritonitis, improper fluid balance and possibly a coronary occlusion.

DR. HOPPS: Wouldn't the fact that this patient seemed to be doing well and then died suddenly indicate that it was something other than peritonitis?

DR. PATZER: Yes, that would lead us to believe it a cardiac lesion.

QUESTION: Just where was this mass that was felt retroperitoneally?

DR. PATZER: I don't know, but that would be another thing which would lead me to consider carcinoma of the pancreas.

QUESTION: How do you account for the initial erythrocyte count of seven million?

DR. PATZER: I believe this was due to dehydration.

QUESTION: Could this have been a tumor of the kidney?

DR. PATZER: I've never seen intestinal obstruction caused by a tumor of the kidney except in infants or children with a massive Wilm's tumor.

ANATOMIC DIAGNOSIS

DR. HOPPS: The first question we tried to answer at necropsy was the exact basis for the intestinal obstruction. This had been somewhat relieved by surgical treatment so that at necropsy there was no ladder pattern apparent and the obstruction was not of extremely high grade. We found a tumor mass within the cecum which was 3 cm. in diameter and which had produced partial obstruction. A similar tumor mass was found at the hepatic flexure which was producing moderate obstruction, but the colon was not particularly distended proximal to this. The mass at the cecum was the major functional obstruction. Grossly it was evident that these were metastasic lesions. They were located within the wall of the bowel and did not interrupt the mucosa. We found no lesion that would have resulted in blood in the stools, i.e., we found no ulcerating lesion of the gastro-intestinal tract. In addition to these tumor masses within the colon the peritoneum was studded with small grey-white

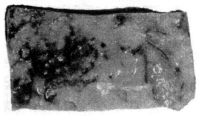

FIGURE II: *Parietal Peritoneum.* Illustrating peritoneal carcinomatosis.

nodules and plaques of firm fleshly tissue 2 to 4 mm. in diameter. Thus this patient had peritoneal carcinomatosis. In addition there was a rather large retroperitoneal mass in the region of the pancreas. Before we dissected this mass it was impossible to make out the pattern of the pancreas. Upon careful dissection, however, it was apparent that the primary neoplasm was in the pancreas. The bulk of the neoplasm was contained in peripancreatic lymph nodes. With this tumor mass, the pancreas weighed only 170 Gm. so that there was only 70 Gm. of tumor at the original site. The metastasic tumor tissue was much more abundant than this. The neoplasm was primary at the *head* of the pancreas and it did not produce painless and progressive jaundice. This is a very unusual

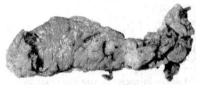

FIGURE I: *Carcinoma of the Head of the Pancreas.* Note the relatively small size of this primary neoplasm.

case in this respect and may be related to the fact that this particular neoplasm did not metastasize in the ordinary fashion. Usually there is early and extensive metastasis to regional lymphnodes so that before long the common and/or hepatic bile duct becomes obstructed. This man had such a process, but it was limited to the *cystic* duct. This duct was almost completely obliterated by an infiltration of neoplastic tissue. The obstruction was not of long duration, however, in that the gallbladder contained only about 5 cc. of dark green bile. Obviously involvement of the cystic duct alone would not result in jaundice. In addition to the peritoneal metastasis and the two masses in the intestine there was metastasis to a suprarenal gland.

Additional findings included marked prostatic hyperplasia. Actually the patient suffered very little from urethral obstruction even though his prostate weighed 110 gms. The bladder wall was but slightly thickened. The region involved in the hyperplasia is the important thing as this case illustrates. In this case the hyperplasia was more or less diffuse and there were no bulky nodules in the median bar or other regions bordering on the prostatic urethra to obstruct this passageway.

The cause of death was *pulmonary embolism.* There were seven fragments of thrombus which average about 1 cm. in diameter

so that they must have come from the femoral vein. These seven fragments had a combined length of approximately 25 cm. They lay, for the most part, in the pulmonary artery and its major branches. With a history of this sort it seems that pulmonary embolism should have been a major consideration. Why wasn't there clinical evidence of thrombosis of the femoral vein? *Phlebothrombosis* is usually silent and it is thrombosis without phlebitis that usually results in embolism. It is usually *thrombophlebitis* which causes pain and edema.

Getting back to the subject of carcinoma of the pancreas, this is a condition which has aroused considerable interest for many years. It is one of the relatively common carcinomas. In one series of 386 cases which have been reported, carcinoma was limited to the head in 40 per cent, and in an additional 40 per cent there was diffuse involvement at the time of inspection so that the origin could not be determined. Actually carcinoma of the pancreas was localized to the body in only 6 to 7 per cent. Carcinoma confined to the tail occurred in only 1 or 2 per cent. The patient which we have presented today did not exhibit metastatic lesions in the liver. This is another unusual feature since the liver is usually the first point of distant metastasis. There is a point of diagnosis which may be of value concerning metastasis in the liver. In the case of carcinoma of the stomach, hepatic metastasis are usually very large. Often they can be palpated in the enlarged liver. Carcinoma of the pancreas on the other hand usually gives multiple small metastatic nodules which do not result in a comparable degree of hepatomegaly. Occasionally in carcinoma of the tail of the pancreas glucose tolerance tests are helpful because the majority of islets of Langerhans are contained in the tail and may be destroyed by neoplastic involvement.

DISCUSSION

QUESTION: Was there any gross evidence of kidney involvement?

DR. HOPPS: There was some evidence indicative of hypertension; the kidneys showed mild arteriolosclerosis. There was no tumor nor evidence of infection.

DR. PATZER: Surgically it is often hard to diagnose carcinoma of the pancreas. When we palpate the pancreas and feel hard nodules we often find that it is only chronic pancreatitis.

DR. HALPERT: Two things may be mentioned as to the frequency of carcinoma of the pancreas in whites and negroes. We reviewed the carcinomas that were observed in the Charity Hospital in 6,000 necropsies and there were 40 cases of carcinoma of the pancreas. Among those 40 about half were in negroes and half in whites. The proportion of males to females was about 5 males to 1 female. The peak age incidence is usually given as the sixth decade. Over one-half of those cases observed at New Orleans, however, were in the seventh decade.

DR. HOPPS: Regarding the etiology of carcinoma of the pancreas we do know of one factor which predisposes to this. Patients with diabetes mellitus have 6 to 8 times more carcinomas of the pancreas than do patients without diabetes. The basis for this relationship is not proved, but it may be related to chronic irritation.

Every library should try to be complete on something, if it were only the history of pin-heads.—*Holmes. The Poet at the Breakfast-Table.*

The finer the nature, the more flaws it will show through the clearness of it; and it is a law of this universe, that the best things shall be seldomest seen in their best form.—*Ruskin.*

ANNOUNCEMENT

The next written examination for candidates of the American Board of Obstetrics and Gynecology (Part I) will be held in various cities on February 7, 1947, 2:00 P.M. Part II of the examination will be held later in the year. All applications must be in the office of Paul Titus, M.D., Secretary, 1015 Highland Building, Pittsburgh 6, Pa., by November 1, 1946.

There are a number of changes in the Board regulations and requirements. For further information address the secretary, Dr. Paul Titus.

THE
MARY E. POGUE
SCHOOL

For Retarded Children and
Epileptic Children

Children are grouped according to type and have their own separate departments. Separate buildings for girls and boys.

Large beautiful grounds. Five school rooms. Teachers are all college trained and have Teachers' Certificates. Occupational Therapy. Speech Corrective Work. The School is only 26 miles west of Chicago. All west highways out of Chicago pass through or near Wheaton. Referring physicians may continue to supervise care and treatment of children placed in the School. You are invited to visit the School or send for catalogue.

30 Geneva Road, Wheaton, Ill.
Phone: Wheaton 319

24th Annual Fall Clinical Conference
The Kansas City Southwest Clinical Society
Municipal Auditorium, Kansas City, Missouri
October 7, 8, 9, 10, 1946

GUEST SPEAKERS

E. T. BELL, M.D., Pathology, Minneapolis
LOUIS A. BUIE, M.D., Proctology, Rochester
RICHARD B. CATTELL, M.D., Surgery, Boston
WARREN H. COLE, M.D., Surgery, Chicago
CHARLES A. DOAN, M.D., Int. Med. and Research, Columbus
A. I. FOLSOM, M.D., Urology, Dallas
L. H. GARLAND, M.D., Roentgenology, San Francisco
TINSLEY R. HARRISON, M.D., Cardiology, Dallas
PAUL H. HOLINGER, M.D., OORL and Bronchology, Chicago

JOHN S. LUNDY, M.D., Anesthesiology, Rochester
PAUL B. MAGNUSON, M.D. Orthopaedics, Washington
WALTER L. PALMER, M.D., Gastroenterology, Chicago
HERBERT E. SCHMITZ, M.D., Obstetrics and Gynecology Chicago
R. GLEN SPURLING, M.D., Neurosurgery, Louisville
WILLARD VAN HAZEL, M.D., Surgery, Chicago
E. H. WATSON, M.D., Pediatrics. Ann Arbor

DAILY FEATURES: Radio Broadcasts — Round Table Luncheons — Scientific Exhibits and Movies — Technical Exhibits — Women's Entertainment.

SPECIAL FEATURES:

Monday evening — Clinicopathologic Conference.
Tuesday evening — Stag Dinner with Entertainment.
Wednesday evening — Alumni Dinners.

SEE KANSAS CITY MEDICAL JOURNAL FOR COMPLETE PROGRAM

THE PRESIDENT'S PAGE

The Secretaries Conference which will be held this month (September) will be most important and every officer of a County Medical Society should attend as at this time information will be imparted which will mean much to the County Societies and the entire membership.

The Standing and Special Committees will convene at the same time. It is also important that the members of these committees attend as they will receive much valuable information which will greatly facilitate the committee work.

Two activities of the Association which will be discussed embrace the medical care program for veterans, wherein the veteran will be allowed to select the physician of his choice, and the other a complete and visual explanation of the publicity campaign for which the special assessment will be levied.

Obviously it is important that the officers of the County Societies have complete informaton concerning these two activities as each program will be a current topic of conversation within the individual county society.

President.

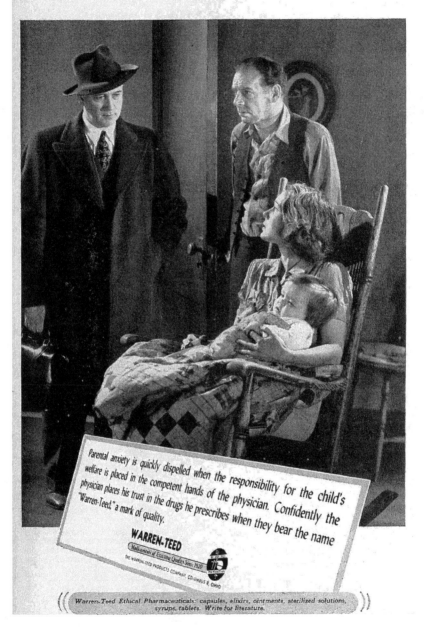

Parental anxiety is quickly dispelled when the responsibility for the child's welfare is placed in the competent hands of the physician. Confidently the physician places his trust in the drugs he prescribes when they bear the name "Warren-Teed," a mark of quality.

WARREN-TEED
Medicaments of Exacting Quality Since 1920
THE WARREN-TEED PRODUCTS COMPANY, COLUMBUS 8, OHIO

Warren-Teed Ethical Pharmaceuticals: capsules, elixirs, ointments, sterilized solutions, syrups, tablets. Write for literature.

The JOURNAL Of The
OKLAHOMA STATE MEDICAL ASSOCIATION

EDITORIAL BOARD
L. J. MOORMAN, Oklahoma City, Editor-in-Chief
E. EUGENE RICE, Shawnee   BEN H. NICHOLSON, Oklahoma City
MR. DICK GRAHAM, Oklahoma City, Business Manager
MR. CLAYTON FONDREN, Oklahoma City, Assistant Business Manager

CONTRIBUTIONS: Articles accepted by this Journal for publication including those read at the annual meetings of the State Association are the sole property of this Journal.

The Editorial Department is not responsible for the opinions expressed in the original articles of contributors.

Manuscripts may be withdrawn by authors for publication elsewhere only upon the approval of the Editorial Board.

MANUSCRIPTS: Manuscripts should be typewritten, double-spaced, on white paper 8½ x 11 inches. The original copy, not the carbon copy, should be submitted.

Footnotes, bibliographies and legends for cuts should be typed on separate sheets in double space. Bibliography listing should follow this order: Name of author, title of article, name of periodical with volume, page and date of publication.

Manuscripts are accepted subject to the usual editorial revisions and with the understanding that they have not been published elsewhere.

NEWS: Local news of interest to the medical profession, changes of address, births, deaths and weddings will be gratefully received.

ADVERTISING: Advertising of articles, drugs or compounds unapproved by the Council on Pharmacy of the A.M.A. will not be accepted. Advertising rates will be supplied on application.

It is suggested that members of the State Association patronize our advertisers in preference to others.

SUBSCRIPTIONS: Failure to receive The Journal should call for immediate notification.

REPRINTS: Reprints of original articles will be supplied at actual cost provided request for them is attached to manuscripts or made in sufficient time before publication. Checks for reprints should be made payable to Industrial Printing Company, Oklahoma City.

Address all communications to THE JOURNAL OF THE OKLAHOMA STATE MEDICAL ASSOCIATION, 210 Plaza Court, Oklahoma City 3

OFFICIAL PUBLICATION OF THE OKLAHOMA STATE MEDICAL ASSOCIATION
Copyrighted September, 1946

EDITORIALS

A NEW FEATURE

Beginning with this issue of the Journal Dick Graham and the new Associate Executive Secretary, Clayton Fondren, are instituting a column to be known as "Hits, Runs and Errors".

It is anticipated that this column will be interesting reading if for no other reason than keeping track of what these employees of ours are doing with their time. It is hoped, however, that they will be merciful in their comments about their experiences with this profession of ours. This is said because of our own experience in dealing with the profession on matters other than that of scientific medicine.

S. 1606*

Dingell, Dingell, great long bill,
  How I wonder if you will
With a rebuilt face appear
  When the Congress meets next year.

We have information to the effect that the proponents of S. B. 1606 have abondoned hope of securing its passage at this session of the Congress. We trust our information is correct. Likewise we have grapevine information to the effect that, quoting the Bard of Avon, "we have scotch'd the snake, not killed it," but, that the measure will be entirely rewritten so as to meet as many of the objections presented in committee against it as can be eliminated and still retain compulsory sickness insurance. It seems that this socialistic scheme of compulsory governmental sickness insurance may become a perennial legislative weed, a stinkweed to cumber indefinitely the soil of the legislative garden in Washington.

*To further a timely warning and to enable the doctors of Oklahoma to "red-letter" the anticipated day we are reproducing the above editorial from the August, 1946 issue of the West Virginia Medical Journal. No doubt this editorial is from the pen of our good friend, Dr. Walter E. Vest, Editor of the West Virginia Medical Journal.

VOCATIONAL REHABILITATION IS GOOD INVESTMENT

There are persons in every community who are unable to work or unable to work efficiently because of arthritis, poliomyelitis, tuberculosis, heart disease, or some other condition brought on by infection or traumatic injuries. Reliable statistics indicate that there are more than one million such persons over sixteen years of age in the United States; and Oklahoma, along with the other states, has her share. The Rehabilitation Service, maintained by the State Board of Education, is returning many of these persons to useful and gainful employment.

Disabled persons are a drain on their communities when they are unable to earn the money with which to procure the necessities of life for themselves and their families and must therefore be dependent upon their relatives or upon relief agencies for support. Such a condition is unhealthful, both for the morale of the disabled person and the economic welfare of the community. Many of these persons have the mental and physical capacity for productive employment, if they had the skill or necessary training for the types of employment compatible with their impairments. If the disabling condition is one that is not progressive (or is very slowly progressive) such persons may be trained by the Rehabilitation Service for a type of work in which their disabilities will not constitute a handicap, or in which the handicap will be greatly minimized. Thus the disabled person is converted from a status of economic liability into one of a self-sustaining and productive citizenship in his community.

In order for rehabilitation to be effective, it must be carried out on an individual basis. It is first necessary to determine the individual's problems and needs, and second to plan and carry out a program designed to meet these needs. His problem may be educational, medical, social, psychological, or vocational in nature. Hence, the planning varies with the individual client.

In evaluating a suitable vocation for a client, trained personnel are used. The counseling is based on known facts revealed by a study of each individual situation. These facts may have been derived from medical information, from intelligence or aptitude tests, from previous employment history, or from apparent personality traits. Thus the individual is guided into the selection of a vocational objective compatible with his intelligence, interests, and abilities, always considering the handicap which must be overcome.

Having determined the vocational objective, the Rehabilitation Service arranges and pays for the training that may be required to prepare the client for it. Counseling and vocational training are provided without reference to the individual's means. If he is unable to support himself during the training period, maintenance may be furnished for him. If tools or training materials are needed, they may be purchased for him. With the completion of training, the client is placed in employment suited to his needs. Even

then, contact is maintained with him for a reasonable period of time, to make sure that a satisfactory adjustment has been made.

In some instances medical or surgical procedures or prosthetic appliances are necessary to prepare the client for employment or for a more suitable type of employment. The Rehabilitation Service can purchase these for the disabled individual if he is unable to pay for them himself. Such services, if provided must be directly related to the vocational objective and must not be available from any other source.

The State Board of Education in order to obtain competent guidance in the medical care phase of the program, which is relatively new, has appointed a Medical Advisory Committee. This Committee was selected from a list of names suggested by the State Medical Association, and is composed of five physicians, one dentist, and one hospital administrator. The Committee meets monthly, or as often as needed. Its functions are briefly as follows: *First*, to interpret to the State Board of Education the thinking and practices of the medical profession of the state with reference to public supported programs of this type; *second*, to advise on the types of conditions that come within the purview of such a program; *third*, to advise with reference to the selection of physicians, and payment of fees for their services; and *fourth*, to interpret the program of rehabilitation to the medical profession of the state. The State Board also employs a trained Medical Social Worker, who supervises the program, and a Medical Consultant on a part-time basis.

The following case is cited, with the permission of the individual concerned, to demonstrate the importance of the physical restoration program:

Allen B. Vollmer is a young man whose vision in the left eye was destroyed by a bean shooter when he was a small boy. While he was still in his teens, a pencil injured the right eye, making him almost totally blind. Allen attended the School for the Blind at Muskogee and completed his high school training. He stayed on at the school and taught other blind children after graduating. His specialties were gymnasium, handicrafts and the work in the broom shop.

Allen left his teaching job after the outbreak of the war, and came to the Vocational Rehabilitation Service for assistance in securing defense work. He was placed on a job at the Douglas Plant as a filer and burrer, a job that is successfully performed by blind workers. At Douglas he met the young lady to whom he is now married. In August, 1944, Allen moved on to a better-paying position at O.C.A.D. and worked there until he was replaced by a veteran.

When Allen came back to the Vocational Rehabilitation Service in 1945, the new physical restoration program had been added to the services available, and he was sent to an ophthalmologist for examination. The ophthalmologist reported that the vision in the left eye was zero and in the right eye, 3/200. He believed that surgery to the right eye would restore it almost to normal. After the surgery had been done, Allen was fitted with glasses. The vision in his right eye was 20/20-2. A new job at the Douglas plant was secured for him, but this time it was work that could be done by a person with vision. In the Production Control Department, Allen classified airplane parts and forwarded them to the proper departments.

At the present time, Allen is employed as a baker's helper. He enjoys baking, and is learning a trade that will be useful to him for the rest of his life. Best of all, he will never be a drain on the resources of any community in which he lives.—Voyle C. Scurlock.

LIKE OLD MAN RIVER

If under the unhappy influence of postwar psychology, influenced by the social and economic unrest dependent upon the present conflict between labor and capital, the plan for compulsory health insurance should be adopted by a vasilating Congress, doctors must calmly and wisely choose their course of action in keeping with medical traditions, knowing that nothing can destroy the innate principles of professional freedom without obvious physical, social, moral, and economic penalties upon the uninformed populace. Soon such penalties would cause liberty loving American people to react with a flood of indignation. They will not sacrifice their American birthright for a song. With the irresistible power of Old Man River, American medicine will keep rolling along.

Medical School Notes

Dean Appointed

Dr. Jacques P. Gray, Dean of the Medical College of Virginia, Richmond, Va., has been appointed Dean of the University of Oklahoma, School of Medicine, effective September 1, 1946. Dr. Gray has had extensive experience in medical education and public health, having served on the faculty of the Stanford University School of Medicine, University of California, and University of North Carolina, and in public health work with the U. S. Public Health Service, California and Michigan State Health Departments and the W. K. Kellogg Foundation. He is a graduate of Johns Hopkins University, School of Medicine, 1928, and Harvard University, School of Public Health, M.P.H. 1935. He is a Fellow of the American Medical Association and the American Public Health Association. Since 1942, Dr. Gray has been Dean of the Medical College of Virginia. He succeeds Dr. Wann A. Langston, Professor of Medicine, who has served as acting Dean since the death of Dr. Tom Lowry, December 11, 1945.

Announcing The Sixteenth Annual Conference of The
OKLAHOMA CITY CLINICAL SOCIETY

OCTOBER 28, 29, 30, 31, 1946

DISTINGUISHED GUEST LECTURERS

Harrison H. Shoulders, M. D., PRESIDENT, THE AMERICAN MEDICAL ASSOCIATION, Nashville, Tennessee.

Charles L. Brown, M.D., MEDICINE, Dean and Professor of Medicine, Hahnemann Medical College, Philadelphia, Pennsylvania.

Samuel A. Cosgrove, M.D., OBSTETRICS, Clinical Professor of Obstetrics, Faculty of Medicine, Columbia University; Medical Director and Superintendent and Chief of the Staff, Margaret Hague Maternity Hospital, Jersey City, New Jersey.

Claude F. Dixon, M.D., SURGERY, Professor of Surgery, Mayo Foundation, Postgraduate School, University of Minnesota., Rochester, Minnesota.

Austin I. Dodson, M.D., UROLOGY, Professor of Urology, Urologist to Hospital Division, Medical College of Virginia, Richmond, Virginia.

Philip S. Hench, M.D., MEDICINE, Consultant and Head of a Section on Medicine, Chief of the Department for Rheumatic Diseases; Associate Professor of Medicine, Mayo Foundation, Postgraduate School, University of Minnesota, Rochester, Minnesota.

Waldo E. Nelson, M.D., PEDIATRICS, Professor of Pediatrics, Chief of the Pediatric Department, Temple University School of Medicine, Philadelphia, Pennsylvania.

Paul Padget, M.D., MEDICINE, Assistant Professor of Medicine, Johns Hopkins University School of Medicine, Veterans Administration, Fort Howard, Maryland.

Walter L. Palmer, M.D., MEDICINE, Professor of Medicine, Department of Medicine, University of Chicago, Chicago, Illinois.

Rowley M. Penick, Jr., M.D., SURGERY, Associate Professor of Clinical Surgery, Tulane University School of Medicine, New Orleans, Louisiana.

Leo G. Rigler, M.D., RADIOLOGY, Professor and Chief of the Department of Radiology and Physical Therapy, University of Minnesota School of Medicine, Minneapolis, Minnesota.

Richard H. Sweet, M.D., SURGERY, Instructor in Surgery, Harvard Medical School, Boston, Massachusetts.

Richard W. Te Linde, M.D., GYNECOLOGY, Professor of Gynecology, Chief Gynecologist, Johns Hopkins University School of Medicine, Baltimore, Maryland.

James E. M. Thomson, M.D., ORTHOPAEDIC SURGERY, Lecturer in Plastic Surgery to the College of Dentistry, University of Nebraska; President American Academy of Orthopaedic Surgeons, Lincoln, Nebraska.

O. E. Van Alyea, M.D., OTOLARYNGOLOGY, Clinical Associate, University of Illinois, College of Medicine, Chicago, Illinois.

Shields Warren, M.D., PATHOLOGY, Assistant Professor of Pathology, Harvard Medical School, Boston, Massachusetts.

Alan C. Woods, Sr., M.D., OPHTHALMOLOGY, Professor of Ophthalmology; Ophthalmologist-in-chief, Johns Hopkins University School of Medicine, Baltimore, Maryland.

GENERAL ASSEMBLIES   ROUND-TABLE LUNCHEONS   DINNER MEETINGS

POSTGRADUATE COURSES   SMOKER   COMMERCIAL EXHIBITS

Registration fee of $10.00 includes ALL the above features.

For further information, address EXECUTIVE SECRETARY, 512 Medical Arts Building, Oklahoma City, Oklahoma

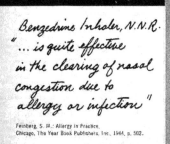

Benzedrine Inhaler, N. N. R.
"... is quite effective
in the clearing of nasal
congestion due to
allergy or infection"

Feinberg, S. M.: Allergy in Practice.
Chicago, The Year Book Publishers, Inc., 1944, p. 502.

Your hay fever patients will be

grateful...particularly between office visits...for the relief of nasal
congestion afforded by Benzedrine Inhaler, N. N. R.
The Inhaler may make all the difference between weeks of acute
misery and weeks of comparative comfort.

Each Benzedrine Inhaler is packed with recemic amphetamine, S.K.F., 250 mg.; menthol, 12.5 mg.; and aromatics.

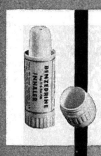

Benzedrine Inhaler
a better means of nasal medication

Smith, Kline & French Laboratories,   Philadelphia, Pa.

SPECIAL TRAIN A SUCCESS

One hundred seven Oklahoma physicians, their families and friends from Kansas, Texas, Missouri, Louisiana, Tennessee, South Dakota and New York, stepped on their Special Train to San Francisco and the A. M. A. convention on June 27 and until their return on July 16, after a post-convention tour through the Pacific Northwest and Canada, the cares of their offices and patients were blissfully forgotten. Probably no group of physicians and their families ever had a more enjoyable trip than this one sponsored by the Association through Mr. Harry Kornhaum of the Rainbow Travel Service. From the time of the first puff of smoke in Oklahoma City until the last grinding stop at the Santa Fe Station upon returning home the weather man gave his benevolent benediction to this group of travelers. Sunshine and moon light was the rule of the day and night, with the exception of one morning's trip to the snow bound Paradise Inn of Mt. Ranier.

The Santa Fe, Southern Pacific, Northern Pacific and Burlington vied with each other in giving to these travelers the most excellent cuiesine that their chefs were able to bring forth. Breakfast, luncheon and dinner were a grandiose experience of adventures in good eating, ranging from the beef of the middle west to the salmon steaks of the northwest. If the delicious food were not enough, there was hardly a time when the panoramic vista which could be viewed from the dining car window did not more than compensate for the relaxing interlude for food.

War time service in traveling was forgotten by the excellent stewards, porters and railway men who at all times gave their every attention to any demands of the Special Train travelers. Mr. Emanuel of the Santa Fe, Mr. Davis of the Southern Pacific, Mr. Cleef of the Northern Pacific and Mr. Ferrell of the Burlington saw to it that their respective roads made the journey of this Special Train one never to be forgotten.

Grand Canyon First Stop

After a two nights' ride the Special Train pulled into the Grand Canyon at 7:00 A.M. where everyone immediately partook of a hardy breakfast, and gave themselves over to the wonderments of the Canyon. As so aptly put by one of the travelers it was "golly, what a gulch". Our Special Train travelers took advantage of tours around the rim and by 5 o'clock were back in their air-conditioned cars for the last lap through Arizona and central California to San Francisco and the five days of the convention.

San Francisco

In as much as true reporting of this trip must be given prime consideration, it must be admitted that the overly crowded conditions in San Francisco made the selection of a hotel for the group extremely difficult. Although the majority of the party found it necessary to commute between Berkeley and San Francisco there were many who thoroughly enjoyed the quietness of Berkeley, the home of the University of California. The Durant Hotel, our headquarters, nestled at one side of the beautiful University of California campus and although there was some inconvenience in having to commute to San Francisco, a daily panoramic view of the Golden Gate and the San Francisco skyline were always sources of enjoyment. Whether or not the Chamber of Commerce of San Francisco made a special request of the weather man is a moot question, but during the time of the meeting old man Sol made his daily pilgrimage from the East to the West in his full regalia bringing with him in the evening cool, refreshing breezes, allowing the investigation of San Francisco's water front, China Town, beautiful homes and drives to be enjoyed to the maximum.

Following five days of unadulterated enjoyment for both the ladies of the train, who enjoyed the shops and stores, and the excellent scientific program available to the physicians, our Special Train was amalgamated with one from Ohio and Indiana and 22 cars pulled out from Berkeley for a non-stop trip to Portland. The ride from Berkeley took our travelers up the Shasta Trail past beautiful Mt. Shasta and into the shadow of Mt. Hood, rising majestically north of Portland, the Columbia River Drive and Multnomah Falls.

The 22 cars arrived in Portland at approximately 4:00 P.M. where there was a scramble to enter our sight seeing buses for the drive along the Columbia River to Multnomah Falls and until such time as all can see this gorgeous wonderment of nature they will not have lived life to the fullest. Leaving Portland the train proceeded to Seattle where two days were spent in enjoying the State of Washington's scenery with a side trip to Victoria, British Columbia, and Burchart's Rose Garden, this garden being far beyond the conception of any botanist who has not reveled in its splendor.

The second day in Seattle was devoted to an all day trip to Paradise Inn, 6,000 feet up the thorny side of 12,000 foot Mt. Ranier, through the pine, spruce, fir and hemlock which tower majestically upward. Certainly it was hard to believe that there could be a lumber shortage in good old Oklahoma. Paradise Inn spread its hospitality to its visitors and it was difficult to think of 100 degree heat in Oklahoma while eating our lunch and gazing through the windows onto four feet of snow.

Seattle was the axis of the trip because from this point we boarded the Northern Pacific with its nose pointed East for Yellow Stone National Park, Cody, Wyoming, Kansas City, Missouri and home.

Yellow Stone National Park

Two and a half days were spent in this never to be forgotten national park where geysers are at every hand and boiling pools give out a multitude of colors and scenic wonderment. Old Faithful Geyser still has its magic draw for both old and young and is still faithfully spewing forth from Mother Earth approximately every 66 minutes, rising to a height of 200 feet. Disappointment was evidenced by some upon arriving at Old Faithful Inn where the afternoon, night and next morning were spent, in that they had as yet seen no bears. Their desires were not long in being fulfilled in as much as the next day, on the trip to the Canyon Hotel, there was an abundance of bear, antelope, deer, buffalo, ducks, pellicans and sea gulls for the amateur and professional photographers in the entourage to photograph to their hearts' content.

The Canyon Hotel will always have a warm spot in everyone's heart because it was at this place that everyone was given a room with bath and the luxury of soaking suds; the celebration of Dr. and Mrs. Joe Kelso's 14th wedding aniversary was a highlight. The following morning a delightful 50 mile bus ride to Cody, Wyoming, through the Shoshone Valley to Billy the Kid's Dam gave a picture of man's supremacy over nature.

Homeward Bound

From Cody, Wyoming, where Dr. Jake Eskridge discovered an old patient, there was an undercurrent of rejoicing that "Oklahoma, here we come" was the theme song, although it was difficult to leave the beautiful Pacific Northwest. As the Burlington drew our new Oklahoma Special Train, having left our Indiana and Ohio friends at Seattle, onto the great plains of Wyoming, Montana, North Dakota, Nebraska and Missouri, home beckoned more strongly. Our Special Train literally flew from Kansas City to Oklahoma City where "finis" was written to 18 days of true good fellowship and scenic beauty.

Oddities

Obviously no trip of this kind could be made without its pathos and its humor. Fortunately there were no injuries or serious illnesses. One member of the party from Kansas was called home due to the untimely death of his associate, but to counteract moments of seriousness there were many interludes of laughter and it will be many a day before those on the trip will cease to inquire of Dr. C. J. Fishman as to just how to find the fire escape in a hotel and return safely to your room, Dr. Sullivan of Carnegie on how best to protect your pocket book and Dr. Renegar of Tuttle as to the necessity for a compass or guide to find your way around the Canyon Hotel. The little side lights and the causes for hilarious moments of laughter are all too numerous to mention. In closing this saga of the trip it can only be said that to know the true delight of such a trip is to make one's plans now for the next Special Train in 1947 when it is tentatively planned to explore our national capitol, the metropolitan city of New York, the New England states, Montreal and Quebec, and to take our wives to see the wonderments of Niagara Falls, though it be a second time.

NORMAN OFFERS BLUE CROSS TO ITS CITIZENS

Nearly 4,000 participants were added to the Blue Cross Plan for hospital care, and 508 persons joined Oklahoma Physicians Service, companion plan to Blue Cross which covers surgical and obstetrical fees, during a two-week community enrollment drive in Norman which ended July 27. Norman is the seventeenth city in Oklahoma to give voluntary sponsorship and guidance in the enrollment of its citizens in this non-profit plan to remove the uncertainty of sickness costs. Organizations sponsoring the drive were the Cleveland County Medical Society, Chamber of Commerce, Lions, Rotary and Kiwanis Clubs, the Municipal Hospital, civic leaders, and business men and women of Norman.

The sequence of events leading up to the successful drive began with the opening of the Norman Municipal Hospital on June 1. The fine 61 bed institution represented a three year struggle to bring adequate health facilities to the city of Norman and stood as a real civic achievement. But the Chamber of Commerce, sensing a responsibility that went beyond ''just building a hospital'', realized that many people in the community could not afford the relatively high cost of hospital care even in a city owned, non-profit institution. Since the hospital had been a project of the Chamber of Commerce, it became their project to make hospital service available to all the people of the community it was built to serve.

After investigation, Charles R. Rayburn, M.D., Chairman of the Health and Hospital Committee of the Chamber of Commerce, invited Arthur Peterman, Enrollment Manager for the Oklahoma City Blue Cross branch, to Norman to explain the Blue Cross Plan and suggest a means of bringing the benefits of Blue Cross to the entire populace of the city. Peterman explained that Blue Cross was essentially a group plan, and in order to be eligible to join, a person must be employed in a group of five or more employees, but under the community enrollment plan, individuals who cannot qualify for membership in a group may come into the plan on an individual basis provided that a responsible col-

lection agency can be established to take care of membership dues. The Chamber of Commerce voted to sponsor a Blue Cross community enrollment in Norman. The Health and Hospital Committee worked out the details as follows: Arranged for Miss Nellie Mae Sloan, admission clerk at the hospital, to spend a week each quarter at the Chamber of Commerce offices to handle collections for members enrolling as individuals; scheduled a banquet for civic leaders and business men and women to hear the details of the plan explained; arranged for a publicity committee to coordinate public education activities; and made plans for a direct mailing piece to be delivered to all of the more than 4,000 mail stops in Norman.

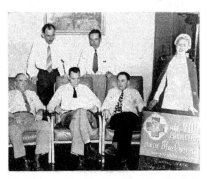

Left to right: T. E. Thompson, City Manager; Lloyd Lamirand, Blue Cross Representative; Paul Smith, Supt., Norman Municipal Hospital; Carl Chaudoin, Secretary and Manager, Chamber of Commerce; James O. Hood, M.D., President, Cleveland County Medical Society.

Mayor H. V. Thornton gave an official indorsement through a proclamation published in the Sunday issue of the Transcript, and the same paper carried a front page story every day on the progress of the drive. A full-page and a quarter-page advertisement were donated by the Chamber of Commerce explaining the benefits and costs of the plan. Radio station WNAD broadcast spot announcements, and Blue Cross posters were placed in many store windows telling how and when to enroll. When the drive started on Monday, July 15, its success was assured by the fine support and sponsorship of a civic-minded, health-minded community.

Other communities who might be interested in such a procedure should contact either Mr. Arthur Peterman, Blue Cross Hospital Plan, First National Bank Bldg., Oklahoma City or the Executive Office.

WILLIAM E. EASTLAND, M.D.
F. A. C. R.

RADIUM AND X-RAY THERAPY
DERMATOLOGY

405 Medical Arts Bldg.

Oklahoma City, Oklahoma   Phone 3-1446

HILL BURTON BILL RECEIVES CONGRESSIONAL APPROVAL

Senate Resolution No. 191, commonly known as the Hill Burton Bill and designed to give to local communities assistance in building hospitals and health facilities, was passed by the House of Representatives in the closing days of the session.

The Bill as passed has had several amendments placed in it by the House of Representatives, the most important amendment being the reducing of the Federal matching grant to a maximum grant of 33 1/3 per cent of the total construction cost.

At the time the Journal went to press, President Truman had not signed the measure but there is little doubt that he will do so as this resolution has full administration backing.

Public Health Department To Consider Applications for Assistance

Under the bill a single state agency will be designated as the administering office. In Oklahoma this will be the State Board of Health and individual communities desiring to inquire as to their eligibility for consideration under the act should write direct to Dr. Grady F. Mathews, Commissioner of Health, Oklahoma City.

Cancer Research Defeated

House Resolution 4502 which would have created a fund of a hundred million dollars for cancer research at government expense, became entwined with last minute congressional maneuvers and did not secure sufficient strength to be passed at this session of Congress.

Leaders in cancer work, both lay and professional, were in favor of the measure and it is anticipated that this legislation will be introduced in the next Congress.

ASSOCIATION TO EXHIBIT AT STATE FAIR

An inovation for both the Association and the State Free Fair in 1945 was the establishing of an exhibit whereby the general public would gain knowledge of the activities of the Oklahoma State Medical Association.

The reception given this booth was so outstanding that the idea will again be followed this year with a general expansion of organizations and agencies participating.

At a called meeting of representatives of the Oklahoma Division of American Cancer Society, Blue Cross and Oklahoma Physicians Service, Crippled Children's Commission, National Foundation for Infantile Paralysis, State Tuberculosis Association, State Hospital Association, State Dental Association, State Pharmaceutical Association, State Nursing Association, State Vocational Rehabilitation, State Public Welfare Department, State Health Department, University of Oklahoma School of Medicine and Veterans Administration in the office of the Association it was unanimously agreed that these agencies would underwrite the rent of a building and participate with exhibits. The building and project will be known as the "Exhibit on Health Education". All physicians who attend the Fair are urged to include the Health Education exhibit in their itinerary.

COUNCIL AUTHORIZES EMPLOYMENT ASSOCIATE EXECUTIVE SECRETARY

The Council, at its last meeting on August 4, approved the appointment of Mr. Clayton Fondren of Oklahoma City as Associate Executive Secretary effective August 20, by the House of Delegates although it was not believed that such an appointment could be made prior to January 1, 1947 when the increase in dues would warrant the employment of an Associate Executive Secretary.

The early appointment was made possible by the approval of the Executive Office for Veterans on-the-job training. Due to an office reorganization there will be no increase in the budget for salaries.

Associate Executive Secretary Will Improve Services of Association

The House of Delegates was motivated to approve the appointment of an Associate Executive Secretary by the

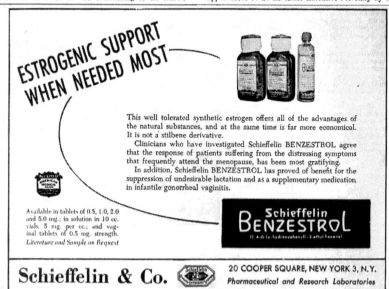

ESTROGENIC SUPPORT WHEN NEEDED MOST

This well tolerated synthetic estrogen offers all of the advantages of the natural substances, and at the same time is far more economical. It is not a stilbene derivative.

Clinicians who have investigated Schieffelin BENZESTROL agree that the response of patients suffering from the distressing symptoms that frequently attend the menopause, has been most gratifying.

In addition, Schieffelin BENZESTROL has proved of benefit for the suppression of undesirable lactation and as a supplementary medication in infantile gonorrheal vaginitis.

Available in tablets of 0.5, 1.0, 2.0 and 5.0 mg.; in solution in 10 cc. vials, 5 mg. per cc.; and vaginal tablets of 0.5 mg. strength. *Literature and Sample on Request*

Schieffelin
BENZESTROL
(2, 4-di (p-hydroxyphenyl) -3-ethyl hexane)

Schieffelin & Co.

20 COOPER SQUARE, NEW YORK 3, N.Y.
Pharmaceutical and Research Laboratories

need for a closer contact between the Executive Office and the membership as a whole. Since the employment of an Executive Secretary eight years ago, the activities of the Executive Office have increased to such a degree that the Executive Secretary has found it virtually impossible to meet with the County Societies and the membership as originally anticipated. Now that the details of the office, committee organizational work and administration of the present activities of the Association will be augmented by the additional help, County Societies will be visited regu'arly by either Mr. Graham or Mr. Fondren in order that the membership may have full knowledge of the program of the Association and its progress. County Societies are urged to avail themselves of the opportunity of learning more about the activities of the Association by keeping the Executive Office informed of their meeting dates.

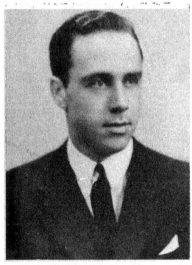

Clayton Fondren

Mr. Fondren is a native of Oklahoma, having been born and raised in Oklahoma City. He is a graduate of the University of Oklahoma with a degree in Business Administration. He served forty-three months with the Army Air Forces and was released from active service in November, 1945. Mr. Fondren is married and has a fifteen month old son.

ANNUAL SECRETARIES CONFERENCE TO BE HELD LATE SEPTEMBER, EARLY OCTOBER

The annual Secretaries Conference which includes all officers of County Societies will be held the last week of September or the first week of October, the date depending upon the action of the Committees on Public Policy and Publicity and Veterans Medical Care in completing their respective work on the publicity campaign, and the agreement between the Veterans Administration and the Association for a medical care program whereby the veteran may select his own physician.

Dr. L. C. Kuykendall, President of the Association, has also announced that he will call together his special

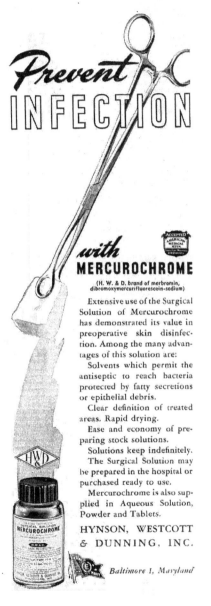

Prevent INFECTION

with MERCUROCHROME

(H. W. & D. brand of merbromin, dibromoxymercurifluorescein-sodium)

Extensive use of the Surgical Solution of Mercurochrome has demonstrated its value in preoperative skin disinfection. Among the many advantages of this solution are:

Solvents which permit the antiseptic to reach bacteria protected by fatty secretions or epithelial debris.

Clear definition of treated areas. Rapid drying.

Ease and economy of preparing stock solutions.

Solutions keep indefinitely.

The Surgical Solution may be prepared in the hospital or purchased ready to use.

Mercurochrome is also supplied in Aqueous Solution, Powder and Tablets.

HYNSON, WESTCOTT & DUNNING, INC.

Baltimore 1, Maryland

and standing committees to work out their programs for 1946-47.

Officers of County Medical Societies should be making plans to attend the Conference as it will be important that each County Society have full information concerning the program of the Association for the coming year.

Program Not Complete

While the program has not been completed for the Conference, it is known that the Veterans Care program and the publicity campaign of the Association will take up a large portion of the Conference's time. Dr. John Burton, Chairman of the Veterans program has indicated that his Committee will try and have all details, including the fee schedule for veterans work, completed in order that the details may be discussed.

The final program will be sent to all officers of the County Societies as soon as possible. In the interim, should any officer desire to suggest a topic for the Conference, please send the suggestion to the Executive Office, 210 Plaza Court, Oklahoma City, at once in order that it may be considered by the Conference officers.

RADIUM

(Including Radium Applicators)

FOR ALL MEDICAL PURPOSES

Est. 1919

Quincy X-Ray and Radium Laboratories
(Owned and directed by a Physician-Radiologist)

HAROLD SWANBERG, B.S., M.D.,Director
W.C.U. Bldg.   Quincy, Illinois

Hits, Runs, Errors

Several members have suggested that the Journal needs more personalizing and, shall be say, light reading! We agree! The Executive Office *dairy** that we are going to try out is a feeble effort to give a day by day account of the many things that come through this office either through the mail, personal calls or a trip on the road. It must of necessity be informal and brief so we hope no one will be offended as we go merrily on our way should a name or city be omitted. Remember we are only human and make mistakes, sometimes too many according to the President and the Council.

(*Original copy in long hand by Dick Graham; ask Dr. James Stevenson how Dick Graham spells ''shining''.)

AUGUST 11: Off for Muskogee at 7:00 A.M. with the Delegate to A. M. A., C. R. Rountree, M.D., and the new hired help, Fondren, to see member of the Board of Health, Charles Ed. White, M.D. Dr. Rountree insisted on driving across the street to park in the sun when shady (‡ ‡ ‡) filling stations lined the right hand side of the highway. Back through Tulsa and we stop to see ''Aunt Nell'' (Mrs. J. Stevenson) and Ralph McGill, M.D., who are in St. Johns and Hillcrest Hospitals respectively. Both on the mend and everyone is pleased.

AUGUST 12: Many visitors today, including Dick Brightwell, M.D., from V. A. in St. Louis who is thinking about coming home to Oklahoma to practice. Line forms at the left. 8:00 P.M. meeting in Council Room with representatives from 14 state organizations dealing in some phase of health concerning a health education exhibit at the State Fair. Everyone in agreement and so —come September 21 the Fair visitors will have a chance to see what medicine is doing for them. Any good ideas from the membership?

AUGUST 13: The morning mail brings a letter from the President with instructions to refer the E. M. T. C. program to the Council so we will once again go over

DIAGNOSTIC CLINIC OF INTERNAL MEDICINE AND ALLERGY

Philip M. McNeill, M. D., F. A. C. P.

General Diagnosis

CONSULTATION BY APPOINTMENT

Special Attention to Cardiac, Pulmonary and Allergic Diseases

Electrocardiograph, X-Ray, Laboratory
and Complete Allergic Surveys Available.

1107 Medical Arts Bldg.
Oklahoma City, Okla.

Phone 2-0277

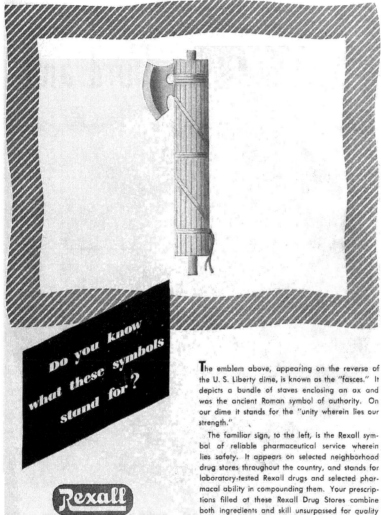

Do you know what these symbols stand for?

Rexall
DRUGS

REXALL FOR RELIABILITY

The emblem above, appearing on the reverse of the U. S. Liberty dime, is known as the "fasces." It depicts a bundle of staves enclosing an ax and was the ancient Roman symbol of authority. On our dime it stands for the "unity wherein lies our strength."

The familiar sign, to the left, is the Rexall symbol of reliable pharmaceutical service wherein lies safety. It appears on selected neighborhood drug stores throughout the country, and stands for laboratory-tested Rexall drugs and selected pharmacal ability in compounding them. Your prescriptions filled at these Rexall Drug Stores combine both ingredients and skill unsurpassed for *quality control.*

UNITED-REXALL DRUG CO.
LOS ANGELES, CALIFORNIA
PHARMACEUTICAL CHEMISTS FOR MORE THAN 43 YEARS

"...Unto the Third and

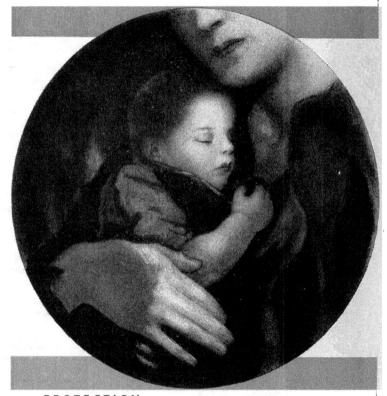

PROTECTION

PROTECTION against congenital syphilis can often be accomplished by treatment of the expectant mother.

Fourth Generation . . . ˮ

Proper antisyphilitic therapy during pregnancy can prevent or control syphilis in the infant . . . lower the mortality rate in fetal syphilis . . . reduce the frequency of premature labor— even if the antisyphilitic course is comparatively short and the child not cured. Syphilis in mothers can be well started toward symptomatic and serologic cure.

MAPHARSEN (meta-amino-para-hydroxyphenyl arsine oxide (arsenoxide) hydrochloride) gives maximum therapeutic effect—rapid disappearance of spirochetes and prompt healing of lesions. Minimal untoward reactions are less severe than those observed after use of arsphenamines.

MAPHARSEN

PARKE, DAVIS & COMPANY

DETROIT 32, MICHIGAN

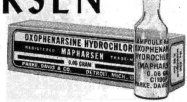

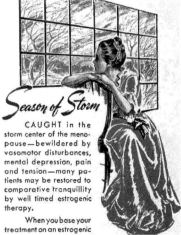

Season of Storm

CAUGHT in the storm center of the menopause—bewildered by vasomotor disturbances, mental depression, pain and tension—many patients may be restored to comparative tranquillity by well timed estrogenic therapy.

When you base your treatment on an estrogenic product of unquestioned **purity and potency, you can feel certain you have given your patient the best assistance possible through medication.**

Physicians using Solution of Estrogenic Substances, Smith-Dorsey, may rest upon that certainty ... for Smith-Dorsey's product is manufactured under rigidly regulated conditions ... to meet the highest standards of the industry.

A reliable product ... judiciously administered ... receding menstrual "storm" symptoms.

SOLUTION OF *Estrogenic Substances*　　SMITH-DORSEY

Supplied in 1 cc. ampuls and 10 cc. ampul vials representing potencies of 5,000, 10,000 and 20,000 international units per cc.

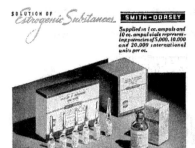

THE SMITH-DORSEY COMPANY

LINCOLN, NEBRASKA · DALLAS · LOS ANGELES

. *Manufacturers of Pharmaceuticals to the Medical Profession Since 1908*

this topic of such controversy. Arranged with E. Eugene Rice, M.D., Shawnee, to have an Editorial Board meeting at his house come Thursday night; the "cokes" will be on the Rice family. Visited with the Editor concerning the paper he will read before the Colorado State Medical Association in September on the "General Practitioner"; an excellent article and it should be read at home. No visitors today so the correspondence got some attention.

AUGUST 14: Jane and the Executive Secretary got involved in trying to figure out the cost per square foot for the exhibit space at the Fair. Too complicated; referred it to the auditors. Comes 11:00 o'clock and two visitors *thinking* about locating in Oklahoma; we work the list. Made a dash for the bus and a luncheon date with Lee Emenhiser, M.D., President of Oklahoma University Medical School Alumni, to discuss things of interest and work to be done for the Alumni organization. Dr. Lee is wondering why his alumni "don't" send in their $100 for life membership so building plans for the Research Institute can get under way. I don't have the answer. It's the greatest thing the Alumni could accomplish. Middle of the afternoon we were off to Stillwater where we took in Dr. Puckett and Dr. Rippy's new office and clinic. It's a beauty; however, the air conditioning unit will help. If any doctor wants to see what's new in offices, stop in; everyone is welcome.

AUGUST 15: This morning is Crippled Children Committee morning. Conversation with the Chairman, Earl McBride, M.D., and then the preparation of the brief for the Committee to study re payment of fee to doctors for care of polio patients. To lunch with Cob Burnside and Dick Woodmansee, a couple of my old K. U. sidekicks. Afternoon conference with W. E. Eberle who carries the Association's mal-practice insurance policy. Too many claims coming up all of a sudden and physicians who are being sued are not reporting claims. Remember, contact your insurance agent if you even *think* you *may* be sued. From Eberle's to Rainbow Travel Service to see Harry Kornbaum about making up another Special Train, this time to Southern Medical in Miami, November 4-7; also trying to figure out if special planes would be better. Everyone will get a letter on this later. No Editorial Board meeing tonight in Shawnee; both Moorman and Nicholson are unable to attend.

AUGUST 16: A telephone conversation with President Kuykendall for last minute instructions before the President leaves on a vacation to the land of wall-eyed pike, bass and pickerel. Result, among other things, is reference of the problem of the government suit against opticians and eye doctors to the Committee on Judicial and Professional Relations. The Coal County Chamber of Commerce invited us down to discuss building of hospitals; we were pleased to go as a hospital is badly needed in that area.

AUGUST 17: This is the day the new Associate Executive Secretary, Clayton Fondren, officially reported for duty. We spent the morning rearranging the office and the *old?* Executive Secretary told lies about the past. Now there is no excuse for the Executive Office's not being able to meet with any County Society any time or any place.

AUGUST 18: An afternoon meeting with Carroll M. Pounder, M.D., and the Executive Committee of Councillor District No. 4, present being Dr. Petty, Guthrie; Dr. Regan, Norman; Dr. Bohlman, Watonga; Dr. Hood, Oklahoma City. A swell meeting and everyone was in favor of the idea of giving the County Societies a closer insight in the work of this office and the Council.,

AUGUST 19: The Associate Executive Secretary spent the day going through the activities of the office, Orene and Jean telling about the Post Graduate course and how the Journal finally gets out. Talked to Dr. Shoemaker at the Medical School concerning refresher courses for doctors who want to prepare for the specialty boards. Attorney General's office called about National Optical Stores in Shawnee and Clinton Gallaher, M.D., Secretary of the Pottowatomie County Medical Society did his usual excellent job of cooperation. Oh, what a "joyus"

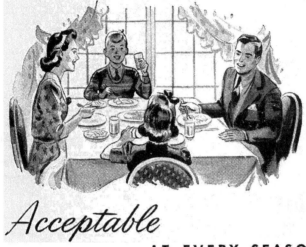

Acceptable

AT EVERY SEASON

Taken cold during the summer months or hot during the wintertime, the delicious food drink made by mixing Ovaltine with milk provides a wealth of essential nutrients in readily digested and assimilated form. Its delicious taste makes it enjoyable at every season. As a supplement to an inadequate diet, in the correction of the milder forms of malnutrition, or when the intake of all essential nutrients must be augmented, it makes a worth-while contribution, as

indicated by its composition shown in the table below. This dietary supplement provides biologically adequate protein, readily utilized carbohydrate, highly emulsified fat, ascorbic acid, B complex and other vitamins, and essential minerals. Its low curd tension makes for rapid gastric emptying and easy digestibility. It is relished by both children and adults, and is unusually acceptable either as a mealtime beverage or with between meal snacks.

THE WANDER COMPANY, 360 N. MICHIGAN AVE., CHICAGO 1, ILL.

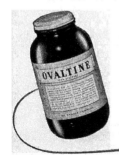

Ovaltine

Three servings daily of Ovaltine, each made of
½ oz. of Ovaltine and 8 oz. of whole milk,* provide:

CALORIES	669	VITAMIN A	3000 I.U.
PROTEIN	32.1 Gm.	VITAMIN B₁	1.16 mg.
FAT	31.5 Gm.	RIBOFLAVIN	1.50 mg.
CARBOHYDRATE	64.8 Gm.	NIACIN	6.81 mg.
CALCIUM	1.12 Gm.	VITAMIN C	39.6 mg.
PHOSPHORUS	0.939 Gm.	VITAMIN D	417 I.U.
IRON	12.0 mg.	COPPER	0.50 mg.

*Based on average reported values for milk.

life if all County Societies were like Pottowatomie. Heard some gossip about Health Department's activities in approving hospitals: Am on the trail of the Chairman of the Board to see what this is all about. Look forward to a good night's sleep after the two inch rain, but woe is me, we will have to start grass cutting again.

AUGUST 20: To Rotary Club and a chance to discuss business with Dr. Ben' Nicholson and Joe Hamilton of the Crippled Children Committee, killing two birds with one stone. Joe Musgrave from Tulsa was in to see us about Mr. Olney Flynn of Tulsa for governor. If everyone were as enthusiastic about his work as Joe Musgrave this would be a busy world. Edward Thorp, M.D., just out of Uncle Sam's Army, was in to discuss locations and we gave "Lecture No. 1" about the advantages of the small community, probably to no effect because of the old bug-a-boo about hospital facilities. We wonder why the medical schools can't teach the young doctors to practice without nurses, technicians, etc.

In love and friendship the imagination is as much exercised as the heart, and if either is outraged the other will be estranged. It is commonly the imagination which is wounded first, rather than the heart, it is so much the more sensitive.—*Henry D. Thoreau.*

CREDIT SERVICE

330 American National Building

Oklahoma City, Oklahoma

(Operators of Medical-Dental Credit Bureau)

★

We offer a dignified and effective collection service for doctors and hospitals located anywhere in the State. Write for information.

★

28 YEARS

Experience In Credit and Collection Work

Robt. R. Sesline, Owner and Manager

Obituaries

A. J. Wells, M.D.
1875-1946

On July 25, Dr. A. J. Wells, Calera, died of a cerebral hemorrhage. Dr. Wells, born in Farmersville, Texas, was the son of a Baptist minister. He began his education in the Kemp schools, completing it with a medical education at the Barns Medical College of St. Louis, Mo., from which he was graduated in 1902.

Dr. Wells was President of Bryan County Medical Society for two years, President of the Southeastern District Association for one year and held many other positions of honor in local organizations.

Surviving Dr. Wells, are his wife, two daughters, Mrs. Blanche McFarland and Mrs. Edith Sandquist, one son, H. C. Wells, four grandchildren and six sisters.

Clinton M. Tracy, M.D.
1875-1946

Dr. Clinton M. Tracy, retired physician, died August 8, 1946 at his home. Dr. Tracy had practiced medicine in Sentinel since 1912. He was a graduate of Gate City Medical College, Dallas, 1906, after which time he practiced in Canton and Woodward. In 1917 he established a hospital in Sentinel which he operated until his retirement in 1933.

Dr. Tracy was a member of the Washita County Medical Society and is survived by his wife, brother and other relatives.

F. Z. Winchell. M.D.
1878-1946

Memorial services were held July 25 for Dr. F. Z. Winchell who died Monday, July 22. Dr. Winchell was born in Marvin County, Mo., February 28, 1878, son of Eugene and Susan E. Winchell.

Dr. Winchell attended the country schools of Missouri as a boy and was graduated from Long Island High School, Long Island, Kansas. He received his medical education for the University of Kansas, graduating in 1902. After his marriage in 1902 to Miss Tilla Johnson, Dr. Winchell located in Agra, Kansas, until coming to Harper County. He was a pioneer doctor and pursued his work from the early days, driving many long miles in horse drawn vehicles.

Dr. Winchell is survived by his wife, one son, one daughter, a grand-daughter, three brothers and two sisters.

John A. Haynie. M.D.
1877-1946

Dr. John A. Haynie died shortly before noon July 29, 1946 .in the Haynie Hospital and Clinic where he was associated with his son, Dr. W. K. Haynie.

He was born in Union County, Miss., in 1877 where he grew up. In 1903 Dr. Haynie married Miss Mary E. Lackey and they later moved to Oklahoma. He received his medical education from the St. Louis College of Physicians and Surgeons and was graduated in 1914. At various times Dr. Haynie was President of the Bryan County Medical Society and has been Councillor of the Tenth District since 1944.

Dr. Haynie is survived by his wife, two sons, Dr. W. K. Haynie and Morris Haynie, three daughters, Mrs. Estella Marxsen, Miss Opal Haynie and Mrs. Lynn Marsh, three brothers, one sister and six grandchildren.

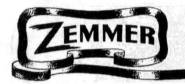

Prescribe or Dispense

Zemmer Pharmaceuticals

A complete line of laboratory controlled ethical pharmaceuticals.   OK 9-46

Chemists to the Medical Profession for 44 years.

The Zemmer Company   Oakland Station Pittsburgh 13, Pa.

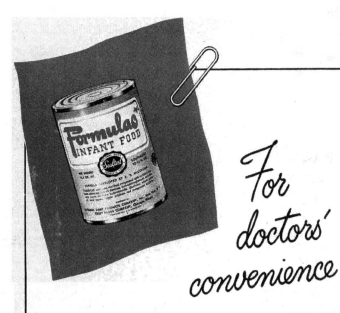

For doctors' convenience—

VITAMIN D CONTENT OF FORMULAC INCREASED FROM 500 TO 800 U.S.P. UNITS

IN LINE with customary usage of vitamin D among pediatricians — and in response to requests from leading practitioners—the vitamin D content of FORMULAC Infant Food has been increased from 500 to 800 U.S.P. units.

FORMULAC originally had a vitamin D content of 500 units, more than adequate for the needs of *average* infants. At the request of pediatricians for added protection to cover even *exceptional* cases (such as prematures and others requiring larger amounts of vitamins in their diet) the vitamin D content has been raised 300 U.S.P. units.

For further information about FORMULAC, and for professional samples of this new vitamin-and-mineral fortified Infant Food, mail a card to National Dairy Products Company, Inc., 230 Park Avenue, New York 17, N. Y.

Distributed by KRAFT FOODS COMPANY

NATIONAL DAIRY PRODUCTS COMPANY, INC.
New York, N. Y.

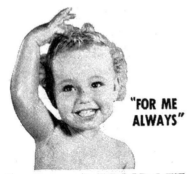

"FOR ME ALWAYS"

Because DARICRAFT

1. is EASILY DIGESTED
2. has 400 U. S. P. Units of VITAMIN D per pint of evaporated milk.
3. has HIGH FOOD VALUE
4. has an IMPROVED FLAVOR
5. is HOMOGENIZED
6. is STERILIZED
7. is from INSPECTED HERDS
8. is SPECIALLY PROCESSED
9. is UNIFORM
10. will WHIP QUICKLY

PRESCRIBED BY MANY DOCTORS
... You also may want to utilize Daricraft as a solution to your infant feeding problems, as well as in special diets for convalescents.

PRODUCERS CREAMERY CO., SPRINGFIELD, MISSOURI

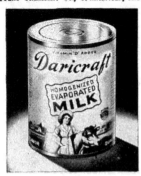

Book Reviews

CORNELL CONFERENCES ON THERAPY. Harry Gold, M.D., Editor. Sixth Edition, 322 pages. The Macmillan Company, New York, N. Y. $3.25.

In 1937 the departments of Medicine and Pharmacology at Cornell University Medical College inaugurated the *Cornell Conferences on Therapy.* In the preface of the book under this title the natural relationship of these two departments is stressed and emphasis placed upon the fact that they are too often widely separated in many medical schools with resulting faculty and student prejudices. Appropriately the volume opens with this motto from Thoreau: "It is never too late to give up our prejudices. No way of thinking or doing, however ancient, can be trusted without proof." Though it is never too late to corroborate and prove, this is a good place to stump the experts.

The preface indicates that the book covers the whole range of therapeutics and that, while originally designed for students, it was found that the discussions were equally valuable to the house staff, the attending staff and visiting physicians.

This useful volume in attractive, comfortable format runs 322 pages, embracing the following interesting chapters: 1. The Doctor's Bag; 2. Use and Abuse of Bed Rest; 3. Hypnotics and Sedatives; 4. Psychologic Aspects of the Treatment of Pain; 5. Surgical Measures for the Relief of Pain; 6. Treatment of Heart Failure, I; 7. Treatment of Heart Failure, II; 8. Digitalis vs. Digitoxin; 9. The Use of the Mercurial Diuretics; 10. Treatment of Subacute Bacterial Endocarditis; 11. Management of Abdominal Distention; 12. Treatment of Some Intestinal Infestations; 13. Treatment of Some Common Diseases of the Eye; 14. Treatment of Poisoning; 15. The RH Factor in Therapy.

Readily it may be noted that with the exception of one or two chapters this is a book for the general practitioner. It is impossible to read any one of the 15 chapters without gleaning helpful knowledge. While much of the knowledge and many of the conclusions have been evolved through team work, laboratory and technical methods, it may be said that facts having once been established, with clear cut criteria, may become practical for the general practitioner. The book is heartily recommended to the doctor in general practice.—Lewis J. Moorman, M.D.

WOMEN IN INDUSTRY. Anna M. Baetjer, Sc.D., Assistant Professor of Physiological Hygiene, School of Hygiene and Public Health, John Hopkins University. First Edition, 344 pages. W. B. Saunders, Philadelphia, Pa. 1946.

This text is not intended to justify the employment of women in industry, nor to condemn it. Rather it is to make available information for the proper placement of women when their service is required.

Anna M. Baetjer, Sc.D., Assistant Professor of Physiological Hygiene, School of Hygiene and Public Health, John Hopkins University, edited the book. It is issued under the auspices of the Division of Engineering and Industrial Research of the National Research Council and prepared in the Army Industrial Hygiene Laboratory. The author believes that it is the physician's role to assist in the proper job assignment to women employees. In order to do this, he must acquaint himself with the various types of jobs available and various factors of job employment as they apply specifically to the female.

A vast amount of information is presented in the form of charts and statistical surveys. Practical information can be gained from their presentation which will aid anyone responsible for proper job assignment for women. Causes for absenteeism in women are discussed, and sensible, rational reasons are presented. Methods to reduce this are given. Women are off work more than men, especially with such problems as illness, home distractions and conditions peculiar to their sex.

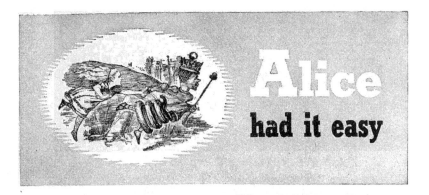

We've come to appreciate Alice's feelings in "Through the Looking Glass" when the Red Queen said,

"... *it takes all the running you can do, to keep in the same place. If you want to get somewhere else, you must run at least twice as fast as that!*"

But we find ourselves in an even more trying predicament.

Production of AMINOIDS* is up more than 100% over last year and still we are not able to keep up with the demand.

We are improving and extending production facilities as rapidly as post-war conditions permit. Meanwhile we are trying to distribute our output as equitably as possible. We hope we shall soon be able to fill every order promptly. Your understanding of our predicament and your continued friendly cooperation will be appreciated.

*The word AMINOIDS is a registered trademark of The Arlington Chemical Company.

THE ARLINGTON CHEMICAL COMPANY

YONKERS 1   NEW YORK

In regards to frequency of accidental injuries, as compared to men, women have no more, if you consider their inexperience in handling hazardous equipment. Some investigators claim that women as a whole are more careful than men. It is to be noted that non-industrial accidents and illnesses far outweigh industrial diseases and injuries in the cause of time loss.

Gynecological and obstetrical problems associated with the employment of women are investigated in detail. The author's conclusions regarding pregnancy of industrial workers are very interesting. One of the most valuable parts of the book is the complete list of all occupations which are suitable for women. With this list is given the normal training period necessary for learning the particular job.

This book is a real aid to anyone whose practice is concerned with the employment of women in industry.—William K. Ishmael, M.D.

Medical Abstracts

HYSTERECTOMY — THERAPEUTIC NECESSITY OR SURGICAL RACKET? Norman F. Miller, M.D., American Journal of Obstetrics and Gynecology, Vol. 51, No. 6, pp. 804-810, June, 1946.
Under this provocative title Dr. Miller analyzes 246 cases of hysterectomies, done in ten different hospitals in ten different localities.

The material used consisted of replies to questionnaires sent to the doctors. Dr. Miller also studied the histories and pathological reports. Attempts were made to (1) determine approximately the number of operations that were justified and (2) attempt to correlate symptoms and physical findings with demonstrable gross and histo pathology. Sixty-seven per cent of the women had justifiable operations. Thirty-three per cent had either no histo pathology or a diagnosis that contra-indicated hysterectomy (e.g. pregnancy, etc.). Seventeen per cent had neither symptoms nor pathology, 19 per cent had neither palpable nor microscopic disease, 17 per cent had neither symptoms, suspected pelvic disease nor histo-pathological changes in the removed organs. Ten per cent were operated because of various "functional" symptoms; e.g. "nervousness", "headache", etc.

Bethel Salomon's statement, as quoted by Dr. Miller in his article, cannot be improved upon: " . . . I would say a gynecologist is not a gynecologist until he ceases to perform unnecessary hysterectomies . . . ".—G.P., M.D.

THE MASKING EFFECT OF SULPHONAMIDE WHEN USED IN THE TREATMENT OF ACUTE OTITIS MEDIA. I. M. Farquharson. The Journal of Laryngology and Otology, Vol. 60, pp. 269-278, July, 1945.
It is now a generally recognized fact that the use of sulfonamide preparations in the course of acute otitis media as a prevention of mastoiditis is very dangerous. The drug, by its marked analgesic and antipyretic properties, tends to obscure the clinical picture, often giving rise to a latent course of the disease and a number of pathological changes. It has a masking effect upon symptoms which would indicate surgical intervention. It is also liable to mask the fever which, as a result of complications, may develop after ordinary operations on the mastoid.

For this reason, therefore, following simple mastoidec-

tomy the drug should not be given in uncomplicated cases. In the case of lateral sinus thrombosis or petritis, the limit of surgical measures must be reached before the drug can be safely given.

The author mentions that in the last eight years appreciable deterioration in hearing has been noticeable in the cases of otitis media, which, in the absence of other factors, must be put down to the masking effect of the drug causing delayed drainage from the middle ear. This may promote an adhesive inflammatory change or may be due to a hydrops of the labyrinth. His impression is that the routine use of sulfonamide in otitis media increased the number of cases which have developed chronic otitis media. Indeed, so much had the whole picture of acute otitis media changed in the last few years that one may justly talk of an "otitis media-sulfonamide syndrome".

This syndrome, or atypical disease, can be recognized by the following features. The aural discharge is variable, scanty or moderate, sometimes sterile, becoming profuse on discontinuing the drug. The tympanic membrane is thickened, with alteration of the usual anatomical landmarks, but the sagging of roof and the herniation of the drum is frequently absent. Tenderness and pain in the mastoid is usually absent. There may be normal temperature, with occasional irregular elevations the cause of which remains to be difficult to discern since it may be due as much to drug sensitivity as to further invasion of infection. The characteristic variations associated with invasion of the meninges and lateral sinus may be absent.

Even the x-ray findings are changed. The appearance of the films indicate that the mastoiditis is not as severe as clinical evidence would suggest. The drug appears to do something to the contents of the cells whereby they become more translucent to the x-rays. Hence, the use of stereoscopic films is essential if any guidance is to be obtained from them.

The final decision as to whether sulfonamide is to be given to a case of acute otitis media should rest on the ability of the otologist to carry out treatment along the following lines: hospitalization, confinement to bed, adequate dosage of the drug, early paracentesis, determination of the patient's immunity to a specific bacterium. If this cannot be assured the drug should be withheld as the risks of turning a simple condition into a dangerous one are too great. General practitioners should not attempt to use sulfonamides in acute otitis unless they can observe the case from day to day on a four-hourly chart.—M.D.H., M.D.

COMPOSITE FREE GRAFTS OF SKIN AND CARTILAGE FROM THE EAR; James Barrett Brown, Bradford Cannon, Surgery, Gynecology and Obstetrics, Volume 82, No. 3, pp. 253-255; March, 1946.
Tissue losses from such areas as the nostril border, tip of nose, and columella require replacement of both cartilage and skin. This article reports a method of accomplishing such replacement by a one stage method in which the required tissues are obtained from the patient's ear. The reported cases show good cosmetic restoration with very little deformity of the ear.—J.F.B., M.D.

KEY TO ABSTRACTORS

G.P., M.D. ....Grider Penick, M.D.
J.F.B., M.D. ....John F. Burton, M.D.
M.D.H., M.D. ....Marvin D. Henley, M.D.

J. E. HANGER, Inc.

ARTIFICIAL LIMBS, BRACES, AND CRUTCHES

Phone: 2-8500   612 N. Hudson

L. T. Lewis, Mgr.   BRANCHES AND AGENCIES IN PRINCIPAL CITIES Oklahoma City 3, Okla.

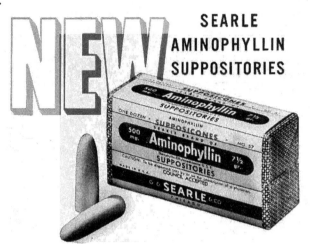

NEW

SEARLE
AMINOPHYLLIN
SUPPOSITORIES

For more convenient and effective rectal administration of
Aminophyllin,* Searle Research has produced

AMINOPHYLLIN SUPPOSICONES
(SEARLE BRAND OF AMINOPHYLLIN SUPPOSITORIES)

Differing from all other types of suppositories, Searle
Aminophyllin Supposicones are molded with a new base
material which liquefies rapidly in the rectum, permitting
complete absorption of the Aminophyllin, but which remains
stable and solid at temperatures up to 130° F. outside the body.

Searle Aminophyllin Supposicones are non-irritating to the
rectal mucosa—require no anesthetic—are of proper
size and shape for easy insertion and retention.
Each Aminophyllin Supposicone contains 500 mg. (7½ grs.)
Searle Aminophyllin. Packaged in boxes of 12.

*Searle Aminophyllin contains at least 80% of anhydrous theophylline
Supposicones is the registered trademark of G. D. Searle & Co., Chicago 80, Illinois

SEARLE
RESEARCH IN THE SERVICE OF MEDICINE

OFFICERS OF COUNTY SOCIETIES, 1946

★

COUNTY	PRESIDENT	SECRETARY	MEETING TIME
Alfalfa	W. G. Dunnington, Cherokee	L. T. Lancaster, Cherokee	Last Tues. each Second Month
Atoka-Coal	J. B. Clark, Coalgate	J. S. Fulton, Atoka	
Beckham	P. J. DeVanney, Sayre	J. E. Levick, Elk City	Second Tuesday
Blaine	W. F. Bohlman, Watonga	Virginia Curtain, Watonga	Third Thursday
Bryan	W. K. Haynie, Durant	Jonah Nichols, Durant	Second Tuesday
Caddo	P. H. Anderson, Anadarko	Edward T. Cook, Jr., Anadarko	
Canadian	G. L. Goodman, Yukon	W. P. Lawton, El Reno	Subject to call
Carter	J. Hobson Veazey, Ardmore	H. A. Higgins, Ardmore	Second Tuesday
Cherokee	P. H. Medearis, Tahlequah	R. K. McIntosh, Jr., Tahlequah	First Tuesday
Choctaw	Floyd L. Waters, Hugo	O. R. Gregg, Hugo	
Cleveland	James O. Hood, Norman	Phil Haddock, Norman	Thursday nights
Comanche	Wm. Cole, Lawton	E. P. Hathaway, Lawton	
Cotton	G. W. Baker, Walters	Mollie Seism, Walters	Third Friday
Craig	Lloyd H. McPike, Vinita	J. M. McMillan, Vinita	
Creek	W. P. Longmire, Sapulpa	Philip Joseph, Sapulpa	Second Tuesday
Custer	Ross Deputy, Clinton	A. W. Paulson, Clinton	Third Thursday
Garfield	Bruce Hinson, Enid	John R. Walker, Enid	Fourth Thursday
Garvin	M. E. Robberson, Jr., Wynnewood	John R. Callaway, Pauls Valley	Wednesday before Third Thursday
Grady	Roy Emanuel, Chickasha	Rebecca H. Mason, Chickasha	Third Thursday
Grant	L. V. Hardy, Medford	F. P. Robinson, Pond Creek	
Greer	J. B. Lansden, Granite	J. B. Hollis, Mangum	
Harmon	W. G. Husband, Hollis	R. H. Lynch, Hollis	First Wednesday
Haskell	Wm. S. Carson, Keota	N. K. Williams, McCurtain	
Hughes	Victor W. Pryor, Holdenville	L. A. S. Johnson, Holdenville	First Friday
Jackson	E. W. Mabry, Altus	J. P. Irby, Altus	Last Monday
Jefferson	F. M. Edwards, Ringling	J. A. Dillard, Waurika	Second Monday
Kay	L. G. Neal, Ponca City	J. C. Wagner, Ponca City	Second Thursday
Kingfisher	John W. Pendleton, Kingfisher	H. Violet Sturgeon, Hennessey	
Kiowa	Wm. Berneli, Hobart	J. Wm. Finch, Hobart	
LeFlore	S. D. Bevill, Poteau	Rush L. Wright, Poteau	
Lincoln	J. S. Rollins, Prague	Ned Burleson, Prague	First Wednesday
Logan	James Petty, Guthrie	J. E. Souter, Guthrie	Last Tuesday
Marshall			
Mayes	L. C. White, Adair	V. D. Herrington, Pryor	
McClain	S. C. Davis, Blanchard	W. C. McCurdy, Purcell	
McCurtain	J. T. Moreland, Idabel	R. H. Sherrill, Broken Bow	Fourth Tuesday
McIntosh	F. R. First, Checotah	W. A. Tolleson, Eufaula	First Thursday
Muskogee-Sequoyah Wagoner	R. N. Holcombe, Muskogee	William N. Weaver, Muskogee	First Tuesday
Noble	A. M. Evans, Perry	Jesse W. Driver, Perry	
Okfuskee	W. P. Jenkins, Okemah	M. L. Whitney, Okemah	Second Monday
Oklahoma	W. F. Keller, Okla. City	John H. Lamb, Okla. City	Fourth Tuesday
Okmulgee	F. S. Watson, Okmulgee	C. E. Smith, Henryetta	Second Monday
Osage	Paul H. Hemphill, Pawhuska	Vincent Mazzarella, Hominy	Third Monday
Ottawa	C. F. Walker, Grove	W. Jackson Sayles, Miami	Second Thursday
Pawnee	H. B. Spalding, Ralston	R. L. Browning, Pawnee	
Payne	F. Keith Oehlschlager, Yale	C. W. Moore, Stillwater	Third Thursday
Pittsburg	Millard L. Henry, McAlester	Edward D. Greenberger, McAlester	Third Friday
Pontotoc-Murray	John Morey, Ada	R. H. Mayes, Ada	First Wednesday
Pottawatomie	F. P. Newlin, Shawnee	Clinton Gallaher, Shawnee	First and Third Saturday
Pushmataha	John S. Lawson, Clayton	B. M. Huckabay, Antlers	
Rogers	W. A. Howard, Chelsea	P. S. Anderson, Claremore	Third Wednesday
Seminole	Clifton Felts, Seminole	Mack I. Shanholz, Wewoka	Third Wednesday
Stephens	Everett King, Duncan	Fred L. Patterson, Duncan	
Texas	Daniel S. Lee, Guymon	E. L. Buford, Guymon	
Tillman	H. A. Calvert, Frederick	O. G. Bacon, Frederick	
Tulsa	John C. Perry, Tulsa	John E. McDonald, Tulsa	Second and Fourth Monday
Washington-Nowata	Ralph W. Rucker, Bartlesville	L. B. Word, Bartlesville	Second Wednesday
Washita	L. G. Livingston, Cordell	Roy W. Anderson, Cordell	
Woods	John F. Simon, Alva	O. E. Templin, Alva	Last Tuesday Odd Months
Woodward	T. C. Leachman, Woodward	C. W. Tedrowe, Woodward	Second Thursday

THE JOURNAL

of the

OKLAHOMA STATE MEDICAL ASSOCIATION

| VOLUME XXXIX | OKLAHOMA CITY, OKLAHOMA, OCTOBER, 1946 | NUMBER 10 |

Pulmonary Sarcoidosis*

HARRY HAUSER, M.D.

CLEVELAND, OHIO

The purpose of this communication is to emphasize the importance of recognizing sarcoidosis as a disease entity particularly by its manifestations in the lungs as observed in the roentgenogram of the chest. In recent years chest radiography was increased to large proportions through greater interest in the value of radiologic findings in general, through tuberculosis surveys of civilian populations and by its routine use in the examination of personnel in industry and in the armed services. Many cases of pulmonary changes in sarcoidosis have been discovered by roentgen examination alone, either by routine or selective studies, and a smaller proportion have had their diagnosis confirmed either by biopsy of a peripheral lesion or by autopsy. Since sarcoidosis is no longer thought of as a rare disease[15], its diagnosis should be readily suspected when the characteristic lesions are present in the radiograph of the chest.

Sarcoidosis, as it is known at the present time, is a generalized disease affecting almost every organ of the body. It has been variously termed lupus pernio of Besnier, multiple benign skin sarcoids of Boeck, Hutchinson's disease, Schaumann's disease or lymphogranuloma benigna, ostitis tuberculosa multiplex cystica (Jungling) and uveo-parotid fever (Heerfordt). According to Hunter[7], the disease was first recognized clinically by Hutchinson as early as 1869 and later described by Besnier[2] as *lupus pernio* in 1889. Boeck[3] was the first to describe the histological features of the skin manifestations and introduced the name *sarcoid* because of the sarcoma-like appearance of the epithelioid connective tissue cells in the perivascular lymph spaces and the occasional giant-cell which was considered to be of sarcomatous type. While Kien-

bock[10] (1902) Kreibich[13] (1904) and Reider[20] (1910) recognized the radiologic appearance of the cystic changes in the small bones of the hands and feet, it was not until 1917 that Schaumann[21] identified lupus pernio and Boeck's sarcoid as the same disease by the microscopic appearance of the lymph nodes and the bone lesions. Again in 1919, Jungling[9] proved the identity of the cystic lesions observed radiographically by biopsy of the soft tissues of a finger, found the characteristic microscopic changes described by Boeck and applied the term *ostitis tuberculosa multiplex cystica* to these bony changes. In 1915 Kutznitsky and Bittorf[14] reported a case of skin sarcoid with pathologic changes occurring in the spleen and lymph nodes and radiologic findings of mottled infiltration in the lungs and enlargement of the hilum nodes. Schaumann[22] (1924) later gave the name of lymphogranuloma benigna to this disease and while it simulated lymphogranuloma maligna (Hodgkin's disease) in its protean manifestations it tended to follow a benign course. *Uveoparotid fever* described by Heerfordt[6] in 1909 was later recognized as another manifestation of Besnier-Boeck's disease by Bruins-Slot[4] in 1936, and 1937 Longcope and Pierson[16] also attributed the uveal tract and parotid involvement to sarcoidosis.

A series of 19 cases of sarcoidosis have been observed on various services at City Hospital and the University Hospitals of Cleveland of Western Reserve School of Medicine in the past decade, 15 of which were proved by biopsy of a peripheral lesion and 4 by autopsy. A number of other cases were also observed in which the diagnosis was made clinically and roentgenologically, but because of lack of histologic proof they are not included in this report. The most striking feature of the 19 cases was the pulmonary

*Delivered before the General Session, Annual Meeting, Oklahoma State Medical Association, May 3, 1946.

and mediastinal lymph node involvement as observed on the chest roentgenogram. Table I includes all the positive findings in the whole series of cases and Table II gives the distribution of the lesions according to anatomical site.

The average age of the series was 29.9 years, the youngest being nine and the oldest sixty-three. There were twelve females and seven males and twelve patients were negro and seven were white. The predominance of negro patients is in accord with the findings of Longcope[15] and Thomas[23].

ETIOLOGY

The etiology of sarcoidosis is not known, most writers on the subject offering no explanation as to causative factors. Pinner[17] holds to the belief that the disease is a form of non-caseating tuberculosis and supports this view mainly on the basis that some of the reported cases have developed a rapidly progressive form of tuberculosis.

The fact that tubercle bacilli cannot be demonstrated in the sections of tissue or following injection of some of the macerated tissues into animals, and that the tuberculin test is negative in the majority of cases has led most students of the subject to discredit tuberculosis as a causative agent. Kissmeyer and Nielson[12] believe, in view of the repeated negative bacteriologic studies, that the disease is due to an unidentified virus. Rabello[19] finds the lesions of cutaneous and osseous sarcoid to resemble leprosy. The latter concept seems unlikely in view of the striking difference of the radiographic appearance of lesions affecting the phalanges in the two diseases.

PATHOLOGY

The lack of caseation and the absence of tubercle bacilli in the histologic section are the two main distinguishing features between the tubercle of sarcoid and that of tuberculosis. The sarcoid tubercle is composed of pale-staining polygonal epithelioid cells with an occasional giant-cell usually of the foreign body type (Figures 7A and 7B). Central necrosis is rarely seen and a peripheral inflammatory reaction is usually absent. In the occasional case there may be a slight degree of central necrosis and a few scattered lymphocytes in the peripheral zone. Giant cells are not always present. Healing may take place by fibrosis and hyalinization. Grossly the lesions are firm, gray "hard" nodules from a few millimeters to about one centimeter in diameter depending upon the extent and the degree of coalescence.

CLINICAL AND ROENTGENOLOGICAL FEATURES

The paucity of clinical signs and symptoms in sarcoidosis is usually the rule. There may be varying degrees of chest findings including cough, expectoration, dyspnea and rales. Examination of the sputum and gastric con-

tents fail to reveal the presence of tubercle bacilli. Fatigue, weight loss and occasionally a low grade fever may be manifestations of the generalized disease. Bizarre phenomena may result from involvement of vital organs such as the case of diabetes insipidus reported by Tillgren[24] in which a focus of sarcoid was found in the pituitary gland. Multiple lesions may occur in the myocardium with changes in cardiac rhythm and evidence of congestive failure[8][1]. External manifestations may present themselves by enlargements of the peripheral lymph nodes, by skin changes of either the Besnier-Boeck or Darier-Roussy types[5], by involvement of the iris, ciliary body, lacrimal, parotid and submaxillary salivary glands, and by enlargement of the spleen, liver or various portions of the skeletal system. The blood cell count is usually within normal limits although polycythemia has been reported. The large monocytes may be increased in number during the active phases of the disease. Eosinophilia is occasionally encountered. Serum globulin is almost always elevated showing a reversal of the A-G ratio. Tuberculin anergy is found in about 70 per cent of the cases. The tuberculin test was positive in four of the present series of 19 cases.

All of the 19 cases reported in this series showed roentgenological changes in the chest consisting of enlargement of the tracheo-bronchial lymph nodes and various forms of pulmonary infiltrations[11]. (Figures 1A and B; Figures 2A and B). The diffuse small nodular and streaked shadows of increased density radiating outwards from the hila are the changes encountered most consistently. Occasionally the closely packed miliary type of nodulations interspersed by thin strand-like infiltration are observed (Figures 4 and 6). The phalanges of the hands and feet were involved in only 1 case in this series (Figures 5A and B). Cystic defects are found in medullary portions of the phalanges without causing destruction of the cortex and without any evidence of surrounding inflammatory changes. Other portions of the skeletal system may be involved by destructive lesions (Figures 3B, C, and D).

Some of the features of sarcoidosis may best be considered by a review of several cases included in this series.

Case No. 2: N. M., a colored female, aged forty-five, was admitted to the hospital on September 26, 1938, complaining of weakness of one year's duration and pain in the left chest for three weeks. Examination revealed rales in both lung bases and the spleen was slightly enlarged. Chest radiography revealed bilateral hilum node enlargement and a slight degree of streaked infiltration in the right base (Figure 1A). A tentative diagnosis of Hodgkin's disease was made. Tuberculin tests down to 1:100 dilutions were negative. Repeated sputum examination including concentration technic were negative for tubercle bacilli. A moderate anemia was present. High voltage roentgen irradiation was administered to the hilum nodes resulting in slight diminution in their size. Biopsy of an axillary node in November and repeated in December was reported as chronic hyperplasia and tuberculosis respectively. An excised skin lesion was reported as, pityriasis rosea. Additional tuberculin tests were performed with P. P. D. and again proved negative. The liver and spleen became palpable a few cm. below the costal margins. The patient was discharged on January 11, 1939, in fair condition but with a poor prognosis and was followed in the Chest Dispensary. She was readmitted on September 15, 1939, with a pleural effusion in the right base, aspiration of which revealed a serous effusion (Figure 1B). Cultures were negative for py-

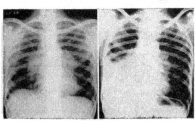

(Figure 1A)   (Figure 1B)

Fig. 1A, Case No. 2. Sept. 27, 1938. Tremendously enlarged hilum nodes, bilaterally. Right paratracheal nodes moderately enlarged. Thickening of interlobar septum on right.

Fig. 1B. Case No. 2. Sept. 18, 1939. Hilum nodes moderately enlarged. Streaked infiltration in right lower lung with large right pleural effuffsion. Autopsy revealed sarcoidosis.

ogenic and tuberculous organisms. Tuberculin tests were again repeated with P. P. D. and a delayed atypical positve reaction was obtained to a double dose of second strength P. P. D. A persistent microscopic pyuria was noted and urinary sediment was negative for tubercle bacilli. The patient gradually became weaker and died on December 26, 1939. Autopsy (Dr. H. H. Macumber) revealed sarcoidosis of the cervical hilum, axillary, portal and superior pancreatic lymph nodes, lungs, liver, spleen and adrenal glands. The spleen weighed 575 grams. Guinea pig inoculation with material from a hilum lymph node yielded negative results.

Comment: The diagnosis of sarcoidosis was not made during life. The clinical picture, the lymphadenopathy, the typical histologic picture of the involved organs, the absence of tubercle bacilli and the anergic reaction to high concentrations of tuberculin are all characteristic features of sarcoidosis.

The effusion in the right pleural cavity was an unusual finding.

Case No. 3: F. A., a 22 year old white male, was admitted to the hospital on July 5, 1939, with marked swelling in both parotid regions and of his eyelids which had first appeared five weeks previously. Examination revealed hard, almost immobile enlargement of both parotid, submaxillary and lacrimal glands. The temperature was 37.2 degrees C. The clinical impression was that of Mickulicz disease. Tuberculin tests were negative with O. T. down to 1:100 dilution and with second strength P. P. D.

A radiograph of the chest on July 13, 1939, revealed "potato-like" enlargements of both groups of hilum nodes (Figure 2A). A biop-

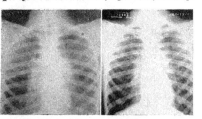

(Figure 2A)   (Figure 2B)

Fig. 2A. Case No. 3. July 15, 1939. Greatly enlarged hilum and paratracheal lymph nodes. Biopsy of parotid gland revealed sarcoidosis.

Fig. 2B. Case No. 3. June 6, 1940. Hilum and paratracheal nodes smaller. Diffusely scattered nodular and streaked pulmonary infiltration.

sy from the left parotid gland revealed hyperplastic tuberculosis but was later considered to be Boeck's sarcoid. Special stains failed to reveal the presence of tubercle bacilli. The patient was discharged from the hospital on July 25, 1939, without having received any active therapy and the prognosis was considered good. A follow-up chest radiograph made on June 12, 1940, showed moderate diminution in the size of the hilum nodes and a diffuse nodular and streaked infiltration throughout both lungs (Figure 2B).

Comment: This case had the clinical features of Mickulicz disease and uveo-parotid fever although there were no eye changes and the temperature was normal. The radiographic features in the hilum nodes and lungs were characteristic of sarcoidosis.

The biopsy from the parotid gland showed microscopic features consistent with a diagnosis of Boeck's sarcoid (Dr. H. Z. Lund).

Case No. 4: B. P., a white female, aged 9, was admitted to the hospital on July 5, 1939, with a history of loss of strength and appetite since August, 1938, and a stiff neck beginning October, 1938. Radiographs of the cervical spine and chest showed destructive

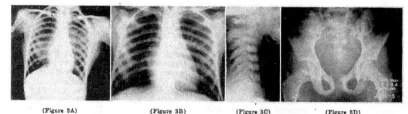

(Figure 3A)   (Figure 3B)   (Figure 3C)   (Figure 3D)

Figure 3A. Case No. 4 July 12, 1939. Slight pulmonary infiltration radiating outwards from left hilum. Destruction of anterior right fourth and fifth ribs and posterior left sixth rib.

Fig 3B. Case No. 4 Dec. 14, 1939 More advanced destruction of anterior right fourth and fifth (biopsy) and posterior left sixth rib due to sarcoid infiltration.

Fig. 3C. Case No 4, Feb. 10, 1941. Mottled appearance of second to sixth cervical vertebrae due to destruction and new bone production by sarcoidosis (Biopsy).

Fig 3D Case No. 4 June 5, 1941. Destruction of pubic bones at symphysis considered to be part of generalized sarcoidosis.

changes from C-1 to C-6 inclusive and destruction in the anterior ends of the right fourth and fifth ribs, (Figures 3B and C), with scattered nodular and streaked infiltration radiating outwards from both hila (Figure 3A). Tuberculin tests down to 1:100 dilution and second strength P. P. D. were negative. For a period of six months there was a gradual increase in visual disturbance with blurring and also the development of some deafness. Diagnoses of primary optic atrophy and chronic serous otitis media with secondary deafness were made. Biopsies were made of the spinous process of the third cervical vertebra, of the posterior portion of the left sixth rib, which were reported as chronic inflammation. Later the patient developed swelling of both sides of the mandible and had difficulty in opening her mouth. Biopsy made of the left mandible was reported as chronic destructive inflammation of bone, non-suppurative.

Radiograph of the pelvis on June 5, 1941, showed irregular destruction of the symphysis pubis (Figure 3D).

All the biopsy material was sent to Dr. Henry L. Jaffe, pathologist for the Hospital for Joint Diseases of New York City, who believed the diagnosis was sarcoid. Additional tuberculin tests were made all of which proved negative. The patient was discharged on June 26, 1941, to the State Institute for the Blind.

Comment: This case presents unusual features in that multiple bones are involved in a similar manner. The repeatedly negative tuberculin tests, the infiltration in lungs, and the opinion of an experienced pathologist in bone diseases augur well for a diagnosis of sarcoidosis. It is not certain that the primary optic atrophy can be accounted for by involvement by sarcoidosis, but it could be a possibility since it is known that nerve tissue may be involved[15].

Case No. 5: O. S., a colored female, gradu-

ate nurse, aged 27, was admitted to the tuberculosis division on July 12, 1940. She gave a history of malaise and mild fatigue of six months duration, followed during the two months prior to admission by progressive dyspnea of such degree that she was conscious of labored respirations when walking. There was also present a hacking cough, usually unproductive, a loss of eight pounds in the six months before admission. She continued to work until three days before entry into the hospital.

Examination revealed a well developed young colored female, dyspneic on exertion but breathing quietly at rest and not appearing seriously ill. The temperature was normal, the pulse rate varied between 80 and 100, and the blood pressure was 112/72. Fine rales were audible in the lower two-

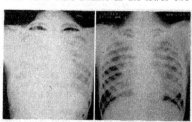

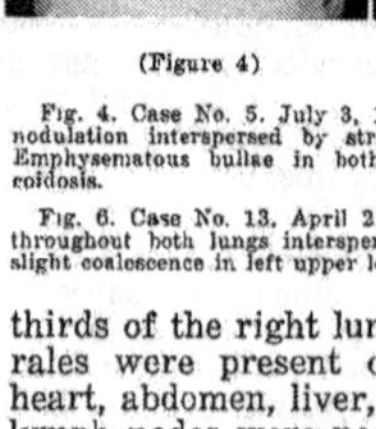

(Figure 4) 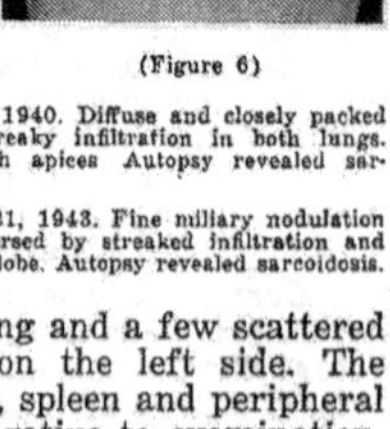   (Figure 6)

Fig. 4. Case No. 5. July 3, 1940. Diffuse and closely packed nodulation interspersed by streaky infiltration in both lungs. Emphysematous bullae in both apices Autopsy revealed sarcoidosis.

Fig. 6. Case No. 13. April 21, 1943. Fine miliary nodulation throughout both lungs interspersed by streaked infiltration and slight coalescence in left upper lobe. Autopsy revealed sarcoidosis.

thirds of the right lung and a few scattered rales were present on the left side. The heart, abdomen, liver, spleen and peripheral lymph nodes were negative to examination. The vital capacity on admission was 1100 cc. or 35 per cent. Hemoglobin, blood cell count and urine were within limits of normal. Tuberculin tests with P. P. D. were negative using first and second strengths, but a positive test was obtained using a double dose of second strength material. The sputum was mucoid in character and repeated examinations of sputum and gastric contents for tubercle bacilli and fungi were negative.

The chest radiograph revealed a symmetrical diffuse nodulation and streaked infiltration of both lung fields sparing the apices, and showed enlargement of the mediastinal lymph nodes (Figure 4).

During her hospital stay the patient developed progressive dyspnea and her par-

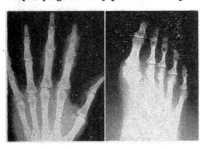

(Figure 5A)　　(Figure 5B)

Fig 5A. Case No. 6. July 3, 1941. Ovoid punched-out areas of destruction involving the phalanges of the hands. Biopsies from skin of nose, arm and back showed Boeck's sarcoid.

Fig. 5B. Case No. 6. July 3, 1941. Punched-out areas of bone destruction of the phalanges of the feet. Biopsies from skin of nose, arm and back showed Boeck's sarcoid.

oxysmal unproductive cough became worse. She was afebrile except late in the course of her disease, but the temperature did not exceed 38 degree C. The urine later contained 1+ albumin and the total white blood

cell count rose to 18,000. Late in the course of her disease she developed two small lymph node enlargements in the left axilla and a small node in the right axilla. She became progressively worse and despite symptomatic treatment and the administration of potassium iodide died on September 16, 1940, of respiratory and cardiac failure.

The autopsy (Dr. A. E. Margulis) revealed Boeck's sarcoid of the lungs, bronchi, pleura, pericardium, spleen, right kidney, and mediastinal, left inferior deep cervical, pretracheal, celiac, hepatic and para-aortic lymph nodes. The right side of the heart was moderately dilated and slightly hypertrophied (cor pulmonale).

Comment: The radiographic appearance of lungs was not unlike that of miliary tuberculosis (Figure 4) with nodular and streaked shadows closely packed except for emphysematous bullae in the apices. With the temperature approximately normal, the absence of tubercle bacilli in the sputum and gastric contents and the tuberculin tests negative in higher dilutions, a diagnosis of tuberculosis seemed unlikely and the final clinical diagnosis was thought to be metastatic neoplasm to the lungs.

Case No. 13: R. J., a colored female, aged 15 years, was admitted to the tuberculosis division of City Hospital on April 17, 1943. Her illness began in June, 1942, with cough productive of small amounts of mucopurulent sputum, weakness and gradual weight loss. Two months later she reported to Children's Health Dispensary and was told she had mumps. She continued to be moderately ill until two weeks before admission when she developed fever, night sweats and moderate dyspnea. Routine fluoroscopy in school revealed a pulmonary lesion. Her total weight loss was 37 pounds.

Examination revealed a poorly nourished, chronically ill young girl in no apparent dis-

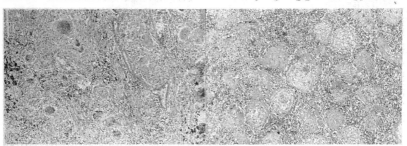

(Figure 7A)　　(Figure 7B)

Fig. 7A. Case No. 13. Photomicrograph (x 160) of section of lung showing epithelioid tubercles and considerable interstitial fibrosis. A few scattered giant-cells are present. No caseation or central necrosis.

Fig. 7B. Case No. 13. Photomicrograph (x 142) of a lymph node showing tubercles formed by pale-staining epithelioid cells. Caseation and necrosis are not present.

TABLE I — PULMONARY SARCOIDOSIS — TABULATION OF FINDINGS IN 19 CASES

Case No. Initials Age / Color	Date Admission	Radiographic Appearance of Lungs	Lymph, Nodes, Radiographic and Clinical	Skin	Other Organs	Globulin Per Cent	Tuberculin Reaction	Remarks
22 B.M. M W	1-20-36	Slight infiltration adjacent to hilum	Hilum bilat.	Eyelid* Leg*			Neg.	
2 N.M. F B	9-26-38	Streaked infiltration right middle and lower lobes	Cervical, hilum, axillary, portal, sup. pancreatic		Spleen, Liver, Adrenals right pleural effusion		Neg.	Autopsy (see case report)
22 F.A. M W	7-5-39	Disseminated nodular and streaked infiltration	Hilum bilat.		Parotid glands*		Neg.	See case report
4 B.P. F W	7-5-39	Scattered nodular and streaked infiltration			Ribs* C-3* left mandible* Symphysis Pubis—Liver	4.2	Neg.	Referred to State Institute for the Blind. Primary optic atrophy
5 O.S. F B	7-12-40	Miliary and streaked infiltration	Mediastinal left inferior deep cervical, pretracheal, celiac, hepatic and para-aortic		Pleura pericardium right kidney	6.0	Neg.	Autopsy (see case report) Tuberculin positive double dose second strength P.P.D.
6 F.W. F B	6-28-41	Slight nodular infiltration	Hilum bilat.	Nose* Arm* Back*	Phalanges of fingers and toes bilat.	4.25	Neg.	Tonsil biopsy showed endothelial hyperplasia
63 A.G. F B	10-4-41	Streaked infiltration right upper and left lower lobes		Right foot*		6.1	Pos.	Tuberculin P.P.D. second strength
32 H.O. M W	10-4-41	Nodular and patchy infiltration	Hilum bilat, right paratracheal	Back* Left knee	Iris		Neg.	Many skin nodules on back
9 C.L. F W	3-20-42	Slight nodular infiltration	Left inguinal* Generalized superficial right paratracheal Hilum bilat.			4.16		Secondary anemia
10 E.M. M B	7-17-42	Nodular and streaky infiltration	Left axillary* right paratracheal Generalized superficial			4.5	Neg.	
11 S.G. F W	8-11-42	Streaked infiltration left lower lobe	Cervical* Paratracheal* and hilum bilat.			4.2	Pos.	Tuberculin P.P.D. second strength Nodes disappeared
13 M.H. M B	12-9-42	Slight infiltration at left hilum	Right supraclavicular* hilum bilat. Right paratracheal		Liver	3.16	Pos.	
13 R.J. F B	4-17-43	Diffuse miliary and streaked infiltration	Cervical Bronchopulmonary		Liver, spleen, kidney, colon, submax. salivary gland, lingual and faucial tonsils	6.0	Pos.	Autopsy (see case report) Tuberculin P.P.D. second strength
14 J.B. F B	5-27-43	Diffuse nodular infiltration	Cervical* Right paratracheal	Chest* Neck*	Iris, lacrimal gland, parotid liver, spleen	3.8	Neg.	All lesions cleared 4-15-46
15 W.P. M R	1-28-44	Streaked infiltration, right upper and lower lobes	Inguinal* Left Epitrochlear*				Neg.	
16 G.A. F R	3-15-44	Nodular and streaked infiltration	Hilum and paratracheal	Abdomen*		6.15	Neg.	Irreg. fever rising to 39.5 degrees C.
7 F.Y. F R	4-18-44	Bilateral infiltration	Mediastinal lymph nodes		Liver			Autopsy Died two days after admission Bronchopneumonia
18 W.S. M B	11-19-44	Miliary and streaked infiltration (Reticulated)	Right inguinal* Generalized superficial Hilum and paratracheal		Uveitis bilat. iris, right	8.85	Neg.	Blood smear showed 30 large monocytes
19 O.C. M B	10-16-45	Diffuse streaked infiltration	Bilat. hilum right paratracheal	Chest* Neck*	Uveal tract parotid		Neg.	

*Biopsy

tress. Abnormal findings were limited to the chest where rales were heard over both lungs. The temperature was 37 degrees C., pulse 90, respirations 22, blood pressure 115/90 and vital capacity 1100 cc. or 33 per cent.

Laboratory studies showed the urine to be normal. Sedimentation rate was 1.33 with hematocritic 41. Blood urea nitrogen was 12.6, total proteins 10.2 grams, albumin 4.2 and globulin 6.0 grams per 100 cc., the A-G ratio being 0.69. Eight sputum concentrations and three gastric washings were negative for tubercle bacilli. Several tuberculin tests were negative, but further testing with second strength P. P. D. was strongly positive. Sputum cultures for fungi and blood cultures were negative.

Roentgen examination of the chest revealed a diffuse miliary nodulation throughout both lung fiields with a tendency towards coalescence in the left upper lobe. A fine streaked infiltration was interspersed between the nodules. The hilum lymph nodes were moderately enlarged. No change took place in the appearance of the lungs and mediastinum during an eight months period (Figure 6).

Throughout the eleven months in the hospital, the patient's fever was low grade in character. She gained a few pounds in weight and had no specific complaints other than cough productive of 50 grams of sputum. During the last several months she had a marked tachycardia and increasing dyspnea. On February 26, 1944, a diastolic gallop rhythm was heard over the apex of the heart. During her last week she developed orthopnea, ascites, hepato and splenomegaly with a total weight gain of 14 pounds. Death occurred on March 6, 1944, the 328th hospital day.

The autopsy (Dr. H. Z. Lund) revealed widespread pulmonary fibrosis, both nodular and reticular consistent with a diagnosis of sarcoidosis (Figure 7A). Characteristic lesions of sarcoidosis were found in the liver, salivary glands, colon, kidneys, spleen, cervical and bronchopulmonary lymph nodes (Figure 7B) and lingual and faucial tonsils. Other findings were relative right ventricular hypertrophy, marked pulmonary emphysema, chronic bronchitis, bronchiectasis, fibrous pleural adhesions and right pleural effusion of 500 cc. A portion of the spleen was macerated, suspended in saline solution and injected into the subcutaneous tissues of a guinea pig. The pig died in three weeks without evidence of tuberculosis or other grossly demonstrable disease.

Comment: The clinical diagnosis was considered to be far advanced pulmonary tuberculosis. Because of experience gained from Case No. 5 and because of lack of change in the character of the lesions over a period of about eight months, the roentgenologic interpretation late in the course of the disease was pulmonary sarcoidosis. In all probability, the earlier diagnosis of "mumps" was in truth sarcoidosis of the parotid glands (uveoparotid fever).

DIFFERENTIAL DIAGNOSIS

The diagnosis of sarcoidosis of the lungs and mediastinum is more often confused with pulmonary tuberculosis than with other diseases. The character of the nodulation and streaked infiltration with hilum and paratracheal node enlargements, the lack of fever, the anergic reaction to tuberculin, the elevated serum globulin fraction with reversal of the A-G ratio are distinguishing clinical features between sarcoidosis and tuberculosis. Hodgkin's disease or some other form of lymphoblastoma may simulate sarcoidosis because of widespread lymph node involvement and a biopsy of the peripheral lesion may be required to determine the correct diagnosis. The fine nodulation in the lung fields is rarely found in Hodgkin's disease and is often observed in sarcoidosis. The history, clinical and roentgenologic features of sarcoidosis usually serve well in differentiation from hilum node tuberculosis, miliary carcinomatosis, erythema nodosum, fungus disease, pulmonary hemosiderosis and silicosis. The absolute diagnosis of sarcoidosis is dependent upon histologic studies of the involved tissues.

TREATMENT

Little can be said regarding specific treatment of sarcoidosis since most of the cases recover spontaneously. Bed rest, arsenic, codliver oil, leprosol, gold salts, hyperpyrexia and ultraviolet light have been advocated at one time or another. Radiotherapy, in the hands of some workers [18] [1], has produced rapid retrogression of some of the lesions. Further experience will be required before the value of roentgen therapy can be established.

SUMMARY

The importance of recognizing pulmonary involvement in sarcoidosis is emphasized. Sarcoidosis is a generalized disease affecting almost every organ and system in the body. In past years various eponyms has been used to designate the disease as it affected different anatomical sites such as skin, bone marrow, lymph nodes, lungs, parotid glands and various structure in and about the eye. Nineteen cases with pulmonary involvement and coexisting lesions have been reviewed. Five case reports are included illustrating clinical, roentgenological and pathological manfestations of the disease. The prognosis is good in most of the cases, three having died of sarcoidosis and one from bronchopneumonia. The etiology, pathology, differential diagnosis and therapy are discussed.

TABLE II—DISTRIBUTION OF LESIONS

Location	Number	Biopsy	Autopsy
Lungs	19		4
Lymph Nodes			
Superficial	10	7	3
Mediastinal	11		2
Bronchial	12		2
Abdominal	2		2
Skin	6	6	
Bones	2	1	
Eyes			
Iris	3		
Uveal tract	2		
Lacrimal Gland	1		
Salivary Glands			
Parotid	3	1	
Submaxillary	1		1
Tonsils	1		1
Liver	5		2
Spleen	2		1
Adrenal Gland	1		1
Pleura	1		1
Pericardium	1		1
Kidney	2		2
Colon	1		1

BIBLIOGRAPHY

1. Bernstein, S. S. and Oppenheimer, B. S. Böeck's Sarcoid: Report of Six Cases With One Necropsy. J. Mt. Sinai Hosp., Vol. 9, pp. 320-343; 1942.

2. Besnier E. Lupus pernio de la face; synovites fongeuses (scrofulo-tuberculeuses) symetriques des extermites superieures. Ann. de dermat. et syph. Vol. 10 (Series II) pp. 333-336; 1889.

3. Boeck, C. Multiple benign sarkoid of the skin. J. Cutan. & G. U. Dis., Vol. 17, pp. 543-550; 1899.

4. Bruins-Slot, W. J.: Besnier-Boecks disease and Uveo-parotid Fever (Heerfordt). Nederl. Aijdschr. V. Gneesk. Vol. 80, pp. 2859; 1936.

Bruins-Slot, W. J. Goedbloed, J., and Goslings, J. Die Besnier-Boeck (Schaumann)-sche Krankheit und die Uveo-Parotitis (Heerfordt) Acta med. Scandinav., Vol. 94, pp. 74-97; 1938.

5. Ernsting, H. C. Boeck's Sarcoid of the Eyelid with Co-existing Darier-Roussy's Sarcoid. Arch. Ophth. Vol. 17, pp. 483-504; 1937.

6 Heerfordt, C. F. Ueber eine Febris uveo-parotidea sub-chronica an der Glandula parotis und der Uvea des Auges localisiert und Laufig mit Parensen cerebrospinalen Nerven komplicirt. Arch. f. Ophth. Vol. 70, pp. 254-273; 1909.

7. Hunter, F.T. Hutchinson-Boeck's Disease (Generalized "Sarcoidosis"). New Eng. J. Med., Vol. 214, pp. 346-352, 1936.

8. Johnson, J. K., and Jason, R. S. Sarcoidosis of the Heart. Am Jlt J., Vol. 27, pp. 246-258; 1944.

9 Jungling, O Ostitis tuberculosa multiplex cystica (eine eigenartige Form der Knochentuberculose). Fortschr. a. d. Geb. der Roentgenstrahlen, Vol. 27. pp. 375-383, 1919.

10 Kienbock, R. Radiographische Anatomie und Klinik der syphilitischen Knochenerkrankungen an Extremi-taten. Zischr. f. Heilk, Vol. 23 (Abth. f. Chir.), pp. 130; 1902.

11 King, D. S Sarcoid Disease as Revealed in the Chest Roentgenogram Am. J. Roentgenol. & Rad Therapy, Vol. 45, pp. 505-512; 1941.

12. Kissmeyer, A., and Nielson, J. Notes sur l'etiologie des sarcodes de Boeck. Acta dermat., Vol. 14, pp. 283-286; 1933.

13. Kreibich, K. Uber lupus pernio. Arch. f. Dermat. u Syph., Vol. 71, pp. 3-18, 1904.

14. Kuznitsky, E., and Bittorf, A. Boeckisches Sarkoid mit Beteiligung innerer Organe. Munchen med. Wchnschr., Vol. 62, pp. 1349-1353; 1915.

15. Longcope, W. T. Sarcoidosis or Besnier-Boeck-Schaumann Disease. J. Med. Am Assn., Vol. 117, pp. 1321-1327; 1941.

16. Longcope, W. T. and Pierson, J. W. Boeck's Sarcoid (Sarcoidosis Bull. Johns Hopkins Hosp., Vol. 60, pp. 223-296; 1937.

17 Pinner, M Noncaseating Tuberculosis, Am Rev. Tuberc., Vol. 37, pp. 690-728; 1938.

18. Pohle, E. A., and Paul, L. W., and Clark, E. A. Roent-gen Therapy of Boeck's Sarcoid. Am. J. Med. Sc., Vol 209, pp. 503-513; 1945.

19. Rabello, J. Donees nouvelles pour l'interpretation de l'affection de Besnier-Boeck role de la lepre. Ann. de dermat. et syph., Vol. 7, pp. 571-597; 1936.

20. Reider, H. Uber Kombination von chronischer Osteo-myelitis (Spina Ventosa) mit Lupus pernio. Fortschr. a. d. Geb. d. Roent., Vol. 15, pp. 125-135; 1910.

21 Schaumann, J Etude sur le lupus pernio et ses rapports avec les sarcoides et la tuberculose. Ann. de dermat. et syph., Series V, Vol. 6, pp. 357-373; 1917.

22. Schaumann, J. Benign lymphogranuloma and its cutan-eous manifestations. Brit. J. Derm. and Syph., Vol. 36, pp. 515-544; 1924.

23. Thomas, C. C. Sarcoidosis (including 15 cases, 12 in Negroes). Arch. Dermat. & Syph., Vol. 47, pp. 58-73; 1943.

24. Tillgren, J. Diabetes Insipidus as Symptom of Schau-mann's disease. Brit. J. Dermat., Vol. 47, pp. 223-229; 1935.

Announcement

The $34,000 prize contest for physicians' art work on the subject of "Courage and Devotion Beyond the Call of Duty" will be judged at the Atlantic City Centennial Session of the A.M.A. at Atlantic City June 9-13, 1947; closing date is May 15, 1947.

Art works on other subjects may also be submitted for the regular cups and medals.

For full information, write Dr. F. H. Redewill, Secre-tary, American Physicians Art Association, Flood Build-ing, San Francisco, Calif., or to the sponsor, Mead Johnson and Company, Evansville 21, Ind., U.S.A.

Genius in poverty is never feared, because nature, though liberal in her gifts in one instance, is forgetful in another.—B. R. Haydon.

Whatever government is not a government of laws is a despotism, let it be called what it may.—Daniel Webster.

Men must not be poor; idleness is the root of all evil; the world's wide enough, let 'em bustle.—Farquhar.

Our ideals are our better selves.—A. Bronson Alcott.

---

they leave that safety in any hands but their own.—Daniel Webster.

Ill-humor arises from an inward consciousness of our own want of merit, from a discontent which ever accompanies that envy which foolish vanity engenders.—Goethe.

Babylon in all its desolation is a sight not so awful as that of the human mind in ruins.—Scrope Davies.

In that worthiest of all struggles — the struggle for self-mastery and goodness — we are far less patient with ourselves than God is with us.—Timothy Titcomb.

We get impatient, and there crops out our human weakness.—Timothy Titcomb.

Every subject's duty is the king's; but every sub-ject's soul is his own.—Shakespeare.

RADIUM

(Including Radium Applicators)

FOR ALL MEDICAL PURPOSES

Est. 1919

Quincy X-Ray and Radium Laboratories
(Owned and directed by a Physician-Radiologist)

HAROLD SWANBERG, B.S., M.D., Director

W.C.U. Bldg.   Quincy, Illinois

The Rh Blood Factors*

HOMER F. MARSH, PH.D.

Oklahoma University School of Medicine

OKLAHOMA CITY, OKLAHOMA

In view of the apparent confusion concerning the Rh factors of human blood, it seems timely to attempt a general account of the nature of these factors, the tests used in detecting them, and their significance in clinical and medico-legal applications.

HISTORICAL

Since some animal bloods contain antigens which are similar to certain of those found in human bloods, Landsteiner and Wiener, in 1937, used blood from the rhesus monkey to inject guinea pigs and rabbits in an attempt to produce antisera with which further studies of the M antigen could be made in human bloods. In the course of their experiments, there was discovered in human blood an antigen unlike the M, N, or P antigens which had been previously known. In a series of tests it was found that this new antigen occurred in about 85 per cent of the bloods of white persons tested and was entirely absent from 15 per cent of the bloods tested[1]. Because of the source of the material used in preparing these antisera, namely, the blood of the rhesus monkey, they named the newly discovered antigen Rh (rhesus).

The clinical importance of the antigen was soon demonstrated by Wiener and Peters[2] who observed three cases of transfusion reactions which could not be attributed to reactions between the ordinary antigens, i.e., A, B, or AB but which, in each case, was related to the presence of the Rh antigen in the donor's corpuscles. Landsteiner and Wiener, therefore, published their original findings in regard to the Rh antigen in 1940 and within the following year, Wiener[3] saw ten additional instances of intragroup transfusion reactions which could be traced to the presence of the Rh antigen.

NATURE OF THE RH ANTIGENS

The antigen is not a single entity. Following the work of Landsteiner and Wiener it seemed apparent that a simple test for detecting the Rh antigen in human blood lay in the use of anti-Rh serum produced in the guinea pig. Further work, however, revealed at least two difficulties. In the first instance

it is extremely difficult to produce a potent antiserum in animals for testing. It is also now known that all bloods from infants, regardless of whether they are Rh positive or Rh negative, will be acted upon by guinea pig antiserum[4].

It was observed that human serum from Rh negative individuals who had received multiple transfusions of Rh positive blood contained antibodies against the antigen and it was only natural to try this antiserum for testing unknown bloods. Again, however, difficulties were encountered. It was found that the results obtained with such antisera did not coincide with the results observed by Landsteiner and Wiener in their studies on the distribution of the antigen when guinea pig antiserum was used as test material. Three different distribution figures were obtained when human antisera were used[5]. With some human antisera it was found that 87 per cent of the bloods tested were Rh positive, with another antiserum only 70 per cent were positive and with a third antiserum only 80 per cent were positive.

From this evidence it is concluded that the Rh factor is made up of at least three distinct antigens which may occur alone or in combination with one or both of the other antigens in human bloods. These antigens have been named Rh_0, Rh^1, and Rh^{11} and combinations of these give rise to seven types of bloods which are Rh positive, namely Rh_0, Rh^1, Rh^{11}, $Rh^1 Rh^{11}$, Rh_1, Rh_2, and $Rh_1 Rh_2$. The absence of any Rh antigen gives an Rh negative type.

Importance of the various antigens. From the clinical standpoint, only the Rh_0 antigen need be considered. Of all persons having some Rh antigen in the blood, 85.9 per cent will have Rh_0 alone or in combination with Rh^1 or Rh^{11}. Only 1.2 per cent will have either Rh^1 or Rh^{11} in the absence of Rh_0 antigen. By testing for the Rh_0 antigen, therefore, practically all Rh positive individuals will be detected.

Antigenicity of the antigens. Of the three antigens, Rh_0 is apparently most antigenic in the sense that it can stimulate the formation of antibodies when injected. Even with this antigen, multiple transfusions are necessary before a dangerous level of antibodies

*Delivered before the Section on Public Health, Oklahoma State Medical Association Annual Meeting, May 2, 1946.

is reached. It is extremely rare that either Rh[1] or Rh[11] antigen is responsible for transfusion accidents and hence, these two antigens need not be considered in routine clinical studies.

Inheritance of the antigens. The Rh antigens are inherited according to a Mendelian pattern and offspring from Rh positive parents will be Rh positive. Naturally, offspring from Rh negative parents will be Rh negative.

Racial distribution of the antigens varies somewhat as shown by investigators[6][7][8]. As previously remarked, about 85 per cent of the white population tested is Rh positive. Chinese, Japanese, and full blooded American Indians are approximately 99 per cent Rh positive while about 91 per cent of the negroes in this country are Rh positive.

TESTING FOR RH ANTIGENS

The usual test for these antigens consists in a hemagglutination test similar to that used for detecting the A, B, AB, and O groups. The test is not difficult to set up but some skill is needed for correctly interpreting the results.

Testing serum. As in all serologic tests, some starting point must be known. In these tests the individual having no known antiserum with which to start may obtain such commercially. Once tests have been started individuals will be found who, by fortuitous circumstances, have anti-Rh antibodies in the serum. These may be bled for a small amount of blood and their serum used for further tests. It is to be remembered, however, that such antisera should be treated to remove the alpha and beta antibodies of groups A and B; otherwise, unless the individual whose blood is being tested belongs to group O, reactions with the A or B antigen will be encountered. These may be absorbed with A and B corpuscles to remove the alpha and beta agglutinins. By following such procedures any hospital laboratory should be able to maintain sufficient stocks of testing sera.

Corpuscle suspension. Since the Rh antigen occurs in the red corpuscles, suspensions of these are used for testing. A few drops of blood from the ear or finger may be caught in saline and will be sufficient for testing. As a rule, better results will be obtained if the corpuscles are washed with saline and made into a 2 per cent suspension. Fresh blood will give better results than old suspensions.

Test proper. To set up the test, one drop of the corpuscle suspension is mixed with one drop of the testing serum in a small test tube and incubated in a water bath at 37° C. until the corpuscles settle out. This usually requires from 30 to 60 minutes. If a more rapid test is desired the tubes may be lightly centrifuged after a 30 minute incubation

period to facilitate agglutination. If the blood is Rh positive agglutination will be evident. Controls of known Rh positive and known Rh negative corpuscle suspensions must be included in the protocol.

While it is not advisable to attempt tests on the open slide because of erratic results, a recent report has indicated that such tests may be set up if antiserum having an anti-Rh titre of 1:1000 or more is available[9].

When known Rh positive bloods are available, tests may be run on sera for anti-Rh antibodies. This test is set up much the same as the one above except the patient's serum is made up in serial dilutions and tested against the known Rh positive corpuscle suspension for agglutination.

It may be mentioned here that a supplementary test for compatibility of bloods as regards the Rh antigens has been used by Wiener[10]. This is a biological test and is not to be used to supplant the regular test for the Rh antigens. Briefly, it consists in drawing 10 cc of the patient's blood, 5 cc of which is allowed to clot and 5 cc of which is citrated. Fifty cubic centimeters of the prospective donor's blood then is injected intravenously into the patient. After one hour, another 10 cc sample of the patient's blood is drawn and treated as before. The citrated samples are then centrifuged at once and the color of the sera in the two tubes is compared. The clots in the clotted samples are separated and the sera are examined for any change in color. If there is any evidence of hemolysis in any of the tubes, this is evidence of the incompatibility of the donor's and recipient's bloods. If no change occurs, the transfusion may be given carefully, watching for any signs of reaction in the patient.

CLINICAL SIGNIFICANCE

From the clinician's point of view, two conditions in which the Rh antigen is significant present themselves.

Early in the work with the Rh antigen, it was noted that transfusion reactions due to this antigen were seen in two types of cases: 1. Those in which Rh negative patients had received multiple transfusions with Rh positive blood and 2. those in women who showed a reaction on primary transfusion.

Multiple transfusions. This situation may be easily clarified. Since the Rh antigens are antigenic and will cause the formation of anti-Rh antibodies during a series of transfusions, multiple transfusions from an Rh positive donor may lead to the immunization or sensitization of an Rh negative patient so that a subsequent transfusion with Rh positive blood produces severe hemolytic reactions. The occurrence of such type reactions is not high, however. There is an apparent difference in the ease with which Rh negative individuals may be sensitized to these antigens and it is estimated that not more than 2 per cent to 4 per cent of those receiving from 10 to 20 transfusions will be sensitized.

Iso-immunization and erythroblastosis fetalis. The second set of reactions were found to occur in whomen who had recently been pregnant, delivering eighter a normal infant or one who had erythroblastosis fetalis. Further study of these cases lead Levine, Katzin, and Burnham[11] to suggest that this situation is due to iso-immunization of an Rh negative woman carrying an Rh positive fetus. In some as yet unexplained manner, antigen from the fetus goes across the placental barrier to cause the formation of anti-Rh antibodies in the maternal circulation and when the antibody titre becomes high enough, the antibodies pass from the mother to the fetus leading to severe reactions in the fetus or even death. In addition to the possible danger to the infant or fetus, the mother, being sensitized to the Rh antigen, is susceptible to a severe reaction if transfused with Rh positive blood.

In these cases, sensitization of the mother or fetus probably occurs in not more than one in 500 pregnancies. The condition usually does not occur in primiparas, probably because the antibody titre does not reach a dangerous level during a single pregnancy. In multiparas, however, the danger is greater because of the cumulative effect of sensitization instituted during a former pregnancy.

Transfusion in the Rh sensitized individual. In all the conditions described above, whether an Rh negative individual becomes sensitized through multiple transfusions, through carrying an Rh positive fetus, or in the case of the infant, through the transfer of antibodies from the mother, transfusions should be made with Rh negative blood. To do otherwise may result in a severe or even fatal accident. It is well to remember also that Rh antibodies have been shown to be transferred in breast milk[12] and infants exhibiting any signs of erythroblastosis should not be fed mother's milk.

It has been suggested in following the course of a pregnancy, especially in those in which the fetus may be Rh positive and the mother Rh negative, titrations of the maternal serum should be made at intervals. If the titre of anti-Rh antibodies rises higher than 1:10, preparations should be made to have known Rh negative blood available for transfusions if needed. It has further been suggested that if the titre goes above 1:10 at or about the eighth month of pregnancy, labor may be induced to save the infant from severe erythroblastosis fetalis.

Erythroblastosis fetalis due to the Hr antigen. While the conditions described above will account for over 90 per cent of the cases of erythroblastosis fetalis, it may be expedient to interject a few words concerning another cause of this condition.

Levine, Javert, and Katzin[13] called attention to a case which did not follow the usual conditions seen in other cases. They observed a case which occurred in an infant of Rh positive type and whose mother was also of Rh positive type, a situation contrary to that expected. They showed, furthermore, that serum from the mother contained hemagglutinins active against an antigen in all Rh negative bloods and those Rh positive bloods which did not contain the Rh[1] antigen. It was apparent that the case was one involving an antigen distinct from the Rh antigen and due to its peculiar distribution, occurring as it did in all Rh negative bloods, they named the new antigen Hr in contra-distinction to Rh.

Race and his co-workers[14] in England also pointed out the occurrence of this antigen and through their work which was more accurate than that of Levine by virtue of the use of a more potent antiserum, it is now concluded that all individuals including those who are Rh negative are Hr positive except those who are of Rh[1] or Rh₁ type. In view of the rarity of the Rh' type, to all practical intents, only persons who are Rh₁ type are Hr negative.

In cases of erythroblastosis fetalis due to the Hr antigen, the mother must necessarily be of Rh[1] or Rh₁ type, but the fetus may be of any Rh type except Rh₀, Rh₂, or Rh².

Just as in cases of erythroblastosis fetalis due to the Rh antigen, a store of known Hr negative blood should be at hand in the event transfusions are needed. The blood must necessarily be of Rh[1] or Rh₁ Hr negative type.

MEDICO-LEGAL APPLICATIONS

Little need be said concerning the value of blood grouping tests in medico-legal applications. In general, such tests are applicable in cases of disputed parentage, identification, and criminal cases. While excellent results have been obtained through tests for A, B, M, N, and P antigents, the addition of tests for the Rh antigens further enhances the value of such tests.

Cases of disputed parentage. Inasmuch as the Rh antigens are inherited, two general laws can be applied in cases of disputed parentage. These are 1. The antigens Rh₀, Rh[1] or Rh[11] cannot appear in the blood of an infant unless present in the blood of one or both parents and 2. A type Rh₀ or Rh negative parent cannot have a child of Rh₁Rh₂ or Rh[1]Rh² type, neither can a parent of Rh_1Rh_2 or Rh^1Rh^{11} type have a child of Rh_0 or Rh negative type.

Identification tests. On the basis of the heredity of the Rh antigens, an individual will carry a certain blood group antigen pattern through life, thus it would be impossible for him to completely change his identity. While it is not possible to identify an individual on the basis of his blood group antigen pattern, it is possible to exclude others not having the same pattern. Thus, illegal claimants to estates or infants interchanged inadvertently in the hospital may possibly be detected by the application of the blood group tests including the Rh antigen determinations.

Exclusion in criminal cases. The study of blood stains found at the scene of a crime or on the person of the victim will often do much toward excluding certain suspects. If accusations are made and the blood stains can be shown to be of different antigenic make-up from that of the victim and also from that of the accused, there can be no case against the accused.

In all the applications above, however, one must keep in mind that such applications can be used only as exclusion tests and not as positive proof of identity.

SUMMARY

1. About 85 per cent of the bloods of the white population contain an antigen known as the Rh antigen.

2. While this antigen is composed of at least three antigens in combination or alone, only the Rh_0 antigen is of great clinical importance.

3. The Rh antigens are inherited.

4. Blood grouping tests to study the Rh antigen should be done in the following cases:

a. The individual has received multiple transfusions and thus may have become sensitized to the Rh antigen.

b. A woman has borne children or is pregnant and is to receive a blood transfusion.

c. A newborn infant exhibits jaundice or edema. The blood of the mother and father in this case should also be studied in order to exclude or ascertain the possibility of erythroblastosis fetalis.

5. If, in the conditions described above, the individual is found to be Rh negative, only Rh negative blood should be used in transfusions to the individual. This applies as well to the Rh positive infant who is suffering from erythroblastosis fetalis and who requires blood transfusions during the first few weeks of life. Obviously in the latter case, transfusions with his mother's blood is absolutely contraindicated.

6. In cases of early pregnancy or in a woman who is anticipating pregnancy the blood of both the husband and the wife should be examined for the Rh antigen. In the event that the husband is Rh positive and the wife is Rh negative, the possibility of erythroblastosis fetalis must be recognized. The first pregnancy carries little danger to the fetus, but subsequent pregnancies should be closely followed.

7. Periodic examinations for quantative determinations of anti-Rh antibody in the maternal circulation may give some indication for section at about the eight month to protect the infants against erythroblastosis.

8. In the event that Rh testing facilities are not available, remember that a·pregnant woman who is possibly sensitized to the Rh antigen and needs a transfusion should not be transfused with the blood of the husband even if it is of the same blood group. In such a case, if the woman has become sensitized through pregnancy, the husband will be Rh positive in 100 per cent of the cases. In the population as a whole, only 85 per cent are Rh positive and the mother would have one chance in seven of receiving Rh negative blood from anyone else than the husband.

9. In a few cases of erythroblastosis fetalis, the explanation lies in the occurrence of a distinct antigen in all Rh negative individuals and in most Rh positive individuals. This antigen is designated as the Hr antigen.

BIBLIOGRAPHY

1. K. Landsteiner and A. S. Wiener: An Agglutinable Factor in Human Blood Recognized by Immune Serum for Rhesus Blood. Proceedings of the Society for Experimental Biology and Medicine, Volume No. 43, page 223; 1940.

2 A. S. Wiener and H. R. Peters: Hemolytic Reactions Following Transfusion of Blood of the Homologous Group, with Three Cases in Which the Same Agglutinogen Was Responsible. Annals of Internal Medicine, Volume No. 13, page 2306; 1940.

3. A. S. Wiener: Hemolytic Reactions Following Transfusion of Blood of the Homologous Group. II. Further Observations on the Role of Property Rh, Particularly in Cases Without Demonstrable Iso-antibodies. Archives of Pathology, Volume No. 22, page 227; 1941.

4. R. T. Fisk and R. G. Foord: Observations on the Rh Agglutinogen of Human Blood. American Journal of Clinical Pathology, Volume No. 12, page 545; 1942.

5. I. Davidsohn and B. Toharsky: The Rh Factor, An Antigenic Analysis. American Journal of Clinical Pathology, Volume No. 12, page 434; 1942.

6. R. K. Waller and P. Levine: On the Rh and Other Blood Factors in the Japanese. Science, Volume No. 100, page 453; 1944.

7. A. S. Wiener, E. Sonn and C L. Yi: Blood Groups, Subgroups M—N and Rh Types of Chinese. American Journal of Physical Anthropology, Volume No. 2, page 267; 1944.

8. K. Landsteiner, A. S. Wiener and G. Matson: Distribution of the Rh Factor in American Indians Journal of Experimental Medicine, Volume No. 76, page 73; 1942.

9. L. H. Tisdall and D. M. Garland: Large Scale Testing for Rh Negative Blood. Journal of American Medical Association, Volume No. 129, page 1079; 1945.

10. A. S. Wiener, I. J. Silverman and W. Aronson: Hemolytic Transfusion Reactions. II Prevention, With Special Reference to the Use of a New Biological Test. American Journal of Clinical Pathology, Volume No. 12, page 241; 1942.

11. P. Levine, E. M. Katzin and L. Burnham: Iso-immunization in Pregnancy; Its Possible Bearing on the Etiology of Erythroblastosis Fetalis. Journal of the American Medical Association, Volume No. 116, page 825; 1941.

12. E. Witebsky, G. Anderson and Anne Heide: Demonstration of the Rh Antibody in Breast Milk. Proceedings of the

Society for Experimental Biology and Medicine, Volume No. 49, page 179; 1942.
13. P. Levine, L. Burnham, E. M. Katzin and P. Vogel: The Role of Iso-immunization in the Pathogenisis of Erythroblastosis Fetalis. American Journal of Obstetrics and Gynecology, Volume No. 42, page 925; 1941.
14. R. R. Race, G. L. Taylor, D. F. Cappell and M. N. McFarlane: Recognition of a Further Common Rh Genotype in Man. Nature, Volume No. 153, page 52; 1944.

DISCUSSION

CARROLL M. POUNDERS, M.D.

OKLAHOMA CITY, OKLAHOMA

Doctor Marsh has given us a splendid discussion of a subject which is important to us all and about which we know too little. It is important because of the serious consequences which can result from a lack of understanding of the factors involved.

Without attempting to add to what has been said I shall only try to emphasize some of the most important points. As was pointed out the Rh factor is not composed of one single substance but has several components. However, in this discussion we shall speak of it as a single item. It is something that is present in the blood of 85 per cent of our population and absent in that of the other 15 per cent. That should cause us no more concern than the fact that a certain per cent of the people have blue eyes and another per cent have brown eyes were it not for the discovery that this substance possesses antigenic properties. In other words if it happens to get into the blood of an individual who does not normally possess it, the formation of protective antibodies may be stimulated and this antigen antibody reaction may be so violent as to produce harmful or even fatal results.

There are two methods by which this Rh factor may get into the circulation of Rh− individuals in such a way as to cause reactions. First of all it may happen by giving repeated transfusions of Rh+ blood to an Rh− individual. Reactions do not by any means always follow for as Doctor Marsh pointed out, even after as many as 15 or 20 such transfusions, reactions will be seen in only from four to eight per cent of the recipients.

The other instance in which such reactions may arise is when an Rh− woman is pregnant with an Rh+ baby. By some means the Rh factor passes the placental barrier into the mother's blood and stimulates the formation of antibodies. These find their way back into the baby's circulation and by their action against his blood, injure or destroy him. As was pointed out such reactions by no means invariably take place and when they do show up it is not apt to be in the first pregnancy but in subsequent ones.

Now why do such reactions not take place when the first Rh+ blood is transfused into an Rh− individual and often not when any number of such transfusions take place? Likewise, why is the firstborn child pretty sure to escape having erythroblastic anemia while those of later pregnancies may have it? The reason is, of course, that it takes time for the antibodies to be formed and even then the formation of protective antibodies may be such an orderly process that no severe reaction takes place. As a matter of fact, the individual has, since the time he first began to ingest food, and to come into contact with various antigenic substances, had to be manufacturing various protective antibodies. This process generally goes on in such a quiet way that no particular disturbance is caused. But a certain per cent of people do this in an abnormal, sort of way or, speaking more correctly, they overdo the process, so that there comes to be such a violently antagonistic antigen antibody reaction as to cause disturbing symptoms. Such persons may have what we call allergic reactions. If one of these is Rh− and he gets repeated transfusions with Rh+ blood he may show transfusion reactions. Or if the individual be an Rh− woman and she have repeated pregnancies with Rh+ babies, erythroblastic anemia may show up. The 4 to 8 per cent of individuals who show reactions after repeated transfusions might compare fairly closely with the percentage of persons who would show symptoms of hay fever after repeated exposures to massive doses of ragweed pollen.

So where an individual must receive repeated blood transfusions and we make use of this knowledge concerning the Rh factor we may be able to avoid reactions or even deaths. Also, if the Rh factor of both parents is known we may be forewarned and forearmed against erythroblastosis fetalis. This knowledge is more valuable if supplemented by a careful history concerning any past allergic reactions in the persons involved.

Classified Advertisements

FOR RENT: Doctor's three-room office, $40 per month. Office equipment optional. Good location in college town of 3,000. Agriculture. Prospects for oil good. Residence may be purchased. Available November 1. N. E. Ruhl, M.D., 114 West Main Street, Weatherford, Oklahoma.

NEUROLOGICAL HOSPITAL

Twenty-Seventh and The Paseo
Kansas City, Missouri

Modern Hospitalization of Nervous and Mental Illnesses. Alcoholism and Drug Addiction.

THE ROBINSON CLINIC

G. WILSE ROBINSON, M.D.
G. WILSE ROBINSON, Jr., M.D.

X-Ray In Evacuation Hospitals*

EDWARD D. GREENBERGER, M.D.

MCALESTER, OKLAHOMA

I wish to present a brief outline of the organization and operation of the x-ray department in an evacuation hospital in the European Theatre, discuss some of the problems encountered, and cite a few case histories.

My unit was the 109th Evacuation Hospital, attached to the Third Army. We were in continuous operation during General Patton's five big campaigns on the Continent. Over 25,000 patients were admitted to our 400 bed hospital from D-Day to our inactivation in Czechoslovakia; 11,000 patients required x-ray studies. The evacuation hospital was the first hospital in the chain of evacuation from the fluid front lines where x-ray services were available to the soldier and the field medical officers.

The personnel of the x-ray department, as established by the Table of Organization, consisted of one medical officer, three technicians and a clerk. This set-up was inadequate in combat when the x-ray department was required to function continuously. Many of the x-ray departments acquired an additional medical officer and six to ten additional technicians or assistants, employing prisoners of war when available. I was unable to obtain a medical officer, but did acquire two additional enlisted men for our x-ray department. My duty hours were, therefore, determined by the volume of work in the hospital.

The most efficient x-ray team during combat consisted of four men. One technician set the portable x-ray in position and controlled the exposures. The second technician handled the cassettes and positioned the part to be x-rayed. The third technician processed, washed and dried the x-ray films and assisted the medical officers in their wet film readings. The clerk made daily entries, printed the identification slips for each individual film, filed the films of soldiers returned to duty and distributed the films of soldiers being evacuated to their respective wards or to the evacuation officer.

The equipment in the x-ray department consisted of:

(1) Two mobile Picker x-ray units with

*Delivered before the Section on Dermatology and Radiology, Oklahoma State Medical Association Annual Meeting, May 3, 1946.

air cooled tubes. One of the units was used with the Westinghouse portable fluoroscopic table and screen.

(2) Westinghouse 5 gallon developing-fixing film tank with cooling-heating unit and an auxiliary wash tank, all housed in a portable dark room tent 9 x 12 feet.

(3) Two small gasoline generators to activate the x-ray machines and dark room equipment, placed outside the ward tent.

The civilian roentgenologists during the war were handicapped by the lack of sufficient x-ray films and an increased case load. The evacuation hospitals obtained all the x-ray films they required and desired, but we were unable to obtain x-ray accessories. We operated our x-ray department almost through the entire war with six cassettes, two of each standard size, and six corresponding film hangers for the three sizes of film. The exposed films were processed in the small, stuffy, hot, dark room. Wash water for films was delivered to us by our unit 700 gallon water tank every second to fifth day, depending on the source of the available water supply. The auxiliary wash tank in my unit was outside the dark room tent which permitted routine wet film readings. We did not have a regular film dryer, but we improvised drying units, built film racks which were placed near the stove, or we suspended films on wires above the stove and thus dried our films rapidly.

Fluoroscopy for localization of foreign bodies was very seldom employed in the evacuation hospitals of the Third Army. When we functioned as a station hospital, the surgeons occasionally reduced their fractures under fluoroscopic control. In the months before and after the Belgium Bulge, I employed the fluoroscope often on soldiers with peptic ulcer syndrome. The x-ray findings in the majority of these patients were negative, so that these soldiers were able to return promptly to their combat units. If the medical officer in charge of the x-ray department were not competent to do gastro-intestinal work, these soldiers were evacuated to the general hospitals for such diagnostic study and the soldiers were thus lost to their units for several weeks.

Superficial x-ray therapy in evacuation hospitals was discouraged by the army. The primary reason was that many of the officers were not trained in therapy. Second, machines were not calibrated in "r" units. I employed x-ray therapy for acute skin infections and skin lesions only on the personnel in our own organization or attached units. We had many cases of gas gangrene in our evacuation hospital that I would like to have treated with the mobile x-ray unit, but the army surgeons accepted the experimental findings of a group of American doctors who reported that x-ray therapy applied to B. Welchi organism in vitro was not of therapeutic value. They disregarded the mass of clinical evidence, the findings of Dr. Kelley and others, who showed that x-ray is the most valuable agent in the treatment of gas gangrene.

I would like to describe the operation of the x-ray department in an evacuation hospital during the periods of battle activity. The ambulances deposited their wounded at our receiving ward, often as many as two hundred casualties a day. The ward surgeons requisitioned x-ray studies on their first examination of most casualties in order to better determine the treatment and priority for surgery and to make assignments of these patients to the proper surgical teams. The assigned litter bearers therefore continued their trek back and forth from these wards to the x-ray department, until all x-ray requests were filled. During such periods of battle activity, sixty to eighty severely wounded patients, many with multiple injuries, would be x-rayed within a twelve-hour period.

There were several other factors other than the volume of work that made the x-ray technique and film interpretation of battle casualties more difficult than in the Army General or civilian hospitals. The wounded soldier was usually brought into the x-ray department before his blood stained, debris covered uniform was removed. X-ray studies were made with the patient on the sagging litter, through his clothes and the fracture immobilization device. Often the soldier had multiple injuries that prevented proper positioning of the part to be x-rayed. My technicians became very adept in angulating the stretcher and patient and tube in such cases to obtain a satisfactory roentgen study. They also became efficient in deciding the minimum number of x-ray exposures and views that were needed for the proper diagnosis and treatment of the patient in the evacuation hospital.

The following are examples of special technique that we necessarily employed in our evacuation hospital:

(1) Hemo pneumothorax, rupture of hollow viscus, or rupture of diaphragm were often diagnosed from x-ray films taken with patient in lateral decubitus position.

(2) Fractures of mandible, bones of the face and the skull were often made with the patient lying on his back, the tube directed from the side and below the stretcher.

(3) Lateral views of extremities for fractures and missiles, and lateral views of cervical, dorsal and lumbar spines were often necessarily taken with the tube in a horizontal position, rather than move the patient. Elevating the injured limb or arching the spine above the handles or metal parts of the stretchers was often difficult and time consuming.

(4) We resorted to the use of tangental views often to determine whether a missile was in the scalp or within the skull; in the lateral abdominal wall or within the peritoneal cavity; in the lateral chest wall or within the pleural cavity, etc. Stereoscopic equipment was not available in evacuation hospitals.

(5) Neither was Bucky Diaphragm available. Satisfactory diagnostic films were obtained with Lysholm grid.

(6) The unpredictable course of a missile demanded x-ray studies far from the site of entrance. For example, if missile entered shoulder, the dorsal spine or chest was x-rayed. If the missile entered the upper thigh, the abdomen was included in the x-ray studies.

The technique that I employed in our unit was that advocated by Mr. Fuch of Eastman Kodak Company; that is, the optimum voltage technique, the milliampere seconds being the variable. This technique is especially suited for rapid roentgen studies as required in the evacuation hospital. I continue to use this technique often in my practice in McAlester where I am in charge or four different x-ray departments.

The roentgenologist in an evacuation hospital was required to know x-ray technique. A roentgenologist can fool his colleagues in private practice about his x-ray technical ability, but he cannot deceive his army technicians who expect their medical officer to know all about x-ray and therefore consult him freely and often on technique. The medical officer who did not know technique rapidly lost the confidence and respect of his enlisted men, and the control of his department.

CASE HISTORIES

1. X-ray studies of the base of the skull of a twenty year old soldier revealed a 2 x 1 cm. missile projecting into the medial edge of the left jugular foramen. The site of en-

trance of the missile was below the left inferior orbital rim. The soldier experienced pain on flexion of neck, deviation of tongue, syncope in upright position, slow unstable pulse, and a low unstable blood pressure. The neuro surgeon obtained a good exposure of the area by cutting sterno-mastoid muscle, but he could not locate the missile. The x-ray was brought into the operating room. The film showed the guide forceps on atlas instead of base of skull. The missile was found as diagnosed by x-ray. This was the first and only occasion that x-ray was carried into operating room in our hospital.

2. From routine A.P. and Lat. views of the chest of a battle casualty I localized an intact 45 cal. bullet within the right sterno-clavicular joint. I was called to the operating room to justify my diagnosis after the surgeon failed to find the bullet. The bullet had entered high on the left lateral side of neck and its path was traced behind the manubrium. I requested that the surgen re-expose the right sterno-clavicular joint and that he open the capsule of this joint. The bullet was found imbedded within the joint in articulating surface of the clavicle.

3. A 21 year old S/Sgt. entered the hospital with a one cm. wound to the left side of his neck at the level of thyroid cartilage, and another 3 cm. wound to left of spine of second dorsal vertebra. The ward surgeon considered these two wounds due to a penetrating missile. X-ray of chest did not reveal any missile or pneumo hemothorax. Two days later the soldier developed athetoid movements and disorientation and on the fourth day paralysis of lower extremities. He died on the fifth day. The spinal cord injury was not suspected early because the ward surgeon was mislead by the course of the missiles. Post mortem examination revealed a fracture of arches and laminae of left side of second and third dorsal vertebrae with depression of the cord. A niche in the dura and hemorrhage was found at the fracture site, but the cord was intact.

4. A soldier assigned to a tank unit entered the hospital with paralysis below level of second lumbar vertebra. The site of entrance of missile was on right side of upper back. The missile was located by x-ray outside the spinal canal over the first sacral vertebra. X-ray of spine revealed a complete absence of entire right lamina and inferior articular process of third lumbar vertebra. The cord was found crushed at level of twelfth dorsal. Review of films showed that the absence of lamina of the third lumbar was due to developmental anomaly.

5. An irregular 1.5 cm. missile fractured right eighth rib posteriorly, penetrated chest, and was located by x-ray in the left posterior axilla at level of sixth rib. The soldier was observed for two days in clearing hospital because of bilateral paresis of lower extremities which disappeared on admission. X-rays revealed bilateral pneumothorax, both lungs collapsed equally about 50 per cent, small amount of fluid at bases. Fluoroscopy revealed elevation of left diaphragm in inspiration. In expiration the diaphragm and fluid in both sides of chest were at same level. Aspiration of over 2,000 cc of air from right chest produced no change whatever in x-ray picture or patient's condition. The soldier had a perforation in posterior mediastenum. He recovered.

We had a similar case the next day. In this case the missile severed the cord at the level of the twelfth dorsal vertebra.

6. A 20 year old well developed soldier entered the hospital because of an erysipelas-like rash in right shoulder and axilla 24 hour duration. History of mild injury three days prior to admission. A single circular erythematous patch about 3 cm. in diameter was noted on his left arm. His temperature was 104°. He was placed on sulfa therapy. Within twelve hours he developed generalized petechial rash, athetoid movements and became semi-comatose. Some stiffness of neck was now observed. Temperature 105°, blood pressure 60/40. Patient died within 24 hours. Post morem revealed petechial hemorrhages in all organs of body and body cavities. The generalized petechial hemorrhage in adrenals explained the rapid fall in blood pressure and shock.

The designated name for this type of meningococcemia is Waterhouse-Friedrich syndrome.

CONCLUSIONS

I have recorded in my personal files, a few hundred case histories of unusual injuries and clinical findings resulting from missiles. It is difficult to convey to you the medical-surgical interest in these cases, or the emotional reaction that I experienced by contact with these battle casualties who came to our hospital within a few hours after they received their injuries. In this dramatic setting, x-ray work in a field hospital was always interesting, and the results of our efforts were most gratifying.

Joy is more divine than sorrow; for joy is bread and sorrow is medicine.—*Henry Ward Beecher.*

Silence is the perfectest herald of joy: I were but little happy if I could say how much.—*Shakespeare.*

Nothing is so envied as genius, nothing so hopeless of attainment by labor alone. Though labor always accompanies the greatest genius, without the intellectual gift, labor alone will do little.—*B. R. Haydon.*

Clinical Pathological Conference

University of Oklahoma School of Medicine

Presented by the Departments of Pathology and Medicine

ROBERT H. BAYLEY, M.D.—BELA HALPERT, M.D.

OKLAHOMA CITY, OKLAHOMA

DR. HALPERT: The patient whose story we are presenting today gave opportunity for very thorough clinical study. Because of this, clinicopathologic correlation should be of more than usual interest. Dr. Bayley will present the clinical aspects of this case.

PROTOCOL

Patient: O. B. D., white female, age 40; admitted August 6, 1945, died November 2, 1945.

Chief Complaints: Weakness, loss of weight, and fever.

Present Illness: The patient was well until September, 1944, when, following the removal of several teeth, she developed weakness and pain in the joints of her arms and legs. The joint pain was severe; however, she noticed no redness, swelling, or increased heat. One month later she noted that she was having a continuous low-grade fever. She went to the Duncan Hospital at this time and has been bedfast since. During hospitalization she heard her doctors remark that her heart "was bad". The weakness, low-grade fever, and lassitude have continued to the present time. She lost about thirty pounds of weight. There has been dyspnea and precordial aching with some palpitation. There is no history of cough, expectoration, hemoptysis or pleurisy. The remainder of the history is noncontributory.

Past and Family History: Noncontributory except for the usual childhood diseases and one miscarriage.

Physical Examination: The patient was emaciated and had many carious teeth. Cooperation was poor. The skin was very loose and dry and presented a very light brown pigmentation. The pupils were equal in size, reacted to light and accommodation. There were a few small petechial hemorrhages in the conjunctiva. The fundi were negative. There was slight cheilosis. Mucous membranes exhibited moderate pallor. There was no lymphadenopathy. The lung fields were clear. The cardiac apex impulse was approximately 8 cm. to the left of the midline and of increased forcefulness. A rather loud apical systolic murmur was heard. Blood pressure was 115/65 and pulse rate 100. The liver was not palpable. The spleen extended two finger breadths below the costal margin on deep inspiration; its edge was firm, its surface smooth and non-tender. There was no edema of the feet or ankles. Fingers exhibited moderate clubbing. Examination of genitalia revealed a cervical and vaginal discharge, also a purulent urethral discharge. A cystocele and rectocele were present.

Laboratory Data: During her two months hospitalization, urinary specific gravity varied from 1.008 to 1,014, proteinuria from 0 (once 3 plus). No red blood cells were found. The red blood count ranged from 2.2 to 3.7 million; hb. varied from 5 to 9 grams. Leukocytosis was usually present, averaging 16,000 with 82 per cent polys. Spinal fluid was negative. Three Mazzini tests were: 3 plus, 2 plus, and negative. Two Kolmer reactions were negative. Cervical and urethral smears revealed intracellular Gram negative diplococci on four occasions. On two additional occasions mixed flora were found. On one occasion a culture of gonococci was negative. Two blood cultures were negative. An electrocardiogram was reported as negative. A requested sound tracing was not done because the apparatus was not available. It was stated, however, that there was a 3 plus accentuation of the mitral first sound, followed by 3 plus systolic murmur, and preceded by a diastolic rumble. An aortic diastolic murmur was also present along the left border of the sternum at the third and fourth I.C.S. There was no evidence of free aortic insufficiency, rheumatic. On the eighth hospital day, penicillin was given, 50,000 units every three hours for three doses, then 25,000 units every three hours for five doses. Sulfathiazole, which had been started two days before the penicillin, was discontinued on the 20th

LIBRARY OF THE
COLLEGE OF PHYSICIANS

day. A psychiatric consultant stated that no psychopathic condition was present, but that the negativistic reaction was probably a part of her gradually developed personality since childhood. On the 3rd hospital day penicillin was given again, 25,000 units every three hours for 72 hours. On the 57th hospital day an arterial blood culture showed growth of a nonhemolytic staph aureus in both tubes. X-ray taken on August 8, 1945, showed heart and lungs normal except for quite a prominent pulmonary conus. A second x-ray, taken on September 26, 1945, suggested cardiac enlargement and pulmonary congestion.

Clinical Course: Low grade fever continued with septic spikes, occasionally up to 103 degrees. She was often uncooperative and refused medication on several occasions. Sulfathiazole was started August 12, 1945. On August 14, 1945, penicillin was given which was repeated at intervals through the course of the disease. On November 2, 1945, the patient complained of severe abdominal pain. Examination showed marked abdominal distention, rigidity and absence of borborygmus. A Wangensteen tube was ordered. There was blood in the stools and she vomited blood once. She died on November 2, 1945.

CLINICAL DIAGNOSIS

DR. BAYLEY: Our case today is that of a white female, aged 40, who was admitted to and died on the Medical Service. Her chief complaints of weakness, loss of weight and fever immediately suggested some infectious process. Tuberculosis would be a distinct possibility in view of the general appearance which the patient presented and the rather insidious onset of symptoms. The onset of her present illness was characterized by joint pains and this was soon accompanied by low grade fever. Such an onset suggests undulant fever, rheumatic fever, or perhaps rheumatoid arthritis. She is a little advanced in age for this latter, but we do sometimes see rheumatoid arthritis beginning at this age. During her initial hospitalization she overheard her doctor remark that she had a bad heart. It is difficult to interpret such a statement from the patient. Knowledge of the exact status of things at this point would be very helpful. This does further our consideration of rheumatic fever, however. We know that patients with subacute bacterial endocarditis have insidious onset, loss of weight, fever and joint pains, so that we must include this in our differential diagnosis. The fact that her joints were not swollen or reddened would be evidence for bacterial endocarditis, rather than active rheumatic fever. There is also a history of some precordial pain. This is difficult to evaluate but would be compatible with either condition. There is no history of hemoptysis. The patient's past history does not contribute much of value.

Before we review the physical examination it might be interesting to anticipate some of the possible findings. Since we have considered tuberculosis, we should expect to examine the lungs thoroughly — similarly with the heart since we are considering rheumatic fever also. As a rule, cardiac murmurs which appear during the course of active rheumatic fever disappear by the end of the acute attack. It may be six months later before "residual murmurs" develop. We should carefully examine the joints for redness, etc., because this would definitely point toward rheumatoid arthritis. If this were rheumatoid arthritis, we should find little change in the heart. Splenomegaly does not accompany rheumatic fever, but occasionally does characterize rheumatoid arthritis (Felty's syndrome). The patient had moderate anemia. This is often seen in rheumatic fever and is an invariable accompaniment of subacute bacterial endocarditis. The loose dry skin may be interpreted as a manifestation of dehydration. The diffuse, light brownish pigmentation would fit in with subacute bacterial endocarditis. Conjunctival hemorrhages (petechial), such as were recorded here, should be carefully inspected because often examination may reveal a white center. Such lesions may be found in the occular fundi when they appear nowhere else. These, of course, would represent tiny septic infarcts and would be pathognomonic of subacute bacterial endocarditis. Now to consider the heart —this was not appreciably enlarged although pulsations were of increased forcefulness. As a rule, in subacute bacterial endocarditis, the heart shows little enlargement. It is an interesting point that those patients who have repeated attacks of rheumatic fever (and cardiac enlargement) are the very group who do not develop bacterial endocarditis. Dr. Levine has pointed out that the onset of subacute bacterial endocarditis after the last attack of rheumatic fever is, on the average, about 17 years. Subacute bacterial endocarditis has been noted to occur, however, during an attack of rheumatic fever. Here we are up against the problem of differentiating between rheumatic fever and subacute bacterial endocarditis. We know that in both cases there are joint pains and fever. Those patients having rheumatic fever usually have striking cardiac enlargement; with subacute bacterial endocarditis there is no such enlargement. In rheumatic fever, splenomegaly is not characteristic. The splenomegaly which this patient exhibited is typical of subacute bacterial endocarditis. Here in examination of the heart there was a diastolic and presystolic murmur. The apical systolic murmur may have been hemic in origin. The blood pressure was 115/65 and the pulse rate 100.

All of these findings point toward bacterial endocarditis. We have also the history that just before onset of this present illness the patient had several teeth removed. Not infrequently the extraction of infected teeth causes a bacteremia which, in turn, leads to subacute bacterial endocarditis. I saw this patient clinically; the diagnosis of subacute bacterial endocarditis was entertained throughout her hospital course.

Regarding the laboratory findings, the leukocytosis observed is quite compatible with bacterial endocarditis.

I believe that the positive Mazinni tests were not significant because of the septic state. Subacute bacterial endocarditis is rarely superimposed upon a luetic lesion, but this can occur. The vaginal and urethral discharge, with demonstrable gram negative intracellular diplococci should make the diagnosis of gonorrhea — this infection I believe was incidental. Gonococcal endocarditis does rarely occur, but usually involves the pulmonic valves. All evidence here points to involvement of the left heart. Venous blood cultures were negative upon two occasions. In most instances subacute bacterial endocarditis is limited to the left side of the heart. Because of this, bacterial emboli are filtered out in large measure before ever reaching the venous system. Often in these patients venous blood cultures will be negative whereas arterial blood cultures, taken at the same time, may be positive. In this case a culture of arterial blood was positive for nonhemolytic Staph. aureus. This is a very unusual organism to cause subacute bacterial endocarditis. The same organism was recovered in two culture tubes which would be strong evidence that this was not a laboratory contamination. It is possible, however, that the blood was contaminated at the time it was drawn. At any rate this lends much additional support to our diagnosis. To consider the precise character of this lesion in the heart we must consider again the physical findings. From the type of cardiac murmurs heard it was my opinion that this patient had vegetative lesions of both the mitral and aortic valves. On the basis of this diagnosis, one expects a wide variety of embolic phenomena. It may have been on the basis of tiny cerebral embolic lesions that psychic disturbances were manifest.

Regarding treatment it must be said that in the light of recent clinical studies the amount of penicillin which this patient received was certainly very small in comparison with the relatively enormous doses necessary to effectively treat this condition.

CLINICAL DISCUSSION

QUESTION: Do you think that, from the clinical evidence, the rheumatic process was active at the time of death?

DR. BAYLEY: That is possible, but it is unusual in subacute bacterial endocarditis and there is no clinical basis for a diagnosis of active rheumatic fever.

QUESTION: Could some anomaly, such as a bicuspid aortic valve, rather than a rheumatic lesion, have been the underlying basis for this bacterial endocarditis?

DR. BAYLEY: I doubt it. In the first place, rheumatic fever is much the more common predisposing factor and secondly, we have evidence that suggests involvement of the mitral valve in addition to the aortic valve.

DR. HALPERT: Perhaps we should review the x-ray studies on this patient.

DR. SHRYOCK: These roentgenograms show no cardiac enlargement although there is a marked fullness and prominence of the pulmonary conus. There is also increased hilar vascular markings in the lungs.

DR. BAYLEY: Would these findings be compatible with bronchopneumonia?

DR. SHRYOCK: I can see no definite evidence of cellular infiltration.

QUESTION: Is the pulmonary osteo-arthropathy related to rheumatic fever?

DR. BAYLEY: No, rheumatic fever does not cause clubbing of the fingers. Subatcute bacterial endocarditis, on the other hand, frequently leads to this.

ANATOMIC DIAGNOSIS

DR. HALPERT: At necropsy this woman showed evidence of marked emaciation; she was 61 inches tall and weighed less than 100 pounds. The skin presented purple blotches which faded on pressure. No petechiae were noted. The abdomen was moderately distended and there was approximately 400 cc. of bloody fluid in the peritoneal cavity. A layer of fibrinopurulent exudate covered the surface of the liver. The mesenteric vessels were firm and an embolus occluded the superior mesenteric artery for a length of 4 cm. There was an aneurysm of the inferior mesenteric artery a few cm. from its origin. The sudden occlusion of the superior mesenteric artery had resulted in infarction of a large segment of ileum. This portion of bowel was distended with gas, discolored reddish brown and covered with fibrinopurulent exudate. No definite point of perforation was observed. There is little question but that the peritonitis resulted from passage of bacteria through the wall of this markedly altered ileum. Both pleural cavities contained serous fluid, the left approximately 100 cc., the right, 800 cc. The heart was slightly enlarged, the result of dilation. It measured 12 cm. from base to apex and 12 cm. across the base; it weighed

325 Gm. The mitral and aortic valve cusps exhibited nodular areas of fibrous tissue at the line of closure and there was moderate thickening of the valves themselves. Friable granular vegetations were present on both the mitral and aortic valves. The myocardium was light tan and flabby, particularly on the right side. The lungs were moderately increased in weight and there was an area of lumpy consolidation in the right upper lobe with some hemorrhage. The spleen, although palpable during life and estimated to be quite large, weighed only 220 Gm. The liver was somewhat decreased in size and weighed 1100 Gm. The kidneys weighed 100 Gm. each. No areas of interstitial hemorrhage were discernible. Minute foci of hemorrhage were apparent on microscopic examination however, and the picture was actually that of embolic glomerulonephritis. Cultures from the valvular vegetations were not taken at necropsy. In the spleen there were numerous scars which were quite characteristic of old infarcts. There were no recent infarcts.

DISCUSSION

QUESTION: What was the extent of the gonorrheal infection?

DR. HALPERT: This was limited to the cervix and was minimal at time of death. It is probable that the penicillin therapy had resulted in an almost complete cure.

QUESTION: What caused the splenomegaly which was so evident clinically?

DR. HALPERT: This is readily accounted for on the basis of septicemia. Occasionally in cases of this sort the spleen becomes smaller in the terminal stages.

DR. BAYLEY: In people with subacute bacterial endocarditis the temperature goes down and the spleen reduces during treatment, but when therapy is discontinued or becomes ineffective, the spleen enlarges again.

DR. HOPPS: At the University of Chicago we were quite impressed by the rather high percentage of persons with subacute bacterial endocarditis whose onset of illness followed tooth extraction. Just recently, experimental studies carried out by the Zollar Dental Clinic demonstrated that transient bacteremia occurs in almost 100 per cent of patients following the extraction of a tooth. Particularly, in patients with a history of previous rheumatic fever, I believe that sufficient sulfonamides should be given to maintain a rather high blood level during the actual time of tooth extraction and for a period of twelve to twenty-four hours afterwards.

DR. BAYLEY: I agree with Dr. Hopps except that I believe penicillin would be the drug of choice. This would necessitate, however, an intramuscular injection.

Announcing The Sixteenth Annual Conference of The
OKLAHOMA CITY CLINICAL SOCIETY

OCTOBER 28, 29, 30, 31, 1946

DISTINGUISHED GUEST LECTURERS

Harrison H. Shoulders, M. D., PRESIDENT, THE AMERICAN MEDICAL ASSOCIATION, Nashville, Tennessee.

Charles L. Brown, M.D., MEDICINE, Dean and Professor of Medicine, Hahnemann Medical College, Philadelphia, Pennsylvania.

Samuel A. Cosgrove, M.D., OBSTETRICS, Clinical Professor of Obstetrics, Faculty of Medicine, Columbia University; Medical Director and Superintendent and Chief of the Staff, Margaret Hague Maternity Hospital, Jersey City, New Jersey.

Claude F. Dixon, M.D., SURGERY, Professor of Surgery, Mayo Foundation, Postgraduate School, University of Minnesota., Rochester, Minnesota.

Austin I. Dodson, M.D., UROLOGY, Professor of Urology; Urologist to Hospital Division, Medical College of Virginia, Richmond, Virginia.

Philip S. Hench, M.D., MEDICINE, Consultant and Head of a Section on Medicine; Chief of the Department for Rheumatic Diseases; Associate Professor of Medicine, Mayo Foundation, Postgraduate School, University of Minnesota, Rochester, Minnesota.

Walde E. Nelson, M.D. PEDIATRICS, Professor of Pediatrics, Chief of the Pediatric Department, Temple University School of Medicine, Philadelphia, Pennsylvania.

Paul Padget, M.D., MEDICINE, Assistant Professor of Medicine, Johns Hopkins University School of Medicine; Veterans Administration, Fort Howard, Maryland.

Walter L. Palmer, M.D., MEDICINE, Professor of Medicine, Department of Medicine, University of Chicago, Chicago, Illinois.

Rowley N. Panick, Jr., M.D., SURGERY, Associate Professor of Clinical Surgery, Tulane University School of Medicine, New Orleans, Louisiana.

Leo G. Rigler, M.D., RADIOLOGY, Professor and Chief of the Department of Radiology and Physical Therapy, University of Minnesota School of Medicine, Minneapolis, Minnesota.

Richard H. Sweet, M.D., SURGERY, Instructor in Surgery, Harvard Medical School, Boston, Massachusetts.

Richard W. Te Linde, M.D. GYNECOLOGY, Professor of Gynecology; Chief Gynecologist, Johns Hopkins University School of Medicine, Baltimore, Maryland.

James E. M. Thomson, M.D., ORTHOPAEDIC SURGERY, Lecturer in Plastic Surgery to the College of Dentistry, University of Nebraska; President American Academy of Orthopaedic Surgeons, Lincoln, Nebraska.

O. E. Van Alyea, M.D., OTOLARYNGOLOGY, Clinical Associate, University of Illinois, College of Medicine, Chicago, Illinois.

Shields Warren, M.D., PATHOLOGY, Assistant Professor of Pathology, Harvard Medical School, Boston, Massachusets.

Alan C. Woods, Sr., M.D., OPHTHALMOLOGY, Professor of Ophthalmology; Ophthalmologist-in-chief, Johns Hopkins University School of Medicine, Baltimore, Maryland.

GENERAL ASSEMBLIES	ROUND-TABLE LUNCHEONS	DINNER MEETINGS
POSTGRADUATE COURSES	SMOKER	COMMERCIAL EXHIBITS

Registration fee of $10.00 includes ALL the above features.

For further information, address EXECUTIVE SECRETARY, 512 Medical Arts Building, Oklahoma City, Oklahoma

Special Article

DEAN GRAY

On September 1, Dr. Jacques P. Gray entered upon his duties as Dean of the Medical School. He succeeded Dr. Wann Langston who has served in the capacity of Acting Dean from the time of Dr. Tom Lowry's death.

Dr. Gray is eminently fitted for this position.* Through both education and experience he has become a seasoned administrator. He comes to us with a splendid reputation, academic and administrative, in medical education and public health.

In the last analysis the medical school is the property of the people, the taxpayers. The law says there are two kinds of property, real and personal. To the doctor this ownership should be genuinely personal. While this applies particularly to the Alumni, every doctor in the state should manifest a real interest in the medical school and should

*Dean Appointed, Journal of the Oklahoma State Medical Association, page 376, September, 1946.

exact a certain amount of interest and consideration from the medical school. Working together, the Dean, the faculty and the doctors of the state should see that medicine in Oklahoma comes into its own and that it gives to the medical profession and the people all that the taxpayers have a right to expect, plus a gratuitous bounty in keeping with traditions of medicine.

With the above in view it may be said that every doctor in the state should stand four square behind the Dean. With the present enthusiasm of the Alumni and the growing interest of the public in medical research, Dean Gray comes at a propitious time. The medical school is part of a great university; it does not belong to Oklahoma City. Every doctor in the State should become vitally interested in medical education and scientific research and make his individual contribution by helping the Dean hold the torch high.

THE PRESIDENT'S PAGE

PROFESSIONAL COURTESY

Recently my attention was called to an experience a physician had with a large Clinic. He wrote for an appointment for himself and wife, so that they might have a check up, designating a date twelve days from the date of his letter. In reply he was told he could have an appointment three months from the date the reply was written, unless it was an emergency.

This particular physician was well known to them as he had sent many patients to the Clinic and had himself been a patient. They showed lack of professional courtesy in his case when they did not take into account the fact that he also was a physician.

Then there is the case of the physician who will accept a patient, who is under treatment by another physician, when the patient has not been dismissed by the physician or paid for his services.

It sometimes happens that after a physician is called in Consultation he will accept the patient for treatment without the original physician's knowledge or consent.

All of these constitute lack of professional courtesy and should not be practiced at any time.

L. C. Kuykendall

President.

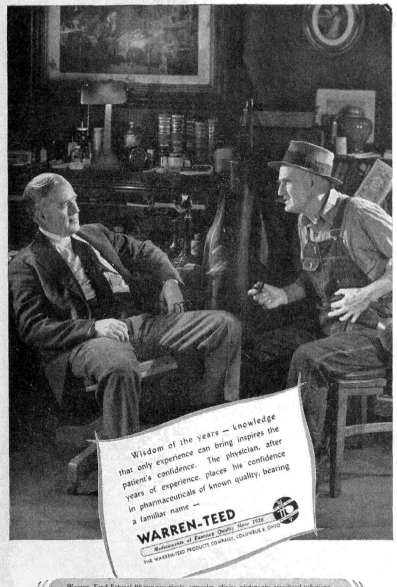

Wisdom of the years — knowledge that only experience can bring inspires the patient's confidence. The physician, after years of experience, places his confidence in pharmaceuticals of known quality, bearing a familiar name —

WARREN-TEED

Medicaments of Exacting Quality Since 1920

THE WARREN-TEED PRODUCTS COMPANY, COLUMBUS 8, OHIO

Warren-Teed Ethical Pharmaceuticals: capsules, elixirs, ointments, sterilized solutions, syrups, tablets. Write for literature.

The JOURNAL Of The
OKLAHOMA STATE MEDICAL ASSOCIATION

EDITORIAL BOARD

L. J. MOORMAN, Oklahoma City, Editor-in-Chief

E. EUGENE RICE, Shawnee   BEN H. NICHOLSON, Oklahoma City

MR. DICK GRAHAM, Oklahoma City, Business Manager

MR. CLAYTON FONDREN, Oklahoma City, Assistant Business Manager

CONTRIBUTIONS: Articles accepted by this Journal for publication including those read at the annual meetings of the State Association are the sole property of this Journal.

The Editorial Department is not responsible for the opinions expressed in the original articles of contributors.

Manuscripts may be withdrawn by authors for publication elsewhere only upon the approval of the Editorial Board.

MANUSCRIPTS: Manuscripts should be typewritten, double-spaced, on white paper 8½ x 11 inches. The original copy, not the carbon copy, should be submitted.

Footnotes, bibliographies and legends for cuts should be typed on separate sheets in double space. Bibliography listing should follow this order: Name of author, title of article, name of periodical with volume, page and date of publication.

Manuscripts are accepted subject to the usual editorial revisions and with the understanding that they have not been published elsewhere.

NEWS: Local news of interest to the medical profession, changes of address, births, deaths and weddings will be gratefully received.

ADVERTISING: Advertising of articles, drugs or compounds unapproved by the Council on Pharmacy of the A.M.A. will not be accepted. Advertising rates will be supplied on application.

It is suggested that members of the State Association patronize our advertisers in preference to others.

SUBSCRIPTIONS: Failure to receive The Journal should call for immediate notification.

REPRINTS: Reprints of original articles will be supplied at actual cost provided request for them is attached to manuscripts or made in sufficient time before publication. Checks for reprints should be made payable to Industrial Printing Company, Oklahoma City.

Address all communications to THE JOURNAL OF THE OKLAHOMA STATE MEDICAL ASSOCIATION, 210 Plaza Court, Oklahoma City 3

OFFICIAL PUBLICATION OF THE OKLAHOMA STATE MEDICAL ASSOCIATION
Copyrighted October, 1946

EDITORIALS

THE FALL CLINICAL CONFERENCE

The Oklahoma City Clinical Society has consummated plans for its great Clinical Conference on October 28, 29, 30, 31.

The first announcement was in the September issue of the Journal, but this late appeal is intended for those who have not "red-lettered" the dates. No honest, ambitious practitioner can afford to miss this opportunity for post-graduate study. Never in the History of Medicine has the need of such refresher studies been so urgent.

Henry Christian has said, "There were two great groups of physicians; those who are learning and those who are forgetting." Will you be there or will you be forgetting?

RESOLUTION ADOPTED BY A.M.A.

At the American Medical Association meeting in San Francisco, July, 1946, the House of Delegates passed the following resolution:

RESOLUTION ON STATEWIDE MENTAL HYGIENE AND MENTAL DISEASE PROGRAM*

"Dr. G. A. Woodhouse, Ohio, presented the following resolution, which was referred to

.... *Proceedings of House of Delegates, American Medical Association, San Francisco, July, 1946.

the Reference Committee on Medical Education.

"WHEREAS, there is an urgent need in most of the states for well organized and adequately financed mental hygiene programs, for research activities in the field of mental disease and for improved institutional care of the mentally ill; and

"WHEREAS, the medical profession should give increased leadership and support to such activities; therefore be it

"RESOLVED, that each state medical association be requested to take the lead in the development of an adequate statewide mental hygiene and mental disease program and to cooperate with other groups in stimulating public support in order that sufficient funds may be secured for the proper operation and maintenance of such activities."

This resolution should have careful consideration by every doctor in Oklahoma. No doctor can escape the responsibility of dealing with the mentally inadequate and the psychologically disturbed. Every patient who seeks medical advice presents a mental threshold which the doctor must measure and beyond which he must go with analytical perception and precision.

Considering the rapid increase in mental diseases and the recent agitation concerning the short comings of institutional management throughout the United States doctors should initiate and actively support a well balanced program for research in mental hygiene and improved institutional care of the mentally ill.

RESEARCH

Soon our boys will go out to raise funds for the University of Oklahoma Research Foundation. When they do we must shell out. The spirit of scientific investigation is more than 2000 years old. We do not need more time to think it over. We must set the example and through our interest and generosity we should not only reach down in our jeans but jar loose some of the wealth of Oklahoma.

After 20 centuries Oklahoma has a chance to come into her own. This is no time for doctors to hesitate. The eyes of the world are upon us. If giving means a sacrifice, it should be remembered that the money will be used to purchase sacrificial service for the purpose of controlling disease and saving life. Who ever knew a bonafide scientific in-vestigator in the field of medicine who was not underpaid.

This is our chance to tie up the general practitioner with the worker in pure science through the medical school teachers as middle men. Only in this way can the medical profession and the medical school keep faith with the people.

Would that this editorial had the fire and thunder from Sinai or at least the persuasive power of the Sermon on the Mount. Even though the stimulus is wanting, let's give.

PUBLIC HEALTH IN OKLAHOMA

Public health in Oklahoma is now 56 years old and has made great strides during the past year. From its humble beginning, as provided by the first territorial legislature in December of 1890, the State Department of Health has grown to assume a protective in-fluence for all citizens of the state.

During the early territorial days, the Superintendent of Public Instruction served as ex-officio president of the Board of Health and was assisted by two staff members, a vice-president who served without pay and a Superintendent of Public Health who received $500 annually for recording the work and acts of the health department.

At this time, the Board of Health was authorized to make and enforce needful rules and regulations for the prevention and cure of disease. In this connection, licenses were issued permitting doctors to practice medicine in the territory.

In early statehood, the Oklahoma State Department of Health was impowered to establish quarantines, to remove the carcasses of dead animals, to condemn and remove any impure or diseased articles of food offered for sale, and to prevent the spread of any contagious, infectious or malarial disease among persons or domestic animals.

The influence of public health has grown. To understand how much it has grown we need only compare the appropriation of $33,600 which was granted public health officials in 1910 to the last appropriation of $549,752 which was granted for the fiscal year ending June 30, 1947. Even this increased appropriation is not sufficient to undertake all authority delegated to the State Department of Health by the twentieth session of the Oklahoma State Legislature.

During the past few years many acts pertaining to public health have been adopted as a culmination and recognition of over 50 years of work by officials of the State Department of Health.

Recent legislation required an examination for syphilis prior to the issuance of a marriage license. Another act created the Board of Health, which is impowered to appoint a Commissioner of Health.

Frozen food lockers are now subject to inspection and regulation, as are all bedding manufacturers in the state. Serological blood tests for syphilis of pregnant women is now a state requirement; and on July 1, the State Department of Health undertook to inspect and license all hospitals and related institutions now operating in the state.

The legislature appropriated $231,000 for the fiscal year ending June 30, 1947, to be used in financing county health departments; and the State Department of Health was authorized to accept grants of money, personnel and property from federal agencies to promote and carry on in Oklahoma a program of public health, maternity and infancy care, venereal disease control, tuberculosis control, malaria control, industrial hygiene and sanitation, urban and rural sanitation and other phases of a general public health program.

Senate Bill 153 provided authority for school districts, boards of education, cities and towns to furnish funds to assist in the operation of local health departments. For the first time in the history of the state money was appropriated for the State Department of Health Tuberculosis Control and Industrial Hygiene Divisions. Tuberculosis Control received $10,000 annually and $5,000 was appropriated for Industrial Hygiene. In addition, Venereal Disease Control was allotted $20,000 for each fiscal year, or an increase of $10,000 annually.

The people of Oklahoma should take notice of the fact that the legislators have recognized the importance of promoting better health and constructed legislation to that end. Much credit for the enactment of these laws belongs to Governor Kerr, who outlined the public health needs in his message to the legislature.

Our thanks should also go to the capable public health workers who have overcome seemingly insurmountable obstacles to render good and efficient service, and to the House of Delegates of the American Medical Association and the Oklahoma State Medical Association for their resolutions endorsing and advocating the establishment of full time local health departments to serve every area and unit of population.—Grady F. Mathews, M.D.

THIS TOTTERING WORLD

Atlas was having a difficult time holding the world aloft until Socrates taught the world to look to reason for stabilization and medicine under the stimulus of Hippocrates, and Socrates initiated the age of enlightenment and helped to bring individual freedom in thought and action.

Under Greek influence, medicine for the first time was free and democratic. With the exception of the mad, and the morons, people learned to keep their heads, their own little worlds, squarely on their shoulders. This individual balance helped to secure collective equilibrium, thus enabling Atlas to hold the world in its appointed place.

The coming of Socialism and Communism in this modern era has robbed Atlas of the steadying influence which came through individual balance and we feel the world swaying on the Titons tired shoulders. With North America looking upon socialistic trends as the way to redemption and the bureaucrats standing ready to rob Atlas of his main stabilizing force — medicine as a free enterprise — we may expect the crash unless we "Wake up America".

If Atlas, created for the task, is having a hard time with the wobbly cockeyed world, how can Mr. Altmier, the Surgeon General of the Public Health Service and their bureaucratic cohorts hope to cope with it after knocking the last prop out.

In the eyes of the thinking citizens of the United States, they are either too busy to look the proposed adventure squarely in the face or they are the world's prize egoists. Perhaps some of the cortex they are counting on may prove to be cheap cork. Shall we be damned by their exaltation or shall we act upon the knowledge at hand and put them in their places.

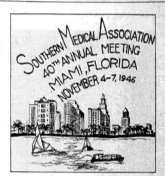

SCIENCE AT THE NATION'S PLAY-GROUND — a top scientific medical meeting amid delightful tropical surroundings with every known recreational facility available — Southern Medical Association, Miami, November 4-7. The Southern Medical Association meetings always have been and always will be the ESSENTIAL medical meetings IN and FOR the South. In its twenty-one scientific sections, the four general clinical sessions, the general public session, the four conjoint meetings and the scientific and technical exhibits, in a streamlined program, one will get the last word in modern, practical, scientific medicine and surgery. And after Miami, Havana and/or Nassau.

REGARDLESS of what any physician may be interested in, regardless of how general or how limited his interest, there will be at Miami a scientific program and recreational facilities to challenge his every interest and make it worth-while for him to attend.

ALL MEMBERS of State and County medical societies in the South are cordially invited to attend. And all members of state and county medical societies in the South should be and can be members of the Southern Medical Association. The annual dues of $4.00 include the Southern Medical Journal, a journal valuable to physicians of the South, one that each should have on his reading table.

SOUTHERN MEDICAL ASSOCIATION
Empire Building
BIRMINGHAM 3, ALABAMA

RESEARCH FOR HUMANITY

John H. Lamb, M.D.

The Oklahoma Medical Research Foundation was formally incorporated on August 3, 1946, at a dinner held at the Skirvin Hotel. Mr. George Lundy of the firm of Marts and Lundy was a guest at this meeting, at which time he outlined plans for a campaign to begin early in October composed primarily of publicity the first two or three months, followed by an intensive financial drive in January or February.

The initiating group was selected by the trustees of the Alumni Association and is made up of twenty directors and twenty laymen. The physician directors were selected from three groups, the State Medical Association, the Alumni Association, and three representatives from the Faculty of the School of Medicine.

It has been an earnest desire on the part of those who established the Foundation to spread their influence over the entire State. Those who were placed on the initiating Board were those who have shown interest in the past several years. By-Laws of the Foundation state that there will be a yearly election, at which time those who have becomes members of the Foundation in the various groups by their contributions will have a vote to elect their respective directors on the Board. It is planned to make the Foundation a state-wide democratic organization so that the entire State will have an interest in Medical Research and the School of Medicine.

This organization has great potentialities, not only to interest the public in endowments for the School of Medicine, but by bringing expert Research Personnel to Oklahoma Medicine, thus medical educaton will be advanced one hundred fold.

It is felt that the motto "Better medical education today means better health tomorrow" would be an excellent theme for the campaign. At the incorporation meeting August 3 the following were elected as Directors of the Foundation:

LAYMEN: Henry S. Griffing, L. C. Griffith, C. R. Anthony, Edgar C. Van Cleef, W. R. Wallace, D. A. Harmon, Roy C. Lytle, Moss Patterson, C. A. Vose, Ancel Earp, Fred Jones, and Robert S. Kerr, of Oklahoma City; Fred L. Dunn, Ralph Talbot, Charles L. Follansbee, of Tulsa; H. B. Alspaugh, Duncan; J. Frank Buck, Shawnee; Doan Farr, Clinton; Clyde Muchmore, Ponca City; and W. Lee Woodward of Alva.

ALUMNI: W. Floyd Keller, M.D., and John H. Lamb, M.D., Oklahoma City; Ralph McGill, M.D., and Fred E. Woodson, M.D., Tulsa; William Finch, M.D., Hobart; John Carson, M.D., Shawnee.

OKLAHOMA STATE MEDICAL ASSOCIATION: Henry C. Weber, M.D., Bartlesville; O. C. Newman, M.D., Shattuck; Paul Champlin, M.D., Enid; Lewis J. Moorman, M.D., and Henry Turner, M.D., Oklahoma City; James Stevenson, M.D., Tulsa.

FACULTY: Everett S. Lain, M.D., Howard C. Hopps, M.D., and L. Chester McHenry, M.D., of Oklahoma City.

It is hoped that the entire medical profession will catch the vision and the possibility of this new organization and support it, not only financially, but by their influence on potential givers throughout the State. There have already been many interesting promises made by several potential donors and it rests with the medical profession to initiate this campaign by every doctor giving $100 or more to raise the $25,000 for the expenses of the first five months of the campaign.

Let's help Oklahoma Medicine advance.

HOSPITAL CONSTRUCTION ACT

The State Commissioner of Health, Dr. Grady Mathews, gave a summarization of Public Law 725, commonly referred to as the Hill-Burton Bill at a meeting of the Woodward County Medical Society in Shattuck, Oklahoma, September 11.

The purpose of the act is to assist the States in planning for and providing the modern hospital and public health facilities needed in order that all people may be served. In order to be eligible to participate in the program, each State must prepare a State plan which conforms with the regulations to be prescribed by the Surgeon General, and approved by the Federal Hospital Council.

Construction application forms will be made available for distribution by the State agency when funds are appropriated by Congress. All applications for individual projects must first be approved by the State agency, and then forwarded to the Surgeon General for his approval.

Congress has authorized the appropriation of $75,000,-000 a year for the next five years. *No money for construction has yet been appropriated.* Such an appropriation is not possible until Congress reconvenes. On the basis of the $75,000,000 authorization, Oklahoma will be entitled to an allotment of approximately $1,640,550 annually for the next five years, beginning with the fiscal year June 30, 1946. From this allotment a payment of one-third of the construction cost will be made to each individual approved project.

Information for Each Application

1. Description of site.

2. Plans and specifications which must meet standards and regulations promulgated by both the State and Surgeon General.

3. Title to site must be vested solely in applicant.

4. Reasonable assurance that adequate financial support will be available for the construction of the project and for its maintenance and operation when completed. (This would seem to indicate that the amount of local money must be sufficient not only to meet at least 66 2/3 per centum of the construction cost, but there must be sufficient reserve to provide for operation and maintenance for at least two years.)

5. Applicant must agree rates of pay for laborers and mechanics will be not less than prevailing local wage rates.

6. Facilities must be available to all without discrimination on account of race, creed or color. (This indicates that in counties with an appreciable negro population, provision must be made for the care of this class of people.

7. Each hospital receiving funds under this law must make provision for those unable to pay therefor. (Perhaps the Surgeon General may in his regulations indicate the amount or per centum to be used for "those unable to pay". If not, you will no doubt need to determine this).

8. All institutions receiving funds under this law must be operated on a non-profit basis.

9. Applicant must agree to reimburse the Federal Government if, at any time within 20 years, the hospital is transferred to a person, agency or corporation not eligible to file application under this Act. Value at time of transfer to be determined by agreement or by action in U. S. District Court.

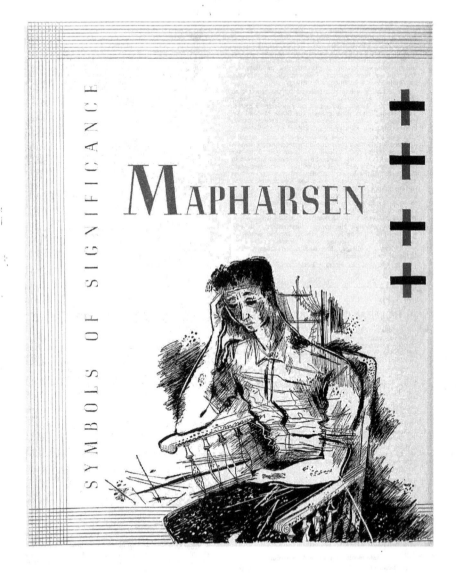

• *"4 plus"* implies exposure, infection and a therapeutic need. MAPHARSEN* has filled the requirement for a relatively safe, antiluetic agent of unquestioned and proved efficacy in case after case, in country after country, in civilian life and for the military services, year in and year out—building an unmatched record of therapeutic performance.

MAPHARSEN is one of a long line of Parke-Davis preparations whose service to the profession created a dependable symbol of significance in medical therapeutics—MEDICAMENTA VERA.

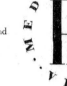

MAPHARSEN (3-amino-4-hydroxy-phenyl-arsineoxide hydrochloride) in single dose ampoules of 0.04 Gm. and 0.06 Gm.; boxes of 10 ampoules. Multiple dose, hospital size ampoule of 0.6 Gm.
*Trademark Reg. U. S. Pat. Off.

PARKE, DAVIS & COMPANY · DETROIT 32, MICHIGAN

SOUTHERN MEDICAL VIA SPECIAL TRAIN

A Special Train to Southern Medical Association, Miami, Florida, and a side trip to Cuba will get under way in November, the details of which are being handled by Mr. Harry Kornbaum. The many doctors and their families who attended the A. M. A. in June will remember Mr. Kornbaum as having conducted the trip through the Northwest, making it a most pleasant and delightful tour.

Transportation

For those who prefer to fly, it is anticipated that there will be a Special Plane leaving Oklahoma City at 5:00 A.M., November 3, making the return trip the afternoon of November 8.

Those going to Miami by train will leave via the Frisco, from Oklahoma City, November 1, 5:50 P.M., picking up Tulsa members of the party at 8:45 P.M. and arriving in Miami November 3 at 5:10 P.M. Hotel reservations for a maximum of 120 doctors and their wives have been made at the famous Robert Clay Hotel, located four blocks from the Convention Hall.

Post Convention Tour to Cuba

A Pan-American Clipper will take members of the party who desire to go to Havana, Cuba, on a post-convention tour. The plane leaves Miami November 8, arriving in Havana after 90 minutes of flying time. Reservations are made at Cuba's "ultra" hotel, the Nacional de Cuba, for four days and three nights. The Clipper returns to Miami November 11, allowing ample time to board the Special Train and head up the seaboard coast for Jacksonville and New Orleans.

Coming Home

The Special will pass through Jacksonville the morning of November 12, turning westward along the Gulf Coast and arriving in New Orleans the following morning, November 13. The party will enjoy a pleasant two-day stopover in New Orleans with sight seeing trips through the many places of interest in this picturesque old town.

At 8:50 A.M., November 15, the party boards the Special Train for the remainder of the trip home. Passing through Memphis at 7:20 P.M. of the same evening, we return to Tulsa November 16 at 9:55 A.M. and into Oklahoma City at 12:40 P.M.

Reservations

The trip to Miami and side tour to Cuba, if elected, is on an all expense basis throughout, except meals. Individual reservations for the return trip for those who do not wish to make the post-convention trip or vacation in Miami, awaiting the return of the Special Train, will be made. There will be available upper berths, lower berths, and compartments. In making reservations, please specify in detail how you wish to travel and whether or not you desire to make the post-convention trip to Cuba. Time is somewhat limited; please make your reservations as soon as possible with Mr. Harry Kornbaum, Rainbow Travel Service, First National Building, Oklahoma City.

PROGRAM FOR VETERANS MEDICAL CARE PROGRESSING RAPIDLY.

As the Journal goes to press the Oklahoma State Medical Association's plan of cooperating with the Veterans Administration to render medical care to veterans is rapidly nearing completion.

Dr. John F. Burton, Chairman of the Committee, studying the plan, and Mr. Dick Graham visited the office of the Kansas plan in Topeka, Kansas, on September 13 and 14. According to Dr. Burton the Kansas plan has progressed more than satisfactorily and their pioneering work has been of great value to other states. Medical fees paid to Kansas physicians during the month of August were approximately $250,000 and gaining each month.

Veterans Administration Representative To Visit Oklahoma

Arrangements have been made for Dr. Thomas Lowry, Director of the Out Patient Department of the Veterans Administration Regional Office in St. Louis, to be in Oklahoma City the latter part of September to meet with the Veterans Medical Care Committee of the Association to discuss fees to be paid for medical services rendered and the method to be selected of approving physicians who will voluntarily agree to participate in the work.

Veterans Regional Office Established In Oklahoma City

With the establishment of a regional office of the Veterans Administration in Oklahoma City, it is anticipated that the operation of the plan will be greatly simplified inasmuch as the Executive Office of the Association will be accessible for coordination of the details.

All members of the medical profession will be contacted directly as soon as the plan is completed and it is contemplated that Councilor District meetings will be held to further explain the plan to the profession.

OKLAHOMA EDUCATION IN HEALTH LEAGUE ORGANIZED

On September 3, 1946, at a meeting held in the offices of the Oklahoma State Medical Association, there was organized the Oklahoma Education in Health League having as its objective "to promote health education to the lay public". The following organizations had representatives attending, which constitute the present membership: American Cancer Society, Blue Cross Hospital Plan and Oklahoma Physicians Service, Oklahoma Society for Crippled Children, National Foundation for Infantile Paralysis, State Tuberculosis Association, State Dental Society; State Pharmaceutical Association, State Vocational Rehabilitation, State Department of Health, University of Oklahoma School of Medicine, Veterans Administration and the Oklahoma State Medical Association. Membership is open to organizations concerned with public health and welfare. Two-thirds vote approval for new members is required.

WILLIAM E. EASTLAND, M.D.
F. A. C. R.

RADIUM AND X-RAY THERAPY
DERMATOLOGY

405 Medical Arts Bldg.

Oklahoma City, Oklahoma   Phone 3-1446

The story of facilities available and the work now being done in the various fields pertaining to health matters, was the objective of the organizations participating in fair exhibition. Considerable effort was expended to make the public conscious of the public health problems and to solicit their cooperation in furthering the improvement of the situation.

The first activity of the League was the "Life Show" presented through the Oklahoma State Fair of 1946. It is anticipated that this is only the first effort to carry out the objective of the organization and that there will be more frequent and larger health educational activities. Considering the broad field of health education, without doubt the opportunities for service by the new league will be innumerable.

V. A. Hospital Construction Program Changes In Oklahoma

The Naval Hospital buildings at Norman have been transferred to V. A. for temporary use as a 750 bed N. P. hospital. A permanent 750 bed N. P. hospital for treatment of cronic cases will be constructed at the Norman site.

A 1000 bed general medical and surgical hospital will be constructed at Oklahoma City, with about 50 beds to be set aside for treatment of acute N. P. cases. This project is subject to a future appropriation.

The Central Oklahoma State Hospital for mental patients being in Norman, and the University of Oklahoma Medical School being in Oklahoma City, make both sites logical locations for V. A. hospitals.

SURPLUS PROPERTY SITUATION, STILL CONFUSING

Through recent correspondence with the War Assets Administration the information has been developed that the program is not so constituted as to give service to the veteran when he is in need of surplus property adaptable to his practice.

It can be seen from the following letter from the W. A. A. that the physician veteran must wait his turn and depend upon being advised at some future date.

"Reference is made to your letter of August 26 regarding availability of 'set aside' items.

"We regret to advise you we do not have any dental or medical 'set aside' items available on our inventory at this time. However, if and when this equipment is available the veterans who are certified will be notified and given an opportunity to purchase.

"If we can be of further assistance to you in this matter kindly advise this office."

RED CROSS REQUESTS DOCTORS TO RETURN OUTDATED PLASMA

Blood plasma which becomes out-dated should not be destroyed, as there are several uses to which it can be put, according to word received at the State Department of Health from Dr. Raymond F. Barnes, director of medical and health services, American Red Cross. Physicians having outdated plasma on hand are requested to send it to the American Red Cross, Midwestern Area Storeroom, 1709 Washington Avenue, St. Louis, Mo.

It has also been noted that a number of physicians have been filling out the report forms found in the boxes of plasma. This is not necessary, Dr. Barnes pointed out, as the army is no longer interested in the questionnaire.

Governor Appoints Committee on Standardization

Governor Robert S. Kerr has made the following appointments to the Committee on Standardization:

Earl McBride, M.D., Oklahoma City, was reappointed to serve as Chairman.

I. F. Stephenson, M.D., Alva, Vice Chairman.

Mr. Joe N. Hamilton, Oklahoma City, appointed Secretary.

Committee members appointed as follows: J. F. Park, M.D., McAlester; E. Eugene Rice, M.D., Shawnee; Floyd Newman, M.D., Shattuck; and M. M. Williams, D.D.S., Chickasha.

DIAGNOSTIC CLINIC OF INTERNAL MEDICINE AND ALLERGY

Philip M. McNeill, M. D., F. A. C. P.

General Diagnosis

CONSULTATION BY APPOINTMENT

Special Attention to Cardiac, Pulmonary and Allergic Diseases

Electrocardiograph, X-Ray, Laboratory
and Complete Allergic Surveys Available.

1107 Medical Arts Bldg.
Oklahoma City, Okla.   Phone 2-0277

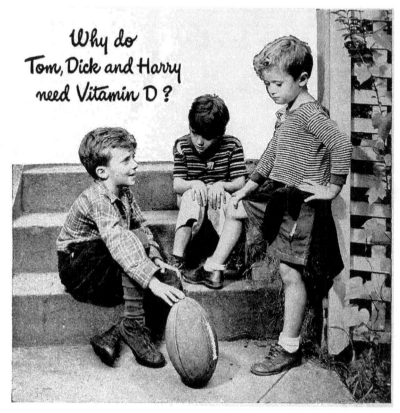

Why do Tom, Dick and Harry need Vitamin D?

Growing children require vitamin D mainly to prevent rickets. They also need vitamin D, though to a lesser degree, to insure optimal development of muscles and other soft tissues containing considerable amounts of phosphorus ... Milk is the logical menstruum for administering vitamin D to growing children, as well as to infants, pregnant women and lactating mothers. This suggests the use of Drisdol in Propylene Glycol, which diffuses uniformly in milk, fruit juices and other fluids.

DRISDOL IN PROPYLENE GLYCOL

TRADEMARK REG. U S. PAT. OFF. & CANADA
Brand of Crystalline Vitamin D₂ (calciferol) from ergosterol

MILK DIFFUSIBLE VITAMIN D PREPARATION

Odorless
Tasteless
Economical

Average daily dose for infants 2 drops, for children and adults 4 to 6 drops, in milk.

Available in bottles of 5, 10 and 50 cc. with special dropper delivering 250 U.S.P. units per drop.

WINTHROP CHEMICAL COMPANY, INC.
Pharmaceuticals of merit for the physician • New York 13, N. Y. • Windsor, Ont.

Have You Heard That...

At the Annual Meeting of the American College of Chest Physicians held at San Francisco June 27-30, 1946 *Dr. Robert M. Shepard*, Tulsa, was re-elected Governor of the College for the State of Oklahoma.

Dr. Ben Bell, having served over three years in the Navy as a Neuro-psychiatrist, has recently returned to the Coyne Campbell Sanitarium.

Dr. G. F. Mathews, Commissioner of Health, announced the appointment of *Dr. S. S. Kirkland* of Sallisaw, as County Health Superintendent of Sequoyah County, effective September 6, 1946.

Dr. Harvey Roys of Norman, recently released from the service, has entered into practice with his brother in Seattle, Washington.

Drs. Thomas H. Briggs and Joseph S. Fulton of Atoka recently attended a meeting of the Chamber of Commerce of Coalgate concerning the construction of a hospital in that City.

Dr. C. E. Northcutt of Ponca City, member of the Council, is now back to his practice after having been hospitalized by an automobile accident.

Dr. Vance F. Morgan has announced the opening of his office at 113 W. Oklahoma Avenue in Guthrie. Dr. Morgan is an O. U. graduate and in addition to serving an internship at University Hospital in Oklahoma City has completed post graduate work at Johns Hopkins and Vanderbilt Universities.

Dr. Howard F. Turner, Tulsa, has been named medical director for the American Airlines in Tulsa.

A former Picher physician, *Dr. Calmes P. Bishop*, is the new director of the Muskogee city-county health unit.

A corporation has been formed in McAlester to build a new Medical Arts Building. *Dr. T. H. McCarley* is president; *Dr. F. T. Bartheld*, Vice-President; and *Dr. E. D. Greenberger*, Secretary-Treasurer.

Dr. Ralph McGill, Tulsa, has returned to his home in the Mayo Hotel after quite a long siege in the hospital.

It looked like a conclave of old grads when recently *Dr. James Stevenson*, Tulsa. *Dr. V. C. Tisdal*, Elk City, and *Dr. Charlie Rountree*, Oklahoma City, arrived simultaneously in the Executive Office, each without knowing the others were present.

Latimer County has welcomed *Dr. G. R. Booth, Jr.*, who has recently opened his office in the Donathan Building in Wilburton, following his release from the armed forces.

Dr. James Hood, Norman, has been appointed as Director of Student Health Service at the University, having succeeded *Dr. John Y. Battenfield* who will go to Liberia in the employment of Firestone Tire and Rubber Co.

Dr. Edward Thorp, a graduate of the University of Oklahoma in 1942, has opened offices in Cushing.

Dr. Morris Smith has resumed his practice in Guymon after a number of months rest. He has entered into partnership with *Dr. E. L. Buford*, who had had his office in the Smith Clinic Building for several months.

The appointment of *Dr. P. H. Anderson* of Anadarko, effective September 15, 1946, as County Superintendent of Health of Caddo County, has been made by Dr. Grady F. Mathews, Commissioner of Health.

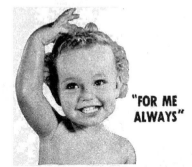

"FOR ME ALWAYS"

Because DARICRAFT

1. is EASILY DIGESTED
2. has 400 U.S.P. Units of VITAMIN D per pint of evaporated milk.
3. has HIGH FOOD VALUE
4. has an IMPROVED FLAVOR
5. is HOMOGENIZED
6. is STERILIZED
7. is from INSPECTED HERDS
8. is SPECIALLY PROCESSED
9. is UNIFORM
10. will WHIP QUICKLY

PRESCRIBED BY MANY DOCTORS
...You also may want to utilize Daricraft as a solution to your infant feeding problems, as well as in special diets for convalescents.

PRODUCERS CREAMERY CO., SPRINGFIELD, MISSOURI

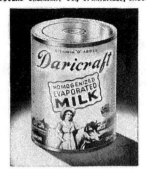

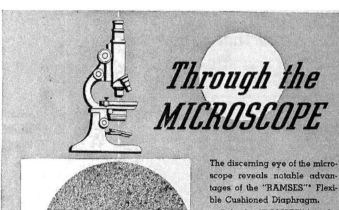

Through the
MICROSCOPE

The discerning eye of the microscope reveals notable advantages of the "RAMSES"* Flexible Cushioned Diaphragm.

Only the "RAMSES" has the patented rim construction which provides both a wide, unindented area of contact with the vaginal walls, and a cushion of soft rubber to buffer spring pressure.

The pure gum rubber used in the dome is prepared by an exclusive process which imparts lightness, strength, velvet smoothness, and long life.

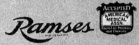

Ramses

FLEXIBLE CUSHIONED DIAPHRAGM

Manufactured in gradations of 5 millimeters in sizes ranging from 50 to 95 millimeters, inclusive. Available through all recognized pharmacies.

gynecological division

JULIUS SCHMID, INC.

423 West 55th St., New York 19, N. Y.

*The word "RAMSES" is a registered trademark of Julius Schmid, Inc.

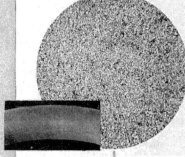

No. 1 Unretouched photomicrograph of the dome (enlarged 10 diameters) and the rim (inset) of a "RAMSES" Flexible Cushioned Diaphragm.

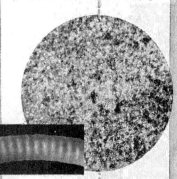

No. 2 Unretouched photomicrograph of the dome (enlarged 10 diameters) and the rim (inset) of a conventional-type diaphragm.

quality first since 1883

Hits, Runs, Errors

AUGUST 21: The highschool All Stars are in town and these boys are certainly a credit to the many cities from which they come. Give them a hand when they get home. Bill Harkey, attorney for the Medical Boards, called and there is a conference over the Optical Store situation. Seems they are only now operating in Okmulgee and Ada, also looks as if the Attorney General is going to take action. Haskell Newman, M.D., in from Shattuck, but not flying his airplane. Who said county practice can't be wonderful? Dr. Coyle from Chandler, we forgot his first name, wanted to know about locations. He is just out of the army. We gave him the list and he will be back. The program for the County Medical Societies Officers' Conference is about complete and with pardonable pride may we say it looks like the best we have ever had.

AUGUST 22: Word from Dr. Day that Dr. Clulow passed away in Tulsa. We will try to get some help for the hospital. Lunch and afternoon conference with Attorney for London and Lancashire who carry our Malpractice Insurance. More correspondance and telephone conversations about On-the-Job training. Now we are discussing interns and residents.

AUGUST 23: Frankly, this was a lazy day. The Journal did get some attention and we are now going to analyze the advertising for the past five years and see if we can arrive on a formula for the number of pages to be printed in ratio to pages of ads. Try this sometime; its fun. Fondren inherits this little problem. North All-Stars beat the South 32-6 and I watched the game on a free ticket from Dr. C. R. Rountree and family.

AUGUST 24: The mail brought a letter from the A. M. A. on their radio program for 1947, the Centennial year. Each state will have its history of medicine dramatized. A note from the President finds Dr. Kuyrkendall in Minneapolis and we are now looking for a box of iced fish. Dr. Northcutt of Ponca City writes that he is on the mend following an accident and invites us to Ponca City on the 12th of September. We are going.

AUGUST 6: First returns received on survey concerning Special Train to Southern Medical Meeting. Looks good. Fondren has a meeting with the groups who will exhibit at the State Fair and things are moving along. William Brooksher, M.D., Secretary of Arkansas Society called concerning Veterans Fee Schedule and suggested Oklahoma and Arkansas try and work together. Of course, this is agreeable.

AUGUST 27: To Rotary for lunch with Dr. John Lamb and President Cross of the University of Oklahoma and a visit about the many new plans for the Medical School. A great day is dawning and everyone must help. A letter from a secretary of a chamber of commerce concerning building a hospital. It seems, according to the letter, that the doctors in the town have to take all of their "obesity" cases to another town for delivery. Something new in medicine.

AUGUST 28: Our genial Secretary, Dick, is on "tour" (???) today — out in West Indian Territory, so pinch-hitter Fondren is the "batter-up". An early caller of the morning was Dr. Brooks of Phillips, Texas. The doctor was in town on business with the Medical School, but also gave us a "hello". The mail brought in increasing data from the various organizations participating in the Health Show of the coming State Fair. Big meeting for all exhibitors scheduled for next Tuesday night, September 3, at which time final arrangements on this Fair Business will be culminated. All signs indicate that some very interesting displays are to be presented at the Fair this year. By the time this is in print, perhaps you will have seen the exhibits — please let us have your comments. Constructive criticism will help us to do a better job next year.

AUGUST 29: Fondren swinging at the ball again today — Dick did return to the office this morning — reported considerable rain on his round trip to western Oklahoma. Luncheon with Dr. John Burton and round tab'e discussion of the Veterans Care problem. Secretaries planned trip to Tulsa tomorrow to start surveying the Annual Meeting situation.

AUGUST 30: Off to Tulsa at 7:00 A.M. First stop — Mayo Hotel to see Manager, Mr. Bentley about the Annual Meeting. From there to Jack Spear's Tulsa County Medical Society Office. Dr. James Stevenson graciously invited us to lunch following which we attended latter part of Tulsa County Medical Society's Board of Trustee meeting. Then to Chamber of Commerce Convention Chairman's and Mr. Bethel at Blue Cross for an interesting and instructive tour of Blue Cross Headquarters.

AUGUST 31: Nothing of interesting news value this Saturday A.M.

SEPTEMBER 2: Since each organization and person consulted planned no operations, the Association's office did not open this Labor Day.

SEPTEMBER 3: Paul B. Champlin, M.D., James Stevenson, M.D., F. Redding Hood, M.D., McClain Rogers, M.D. and Dick Graham departed last evening for St. Louis to attend National Physicians Committee meeting. Final Fair meeting in Library at 8:00 P.M.

SEPTEMBER 4: State Fair meeting last night, 13 participating organizations represented. "Oklahoma Education in Health League" created. Crippled Children's Committee meeting scheduled for today postponed — not enough members could attend.

SEPTEMBER 5: Dick Graham back from trip to St. Louis. Discussion with Dr. John Burton on coming Veterans Care Committee meeting. Had a visit from Dr. Talley concerning a location for a physician.

SEPTEMBER 6: Telephone conference with Harry Kornbaum concerning Special Train to Southern Medical. Tried to talk to Warren Humphreys of Erwin-Wassey on advertising program. Too many people still

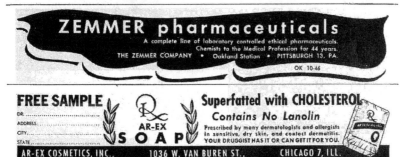

ZEMMER pharmaceuticals

A complete line of laboratory controlled ethical pharmaceuticals.
Chemists to the Medical Profession for 44 years.

THE ZEMMER COMPANY • Oakland Station • PITTSBURGH 13, PA.

OK 10-46

FREE SAMPLE

DR.
ADDRESS
CITY
STATE

AR-EX SOAP

Superfatted with CHOLESTEROL

Contains No Lanolin

Prescribed by many dermatologists and allergists in sensitive, dry skin, and contact dermatitis.
YOUR DRUGGIST HAS IT OR CAN GET IT FOR YOU.

AR-EX COSMETICS, INC.,   1036 W. VAN BUREN ST.,   CHICAGO 7, ILL.

taking vacations. Exhibit program at State Fair causing trouble — too many people with different ideas.

SEPTEMBER 7: Telephone conversation with Dr. Collier on Venereal Disease problem. Talked to Dr. Newman concerning Woodward County Medical Society meeting scheduled for September 11. Muriel Waller called in regard to the Association's Special Assessment. Dr. Coyle in the office to find out about insurance and procedure for joining the Association after he establishes his new location.

SEPTEMBER 8: To Shawnee for a meeting of the Executive Committee of the Seventh Councilor District. Clinton Gallaher, M.D., Councilor, and Mrs. Clint had a wonderful buffet for those in attendance. All but two counties represented, and we were glad to again visit with Dr. Rollins of Prague, Dr. Felts of Seminole, Dr. Robberson of Wynnewood, Dr. Hicks of Holdenville, Dr. Morey of Ada and Dr. Newlin of Shawnee.

SEPTEMBER 9: Dr. Hackler in office this A.M. to help iron out a few more Fair problems and discuss publicity angle. Dr. Rountree dropped in to catch up on current matters — the doctor just returned from Colorado vacation. Harry Kornbaum, our travel expert, called to discuss proposed Southern Medical Meeting trip.

SEPTEMBER 10: Southern Medical Trip plans discussed at great length with Harry Kornbaum of Rainbow Travel Service. Meeting this evening with Harry and Dr. Carroll Pounders. Trip promises to be a great one.

SEPTEMBER 11: Dean Gray, Dr. Lamb, Dick and I went out to Shattuck to attend the Woodward County Medical Society meeting. State Commissioner of Health, Dr. Grady Mathews, was also there to comment on Hospital Construction Act. Dean Gray found his first trip to Western Oklahoma very interesting.

SEPTEMBER 12: Late arrival this A.M. — up late last night because of return trip from Shattuck. Many telephone conversations with organizations participating in Fair program. Dick making arrangements to go to Topeka tomorrow in connection with Veterans Care Program.

SEPTEMBER 13: Dr. Hewitt from Muskogee in office early to discuss available opportunities for returning veteran doctors — gave him list made from survey before his departure. Trying desperately to get articles for Journal lined up; already two days past deadline. Oklahoma Executive Council luncheon at noon — must see the printer this afternoon and work on Journal mailing list problem which is always with us.

SEPTEMBER 14: Dr. Ellis in office to recheck location list. Dr. Stevenson called from Tulsa to arrange meeting of his Medical Education and Hospital Committee. Still trying desperately to get Journal articles assembled for October issue. Working on Dr. McBride's Committee meeting, scheduled for tomorrow morning.

SEPTEMBER 15: Dr. Earl D. McBride held meeting of the Crippled Children's Committee this morning in the Executive Office to discuss fee question for polio patients.

SEPTEMBER 16: Fair Exhibit from A. M. A. arrived this morning. Dick went to McAlester to see Dr. Kuyrkendall and on to Coalgate for hospital meeting.

SEPTEMBER 17: Dr. Glissman paid us a visti this A.M. Dick back from McAlester and Coalgate. Secretaries Conference to be September 29th.

SEPTEMBER 18: Conference with Advertising Agency concerning ads this A.M. Visited the Cancer Society headquarters to see their program for the big meeting the 27th.

SEPTEMBER 19: A busy day. To Chickasha for a 9:00 o'clock meeting with the Chamber of Commerce, and back to the office for a meeting of Dr. Stevenson's Medical Education and Hospital meeting and at 2:30 to Ponca City with Dr. Lingenfelter and Dean Gray. At Ponca City we saw the joining together of Kay and Noble County Medical Societies and a steak dinner to boot. Haskell Smith of Stillwater says this column is well named as our "errors" are more than our hits. We admit we don't know the name of the damn at Cody, Wyoming.

SEPTEMBER 20: This is the day before the Fair and everyone is busy preparing booths for the gala opening tomorrow.

$\mathcal{M}$etrazol – Powerful, Quick Acting Central Stimulant
COUNCIL ACCEPTED

ORALLY - for respiratory and circulatory support
BY INJECTION - for resuscitation in the emergency

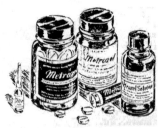

INJECT I to 3 cc. Metrazol as a restorative in circulatory and respiratory failure, in barbiturate or morphine poisoning and in asphyxia. PRESCRIBE I or 2 Metrazol tablets for a stimulating-tonic effect to supplement symptomatic treatment of chronic cardiac disease and fatigue states.

AMPULES - I and 3 cc. (each cc. contains 1½ grains.)
TABLETS - 1½ grains.
ORAL SOLUTION - (10% aqueous solution.)

Metrazol, pentamethylentetrazol, Trade Mark Bilhuber.

Bilhuber-Knoll Corp. Orange, N. J.

advantages
of the
PERENNIAL
METHOD
of treating
HAY
FEVER

AMONG the advantages of the perennial method of treating hay fever are:

CONVENIENCE. Perennial treatment may be started at any time during the year and it is often more convenient for the patient to come to the physician's office at less frequent intervals than is necessary during preseasonal and coseasonal treatment.

EFFECTIVENESS. Greater probability of permanent immunity with this method than with either the preseasonal or coseasonal method.

SIMPLICITY. The perennial method is the one of choice where symptoms of hay fever continue through more than one season. In treating such cases, pollens of all seasons during which the patient is affected may be combined without loss of effectiveness.

CONTROL. This method also enables the physician to keep a much closer check on the patient's general physical condition throughout the entire year.

Physicians may order a complete diagnostic pollen set for testing any individual patient for $1.00 irrespective of the number of pollen allergens it is necessary to include. In ordering these sets, dates of onset and termination of attack are required.

The staff of the Biological Division will be most happy to extend their cooperation and suggestions on any of your allergy problems.

A copy of the treatise, "Advantages of the Perennial Method of Treating Hay Fever", will be sent to physicians upon request.

THE ARLINGTON CHEMICAL COMPANY
YONKERS 1   NEW YORK   Arlington

Book Reviews

PERIPHERAL VASCULAR DISEASES. Edgard V. Allen, B.S., M.A., M.D., M.S. in medicine, F.A.C.P. Division of Medicine, Mayo Clinic, Associate Professor of Medicine, Mayo Foundation, Graduate School, University of Minnesota; Diplomate of the American Board of Internal Medicine; Nelson W. Barker, B.A., M.D., M.S. in Medicine, Mayo Clinic, Associate Professor of Medicine, Mayo Foundation, Graduate School, University of Minnesota, Diplomate of the American Board of Internal Medicine; Edgar A. Hines, Jr., M.D., B.S., M.A., M.S. in Medicine, F.A.C.P., Division of Medicine, Mayo Clinic, Associate Professor of Medicine, Mayo Foundation, Graduate School, University of Minnesota. First Edition, 386 illustrations, eleven colaborators, 871 pages. W. B. Saunders Company, Philadelphia, Pa.

This is an entirely new book. The authors are all competent men, having had extensive experience in the field of peripheral vascular diseases. Eleven of the authors' colleagues have contributed to the book, which is dedicated to Dr. George Elgie Brown, who is credited with doing much of the original work and inspiring these authors to write this book.

A discussion of hypertension and vascular diseases of certain viscera have been omitted. There is no attempt to cover the technical aspects of sympathetic nervous system surgery.

Other than the above omissions, the field of peripheral vascular diseases, including disorders of lymph vessels and veins, is well covered in a clear, concise manner. The authors have expressed their own opinions freely on many controversial matters, and have done an excellent job of avoiding cumbersome repetition, and have wisely omitted burdening their book with researches which do not have a direct clinical bearing.

The book attempts to clarify much of the confusing terminology by devoting the first chapter to a definition of terms.

In reading through this book, one is particularly struck by the open-minded manner, and complete lack of prejudice, with which the authors approach the subject. Simplicity with a thorough understanding and reliance on basic physiologic principles, both as regards diagnosis and treatment, is shown throughout the book. The authors do not rely on any single method or type of treatment (such as alternating suction and pressure, intermittent venous occlusion, contrast baths, sympathetic surgery, intravenous typhoid, etc.) in the care of occlusive vascular disease. Rather, they rely on a combination of several methods of treatment as illustrated by the outline for handling thrombo-angitis obliterans. (Pages 469-70).

I believe that this book is a very worthwhile contribution to a widely neglected field of medicine and that it will go far toward bringing an unanimity of opinion in the proper care of patients afflicted with peripheral vascular diseases.—Turner Bynum, M.D.

GRACIAN'S MANUAL. Martin Fischer, a doctor and professor in the University of Cincinnati. Second and revised edition. 300 pages. Charles C. Thomas, Springfield, Illinois.

"Gracian wings across some fifty odd years of history like the flight of a Mother Carey's chicken. Out of a gray obscurity, he flashes into the visible sky—black, swift, unafraid, screaming his song," Gracian lived in the first half of the seventeenth century.

The following statement taken from the jacket of this volume stimulates the reader, and a first reading justifies the statement:

"This is not a sweetmeat for children, but a volume for men of this world—and but few of them. A new translation into English of the famous Spanish classic of Padre Balbasar Gracian. A practical manual of self-instruction, absolutely unique, and peculiarly appropriate to the thinking man of these perilous times."

Each paragraph is marked by scarlet numerals. While the "art of worldly wisdom" appears on every page, this is not a book to be read at a single sitting, but to be placed at the bedside or in the traveling bag for periodic perusal in small doses during periods when the time is propitious. It would be difficult to find in any other single volume so much sound unobtrusive advice.

This book is heartily recommended to doctors who find it easy to develop the habit of thinking there is no time to read outside the field of medicine. This is a book offering genuine reward in return for spare moments.—Lewis J. Moorman, M.D.

MODERN MANAGEMENT IN CLINICAL MEDICINE. Frederick K. Albrecht, M.D., S. A. Surgeon, ...U. S. Public Health Service Kansas State Tuberculosis Consultant; Formerly Clinical Director, U. S. Marine Hospital, Baltimore, Maryland. 1,238 pages. 1946. The Williams and Wilkins Company. $10.00.

This book was obviously conceived by the author as a volume intended for the doctor's office. A tremendous amount of material has been compiled with the objective of bringing to the medical practitioner a readily available wealth of known facts, as well as new facts. It has been accomplished in such a clever way that the reader need consume only a minimum of time in obtaining necessary information on a particular subject. Excellent photographs and x-ray plates representing disease entities are presented throughout the book.

For those who wish to do more reading on any particular subject or desire more complete information, Dr. Albrecht has included at the end of each chapter, a bibliography of the latest references on each subject.

J. E. HANGER, Inc.

ARTIFICIAL LIMBS, BRACES, AND CRUTCHES

Phone: 2-8500

612 N. Hudson

L. T. Lewis, Mgr.

BRANCHES AND AGENCIES IN PRINCIPAL CITIES   Oklahoma City 3, Okla.

POST-OPERATIVE RECTAL DISCOMFORT

if often alleviated with the use of   **YOUNG'S DILATORS**

Due to post-operative reaction, the anal ring often becomes quite firm, but regular use of the dilators makes the ring pliable with good muscle tone. A valuable adjunct also in constipation, rectal neurosis, puritus ani, etc.

Sold only by prescription. Obtainable at your surgical supply house; available at ethical drugstores. Set of 4 graduated sizes, adult $4.75; children $4.50. Write for brochure.

F. E. YOUNG & CO.   424 E. 75th St.   Chicago 19, Illinois

The most recent developments and discoveries in diagnostic procedures, special techniques and therapy are presented in a readily available form. Such procedures as hepatosplenography, peritoneoscopy, and electroencephalography are discussed. There are excellent chapters on vitamin deficiencies, tropical diseases of postwar importance, chemotherapy and geriatrics. Therapy in all subjects, not only includes recent discoveries, but the common trade names of drugs and pharmaceutical preparations are included which should eliminate difficulty in obtaining and prescribing the proper drugs.

The Appendix includes illustrations and descriptions of procedures such as thoracentesis, sternal bone marrow cavity of administration of fluid and tidal bladder drainage apparatus. The desire of the author to make this book a complete reference for the busy physician is further manifest by his brief but concise description of the preparation of counter irritant such as poultices, hot and cold packs and even the placing of a patient in a wheel chair is not omitted.

The last 11 pages of the Appendix are devoted to the various types of diet, completely described in outline form. Reduction diets, high caloric diets and those of Karrell and Mueleugracht are only a few of those included.—George S. Bozalis, M.D.

NEW AND NONOFFICIAL REMEDIES. 1946 edition. 770 pages. 24 chapters. Council on Pharmacy and Chemistry, American Medical Association.

"This book is published by the Council on Pharmacy and Chemistry which is a standing committee appointed by the Board of Trustees of the American Medical Association, to consider medical preparations offered by pharmaceutical manufacturers for prophylactic and therapeutic use by the physicians." The Council is composed of eighteen members and forty consultants, whose hallmark of approval should be unquestioned. This publication not only lists and describes the product, but also (which is quite essential) lists the manufacturers which put out the product. Manufacturers put out so many specifics that only cure for two or three months and detail men with highpressure salesmanship flood the market with these nostrums that are either inert or possibly toxic (Messengil sulph solution an example). Research facilities should preceed all new products and hence the desirability of this to me, to see if the stamp of approval has to be given by this group of financially disinterested and scientifically interested scientists recommend it. There is a voluminous bibliography on products not acceptable, and show the source of information about such articles.

The Oklahoma University School of Medicine furnishes each graduate with one of these valuable and up-to-date books for perusal. Each physician should have one at his elbow for a check up on the claims of products made more for financial gain and beating their competitors to it, than for the humanitarian aspect. These acceptable products are approved for only three years, and if unwarranted claims of efficiency or change in the formulary, thereby it is a just cause for its being dropped. Since the metric system has displaced the apothecaries weights and measures, there is a chapter and table of equivalents for those not used to the new system.

Addend: Revision of the Rules of the Council on Pharmacy and Chemistry, J.A.M.A., 131-215-219, May 18, 1946, curtails the firms from exploiting remedies for profit, using a few better articles for "window dressing" than for serious promotion. The Council aims to insist that the major business of a firm should be in acceptable articles before any of its products would be accepted by the Council. This, of course, is aimed for the protection of the physician as well as the buying public.
—Lea A. Riely, M.D.

THE TABLET METHOD FOR DETECTING URINE-SUGAR

CLINITEST

offers these advantages to physicians, laboratory technician, patient:

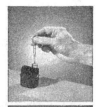

ELIMINATES
Use of flame
Bulky apparatus
Measuring of reagents

PROVIDES
Simplicity
Speed
Convenience of technic
Simply drop one Clinitest Tablet into test tube containing proper amount of diluted urine. Allow time for reaction, compare with color scale.

FOR OFFICE USE Clinitest Laboratory Outfit (No. 2108) includes — Tablets for 180 tests, test tubes, rack, droppers, color scale, instructions. Additional tablets can be purchased as required.

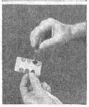

FOR PATIENT USE Clinitest Plastic Pocket-Size Set (No. 2106) includes — All essentials for testing — in a small, durable, packet-size case of Tenite plastic.

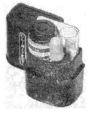

Order from your dealer.
Complete information upon request.

AMES COMPANY, Inc., Elkhart, Ind.

Medical Abstracts

ATOPIC CATARACTS. Frederick C. Cordes and Rafael Cordero-Moreno. American Journal of Ophthalmology. Vol. 29. pp. 402-407. April. 1946.

The association of skin diseases with cataract formation is a generally recognized fact. Cataract may develop in the course of neurodermatitis, poikiloderma atrophicans vasculare, and scleroderma. Cataracts have been also associated with keratosis follicularis, telangiectasis, myxedema, and certain abnormities of the hair (alopecia, aplasia pilaris, etc.)

The dry form of neurodermatitis has been also designated as atopic dermatitis. Atopy is a form of allergy, and includes hayfever, asthma and eczema. It occurs in the presence of specific reagins in the blood stream. These reagins enter the body during embryonic life, and the sensitivity thus transferred will remain until about the middle life. During infancy it is manifested on the skin by eczematous lesions of the weeping, crusty type. In childhood, papular eruption is present, which may or may not be accompanied by asthma. In adult life, the lesions consist of elevated papules and dry, scaly, lichenified plaques. The course of the disease is chronic.

Cataract formation as part of the picture of neurodermatitis or atopic dermatitis may begin at any time. A typical atopic cataract is a white milky plaque in the pupillary area, localized either on the anterior or on the posterior pole of the lens, involving the superficial layers of the lens cortex. The early changes are granular deposits in the anterior capsule, and an increase in the prominence of the Y suture lines. The mature cataract appears gray or light cream in color. Striation of the lens fibers is often present as are small punctate opacities and iridescent crystals. Later, these small opacities will coalesce.

The incidence of cataract in atopic patients is not determined. Some authors mention 10 per cent, which is a rather high rate. The cataract is apt to appear in puberty and young adult life. Sex has no apparent influence in the incidence of atopic cataract.

The mechanism of the formation of the lens opacities is not certain. It may be that lens opacities are but manifestations of an ectodermal disease. It is possible that in the course of allergy the lens may become a so-called shock organ, i.e., an organ which is specially sensitive against the reagins of the blood.

The treatment of such cases is surgical. Most of the patients fall in an age group wherein intracapsular extraction is not recommended since there is a tendency in the capsule to rupture.

The authors report four cases: all of them showed atopic dermatitis with cataract formation. One patient was a 15-year old boy whose father had had asthma for many years and one brother had hayfever; he himself suffered from asthma and eczema; his cataract was bilateral subcapsular. A 17-year old girl had a type of skin disease which was a mild eczema of the face; her cataract was also bilateral, and was complicated by retinal detachment.—M.D.H., M.D.

SOME CONTRIBUTIONS OF ENDOCRINOLOGY TO OBSTETRICS AND GYNECOLOGY. E. C. Hamblen, M.D., American Journal of Obstetrics and Gynecology. Vol. 51. No. 6. pp. 796-803. June. 1946.

Dr. Hamblen briefly reviews endocrinology, with especial reference to the ovary, from the pioneer work of Allen, Loeb, and others to the present time. He then discusses various technical phases of present day conceptions. He states that the climateric patient is too often the victim of very poor therapy. Quoting from his article " . . . In the climateric woman estrogen therapy has often been too frequent and too uncritical . . . ". "Few climateric women require estrogens . . . ". " . . . Injectional therapy is not necessary—its psychologic approach is unhealthy . . . ", "Infrequent injections of large amounts (of estrogen) are an ideal formula for .

C. A. GALLAGHER, M. D.

CURT VON WEDEL, M. D.

(Consultant)

PLASTIC and RECONSTRUCTION
SURGERY

610 N. W. Ninth Street

Oklahoma City, Oklahoma

Office 2-3108

keeping the entire endocrine system in a state of flux and chaos. . . . '' ''If estrogens are necessary, the daily dose should not be larger than .5 mg. of Stilbestrol, or its equivalent.''

To the above might be added that estrogens are potentially dangerous to women who have certain breast tumors, or women who have a family history of cancer. —G.P., M.D.

ROENTGENOGRAPHIC INTERPRETATION OF WHAT CONSTITUTES ADEQUATE REDUCTION OF FEMORAL NECK FRACTURES: Robert T. McElvenny, Surgery, Gynecology and Obstetrics. Vol. 80. pp. 97-106; 1945.

The author has evaluated from his own experience various ways of dealing with intracapsular fractures of the hip. Certain facts have been obtained from his study of failures, and these facts are used in formulating criteria of roentgenographic interpretation at the time of reduction and nailing of fractures. All failures have occurred in hips which have been reduced imperfectly — that is, the neck fragment has not been placed well under and well inside the head fragment. McElvenny feels that accurate placement is absolutely necessary in order that fixation may act as a guide to allow the head to settle on the neck in a position in which the weight thrust is applied directly to the fracture site, without shearing or torsion forces being exerted on the fixation material.—E.D.M., M.D.

TREATMENTS OF TUBERCULOSIS OF THE LARYNX WITH STREPTOMYCIN: REPORT OF CASE. Frederick A. Figi, M.D., Section on Laryngology, Oral and Plastic Surgery, H. Corwin Hinshaw, M.D., Ph.D., Division of Medicine and William H. Feldman, D.V.M., M.S., Division of Experimental Surgery and Pathology. Mayo Foundation.

Case report of a thirty-two year old married woman, first seen at the Clinic March 16, 1945, because of hoarseness of one year's duration, progressively worse. Physical examination revealed nothing of significance, except a laryngeal picture typical of papillary tuberculous laryngitis, confirmed as such by biopsy. X-ray showed some accentuation of the right hilar shadow. Acid fast bacilli were demonstrated in the suptum.

Streptomycin was administered for forty-five days, a total of thirty-four grams was given parenterally. Nebulization with streptomycin was also used. Definite improvement of the laryngeal lesion was noted by the tenth day, and the lesion had improved 75 per cent by the twenty-fifth day of treatment. After the twenty-seventh day, all subsequent biopsys, cultures, smears from the lesion were negative for acid fast bacilli. By the forty-fifth day, the lesion was practically healed. After six months there had been no recurrence, and the patient's voice remained normal.

The authors feel that streptomycin was of definite value in the treatment of this case. However, they do not necessarily anticipate the same favorable results in the usual cases of laryngeal tuberculosis which are associated with extensive, destructive, and often fulminating pulmonary tuberculosis.—H.J., M.D.

RAPID REPAIR OF DEFECT OF FEMUR BY MASSIVE BONE GRAFTS AFTER RESECTION FOR TUMORS. Dallas B. Phemister, Surgery, Gynecology and Obstetrics. Vol. 80, pp. 120-127, 1945.

By means of bone grafting, amputation was avoided in two cases of locally resected bone tumors of the lower end of the femur. Two tibial grafts, each between two-fifth and one-half the circumference of the shaft and from seven to eleven inches in length, were used to bridge the defect. The grafts were part onlay and part intramedullary, with fixation by threaded wires at each end. Firm bony union was obtained in about twelve weeks in one case and in five months in the other case. At the end of three and one-half years, both grafts had been transformed into tubular bone.—E.D.M., M.D.

The
BROWN SCHOOL
For Exceptional Children

Four distinct units. Tiny Tots through the Teens. Ranch for older boys. Special attention given to educational and emotional difficulties. Speech, Music, Arts and Crafts. A staff of 12 teachers. Full time Psychologist. Under the daily supervision of a Certified Psychiatrist. Registered Nurses. Private swimming pool, fireprof building. View book. Approved by State Division of Special Education.

•

BERT P. BROWN, Director
PAUL L. WHITE, M.D., F.A.P.A.,
Medical Director
Box 3028, South Austin 13, Texas

CREDIT SERVICE
330 American National Building
Oklahoma City, Oklahoma
(Operators of Medical-Dental Credit Bureau)

We offer a dignified and effective collection service for doctors and hospitals located anywhere in the State. Write for information.

28 YEARS
Experience In Credit and Collection Work
Robt. R. Sesline, Owner and Manager

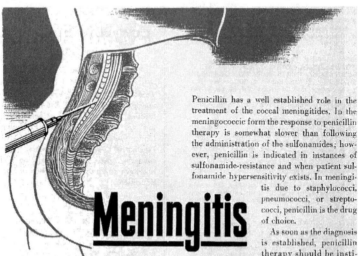

Meningitis

No. 4

IN SCHENLEY LABORATORIES CONTINUING SUMMARY OF PENICILLIN THERAPY....

BEFORE YOU DECIDE ON THE PENICILLIN OF YOUR CHOICE

For many years, Schenley has been among the world's largest users of research on mycology and fermentation processes. In addition, Schenley Laboratories manufactures a complete line of superior penicillin products — products thoroughly tested for potency and quality. These two important facts mean you may give your patients the full benefits of complete penicillin therapy.

Penicillin has a well established role in the treatment of the coccal meningitides. In the meningococcic form the response to penicillin therapy is somewhat slower than following the administration of the sulfonamides; however, penicillin is indicated in instances of sulfonamide-resistance and when patient sulfonamide hypersensitivity exists. In meningitis due to staphylococci, pneumococci, or streptococci, penicillin is the drug of choice.

As soon as the diagnosis is established, penicillin therapy should be instituted in doses of 20,000 to 40,000 units every two to three hours by the intramuscular route. Treatment should be thorough, and should be continued until all signs and symptoms of the infection have been absent for seven to ten days. Since penicillin administered systemically does not penetrate the subarachnoid space, intrathecal (intraspinal, intracisternal, intraventricular) administration is also required. Ten thousand units in 10 cc. of isotonic solution of sodium chloride should be injected (after withdrawal of an equal volume of fluid) once or twice daily until the spinal fluid is clear, and for four days thereafter.

When concurrent sulfonamides are indicated, they should be administered in a dosage sufficient to establish a blood level of 15 mg. per cent.

Surgical, supportive, and other measures should be employed when indicated.

PENICILLIN SCHENLEY

a product of

SPINK, W. W., and HALL, W. H.: *Penicillin Therapy at the University of Minnesota Hospitals* 1942-1944, Ann. Int. Med. 22:510 (April) 1945.

WHITE, W. L.; MURPHY, F. D.; LOCKWOOD, J. S., and FLIPPIN, H. F.: *Penicillin in the Treatment of Pneumococcal, Meningococcal, Streptococcal, and Staphylococcal Meningitis*, Am. J. Med. Sc. 210:1 (July) 1945.

SCHENLEY LABORATORIES, INC. Executive Offices: 350 Fifth Avenue, New York City

MANDIBULAR TUMORS. A Clinical, Roentgenographic and Histopathologic Study. Louis T. Byars and Bernard G. Sarnat. Surgery, Gynecology and Obstetrics. Vol. 83, No. 3, pp. 355-364; September, 1946.

This is a timely article and well worth reading by not only the surgeon but by the dentist and the radiologist. It reiterates a cardinal principle in the treatment of malignancy — namely, that a correct diagnosis is to only be made by microscopic study of the involved tissue.

"Because the ameloblastoma is generally considered to be a benign tumor, and because the roentgenographic pictures may be similar to malignant lesions primarily or secondarily in the jaw, it is of paramount importance to make an early correct diagnosis."

"The primary value of the roentgenogram is to demonstrate the site and extent of the multilocular lesions of the mandible."—J.F.B., M.D.

ASEPTIC NECROSIS OF THE CAPITAL FEMORAL ADOLESCENT EPIPHYSEOLYSIS. Robert D. Moore. Surgery, Gynecology and Obstetrics. Vol. 80, pp. 199-204, 1945.

Moore reviews the literature dealing with descriptions of femoral epiphyseal pathological lesions and gives a detailed account of the macroscopic and microscopic findings in two cases of slipped femoral epiphysis. The article is a purely descriptive recording and offers no explanation as to cause.

This paper may be summarized briefly, as follows: After interruption of the blood supply to the epiphysis in adolescents, the overlying articular cartilage may remain viable or may undergo partial or complete necrosis. In either case, subsequent degenerative and reparative changes apparently result in reduction of the depth of the articular cartilage, as occurs in the adult with aseptic

necrosis of the head, following fracture of the neck of the femur. This is in contrast to the changes seen in Legg-Perthes disease, where rapid growth of the living articular cartilage compensates for any absorption or ossification of the cartilage which takes place after revascularization of the ossification center. Under these circumstances, the depth of the articular cartilage usually increases.—E.D.M., M.D.

TRAUMATIC OSTEOMYELITIS: THE USE OF SKIN GRAFTS—PART 1. TECHNIC AND RESULTS. Robert P. Kelly, Louis M. Rosati, and Robert A. Murray. Annals of Surgery. Vol. 122, pp. 1-11, 1945.

These authors report on the satisfactory use of skin grafting in the treatment of osteomyelitis. The technique is fully described. Emphasis is given to the need for a thorough preliminary saucerization and the equal need for applying the grafts so that compression can be distributed evenly to all of them. On the bases of approximately one hundred cases treated by the method described, it is believed that this is a safe form of treatment and that it will give beneficial results in the majority of instances. While occasional reports of the successful use of skin grafts in the treatment of osteomyelitis have appeared in the literature for many years, the method has not received wide use. The authors hope that this encouraging report will stimulate others to apply this treatment.—E.D.M., M.D.

KEY TO ABSTRACTORS

M.D.H., M.D.	Marvin D. Henley, M.D.
G.P., M.D.	Grider Penick, M.D.
E.D.M., M.D.	Earl D. McBride, M.D.
H.J., M.D.	Hugh Jeter, M.D.
J.F.B., M.D.	John F. Burton, M.D.

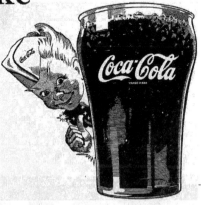

Have a Coke

When you laugh, the world laughs with you, as they say—and when you enjoy *the pause that refreshes* with ice-cold Coca-Cola, your friends enjoy it with you, too. Everybody enjoys the friendly hospitality that goes with the invitation *Have a Coke.* Those three words mean *Friend, you belong —I'm glad to be with you.* Good company is better company over a Coca-Cola.

Obituaries

George H. Clulow, M.D.
1880-1946

George H. Clulow, M.D., passed away on August 17 at the Hillcrest Memorial Hospital of Tulsa following an illness of only a few days.

Since coming to Oklahoma in 1913 Dr. Clulow had practiced in Tulsa until January 1 of this year when he accepted a position on the staff of the Western Oklahoma State Hospital at Fort Supply.

A native of Pennsylvania, Dr. Clulow was born January 15, 1880, and received an A. B. degree from Allegheny College in Meadville, Pennsylvania, in 1909 and an M. D. degree from the Western Reserve Medical School of Cleveland in 1912.

In World War I Dr. Clulow served two years with the 3rd Division and was retired with the rank of Major. He was a member of the Woodward County Medical Society, the Oklahoma State Medical Association and the American Medical Association.

Survivors include Dr. Clulow's wife, Anna, Fort Supply; a son, Mack, Tulsa, and a daughter, Doris, Tulsa.

T. D. Rowland, M.D.
1870-1946

T. D. Rowland, M.D., Shawnee physician since 1902, died in a hospital there September 3.

A native of Tippah, Mississippi, Dr. Rowland came to Shawnee after graduation from the Memphis Hospital Medical College in 1902. He was born November 3, 1870.

Dr. Rowland served overseas for one year during World War I. He was a member of the First Christian Church, the Masonic Lodge and the American Legion. He also held membership in the American Medical Association, the Oklahoma State Medical Association and the Pottawatomie County Medical Society, which he had served as president.

E. K. Collier, M.D.
1903-1946

E. K. Collier, M.D., of Tipton died August 9 in a Norman hospital.

Dr. Collier was born March 25, 1903, near Elmer, Oklahoma, and was reared in Tipton, attending Marion Military University in Alabama, Georgetown University in Texas, the University of Texas, and was graduated from the University of Oklahoma with a B. S. degree and Tulane University with an M. D. degree. His practice in Tipton had extended over a period of 15 years.

Surviving Dr. Collier are his mother, Mrs. Mabel Norfleet Collier; a son, Robert John; a brother, Dr. Roy Collier, and two sisters, Mrs. Helen Anderson and Mrs. Miriam Christian.

Elsie Specht, M.D.
1883-1946

Elsie Specht, M.D., died August 20 in an Enid hospital at the age of 63.

Forty-one years of medical practice in Fairview had been completed by Dr. Specht. She was a member of the Methodist Church in Fairview, the Garfield County Medical Society, the Oklahoma State Medical Association, and the American Medical Association.

L. C. Vance, M.D.
1894-1946

L. C. Vance, M.D., of Ponca City died September 7th of a heart attack. Services were conducted September 9th in the First Baptist Church of Ponca City.

Dr. Vance maintained offices in Ponca City from 1921 until the time of his death, during which time he had been active in many civic organizations and activities. He was a member of the Kay County Medical Society, the Oklahoma State Medical Association, and the American Medical Association.

He is survived by a daughter, Mary Ann, a son, Tex, and two sisters.

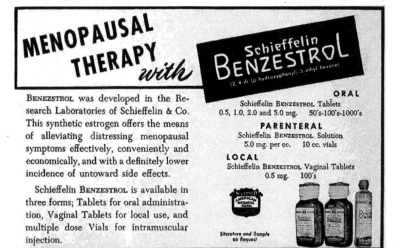

MENOPAUSAL THERAPY with Schieffelin BENZESTROL
(2, 4-di (p-hydroxyphenyl); 3-ethyl hexone)

BENEZSTROL was developed in the Research Laboratories of Schieffelin & Co. This synthetic estrogen offers the means of alleviating distressing menopausal symptoms effectively, conveniently and economically, and with a definitely lower incidence of untoward side effects.

Schieffelin BENZESTROL is available in three forms; Tablets for oral administration, Vaginal Tablets for local use, and multiple dose Vials for intramuscular injection.

ORAL
Schieffelin BENZESTROL Tablets
0.5, 1.0, 2.0 and 5.0 mg.   50's-100's-1000's

PARENTERAL
Schieffelin BENZESTROL Solution
5.0 mg. per cc.   10 cc. vials

LOCAL
Schieffelin BENZESTROL Vaginal Tablets
0.5 mg.   100's

Literature and Sample
on Request

Schieffelin & Co.   Pharmaceutical and Research Laboratories
20 Cooper Square   New York 3, N. Y.

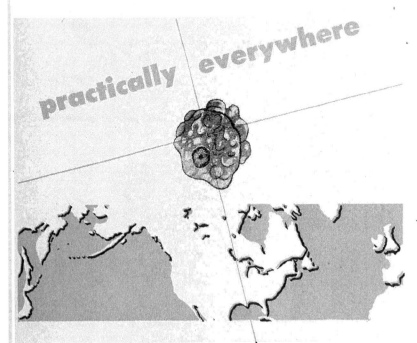

practically everywhere

... including the temperate zones, an
unexpectedly high percentage of carriers of
Endamoeba histolytica is to be found.

DIODOQUIN

(5,7-diiodo-8-hydroxyquinoline)

—potent amebicide—can be used in suspected
as well as proved cases of amebiasis.
Accepted by the Council on Pharmacy and Chemistry
of the American Medical Association.

Diodoquin is the registered trademark of
G. D. Searle & Co., Chicago 80, Illinois

SEARLE

RESEARCH
IN THE SERVICE
OF MEDICINE

Doctor—Judge

PHILIP MORRIS suggests *you* judge . . . from the evidence of your own *personal* observations . . . the value of PHILIP MORRIS Cigarettes to your patients with sensitive throats.

PUBLISHED STUDIES* SHOWED WHEN SMOKERS CHANGED TO PHILIP MORRIS SUBSTANTIALLY EVERY CASE OF THROAT IRRITATION DUE TO SMOKING CLEARED COMPLETELY, OR DEFINITELY IMPROVED.

But naturally, no published tests, no matter how authoritative, can be as completely convincing as results you will observe for yourself.

PHILIP MORRIS

PHILIP MORRIS & CO., LTD., INC.
119 FIFTH AVENUE, NEW YORK, N. Y.

*Laryngoscope, Feb. 1935, Vol. XLV, No. 2, 149-154.
Laryngoscope, Jan. 1937, Vol. XLVII, No. 1, 58-60.

TO THE DOCTOR WHO SMOKES A PIPE: We suggest an unusually fine new blend— COUNTRY DOCTOR PIPE MIXTURE. Made by the same process as used in the manufacture of Philip Morris Cigarettes.

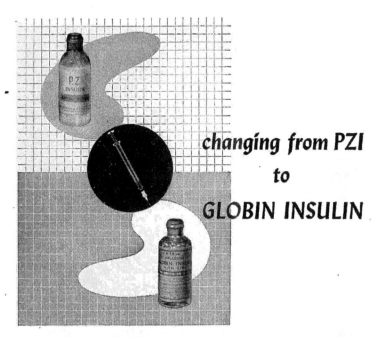

changing from PZI
to
GLOBIN INSULIN

When protamine zinc insulin treatment is complicated by post-prandial hyperglycemia, nocturnal insulin reaction, protamine sensitivity, or other difficulties, a change to Globin Insulin often results in the desired improvement. The change is achieved in three steps:

1. THE INITIAL CHANGE-OVER DOSAGE: The first day, 30 minutes or more before breakfast, give a single dose of Globin Insulin, equal to ½ the total previous daily dose of protamine zinc insulin or of protamine zinc insulin combined with regular insulin. The next day, dose may be increased to ⅔ former total.

2. ADJUSTMENT TO 24-HOUR CONTROL: Gradually adjust the Globin Insulin dosage to provide 24-hour control as evidenced by a fasting blood sugar level of less than 150 mgm. or sugar-free urine in the fasting sample.

3. ADJUSTMENT OF DIET: Simultaneously adjust carbohydrate distribution of diet to balance insulin activity; initially 2/10, 4/10 and 4/10. Any midafternoon hypoglycemia may usually be offset by 10 to 20 grams carbohydrate at 3 to 4 p.m. Base final carbohydrate adjustment on fractional urinalyses.

Most mild and many moderately severe cases may be controlled by *one daily injection of 'Wellcome' Globin Insulin with Zinc.* Vials of 10 cc.; 40 and 80 units per cc. Developed in The Wellcome Research Laboratories, Tuckahoe, New York. U.S. Pat. 2,161,198. Literature on request.

'Wellcome' Trademark Registered

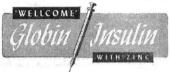

BURROUGHS WELLCOME & CO. (U.S.A.) INC., 9 & 11 EAST 41ST STREET, NEW YORK 17, N.Y.

OFFICERS OF COUNTY SOCIETIES, 1946

★

COUNTY	PRESIDENT	SECRETARY	MEETING TIME
Alfalfa	W. G. Dunnington, Cherokee	L. T. Lancaster, Cherokee	Last Tues. each Second Month
Atoka-Coal	J. B. Clark, Coalgate	J. S. Fulton, Atoka	
Beckham	P. J. DeVanney, Sayre	J. E. Levick, Elk City	Second Tuesday
Blaine	W. F. Bohlman, Watonga	Virginia Curtin, Watonga	Third Thursday
Bryan	W. K. Haynie, Durant	Jonah Nichols, Durant	Second Tuesday
Caddo	P. H. Anderson, Anadarko	Edward T. Cook, Jr., Anadarko	Third Thursday
Canadian	G. L. Goodman, Yukon	W. P. Lawton, El Reno	Subject to call
Carter	J. Hobson Veazey, Ardmore	H. A. Higgins, Ardmore	Second Tuesday
Cherokee	P. H. Medearis, Tahlequah	R. K. McIntosh, Jr., Tahlequah	First Tuesday
Choctaw	Floyd L. Waters, Hugo	O. R. Gregg, Hugo	
Cleveland	James O. Hood, Norman	Phil Haddock, Norman	Thursday nights
Comanche	Wm. Cole, Lawton	E. P. Hathaway, Lawton	
Cotton	G. W. Baker, Walters	Mollie Seism, Walters	Third Friday
Craig	Lloyd H. McPike, Vinita	J. M. McMillan, Vinita	
Creek	W. P. Longmire, Sapulpa	Philip Joseph, Sapulpa	Second Tuesday
Custer	Ross Deputy, Clinton	C. J. Alexander, Clinton	Third Thursday
Garfield	Bruce Hinson, Enid	John R. Walker, Enid	Fourth Thursday
Garvin	M. E. Robberson, Jr., Wynnewood	John R. Callaway, Pauls Valley	Wednesday before Third Thursday
Grady	Roy Emanuel, Chickasha	Rebecca H. Mason, Chickasha	Third Thursday
Grant	I. V. Hardy, Medford	F. P. Robinson, Pond Creek	
Greer	J. B. Lansden, Granite	J. B. Hollis, Mangum	
Harmon	W. G. Husband, Hollis	R. H. Lynch, Hollis	First Wednesday
Haskell	Wm. S. Carson, Keota	N. K. Williams, McCurtain	
Hughes	Victor W. Pryor, Holdenville	L. A. S. Johnston, Holdenville	First Friday
Jackson	E. W. Mabry, Altus	J. P. Irby, Altus	Last Monday
Jefferson	F. M. Edwards, Ringling	J. A. Dillard, Waurika	Second Monday
Kay	L. G. Neal, Ponca City	J. C. Wagner, Ponca City	Second Thursday
Kingfisher	John W. Pendleton, Kingfisher	H. Violet Sturgeon, Hennessey	
Kiowa	Wm. Bernell, Hobart	J. Wm. Finch, Hobart	
LeFlore	S. D. Bevill, Poteau	Rush L. Wright, Poteau	First Wednesday
Lincoln	J. S. Rollins, Prague	Ned Burleson, Prague	Last Tuesday
Logan	James Petty, Guthrie	J. E. Souter, Guthrie	
Marshall			
Mayes	L. O. White, Adair	V. D. Herrington, Pryor	
McClain	S. C. Davis, Blanchard	W. C. McCurdy, Purcell	
McCurtain	J. T. Moreland, Idabel	R. H. Sherrill, Broken Bow	Fourth Tuesday
McIntosh	F. R. First, Checotah	W. A. Tolleson, Eufaula	First Thursday
Muskogee-Sequoyah			
Wagoner	R. N. Holcombe, Muskogee	William N. Weaver, Muskogee	First Tuesday
Noble	A. M. Evans, Perry	Jesse W. Driver, Perry	
Okfuskee	W. P. Jenkins, Okemah	M. L. Whitney, Okemah	Second Monday
Oklahoma	W. F. Keller, Okla. City	John H. Lamb, Okla. City	Fourth Tuesday
Okmulgee	F. S. Watson, Okmulgee	C. E. Smith, Henryetta	Second Monday
Osage	E. O. Keyes, Hominy	Vincent Mazzarella, Hominy	Third Monday
Ottawa	C. F. Walker, Grove	W. Jackson Sayles, Miami	Second Thursday
Pawnee	H. B. Spaulding, Ralston	R. L. Browning, Pawnee	
Payne	F. Keith Oehlschlager, Yale	C. W. Moore, Stillwater	Third Thursday
Pittsburg	Millard L. Henry, McAlester	Edward D. Greenberger, McAlester	Third Friday
Pontotoc-Murray	John Morey, Ada	R. H. Mayes, Ada	First Wednesday
Pottawatomie	F. P. Newlin, Shawnee	Clinton Gallaher, Shawnee	First and Third Saturday
Pushmataha	John S. Lawson, Clayton	B. M. Huckabay, Antlers	
Rogers	W. A. Howard, Chelsea	P. S. Anderson, Claremore	Third Wednesday
Seminole	Clifton Felts, Seminole	Mack I. Shanholz, Wewoka	Third Wednesday
Stephens	Everett King, Duncan	Fred L. Patterson, Duncan	
Texas	Daniel S. Lee, Guymon	E. L. Buford, Guymon	
Tillman	H. A. Calvert, Frederick	O. G. Bacon, Frederick	
Tulsa	John C. Perry, Tulsa	John E. McDonald, Tulsa	Second and Fourth Monday
Washington-Nowata	Ralph W. Rucker, Bartlesville	L. B. Word, Bartlesville	Second Wednesday
Washita	L. G. Livingston, Cordell	Roy W. Anderson, Cordell	
Woods	John F. Simon, Alva	O. E. Templin, Alva	Last Tuesday Odd Months
Woodward	T. C. Leachman, Woodward	G. W. Tedrowe, Woodward	Second Thursday

THE JOURNAL
of the
OKLAHOMA STATE MEDICAL ASSOCIATION

| VOLUME XXXIX | OKLAHOMA CITY, OKLAHOMA, NOVEMBER, 1946 | NUMBER 11 |

Erythema Multiforme, With Unusual Manifestations*

JAMES STEVENSON, M.D.

TULSA, OKLAHOMA

Erythema multiforme is an acute, inflammatory eruptive disease, of unknown cause, ordinarily running a mild uneventful course. The skin lesions are varied in appearance consisting of erythematous macules, papules, nodules, and bullae. Color changes resembling purpura, or hemorrhage into bullous lesions (iris lesions) are common. The distribution is generally characteristic, the lesions occurring chiefly on the dorsum of the hands, the extensor surfaces of the extremities, face, neck and the buccal mucosal membranes. The condition is sometimes recurrent, with attacks occurring usually in the spring or fall months.

The disease is simulated by other conditions and at the onset a difficult diagnostic problem may present itself. The various forms of purpura, bullous impetigo, pemphigus vulgaris and certain drug eruptions (the sulfonamides, the halogens, salicylates, barbiturates and phenolphthalein) often simulate erythema multiforme.

The treatment in the past has been largely empiric and extremely varied. As ordinarily the disease runs a self limited and mild course this does not seem important. Recently, in a severe case, with involvement of the mucous membranes, H. C. Robinson[1] used penicillin. Weisberg and Rosen[2] believe large doses of nicotinic acid (100 milligrams, four times daily) of great benefit. Occasionally, erythema multiforme assumes a febrile course and the symptoms of a prostrating toxemia. In these cases the mucous membranes are largely involved with bullous lesions, as well as the usual cutaneous lesions. Osler[3] reported 29 cases of erythema multiforme with visceral complications. There

*Presented before the Section on Dermatology and Radiology, Oklahoma State Medical Association Annual Meeting, May 1, 1946.

were seven deaths in this group. Later, in 1914[4] he reported these cases as purpura. Another early case[5] reported by de Amicis appears also to be a case of Henochs purpura rather than erythema multiforme.

LESIONS OF THE MUCOUS MEMBRANES

1. Lesions of the Oral and Laryngeal Mucosa:

Oral lesions are usually bullous from the onset. The bullae rupture early, leaving crusted erosions. The lips, tongue and gums may be swollen.

Rendu[6], and later Rendu and Fiessinger, thought they were dealing with a new disease and termed it ectodermosis erosiva pluriorificialis. Some subsequent French and German writers, in reporting cases, also believed they were treating new diseases. Later reporters of this syndrome firmly established this condition as erythema multiforme of an unusually severe type.

2. Conjunctival Lesions:

The mildest and by far the most common form of conjunctival involvement is the catarrhal form. This form usually heals in a few weeks, and causes no permanent damage to the eyes. Another form, the purulent type may lead to corneal ulceration with subsequent corneal perforation and panophthalmitis. Such destructive complications were first reported by Stevens and Johnson[7]. A third form, the pseudo-membraneous, also may appear, and if severe, may be chronic, the clinical picture being identical with that observed in the third stage of trachoma[8].

3. Lesions of the Glans Penis and Anal Mucosa:

While lesions of the anal mucosa and glans penis have been observed, in only one case has there been a serious complication — in that, there occurred prolapse of the anal mucosa, and subsequent sloughing.

4. Tracheal and Bronchial Lesions:

While not described in the textbooks,·a number of cases of tracheo-bronchitis appear in the literature, with sometimes broncho-pneumonia as a sequel.

REPORT OF A CASE

P. T., an American white girl, aged 10, on November 3, 1941, was at a picnic. November 4 she complained of a headache, and had an urticarial eruption on her left fore-arm. During the next few days similar lesions appeared on her abdomen, and she had a temperature of 100 degree, for which aspirin was taken. On November 8 the skin eruption suddenly became generalized, sparing the scalp, palms and soles, her lips were swollen and she complained of photophobia. It was thought she had measles. That night blebs first appeared on her chest, tongue and oral mucous membrane, and the photophobia became marked. November 9 blebs appeared on the palms and soles, and the lips, tongue and oral mucous membrane became so "raw and sore" that the child took food and water with great effort, and she became alarmingly ill, following a shower of blebs appearing on her chest and abdomen.

On admission to the hospital at 9:00 P.M. on November 10, the child appeared acutely ill. Her temperature was 101.2 degrees. Marked photophobia was noted, the conjunctivae were much injected, the eyelids edematous and the eyelashes matted together from a purulent exudate. The lips were swollen and covered with thick crusts. The tongue and oral mucous membrane showed many erosions from ruptured bullae. The skin of the entire body, sparing only the scalp, was involved in a maculo-papular eruption. On the chest, abdomen and extremities were numerous bullae, the largest measuring 15 x 8 cm. Where there were no bullae, the skin could be removed easily (Nikolsky sign). The vulvae and vaginal mucous membranes were red, tender, and raw from ruptured bullae and bathed in a purulent discharge.

.On November 11 the temperature reached 103.2 degrees and on November 12, 104.8 degrees and she appeared to be near death. Numerous new belbs appeared including one involving the entire left palm. A blood transfusion (300 cc) was given at this time. As the child seemed unable to swallow she was given daily infusions intravenously of five per cent glucose in isotonic solution of sodium chloride.

On November 17 a few new blebs appeared on the chest and arms, but the temperature subsided to normal. After six days of an afebrile course, on November 23, the febrile course returned, the temperature reaching 103.4 degrees on the second day, without any change in the cutaneous symtpoms. On November 27 the temperature returned to normal. The skin gradually returned to normal, although some pigmentation remained at the site of the blebs for weeks. The eyes become normal, and there was no impairment of vision. The child made an uneventful recovery and was discharged December 30, 1941.

Laboratory Examination: On the patient's admission to the hospital the Kahn and Kline blood tests were negative. The number of erythrocytes was 5,000,000 and the number of leucocytes 8,050. The hemagloblin content was 14.5 grams (83 per cent). A differential count showed 52 per cent neutrophils, 32 per cent lymphocytes, 14 per cent mononuclears, 1 per cent each eosinophils and basophils. The blood count did not vary notably during her entire illness. A trace of albumin was present in the urine during the height of the disease. Throat cultures showed gram positive diplococci and staphylococci.

TREATMENT

Treatment consisted of one blood transfusion, many intravenous infusions of five per cent glucose in isotonic sodium chloride solution, daily injections of 1 cc. liver extract. Sulfathiazole, grain 7½ every 4 hours was given for a time, but appeared to have no effect upon the disease.

BIBLIOGRAPHY

1. H. C. Robinson; Archives of Dermatology and Syphilology, Volume No. 52, page 91; August, 1945.

2. Capt. Aaron Weisberg and Capt. Emanuel Rosen: Erythema Exudativum Multiforme; Archives of Dermatology and Syphilology, Volume No. 53, page 99; February, 1946.

3. W. Osler: On the Visceral Complications of Erythma Exudativum Multiforme; American Journal of the Medical Sciences, Volume No. 110, page 629; 1895.

4. W. Osler: The Visceral Lesions of the Erythma Group of the Skin Diseases; American Journal of the Medical Sciences, Volume No. 127, page 1; 1904.

5. A. de Amicis: Ein Fall van Erythema Exudativum Multiforme Hemorrhagicum mit Exitus Letalis; Archiv fur Dermatologie and Syphilis.

6. R. Rendu: Six noveau cas d'un Maladie infectiense caracterisee par l'inflammation des muqueuses conjunctival, nasale, bucco-pharyngee et preputinle, et, accessoirement par une eruption vesico-bullense des membres; Presse Medical, Volume No. 35, page 662; 1917.

7. A. M Stevens and F. C. Johnson; A New Eruptive Fever Associated with Stomatitis and Aphthalmia; American Journal of Diseases of Children, Volume No. 24, page 526; December, 1922.

8. W L. Duke-Elder; Textbook of Ophthalmology, Volume No. 2, page 1733; C. V. Mosby Co., St. Louis, Mo.; 1938.

Announcement

The American Academy of Allergy will hold its annual convention at Hotel Pennsylvania, New York City, November 25-27 inclusive. All physicians interested in allegic problems are cordially invited to attend the sessions as guests of the Academy without payment of registration fee. The program has been arranged to cover a wide variety of conditions where allergic factors may be important. Papers will be presented dealing with the latest methods of diagnosis and treatment as well as the results of investigation and research. Advance copies · of the program may be obtained by writing to the Chairman on Arrangements, Dr. Horace S. Baldwin, 136 East 64th Street, New York City, prior to November 10th.

The Value of the Antero-Posterior Lordotic Film of the Chest*

J. R. DANSTROM, M.D.

OKLAHOMA CITY, OKLAHOMA

The purpose of this paper is to describe the antero-posterior lordotic projection in the examination of the lungs, to show the usefulness of this film and to present several cases illustrating its value.

This projection, used to visualize the pulmonary apices, is not a new one. However, that it has been overlooked by, or is not known to, many radiologists is best attested by the paucity of articles on this subject in the medical literature. The method of examination is described in several textbooks on roentgen technique, including those of Sante[1], McNeil[2], and Clark[3]. Cole[4] has used this view in studying the conus arteriosus and the pulmonary artery. Lindblom[5] described its use in pulmonary disease. During the past few years this film was used rather extensively in the services[6][7] and its value in the diagnosis of apical lesions was definitely established.

The routine films of the chest and fluoroscopy and lateral and oblique projections are usually satisfactory for most diagnostic purposes. In some cases special views of the apex are needed.

The apices of the lungs are often poorly visualized and confusing shadows are seen because of the many anatomic structures overlying this small area. These include:

1. Skin, subcutaneous tissue, and muscle.

2. Vascular and nerve structures, including the subclavian artery and vein and branches of the brachial plexus.

3. Bony structures, including the clavicle, the posterior portion of the upper three or four ribs and the anterior portion of the first rib.

Several radiological methods have been used in the attempt to better visualize the apices. The arms have been elevated to displace the clavicles and the tube angled. This method is not satisfactory since too often only the outer portion of the clavicle is displaced and not the obscuring medical portion. Another method[8] is to make the exposure in deep expiration. Here again the visualization

*Presented before the Section on Dermatology and Radiology, Oklahoma State Medical Association Annual Meeting, May 2, 1946.

depends on the movement of the bony thorax. Other methods include over exposure with a Potter-Bucky diaphram and laminagraphy. These methods are of unquestioned value, but laminagraphy is expensive and not available to many of us.

For the past few years we have been using this lordotic film for visualizing the apices. It is an extremely simple method, is inexpensive and requires no special apparatus.

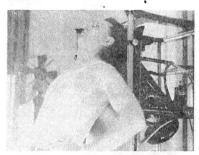

(Figure 1)

A 10 x 12 film is used. The patient faces the tube and leans backward against the cassette with knees slightly bent and the abdomen protruding in extreme lordosis. The central ray of the tube is directed horizontally. The technical factors are the same as for the routine postero-anterior film with the time factor doubled. (Figure 1).

The lordotic projection has been of most value to us in cases of minimal tuberculosis — in discerning the size and character of the lesion and in revealing unsuspected cavitation. It has also been extremely useful in ruling suspicious shadows out of the pulmonary field and proving them to be merely soft tissue shadows. The film has even proven to be helpful in more advanced tuberculosis in showing the extent of cavity formation.

Case 1 (Figure 2) shows a hazy area overlying the right apex. The lordotic film (Figure 3) shows the lung to be entirely clear, demonstrating that the density seen on the PA film was purely a soft tissue shadow and not in the apical lung tissue. It will be noted on the lordotic projection that the clavicle is elevated above the dome of the lung and that the ribs are horizontal.

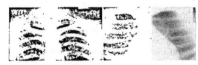

(Figure 2)   (Figure 3)

Case II (Figure 4) shows an infiltrate beneath the first anterior rib on the right with involvement of the apex. The lordotic film (Figure 5) reveals the true size and

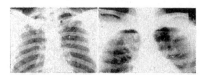

(Figure 4)   (Figure 5)

configuration of this tuberculous lesion and the amount of calcium within it.

Case III (Figure 6) shows what would appear to be a dense solid infiltrate in the right

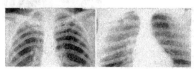

(Figure 6)   (Figure 7)

apex. The lordotic film (Figure 7) beautifully reveals the lesion — a doughnut shaped, fibrous nodule with central cavitation. Thus, an apparently stable appearing lesion on the routine 14 x 17 film is proven to be unstable with cavitation.

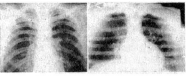

(Figure 8)   (Figure 9)

Case IV (Figure 8) shows a dense calcification near the end of the first rib and

under the clavicle. The lordotic film (Figure 9) proves this to be outside of the lung field and to be densely calcified cartilage at the anterior end of the first rib.

Case V (Figure 10) reveals a moderately advanced tuberculous infiltration in both upper lobes and apices with small cavities vis-

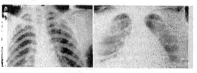

(Figure 10)   (Figure 11)

ualized in both first interspaces. (Figure 11) demonstrates the value of the lordotic film even in more advanced tuberculosis. On this film three separate cavities can be seen in each apex which were not revealed on the 14 x 17 film.

Case VI (Figure 12) shows infiltration in the right apex and first interspace with evi-

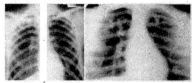

(Figure 12)   (Figure 13)

dence of cavitation in the first interspace. The lordotic film (Figure 13) confirms the cavity seen on the PA film and also shows a thick walled cavity in the apex which was not seen on the 14 x 17 film.

Case VII (Figure 14) reveals a density in the right apex as well as the other fibrous and calcific deposits throughout the lungs.

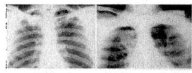

(Figure 14)   (Figure 15)

The lordotic film (Figure 15) proves the apical density to be a tuberculous lesion within the lung and also reveals the presence of a small cavity.

SUMMARY

The antero-posterior lordotic film of the pulmonary apices is described. Its value in the diagnosis of apical lesions is demonstrated by several illustrative cases.

BIBLIOGRAPHY

1. L. R. Sante: Manual of Roentgenological Technique. Edward Bros., Inc., Ann Arbor, Mich.; 1942.
2. C. McNeil: Roentgen Technique. Charles C. Thomas, Springfield, Ill.; 1945.
3. K. C. Clark: Positioning in Radiography. C. V. Mosby, St. Louis, Mo.; 1945.
4. G. C. Cole: The Conus Arteriosus and the Pulmonary Artery; American Journal Roentgenology, Volume No. 45, pp. 32-40; January, 1941.

5. K. Kindblam; Half Axial Projection in Accentuated Lordosis for Roentgen Studies of the Lungs; Acta Radiology, Volume No. 21, pp. 119-125; 1940.
6. G. Haynes and B. Coopleman: The Antero-Posterior Projection in the Roentgenographic Examination of the Lungs. Radiology, Volume No. 43, pp. 135-141; August, 1944.
7. N. E. Bass and S. I. Karperstern: Bulletin, U. S. Army Medical Department No. 84, pp. 102-103; January, 1945.
8. D. Salkin: Expiratory Roentgenograms for Pulmonary Apical Detail; American Journal Roentgenology, Volume No. 39, pp. 363-367; March, 1938.

Fatigue States Associated with Endocrine Disorders*

HENRY H. TURNER, M.D.

OKLAHOMA CITY, OKLAHOMA

Fatigue is, perhaps, the most common, the most baffling and often the most difficult to alleviate symptoms encountered in medical practice. Fatigue in a normal individual responds to average rest. It is a defense mechanism by which the body attempts to keep exertion within the limits of safety. Disregard of this danger signal may result in chronic asthenia. Continuous tiredness not responding to average rest is usually an indication of psychopathology, endocrine dysfunction, or general systemic disease.

Monotony from the repetition of unpleasant routine in office or home is fatiguing. This may also be observed in a precocious child who, because of parental objections to promotion on account of the chronological age of the youngster or because of school requirements, is kept in a grade below his mental capacity. The demands of modern civilization, if it may be called such, in business and in our homes necessitate overstimulation; especially is this true in the urban centers. This is met with more stimulation, sometimes induced by alcohol, or in the more sophisticated by amphetamine, and the end result, is always exhaustion.

Chronic tiredness is almost a constant complaint of those of psychoneurotic temperament. Such individuals fatigue easily and fatigue is conducive to nervousness; hence, a vicious cirle is established.

Though psychogenic factors are the precipitants of fatigue in the majority of instances, endocrine disorders are frequently accompanied by this symptom. This is not surprising when we consider there is likely no bodily function which is not in some manner influenced by the glands of internal secretion. They regulate the electrolyte balance and chemical concentrations in the blood and tissues, and have to do with water, fat, and sugar metabolism. They are concerned in nutrition, growth, sexual development, the regulation of body temperature, sleep, and other

mechanisms of the sympathetic nervous system. There is increasing evidence of their influence on psychic and emotional reactions and the conditioning of moods of elation and depression.

Asthenia of varying degrees is a prominent symptom of Addison's disease, pituitary failure, acromegalia in the regressive state, chronic parathyroid tetany, diabetes mellitus, hypothyroidism, hypogonadism, hyperinsulinism, and other hypoglycemic states.

The pituitary, because of its multiple hormonal effects, relationships with other endocrine glands, and its connections with the diencephalic nuclei, plays an important role in the fatigue syndrome. Through precision in the diagnosis of pituitary disorders is lacking to some extent, sufficient laboratory and clinical evidence of physiopathologic disturbances of the gland has accumulated to warrant the ascription of certain signs and symptoms associated with these changes.

Pituitary cachexia, or Simmonds' disease, is characterized by marked asthenia, loss of weight, a persistent hypotension, slow pulse, frequently hypothermia, intolerance to cold, obstinate constipation, anorexia, and physical and mental sluggishness. Though originally ascribed by Simmonds as being the result of atrophy or destruction of the gland, it is now recognized that the condition may be a functional one, transient or partial, of varying degree, and may be altered according to the intensity of the disturbance.

"One of the most perplexing clinical problems of the day, however, is the differentiation of this condition from that of anorexia nervosa, and in the majority of cases, even after most diligent investigation, the exact diagnosis must usually remain in doubt. It seems rather untenable that two diseases with essentially identical symptom complexes should have a totally different etiology."[1]

There is increasing evidence that continued severe emotional states may have a definite reaction on the gland. As our knowledge of pituitary-hypothalamic interrelation in-

*Presented before the Section on Neurology, Psychiatry and Endocrinology, Oklahoma State Medical Association Annual Meeting, May 1, 1946.

creases, it may help to clarify this baffling etiologic problem.

Asthenia is frequently observed in the so-called "burnt out" cases of acromegalia. It is often encountered in pituitary-hypothalamic syndromes, such as adiposogenitalism and in some instances of pituitary basophilism or Cushing's syndrome.

In hypothroidism, there is a lowering of all metabolic activity and a slowing of all bodily processes; hence, it is commonly the underlying cause of asthenic states. In an analysis of 100 of my patients with actual hypometabolism and other signs of thyroid subfunction, 86 per cent complained of fatigue. The more advanced states of thyroid deficiency are easily recognized, but they are rare in most sections of this country. It is those patients with moderately depressed basal metabolic readings, mild exhaustion, the so-called borderline cases, which are difficult to recognize. As a therapeutic test, it is permissible to note the response of these patients to small doses of thyroid. However, "thyroid deficiency" is now being diagnosed and treated with the same ease, abandon, and recklessness as the menopause. The promiscuous use of thyroid is to be deplored. Too much reliance cannot be placed on basal metabolic determinations since hypometabolism can result from a number of causes and in many cases does not respond to thyroid therapy.

The realization of these individuals with advanced hypothyroidism of their inability to carry on as formerly is often responsible for the development of various neuroses and other disturbed mental states and their complaints interpreted as primarily of neuropsychogenic origin.

Mild hyperthyroidism may also be accompanied by asthenia. These patients, of course, often respond to sufficient rest and sedation.

The parathyroids are definitely concerned with calcium and phosphorus metabolism. Hypofunction of these glands often results in a lowering of the total blood calcium, a rise in the blood phosphorus, and the clinical manifestations of tetany. Easy fatigability and neuromuscular irritability are constantly present in this symptom complex. Treatment may vary with the etiology, but whatever the underlying cause may be, the symptoms of tetany are the result of disturbance in the normal calcium balance of the body. Since the recent introduction of dihydrotachysterol, almost constant and dramatic results have been obtained in the control of chronic tetany associated with hypocalcemia.

Hyperparathyroidism is due to an overactivity of the parathyroid, and is most often associated with tumor or hyperplasia of the gland and accompanied by decalcification and deformities of the bones, hypercalcemia and hypophosphatemia, and increased deposition of calcium in various organs and itssues. Similar conditions may result from the continued injection of excessive amounts of parathyroid extract or the ingestion of overdoses of high potency Vitamin D, at present so commonly used in the treatment of arthritis, and of dihydrotachysterol. The clinical symptoms may vary according to the degree and duration of parathyroid overactivity and the systems affected. There may be general weakness, hypotonia, muscular and joint pain, difficulty in coordination and locomotion, and spontaneous fractures and deformities, due to involvement of the muscles and the skeleton. The most important and only treatment which has given a consistent and permanent result in the cure of hyperparathyroidism is surgical removal of the tumor or hyperplastic gland.

No acceptable data has been presented to account for the function of the thymus. Myasthenia gravis has been associated with thymic tumors, and relief of this most distressing and fata asthenia has followed thymectomy in some instances. However, much additional evidence is necessary before final acceptance of this theory.

The signs and symptoms of pancreatic subfunction, diabetes mellitus, are well recognized and need not be commented upon here.

In recent years, much interest has been evidenced in hyperinsulinism resulting from overactivity of the pancreas. The pathology is usually tumor or hyperplasia of the gland. The complaints are asthenia, faintiness, somnolence, dizziness, tremors, hunger, and at times convulsive episodes. The symptoms may vary with the degree of hypoglycemia. It is important to remember that lowering of blood sugar may result from causes other than hyperinsulinism. Less severe degrees of hypoglycemia may occur in pituitary subfunction, Addison's disease, hyperthyroidism, and certain physiopathologic disturbances of the liver. Surgical removal of the pancreatic tumor or partial resection of hyperplastic tissue when present is indicated. High-fat and low-carbohydrate diets are of value in some instances.

Fatigue, which may be profound, is a primary and constant symptom of adrenal cortical insufficiency. The diagnosis of the advanced Addisonian type of adrenal cortical insufficiency is based upon the severe asthenia, hypotension, pigmentation, gastrointestinal symptoms, and cahcexia. It is further evidenced by the findings of a lowered sodium and chloride concentration in the serum and their increase in the urine. Additional aid may be obtained from the patient's favorable response to injections of adrenal cortical hormone or to increased water and salt intake. Atypical cases or milder degrees of deficiency may not be so easily recognized. Pigmentation is not always present, and sodium and chloride concentrations in the blood and urine may be normal at times. However, the patient's favorable response to injections of the hormone or to high-salt feedings, or the increase of symptoms following reduction of sodium chloride intake would suggest the presence of an adrenal cortical deficiency.

Since the discovery of a synthetic cortical substance and of potent extracts of the gland itself, much controversy has arisen over the existence of subclinical adrenal adrenal cortical insufficiency as a causative factor of the milder degrees of exhaustion. Undoubtedly, many patients have been unnecessarily subjected to a long and expensive therapeutic regime on this assumption. However, it is logical to believe that the degree of adrenal function may vary much the same as that of the thyroid and other glands.

It is well known clinically and has been shown objectively in animal experiments that adrenal insufficiency may primarily affect the neuromuscular system and that these effects in the form of fatigue may occur long before other changes become evident. It is also a well known fact that in pronounced cases of adrenal insufficiency one patient may be adequately maintained by the administration of sodium chloride alone or by cortical extract, another by the synthetic substance desoxycorticosterone, while another may require combinations of these. This may suggest the deficiency of one or more hormones, or may be interpreted as the degree of insufficiency present. It is debatable whether or not extreme exhaustion resulting from undue stresses, infections and shock states is due to adrenal insufficiency though beneficial effects are sometimes obtained from cortical therapy in these conditions.

Fatigue is a prominent symptom of the male and female climacteric, and its alleviation by the administration of natural or synthetic androgens or estrogens is very dramatic at times. However, it is my opinion, which is shared by many others, that "menopause" is too frequently diagnosed and overtreated. Almost any female from 30 to 60 years of age who now-a-days dares complain of fatigue and its concomitants of neckache, tightness in the throat, palpitation, et cetera, is almost certain to be injected with estrogens or given stilbestrol. "Only a minority require any endocrine therapy at this time. Often the subjective symptomatology of these women may be handled more effectively and more economically by measures other than organotherapy. These include reassurance, establishment of a more physiologic hygiene of living, the affording of more rest and relaxation, a long-needed vacation, a more sympathetic attitude of the husband or the family, the dispelling of fears of cancer, the employment of small doses of sedatives, and so on. Sex hormones have a definite place but a limited one in the treatment of the distressing symptoms of the climacteric in both sexes."[1] Testosterone propionate stores nitrogen, inorganic phosphorus and sodium, and therefore may be of definite value in the older age groups of males.

There are many causes of chronic fatigue. Each patient presenting an exhaustion syndrome must be studied from the viewpoint of psychopathology, endocrine imbalance, and general systemic disease. The glands of internal secretion play an important part as the causative factor in many instances. A diagnosis is often difficult, and a careful case history, thorough physical examination, and at times extensive laboratory investigation are imperative. A sympathetic understanding of the patient's problem and common sense are necessary in the treatment. The dismissal of these individuals as "just another case of nerves" is not only poor medical practice, but is unfair to the patient.

BIBLIOGRAPHY

1. Therapeutics of Internal Diseases: Blumer; Diseases of the Endocrine Glands: Turner, Henry H ; D. Appleton-Century Co., Inc.

RADIUM

(Including Radium Applicators)

FOR ALL MEDICAL PURPOSES

Est. 1919

Quincy X-Ray and Radium Laboratories
(Owned and directed by a Physician-Radiologist)

HAROLD SWANBERG, B.S., M.D., Director

W.C.U. Bldg.   Quincy, Illinois

NEUROLOGICAL HOSPITAL

Twenty-Seventh and The Paseo
Kansas City, Missouri

Modern Hospitalization of Nervous and Mental Illnesses, Alcoholism and Drug Addiction.

THE ROBINSON CLINIC

G. WILSE ROBINSON, M.D.
G. WILSE ROBINSON, Jr., M.D.

Pioneer Users of X-Rays in Oklahoma [*]

PETER E. RUSSO, M.D.

OKLAHOMA CITY, OKLAHOMA

During the past year we celebrated the fiftieth anniversary of Roentgen's great discovery, the x-rays. Probably no other single scientific effort has proven so benefical to mankind.

Following Roentgen's work, many additional contributions, such as the Potter-Bucky diaphragm, the cellulose film, the Coolidge tube and many others, have been of considerable aid in the rapid advancement of this relatively new field of science. Medicine from the very beginning has been and still remains its greatest benefactor. Equipped with this new form of radiant energy, medicine has broadened its knowledge of human diseases not only in their diagnosis but likewise in their treatment. Many of the more recent advances in many of the specialties, notably Urology, Gastroenterology, Neuro and Thoracic Surgery can be directly attributed to the utilization of x-rays.

The founders of this new science, today referred to as Radiology, fortunately were men of learning, skill and courage. Often at the risk of life and limb they laid down the basic knowledge upon which was founded this specialty. Heeding their warnings and following their advice Radiology has attained its rightful place among the medical specialties. Today a training period of three years in this type of work is required after completion of a medical education and a recognized internship. In this way we of a later generation doing this line of work may better appreciate and assume the obligations and responsibilities entrusted to us.

There is still some question as to who was the first in America to reproduce x-rays after Roentgen made public his first communication on December 28, 1895. This startling scientific news was cabled to the entire civilized world from London on January 5, 1896. Otto Glasser in a recent publication sets forth the claims of over a dozen American scientists claiming this distinction[2].

However, he arrives at the conclusion that this is a most difficult matter to settle as none of these early x-rays were marked with the date they were taken. Nevertheless we are certain that only a few days and weeks after the announcement of the discovery, American physicians and physicists were making their own x-ray exposures.

So far in this discussion I have mentioned certain facts too well known to all of you, but they serve as a necessary introduction to the subject at hand. The Oklahoma Territory was opened to the white settlers in 1889, the year of the Great Run. Oklahoma City was also founded in that year. However even up to 1907, the year statehood was granted, it consisted of the Indian and Oklahoma Territories. It seems remarkable to learn that x-ray apparatus was used as early as 1901 in this state[3].

Dr. John Reck, a graduate of Marion Sims Medical College of St. Louis, class of 1893, after several years of practice in Missouri opened offices in Oklahoma in 1899. In 1901 he purchased a Waite Bartlett x-ray machine. Dr. Reck recalls that after acquiring this new apparatus it was first used in the successful localization and removal of a piece of sewing needle embedded in the hand of a washwoman. Five years later he sold this equipment when a radiation dermatitis and later burns developed in the skin of his hands and face. However Dr. Reck is still alive and in practice in Oklahoma City.

In the following year, 1902, another progressive Oklahoma City physician purchased his first x-ray machine, Dr. J. M. Postelle[3]. As were all machines of that era, this was a disc type and operated by hand. Two years later Dr. Postelle exchanged his equipment for a later model. This was a Schiedel-Western which featured a Leyden jar and a sulfuric acid pot condenser. However even this newer model had only limited use and often was unreliable and troublesome due to the gas tubes used in those days. Dr. Postelle claims another distinction in that he was the first to operate a chemical and bacteriological laboratory in this state. Dr. Postelle still maintains his office in the Medical Arts Building in Oklahoma City.

A Dr. Wall of Geary, Oklahoma, who practiced here for only a very short time and about whom very little is known also had

[*]Delivered before the Section on Dermatology and Radiology, Annual Meeting, Oklahoma State Medical Association, May 2, 1946.

equipped himself with an x-ray machine in 1902.

Dr. Everett S. Lain, to whom I am indebted for much of this information, located in Weatherford, Oklahoma, in 1902 and bought his first piece of x-ray equipment in 1903[3]. Later he moved his office to Oklahoma City and in 1908 he installed both a disc and coil type of machine which required the extension of a DC line direct to his office. The electric current for the coil apparatus was interrupted by means of a pot of kerosene containing quick silver. At weekly intervals the kerosene oil had to be changed and the mercury cleaned by passing it through a chamois skin. He too passed through the many griefs of the imperfect x-ray gas tubes. Dr. Lain had been inspired to pursue this line of work by a demonstration of an x-ray machine he attended during his senior year at the Medical School of Vanderbilt University in 1900. For two years he gave lectures on skin diseases and x-rays at the old Epworth Medical School. He continued to give lectures on these same subjects when this school became affiliated with the present Medical School of the University of Oklahoma in 1910. Dr. Lain served as head of the Department of Skin, X-ray and Radium for many years.

Dr. Marion M. Roland, now deceased, become affiliated with Dr. Lain in 1910. Later he moved to Muskogee bringing the first x-ray apparatus to that city. In 1915 Dr. Roland rejoined Dr. Lain in Oklahoma City until the beginning of the First World War. Dr. Roland enlisted and taught Roentgenology at an Army school. It was during this period that Dr. John E. Heatley first became interested in x-rays. After the Armistice he opened offices in diagnostic roentgenology with the encouragement of Drs. Roland and Lain. Dr. Heatley has served most ably as head of the x-ray department at University Hospitals for many years.

Dr. Lain was the first doctor in this state to purchase and use radium. His first investment was a 5 mg. plaque, the cost of which in those days was about five times its present value. Dr. Lain recalls that the only filtration used at that time were filters made of aluminum and dental rubber.

Dr. Leroy Long as dean of the Medical School was instrumental in the planning and building of the original University Hospital which included an up-to-date laboratory and x-ray department. The hospital was opened for public use in 1919[1].

We may also mention another distinction for our state. The first x-ray technician to take and successfully pass the examination given by the American Registry of X-ray Technicians in 1922 was Sister Beatrice of St. Anthony's Hospital, Oklahoma City.

As far as I have been able to learn these men were responsible for bringing to the people of Oklahoma the benefits derived from the most recent advances in medical science. It is a credit to these men and to the medical profession of the State. Progress however is a steady march and we of the younger generation must keep pace and continue to give the people of this state the best that medical science has to offer.

With your kind indulgence I would like to propose at this time that the members of this section form a state radiological society. There are listed in the Society Proceedings of the American Journal of Roentgenology about 52 local radiological societies in the large cities and states of this country, exclusive of the national organizations. It has been expressed by many of you present that there is a definite need for such an organization in this State. Medicine in general and our specialty in particular today is confronted by many problems. The proper solution of these problems could more easily be solved by the deliberations of such a group. By inaugurating such a movement at this time we may in a small way make a contribution to those who will follow in our foot-steps to carry on this type of work.

· BIBLIOGRAPHY

1. Hayes, Basil A.: Leroy Long; Norman University Press, 1943.

2. Glasser, Otto: Early American Roentgenograms; American Journal of Roentgenology; pp. 54-590; 1945.

3. Personal communications.

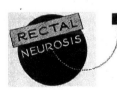

YOUNG'S Rectal Dilators

Rectal disturance is never trivial. Young's Rectal Dilators afford mechanical correction for bowel sluggishness when due to tight sphincter muscles. Effective elimination relieves nervous tension, permitting normal nerve reaction. Sold only by prescription. Obtainable at your surgical supply house; available for patients at ethical drug stores. Adults and children's sizes, in sets of 4 dilators. Write for Brochure.

F. E. YOUNG & CO. 424 E. 75TH STREET, CHICAGO 19, ILLINOIS

Clinical Pathological Conference

University of Oklahoma School of Medicine

Presented by the Departments of Pathology and Medicine

ROBERT H. BAYLEY, M.D. AND HOWARD C. HOPPS, M.D.

OKLAHOMA CITY, OKLAHOMA

DR. HOPPS: Our case for consideration this morning illustrates a disease which is very important in that it is one of the major causes of death. Pathologic findings are of special interest because of their close correlation with clinical manifestations. Dr. Bayley will present the clinical aspects.

PROTOCOL ·

Patient: C. W., colored female, age 64; admitted November 11, 1945, died November 17, 1945.

Chief Complaint: Stupor (few days), dyspnea (two years), swelling of feet (one month).

Present Illness: This patient was apparently in good health until two years prior to her death when she noted vertigo. This was attributed to a "weak heart and high blood pressure". After this she began to tire easily while working, became short of breath and had pain in the left shoulder and arm. She slept on two pillows. She did not consult a physician and apparently got along well until one month prior to death when she noted swelling of the feet and ankles. The sharp pain in the left shoulder radiating down the left arm became exaggerated· and she was unable to "get along" by sleeping on two pillows. She had to sit or stand to obtain relief from the dyspnea. She was seen by a physician. Medication and a special diet was prescribed, but in spite of this she became progressively worse and was admitted to the hospital one month later (six days before death).

Past and Family History: Not significant.

Physical Examination: The patient was a well developed colored woman, semicomatose and unable to cooperate. The respiration was shallow and rapid. The pupils were constricted. There were moist rales in both lungs throughout. The heart sounds were distant and sounded "spongy". The heart was enlarged to the anterior axillary line on the left. A soft mitral systolic murmur was

heard. The abdomen was flat. The liver was palpable three fingers below the costal margin on the right. Three plus pitting edema was present in the lower extermities.

Laboratory Data: On November 11, 1945, the urine was brownish yellow, clear and acid. The specific gravity was 1.024. There was 1 plus albumin, no glucose and no cells or casts. The hemoglobin was 9 Gm., the red blood cell count 2,222,000 and the white blood cell count 10,000 per cubic millimeter with 90 per cent neutrophils (4 per cent immature), 9 per cent lymphocytes, 0.5 per cent eosinophils and 0.5 per cent monocytes. On November 12, 1945, the N.P.N. was 44 mg./100 cc. and the blood sugar 105 mg/100 cc. The Mazzini test was 2 plus, the Kolmer-Wassermann negative. E.C.G. diagnosis on November 12, 1945, was: Large anterior antero-lateral and lateral infarction (extensive) recent (or old with superimposed acute generalized pericarditis). X-ray report on November 12, 1945, was: Increased density of right lung field shows patchy type distribution. Similar change on the left side to a lesser degree. Impression: Bronchopneumonia.

Clinical Course: An E.C.G. was taken to evaluate possible effects of digitalis. No such evidence was apparent so that rapid digitalization was begun. The patient's course was steadily downward, however, and she died on November 17, 1945.

CLINICAL DIAGNOSIS

DR. BAYLEY: The case today is that of a colored female, age 64, who was admitted to the hospital and lived only six days. This history was not obtained directly from the patient because she was in a semi-comatose condition. The patient is said to have had shortness of breath for two years and swelling of feet for one month. She was apparently in good health until this time. She complained also of vertigo and was told by her physician that she had high blood pressure. Hypertension of a severe type usually causes serious consequences before this age (64), more often in the mid-fifties, especially in women. These severe consequences usually relate to some lesion in either the heart, brain or kidneys. Of 100 fatal cases of hypertension, approximately 75 die of cardiac failure; 15 from a cerebrovascular accident and 10 from uremia. Soon after the onset of the present illness this patient began to tire easily, had pain in the shoulder and had to sleep on two pillows. We do not know, but it is reasonable to believe that the dyspnea probably came on after the onset of this pain. It was a sharp pain originating in the left shoulder and radiating down the left arm. If we keep in mind that the patient had hypertension, four common diagnostic possibilities should be considered: first, heart pain, because as hypertension progresses it may be associated with degenerative changes in the coronary arteries which finally lead to *angina pectoris*; second, d e g e n e r a t i v e changes in the walls of the aorta, usually the first portion of the aorta which may lead to extensive medial necrosis and *dissecting aneurysm*. In the majority of instances this dissection first involves the thoracic portion and may stop at the level of the diaphragm. After a time it may then extend into the abdominal aorta so that symptoms can occur in two stages, first thoracic and then abdominal. As this dissection extends it may compress the lumen and symptoms are often those characterized by occlusion of the aorta, numbness of extremities and paralysis. With sharp pain radiating into the arm, we should consider as a third possibility *spontaneous pneumothorax*. With this there is usually also interstitial emphysema and this is sometimes readily apparent in the soft tissues of the neck. The pain may be referred to as pain of the heart. Usually in such cases rupture of the mediastinal pleura occurs giving rise to the pneumothorax with subsequent displacement of the mediastinum and resultant dyspnea. Finally, we should consider as a fourth possibility, *luetic aortitis*, especially since this condition is much more prevalent in the negro race.

If we examine these possibilities carefully, we must conclude that dissecting aneurysm is unlikely because congestive heart failure is not a secondary event in this condition. It is true that many times death in dissecting aneurysm is of cardiac nature, but it is usually sudden, the sequel to rupture of the aorta into the pericardial cavity with resultant cardiac tamponade. Certainly spontaneous pneumothorax would not be expected to produce congestive failure of more than a year's duration. With a negative serology and no roentgenographic evidence of aortic dilatation or aneurysm we are inclined to minimize luetic aortitis as a possibility.

Upon physical examination, we have a slender and well developed patient who is unable to cooperate due to a semicomatose state. Patients with hypertension frequently have cerebrovascular accidents. A state such as this may, however, be related to decreased blood pressure which, together with changes in the cerebral vessels, leads to inadequate cerebral circulation, ischemia and coma. The pupils were described as constricted. This might be given considerable significance were it not that we learned that the patient had been given morphine. We are very interested in the description of the heart. Distant heart sounds are also found in pneumothorax. A soft systolic murmur was heard. With damage to the myocardium and dilatation of the heart, the mitral valve often becomes insufficient and gives such a murmur. There were rales in the lung. We note also that the liver was palpable three fingers below the right costal margin. Here are three items to indicate congestive heart failure.

In reviewing the laboratory findings we observe that the urinary specific gravity was 1.024— in a single specimen. In considering the possibility of renal azotemia, any specific gravity of over 1.020 would be quite unusual because this in itself is strong evidence against marked renal insufficiency; 1 plus albuminuria is quite compatible with congestion of the kidney. Anemia, such as this patient exhibited, frequently accompanies hypertension. There is the possibility too, of poor dietary habits leading to nutritional anemia. The white blood cell count was 10,-000 with 90 per cent neutrophils which is rather high. This was interpreted as possibly indicating pneumonia. Pneumonia. is very common in patients with congestive heart failure. It is often difficult to distinguish between bronchopneumonia and pulmonary congestion in heart failure. Even x-rays may be difficult to evaluate in these cases. The Kolmer-Wassermann test was negative and this helps to rule out our diagnosis of luetic aortitis. Then too, we have no evidence of aortic insufficiency on physical examination. Aortic insufficiency is noted in about 50 per cent of cases with luetic aortic aneurysm. X-ray examination revealed that the heart was markedly enlarged—extending all the way to the chest wall on the left side and 4.5 to 5 cm. from the midsternal line on the right side. The lung fields, particularly the right, revealed increased density especially in the hilar areas. There was no evidence of fluid in the pleural cavities. I believe that with this I would be inclined to a diagnosis of pulmonary congestion and pneumonia. There was no evidence of aneurysm of the heart or aorta. The E.C.G. report describes diagnostic signs of a large infarct on the lateral aspect. There is evidence that this was more recent than six months. These changes could, however, be explained in one other way and that is on the basis of generalized pericarditis complicating an older infarct. I am not sure just how and why pericarditis sometimes comes about following a cardiac infarct. It may be that the infaction brings about a marked decrease in local resistance and, as time goes on, an infection is set up. I think that with the findings at hand we can certainly conclude that this patient did have hypertension and that she developed degenerative arterial changes following which a myocardial infarct occurred. I believe that this infarct was rather large, perhaps 7 cm. in diameter. It probably extended most of the way through the heart wall in spite of the fact that a cardiac aneurysm was not apparent. I do not believe that it involved the septum to any considerable extent. We have no evidence of mural thrombosis with embolic phenomena and no reason to suspect pulmonic infarction. Some of the shadows on the x-ray could be the result of congestion, but I believe that pneumonia was present; this could account for the leukocytosis.

CLINICAL DISCUSSION

QUESTION: What was the cause of the coma?

DR. BAYLEY: This was probably a manifestation of cerebral ischemia—the result of sclerotic vascular changes in association with the decreased blood pressure which accompanied heart failure.

DR. HALPERT: The infarct that you describe appears to include that area supplied by the anterior descending branch of the left coronary. In this case, would you not think that the septum was also involved?

DR. BAYLEY: It is very difficult, from the E.C.G., to determine precisely the area involved. By using different leads we can localize this area fairly well however, and my guess would be that the infarct begins at the front of the heart and goes all the way around to the lateral aspect of the left ventricle.

ANATOMIC DIAGNOSIS

DR. HOPPS: Dr. Bayley was not informed of the final results obtained at necropsy in this case. We usually remove from the chart any evidence that might reveal to the clinician the actual status of things as determined at necropsy. I say this so you may appreciate the fact that Dr. Bayley had no more data than you have upon which to base his diagnosis.

The diagnosis given here was quite correct with the exception of one thing. Dr. Bayley said that that the infarct was 7 cm. in diameter when actually it was but 6 cm. This was an anterior lateral infarct as he had surmised, but did involve approximately half of the septum. The patient had a cardiac infarct which was fairly recent—perhaps eight to ten days old. In addition, there was an area perhaps more recent (two to three days). In retrospect it is difficult to find any incident in the history which points directly to the infarct. The patient's frequent episodes of anginal pain may well have masked that pain associated with the actual infarct.

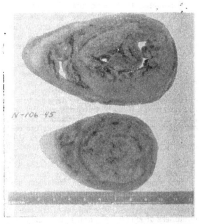

Fig. 1. Note mural thrombus which almost fills the left ventricle, overlying the area of infarction. The right ventricle also contains a mural thrombus which overlies the infarcted portion of the septum.

There was a rather thick mural thrombus in the left ventricle and because of the extensive involvement of the septum, a mural thrombus was also present in the right ventricle. This was of considerable benefit to the patient in that it provided a mechanical reinforcement for the softened necrotic myocardium and prevented cardiac aneurysm and decreased the likelihood of rupture. Such a thrombus is often a two-edged sword, however. In addition to serving as a blow-out patch and preventing marked dilatation and possible rupture, a portion of thrombus may break loose to form a thrombotic embolus. This, depending upon where it lodges, may cause a great deal of damage. In this case we found evidence of such damage in two regions. There was focal necrosis of the pancreas which was practically a terminal affair—not more than 24-36 hours old. That this was an effect of infarction, secondary to embolization, seems the most likely possibility. It has been well established in the last few years that a rather common cause of focal pancreatic necrosis is focal ischemia and necrosis secondary to vascular phenomenon. In addition we found an infarct in the lungs. This was a fairly recent lesion, probably four or five days old. Since the mural thrombus involved both ventricles it was possible for thrombotic emboli to be discharged into both the pulmonic and the systemic circulation. The lungs were moderately increased in weight and exhibited passive congestion. There was a few small focal areas of pneumonia, but these were not significant. There was fairly recent hemorrhagic infarct of the uterus also. Thrombi were demonstrated in both major uterine arteries. It seems unlikely that this was an embolic phenomenon since it would have been necessary for emboli to lodge in both the right and left uterine arteries.

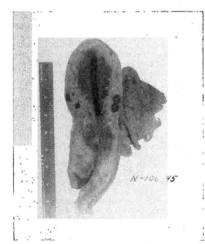

Fig. 2.   Hemorrhagic infarction of the uterus.

DISCUSSION

QUESTION: Did the necropsy findings bring out any reason for the 10,000 white count with 90 per cent neutrophils?

DR. HOPPS: This, I believe, is explained on the basis of cardiac infarction. Unlike most tissue, cardiac muscle, following infarction, elaborates a leukotactic substance which not only causes leukocytic infiltration locally, but also leukocytosis with a relative increase in polys.

QUESTION: What was the explanation for the patient's comatose condition?

DR. HOPPS: We were not permitted to examine the brain. For this reason we do not know whether this resulted, as Dr. Bayley suggested, from generalized ischemia, the result of arteriosclerosis plus a decrease in blood pressure, or whether this might have been the result of an embolic phenomenon.

DR. BAYLEY: Was there enough chronic nephritis to explain the anemia?

DR. HOPPS: No, the kidneys were not remarkable save for passive congestion and slight arteriolonephrosclerosis secondary to hypertension. I should have mentioned before the pathologic evidence for hypertension in this case. The size and shape of the heart were significant in this respect. The heart weighed 480 Gm. and the enlargement (approximately 50 per cent) was predominantly of the left ventricle. This, together with the hyperplastic arteriolosclerosis observed, including arteriolonephrosclerosis, provides an anatomic basis for the diagnosis of hypertension. Dr. McCollum has recently completed a study of those necropsies performed at the University Hospital during the last 10 years which pertain to cardio-vascular disease. Perhaps he will give us some pertinent data concerning hypertensive heart disease.

DR. McCOLLUM: In approximately 1500 necropsies there were 103 cases in which the cause of death could be attributed to hypertension or its effects. We found that of these cases, approximately 41 per cent died of congestive failure, 19 per cent of myocardial infarction, 19 per cent of cerebrovascular accidents and 10 per cent of uremia. Of the miscellaneous conditions w h i c h brought about termination in this group there was one instance of dissecting aneurysm.

One half of the world must sweat and groan that the other half may dream.—*Longfellow.*

Every subject's duty is the king's; but every subject's soul is his own.—*Shakespeare.*

We get impatient, and there crops out our human weakness.—*Timothy Titcomb.*

What's money without happiness?—*Bulwer-Lytton.*

Classified Advertisements

Doctor leaving state, wants to sell hospital equipment and lease building. Approximate value of equipment, $10,000. Physician locating would have to do surgery. 1945 gross income $70,000 cash. Contact Dr. V. D. Herrington, Pryor, Oklahoma.

Special Article

THE MEDICAL SCHOOL AND COMMENCEMENT

The Medical School's obligation to the students does not end with the conferring of a degree and the completion of the graduation festivities. In the eyes of the school authorities the word commencement should take on its true meaning. Webster says it is the act of commencing. The Medical School, supported by the taxpayer's money, should develop ways and means of participating in the graduate's plans in order to see that he makes the most of his education and repays, as far as possible, his community for its support of the medical school. The graduates, after completing their intern service, should be urged to enter medical practice, at least for three to five years valuable experience, not to be had in any other field. As valuable as a hospital service is, it can never take the place of general practice, which presents a cross section of medical problems in the general population. The graduate after completing his intern service should be encouraged to return to his own community for this experience even though he anticipates entering a speciality later. This course would enable him to discharge his obligation to the taxpayers who helped make available his educational opportunity.

In this connection the Medical School should endeavor to make general practice in rural communities more attractive to the young physician. The school should carefully survey its obligation to the physicians and the people of the State and make sure that it fully discharges its duty. It should become the educational center for the general practitioner and keep scientific openhouse all the year round. It should plan periodic refresher courses specially designed for the general practitioner. In order to make such courses more readily available to physicians practicing in rural areas the school should consider the feasibility of sending young staff members to take charge of his practice temporarily, an important phase of the school's educational service, while the physician of the rural area comes to the school to learn and perhaps to teach.

In cooperation with the State Medical Association the University might consider an advisory council with representatives, both lay and professional, from counties and districts throughout the State. Through the aid of such a Council the University might develop a comprehensive program which would inspire an intellectual response resulting in an elevation of cultural and educational advantages, thus encouraging young graduates of medicine to locate in rural communities and to rear their families there. With the advice and aid of the Council the University with the Medical School as its chief agent should survey local medical needs throughout the State to consider the organization of clinics, community hospitals, and laboratories and to supply through the medical school faculty, diagnostic and surgical services and other highly specialized skills not locally available. In addition the University should devise ways and means of engaging the interest of influential lay people in the respective communities and should encourage the investment of local wealth, individual or otherwise, in the provision of adequate facilities for the practice of modern medicine in order to attract and hold qualified generalists in medicine. The provision of such facilities with merited credits toward certification by an American Board on General Practice, which may be expected to follow the establishment of a section on General Practice by the American Medical Association, would go far toward the solution of the present paucity of general practitioners for rural communities. While this plan would require an increase in medical school personnel with additional costs, the obvious benefits to the taxpayers would justify more liberal appropriations for the support of the program. The American people love service and pay generously when anticipated values warrant.

The Medical School is not doing its full duty until its unselfish antennae penetrate every community in the State, seeking opportunities to serve both the physicians and their patients.

Considering local expediency through national policy, the medical organization should contemplate the advocacy of several years in general practice as a requirement for certification by the various speciality boards. Such a ruling would put more physicians in rural communities and ultimately more well rounded men in highly specialized fields.

Obviously, the rural community, to be attractive to the young graduate in medicine, must provide the facilities needed to practice modern medicine, in the form of physical plan and equipment and they then should be provided on a community basis. Something more, however, is needed in the form of community activities which will make living pleasant as well as the practice of medicine attractive. Educational, social, and recreational values are as of great importance to the community's physician as to other members of the group, and to attract a qualified physician, these needs must be respected and met.

The solution of the problem is far from simple, far from easy and far from inexpensive. But the community that wants service and is willing to provide an attractive setting and to pay for the service, can attract the qualified physician and can have good medical care.

THE

MARY E. POGUE SCHOOL

For Retarded Children and Epileptic Children

Children are grouped according to type and have their own separate departments. Separate buildings for girls and boys.

Large beautiful grounds. Five school rooms. Teachers are all college trained and have Teachers' Certificates. Occupational Therapy. Speech Corrective Work. The School is only 26 miles west of Chicago. All west highways out of Chicago pass through or near Wheaton. Referring physicians may continue to supervise care and treatment of children placed in the School. You are invited to visit the School or send for catalogue.

30 Geneva Road, Wheaton, Ill.
Phone: Wheaton 319

Have a Coke

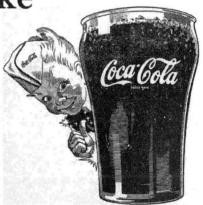

When you laugh, the world laughs with you, as they say—and when you enjoy *the pause that refreshes* with ice-cold Coca-Cola, your friends enjoy it with you, too. Everybody enjoys the friendly hospitality that goes with the invitation *Have a Coke.* Those three words mean *Friend, you belong —I'm glad to be with you.* Good company is better company over a Coca-Cola.

THE PRESIDENT'S PAGE

Possibly in no other profession, at least where the health of the people is concern-ed, have there been the advances, improvements and discoveries made as have been true of the regular medical profession.

This was clearly demonstrated in World War II wherein the loss of life and physi-cal handicaps on account of injury were held at a very low percentage compared with previous wars. Not only was this true in war but in civilian practice as well.

All of this has not come about through selfish financial interests but through the desire to benefit humanity and save human lives. The same cannot be said of any other group or profession.

L. E. Fuykendall

President.

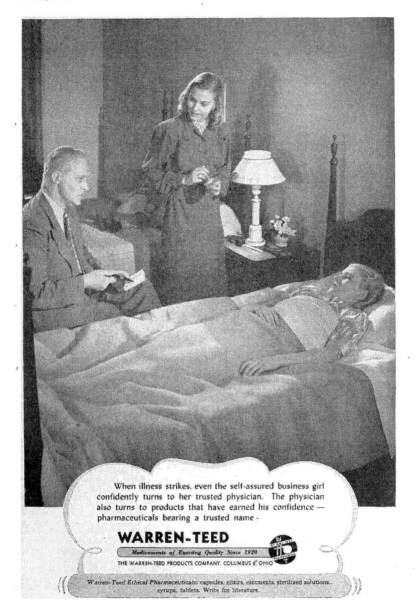

When illness strikes, even the self-assured business girl confidently turns to her trusted physician. The physician also turns to products that have earned his confidence — pharmaceuticals bearing a trusted name ·

WARREN-TEED

Medicaments of Exacting Quality Since 1920

THE WARREN-TEED PRODUCTS COMPANY, COLUMBUS 8, OHIO

Warren-Teed Ethical Pharmaceuticals: capsules, elixirs, ointments, sterilized solutions, syrups, tablets. Write for literature.

The JOURNAL Of The
OKLAHOMA STATE MEDICAL ASSOCIATION

EDITORIAL BOARD
L. J. MOORMAN, Oklahoma City, Editor-in-Chief

E. EUGENE RICE, Shawnee   BEN H. NICHOLSON, Oklahoma City

MR. DICK GRAHAM, Oklahoma City, Business Manager

MR. CLAYTON FONDREN, Oklahoma City, Assistant Business Manager

CONTRIBUTIONS: Articles accepted by this Journal for publication including those read at the annual meetings of the State Association are the sole property of this Journal.

The Editorial Department is not responsible for the opinions expressed in the original articles of contributors.

Manuscripts may be withdrawn by authors for publication elsewhere only upon the approval of the Editorial Board.

MANUSCRIPTS: Manuscripts should be typewritten, double-spaced, on white paper 8½ x 11 inches. The original copy, not the carbon copy, should be submitted.

Footnotes, bibliographies and legends for cuts should be typed on separate sheets in double space. Bibliography listing should follow this order: Name of author, title of article, name of periodical with volume, page and date of publication.

Manuscripts are accepted subject to the usual editorial revisions and with the understanding that they have not been published elsewhere.

NEWS: Local news of interest to the medical profession, changes of address, births, deaths and weddings will be gratefully received.

ADVERTISING: Advertising of articles, drugs or compounds unapproved by the Council on Pharmacy of the A.M.A. will not be accepted. Advertising rates will be supplied on application.

It is suggested that members of the State Association patronize our advertisers in preference to others.

SUBSCRIPTIONS: Failure to receive The Journal should call for immediate notification.

REPRINTS: Reprints of original articles will be supplied at actual cost provided request for them is attached to manuscripts or made in sufficient time before publication. Checks for reprints should be made payable to Industrial Printing Company, Oklahoma City.

Address all communications to THE JOURNAL OF THE OKLAHOMA STATE MEDICAL ASSOCIATION, 210 Plaza Court, Oklahoma City 3

OFFICIAL PUBLICATION OF THE OKLAHOMA STATE MEDICAL ASSOCIATION
Copyrighted November, 1946

EDITORIALS

OUR FRIENDS ARE LEGION AND AMERICAN

At the twenty-eighth convention of the National American Legion the following resolution was unanimously approved. This resolution embodies such a clean cut, verile statement of the undiluted Americanism still animating and motivating the men who have fought our battles that it is receiving this well deserved editorial notice, and is being reproduced for the benefit of our readers.

WHEREAS veterans who have served in the armed forces now have available to them hospital and medical care provided by the United States Government; and

WHEREAS there are countless voluntary health insurance plans now being offered by the physicians and the insurance companies; and

WHEREAS proposed plans of compulsory health insurance would increase the tax burden and bring about regimentation of the medical profession; and

WHEREAS all forms of compulsion are repugnant to our American way of life since our liberties and opportunities would be circumscribed;

NOW, THEREFORE, BE IT RESOLVED: That the National Assembly of the American Legion hereby expresses its opposition to compulsory health insurance.

The members of the State Medical Association should pass this resolution on to their friends and their patients with the request that they compare it with the policies and purposes of certain politicians in Washington who seem to think the American people are incapable of distinguishing between compulsion and freedom.

THE DEMON DEMORAL IN SHEEP'S CLOTHING ALA PAUL de KRUIF

Physicians who have not read the recent controversial correspondence in the American Medical Journal about addiction to Demoral should do so without delay. Those who doubt the habit forming possibilities of this new drug should read the case histories, pages 43-44, Journal of the American Medical Association, September 7 and the letter from Max Samter in the Journal of September 28.

Lay people love to read about medicine and every day they are being misled by false statements appearing in premature lay medical publicity. The Paul de Kruif article about Demoral in the Readers Digest of June, 1946, is a good example. People are falsely informed and physicians must be on guard. Demoral is dangerous if not prescribed with due consideration of the possibility of primary Demoral addiction.

The Readers Digest through de Kruif's unfortunate article has the people falsely informed. It's up to the medical profession to be truely informed in order to protect a trusting public. When may we expect Ph.D.'s and politicians to keep their noses out of our feed bags. Some day they will swallow poison and turn up their toes.

MEETING OF COUNTY SOCIETY OFFICERS

The Sixth Annual Conference of County Medical Society Officers has passed into history. Though the attendance was not as good as anticipated, the spirit of the meeting was commendable, progressive, inspiring and truly representative of medicine's mission in the State.

This Annual Conference not only brings opportunity for exchange of ideas between county officers and suggestions from the Council and Officers of the State Association, but it helps to crystallize policies in the State Office and serves as a great stimulus.

On behalf of the State Association, its officers, council and committees, the editorial staff extends greetings and congratulations to the county officers.

A MESSAGE TO THOUGHTFUL DOCTORS AND HOSPITAL ADMINISTRATORS

This is a message and an appeal especially to the thoughtful doctors and to the wise executives of Oklahoma hospitals. You should be made aware of the fact that increased utilization of the Blue Cross Hospital service contracts and a continually lengthening hospital stay of Blue Cross policy holders is jeopardizing the success of a program which is acknowledged to be the greatest voluntary movement in history — the making available of medical care to the needs of our people. In plain English, it appears that too large a proportion of our policyholders are receiving hospitalization, and for unduly long periods.

Sponsors of the Blue Cross Plan have watched nervously while this tendency grew ever more threatening during the past three or four years — years that saw our reserves being whittled away to pay the costs of unnecessary hospital admissions and unduly prolonged hospital stays. Finally the situation became so dangerous that something had to be done, and the easiest method for most Plans was to increase membership dues. So, after sustained losses over a twelve month period made it clear that this move was absolutely necessary, the Oklahoma Plan was compelled to increase its dues in July of this year. During the year 1945, all moneys paid

in by the members were paid out for hospital care and operating expenses. The same is true also of the first six months of 1946. We have not been able to add any amount to the surplus necessary to guard against contingencies. Our reserves must be increased as the membership increases if the Blue Cross Plan is to continue to function. And the Blue Cross Plan cannot survive if this tendency to over-utilization continues. Hence, this appeal to the hospitals, the doctors, and the members of Blue Cross to cooperate fairly and make this Plan a truly mutual one, working for the benefit of all and not for the selfish few who would abuse it. Even the present small dues paid by the members (individual $.85, man and wife $1.50, family $1.75) will pay for sufficient necessary hospital care, but these present dues, or any increased dues, will not cover continual increasing abuses of the service.

The statistical basis for Blue Cross is the law of averages. It has been found that during the course of a certain period of time, a certain per cent of the population will become ill enough to be hospitalized. The law of averages is actuarially sound and will work unless it is influenced by abuses. During the last year or two, when authorities agree that the health of the American people has been better than at any time in history, the admission rate per member of all Blue Cross Plans jumped from 11.71 per 100 participants in July, 1945, to 12.12 in July, 1946. During the same period, admission rates for the Oklahoma Plan rose from 11.4 to 13 per 100 participants. The national average length of stay for members increased from 7.71 days in July, 1945, to 8.41 days in July, 1946, and this at a time when hospital beds are at a premium, when adequate nursing staffs are difficult to maintain, and when many hospitals have waiting lists of patients in real need of hospital care. It is clear to thoughtful people that this trend must stop if Blue Cross is to grow in range of service, and if it is to fulfill one important mission to which it is dedicated. This purpose is to help forestall Federal compulsory health insurance by giving American people the best possible medical and hospital care at the lowest possible cost through voluntary agencies. The Blue Cross Plan has no desire to withhold any necessary hospital care. Their office is conducted as efficiently and economically as it is possible, but the Blue Cross Plan is not meant to be used unnecessarily.

If all the hospitals and doctors will cooperate honestly with Blue Cross by admitting patients to hospital beds only if bed care is absolutely needed, the doctors treating patients as out-patients whenever possible, seeing to it that patients are not needlessly kept in hospitals longer than necessary, and contributing an all-round awareness of the limitations of the Blue Cross Plan, the Plan will work and continue to give enlarging services. If this cooperation is not given, the Plan will be forced to operate in that precarious zone between safety and danger, and one day will be remembered only as a "noble American experiment". Our appeal to you is to make yourselves acquainted with the basic principles of Blue Cross, with its aims, ideals, and spirit. Play fair with your Blue Cross Plan. Don't "kill the goose that laid the golden egg".—A. S. Risser, M.D.

MEDICAL EXAMINERS SYSTEM BILL

At the last meeting of the Council and at the recent meeting of county medical society officers Dr. Floyd Keller explained the meaning of the proposed bill, Medical Examining System, and emphasized the need of such a bill. The present procedure amounts to an inexcusable farce and brings discredit upon the medical profession and the State of Oklahoma.

Unfortunately, this proposed legislation has been too long delayed. The Council reaffirmed its interest in the proposed legislation and requested that it be placed in the hands of the Public Policy Committee for legislative action.

The members of the medical profession and the people of the State are greatly indebted to Dr. Keller for his research in this field and his untiring efforts in favor of much needed legislation.

ANTIHISTAMINE DRUGS—A WARNING

The recent popularization of antihistaminic drugs for the control of symptoms in allergic conditions is accompanied by certain hazards which deserve careful attention.

The hazards concerning not only the patient but the public as well are due to side effects, particularly drowsiness and dizziness. Statistical studies indicate that these symptoms occur in 50-75 per cent of the cases. Other side reactions are dry mouth, feeling of nervousness, urinary frequency, nausea, vomiting, tinnitus, numbness, and tingling of hands and legs.

These side effects are occasionally accompanied by obvious muscular incoordination. In some cases after a single dose it requires twelve to sixteen hours of sleep and several cups of coffee to make the nervous system click. Doctors prescribing these drugs in a given case for the first time should instruct the patient to the annulling possibilities.

There is not only the danger of falling asleep at the wheel, but the hazards of imperfect coordination in connection with occupations requiring mechanistic precision. The legal responsibilities are to be considered.

PEACETIME CRIMINALS

The greatest menace to our survival is to be found in the ever-present predatory disease producing micro-organisms which, without warning assail our bodies. The greatest human achievement has been the silent march of science against these unseen enemies of mankind. But the task is not finished; we have just begun to make use of the beneficient gift of science.

Not only are we guilty of not making the most of scientific research, we are woefully lagging in our application of knowledge already gained. Perhaps the most outstanding example is our failure to control tuberculosis. Robert Koch gave us the key more than sixty years ago, but like the proverbial efficiency man we know how the job should be done, yet we cannot do it.

At the Annual Meeting of the National Tuberculosis Association last June, James A. Doull of the U. S. Public Health Service, Chief, Office of International Health Relations, gave an estimate of 3,000,000 deaths annually in the world from tuberculosis, with a possible total of 5,000,000. Hitler and his war criminals are charged with a total of only 12,000,000 during the six years of the world's worst war. Based upon the lowest estimate, the tubercle bacillus can cap Hitler's catastrophic record in four years with two to go.

Not only do we need more research for the acquisition of knowledge, but wider dissemination of the knowledge at hand. A realization of this situation should bridge the chasm between the worker in the research laboratory and the general practitioner. The teacher in the medical school should become the middle man and with the help of medical schools and universities the people should be brought up to date on the meaning of medical knowledge and constantly informed of progress in medical science.

The U. S. government instead of taking medicine away from the people might well undertake the task of informing them of its adequacy and their failure to make use of it because of indifference fostered by a lack of knowledge.

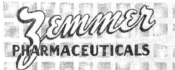

A complete line of laboratory controlled ethical pharmaceuticals.

Chemists to the Medical Profession for 44 years.

OK 11-46 *The Zemmer Company*

Oakland Station • PITTSBURGH 13, PA.

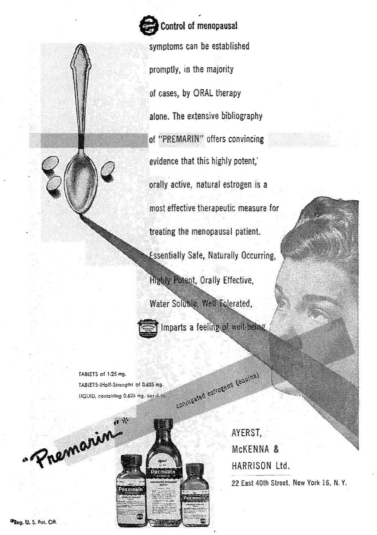

Control of menopausal symptoms can be established promptly, in the majority of cases, by ORAL therapy alone. The extensive bibliography of "PREMARIN" offers convincing evidence that this highly potent, orally active, natural estrogen is a most effective therapeutic measure for treating the menopausal patient.

Essentially Safe, Naturally Occurring,
Highly Potent, Orally Effective,
Water Soluble, Well Tolerated,
Imparts a feeling of well-being

TABLETS of 1.25 mg.
TABLETS (Half-Strength) of 0.625 mg.
LIQUID, containing 0.625 mg. per 4 cc.

conjugated estrogens (equine)

"Premarin"*

AYERST,
McKENNA &
HARRISON Ltd.
22 East 40th Street. New York 16, N. Y.

*Reg. U. S. Pat. Off.

SECRETARY'S CONFERENCE REVIVED

The Annual Conference for County Medical Society Officers, discontinued during the war, was revived this year with a meeting held Sunday, September 29 at the Skirvin Hotel in Oklahoma City.

The Conference began with a Council Meeting at 9:30 A.M., progressing into an important and interesting all day session. At 10:00 A.M. President L. C. Kuyrkendall stated the object of the Conference. Information on the Association's malpractice insurance program was presented by Mr. Roger Bainbridge, representing London and Lancashire Insurance Co. and Dr. V. K. Allen, Chairman of the Insurance Committee. The newspaper publicity campaign and the special assessment program were given in an up-to-date report by Dr. John F. Burton of Oklahoma City who also presented Mr. Warren Humphries of the Erwin-Wasey Advertising Co., who in turn displayed proof copies of the first three ads. It is anticipated that the first ads will appear in the newspapers the latter part of October. Following the report of the Publicity Committee the Chairman of the Postgraduate Committee, Dr. Gregory Stanbro, gave a discussion of the postgraduate education program for 1947. He announced that the 1947 program will be on the subject of Gynecology and the instructor will be Dr. J. R. B. Branch, who is now conducting a similar course in Tennessee.

Buffet luncheon was served at noon by the Association, during which period Dr. McLain Rogers, Clinton, and Dr. Louis Ritzhaupt, Guthrie, spoke on the Association's Public Policy activities.

Dr. John F. Burton, Chairman of Veterans Care Committee, opened the afternoon session with preliminary announcements on the program of medical care for veterans between the State Medical Association and the Veterans Administration. This program is a plan whereby members of the Association will render medical care to male veterans with service connected disabilities and female veterans irrespective of whether or not disabilities are service connected. The program is voluntary on the part of physicians and payment will be made on the basis of a fee schedule established by the Association. At 2:00 P.M. an open forum discussion of activities of the Association and related organizations was conducted. Dr. R. Q. Goodwin spoke in behalf of the Allied Professions Committee. Dr. Kuykendall spoke on councilor district committees and Dr. John Lamb, Secretary of the Oklahoma Medical Research Foundation, told the conference about the Research Foundation. The Hill-Burton Bill and hospital construction was the subject of Dr. C. R. Rountree's discussion. Dr. James Stevenson, treasurer of Oklahoma Physicians Service, spoke on the growing program of O.P.S.

The final portion of the Conference was conducted by Mr. Fred Eakers, Department Service Officer of the State Office of the American Legion, and this program was on the subject of the preparation of medical statements for rating purposes by civilian physicians.

In its entirety, the Sixth Annual Conference was a great success. Newly elected officers are: Dr. Everett King, Duncan, President; and Dr. Ned Burleson, Prague, Secretary.

"WORK SHOP MEETING" — AMERICAN CANCER SOCIETY HELD IN SEPTEMBER

A "work shop meeting" for all county and district commanders of the Field Army, Oklahoma Division of the American Cancer Society, was held September 27 and 28, 1946, at the Skirvin Hotel, Oklahoma City.

Approximately 75 per cent of the counties of the State had representatives in attendance. The meeting, presided over by Mrs. E. Lee Ozbirn, State Commander, laid a foundation for the establishment of permanent local units in each county of the State. It is anticipated that by November 15th all county units will be organized.

Governor Accepts Chairmanship

At the Friday evening dinner meeting, it was announced that Governor Robert S. Kerr had accepted the appointment of State Campaign Chairman for 1947. Governor Kerr succeeds Mr. L. C. Griffith who resigned on the advice of his physician.

In accepting the Chairmanship Governor Kerr stated, "It is but the privilege and duty of every earnest, thinking citizen to pool his God-given talents, whether they be great or small, in a combined effort to stop this insidious killer. With this duty in mind, I humbly take my place alongside the many thousands of veteran workers, who for years past have diligently fought this common enemy."

Members of Cancer Committee Participated in Program

Members of the Association's Committee for the Study and Control of Cancer taking an active part in the program were: Paul B. Champlin, M.D., Joseph W. Kelso, M.D., C. P. Bondurant, M.D., and L. Chester McHenry, M.D.

"THE RELATION OF THE FIELD ARMY TO THE MEDICAL PROFESSION"*

The subject given me for discussion, "The Relation of the Field Army to the Medical Profession", is one of far reaching import. The subect to me actually means the necessity for cooperation between the Field Army and the medical profession in the cancer control program. I might qualify this statement further by saying that the degree of success of an intelligent, carefully planned, long range program depends, absolutely, on the exact degree of cooperation between the Field Army and the Medical Profession.

Thus far, the program as initiated by the Oklahoma Division of the American Cancer Society, generated by the wholehearted cooperative effort of the Field Army and the Medical Profession, has in the words of Dr. C. P. Rhoads, Chairman of our National Committee on Growth, been unique in every respect, and actually has become a model for the entire nation. This enviable record created in less than eight months time is due to the ideal relation between the Field Army and the Medical Profession. It is a perfect example of smoothly working teamwork built on complete understanding.

It is most desirous that the cooperation now existing on a state level be projected to the county and community level.

Let us examine and analyze, if possible, the conditions necessary to preserve a cooperative relationship between the Field Army and the Medical Profession. The conditions are the same for state and local levels. The first requirement is a unity of purpose in the hearts of both the leaders of the Field Army and the leaders of the Medical Profession. That purpose, based on a humanitarian spirit, is: (1) to prevent the ravages of cancer wherever possible, (2) to make possible the means and facilities to save lives of those who may already have the disease, (3) and to help alleviate the suffering of those victims who are beyond known medical and scientific aid. To do these things requires a deep love for humanity in general, which creates unselfish action and effort, as each of you are evidencing by your presence here today. The second requirement of cooperation is a thorough understanding of the fields of endeavor of the two groups. To define this requirement let us substitute the word duty for the word cooperation. First, let us examine the duty of the Medical Profession towards a cooperative relationship. It seems to me this duty includes the following points:

1. A willingness of the Medical Profession to assume the responsibility of formulating medical service plans for the potential and actual cancer patient. Such plans must be acceptable to the Medical Profession as a whole. This duty, this responsibility, has been accepted by the Medical Profession and in order to insure its success all projects having to do with such medical services should be left in the hands of the Medical Profession.

*Address given by Dr. Paul B. Champlin, Enid, Oklahoma, before the Work Shop Meeting of the Field Army, Oklahoma Division, American Cancer Society, Friday Afternoon, September 27, 1946.

By this I do not mean the laity or Field Army should not do any thinking on the subject, but the ultimate method of operation, or the final decision, should be in the hands of the proper medical group. By proper medical group I mean the officers of your County Medical Society or the appropriate medical committee of the Oklahoma Division of the American Cancer Society.

2. Another duty of the Medical Profession in preserving a cooperative relationship, is that of showing a continued interest in all phases of the cancer program, including the educational and fund raising programs. Even though the majority of doctors are intensely busy they will, I am sure, do what they can to aid you in any program you may undertake.

3. A third duty of the medical profession, and one of utmost importance for continued wholehearted cooperation between the laity and the Profession, is the necessity of the Profession to keep pace with the increasing knowledge of the public in relation to cancer. Undoubtedly the Field Army, led by Mrs. Ozbirn, has developed one of the most comprehensive lay educational programs in the nation. Now, it is a challenge to the Medical Profession to avail themselves of the latest medical and scientific knowledge possible regarding the diagnosis and treatment of cancer.

4. It is a further cooperative duty of the Medical Profession to make available to all of the people ethical diagnostic and treatment centers for the cancer patients. To perform this duty in an intelligent manner, and within the scope of legitimate medicine, may require much time, thought, and effort, and the laity should not become impatient for the task is huge.

5. One of the greatest duties, or obligations of the Medical Profession in its relation to the Field Army is the initiation and actual prosecution of research activities. The Field Army has faithfully provided funds for the purpose of research. These funds have been placed at the disposal of the medical and scientific profession without any "strings" attached. It therefore becomes the solemn duty of those charged with the responsibility of directing research, to leave no stone unturned, no avenue with any promise whatever unexplored, in the desperate search to find the cause and cure for cancer. However, this obligation is being, at this moment, fulfilled. The search is going on — and it's being conducted in a highly efficient manner in more than 90 laboratories and research centers throughout the nation. The best scientific brains this nation has ever known are pooled in an effort, which someday, will result in a message of glad tidings to you, and to millions more who live constantly under the shadow of "death from cancer", that the killer's secret has been discovered. When this day will be depends to a large extent on your own faithfulness to the cause. Research costs money — without it the battle may be lost. It's in your hands to accelerate the battle by seeing that sufficient funds are raised each year for the purpose.

May I reiterate, the medical and scientific profession accepts, without reservations, its responsibility to you regarding research.

DR. WU RETURNS TO CHINA

Dr. Patrick P. T. Wu, who has completed an instructorship of a year and a half in the post-graduate course in Surgical Diagnosis, under the auspices of the Post Graduate Committee of the Association, has departed with Mrs. Wu for San Francisco where they are awaiting transportation to return to China.

Dr. Wu is to be the head of the Division of Surgery at the Li Clinic in Honghong, China, with offices in the Bank of East Asia Building.

Physician friends Dr. Wu made throughout Oklahoma will long remember him for his excellent teaching and his energetic and amiable personality.

SCIENTIFIC EXHIBIT

Centennial Session — American Medical Association

At the Centennial Session of the American Medical Association to be held in Atlantic City, June 9 to 13, 1947, the Scientific Exhibit will include both the history of medicine during the past century and the latest developments of medical science.

Application blanks for space are now available. All applicants must fill out the regular form. Applications close on January 13, 1947, after which time the Committee on Scientific Exhibit will make its decision and notify the applicants.

Application blanks for space should be procured as soon as possible. They are available from The Director, Scientific Exhibit, American Medical Association, 535 North Dearborn Street, Chicago 10, Illinois.

RECENT DEVELOPMENTS ON THE HILL-BURTON ACT

The Federal Security Agency of the U. S. Public Health Service has released the following information pertaining to the administration of the Hill-Burton Act.

Formation of a Federal Hospital Council and an advisory committee to assist Surgeon General Thomas Parran of the U. S. Public Health Service in the administration of the Hospital Survey and Construction Act was announced September 12, 1946, by Federal Security Administrator Watson B. Miller. The first meeting of these groups was held September 17 and 18 in the U. S. Public Health Service Building, Washington, D. C.

The purpose of the meeting was to formulate plans for administration of the recently enacted Hill-Burton Act which embodied one important feature of the President's national health program. Mr. Miller characterized this Act as "an epoch in the development of health legislation designed to meet serious and widespread needs", explaining that, "for the first time we are embarked upon a national policy of planning and constructing hospitals and health centers to meet the health needs of all the people. For the first time we are creating new institutes not on a sporadic unplanned basis, but on the basis of a long-range, carefully thought out program, integrated to the role that our hospitals and

WILLIAM E. EASTLAND, M.D.
F. A. C. R.

RADIUM AND X-RAY THERAPY
DERMATOLOGY

405 Medical Arts Bldg.

Oklahoma City, Oklahoma   Phone 3-1446

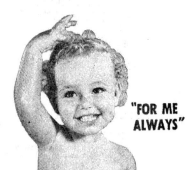

"FOR ME
ALWAYS"

Because DARICRAFT

1. is EASILY DIGESTED
2. has 400 U.S.P. Units of VITAMIN D per pint of evaporated milk.
3. has HIGH FOOD VALUE
4. has an IMPROVED FLAVOR
5. is HOMOGENIZED
6. is STERILIZED
7. is from INSPECTED HERDS
8. is SPECIALLY PROCESSED
9. is UNIFORM
10. will WHIP QUICKLY

PRESCRIBED BY MANY DOCTORS
... You also may want to utilize Daricraft as a solution to your infant feeding problems, as well as in special diets for convalescents.

PRODUCERS CREAMERY CO., SPRINGFIELD, MISSOURI

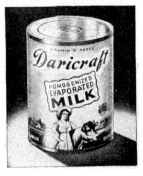

health centers must play in the future.''

To carry out this objective Congress has authorized the appropriation of $3,000,000 for surveys and planning and $75,000,000 for five years annually for construction. Of these sums, $2,350,000 for surveys and planning has been appropriated.

A state will be eligible to receive construction funds after it has developed a State plan for the construction of needed hospital facilities, based on a Statewide survey of existing facilities and existing needs. The state plan will be developed cooperatively by representatives of the state and its local communities and the Federal Government based on general standards formulated by the Surgeon General, with the approval of the Federal Hospital Council and the Federal Security Administrator.

In accordance with the provisions of the Act, the Federal Hospital Council is composed of the Surgeon General, who serves as chairman, ex officio, and eight members appointed by the Federal Security Administrator. Four members are outstanding in health and hospital fields, and four are representatives of the consumers of hospital services.

Members of the Advisory Committee will serve as consultants to the Surgeon General and the Federal Hospital Council, in the administration of the Hospital Survey and Construction Act. To obtain the benefit of as wide representation as possible on the Advisory Committee its membership will be extended as specific needs arise.

The fact was emphasized in announcing the appointment of the Federal Council and Advisory Committee that this program is the direct result of widespread public demand for improved health and hospital facilities. Introduction in the Senate under bi-partisan sponsorship, the bill had the immediate support of the American, Catholic and Protestant Hospital Associations, major labor and farm groups, the American Medical Association, American Public Health Association and numerous other organizations and individuals of national importance. No other important health legislation in recent history has had such universal public support.

COMMITTEE ON MEDICAL EDUCATION AND HOSPITALS STUDY GI TRAINING FOR TECHNICIANS

The Association's Medical Education and Hospital Committee is working with the Oklahoma State Accrediting Agency to enable veterans who aspire to be technicians to receive an ''on-the-job training'' status. Several applications have been made to the State Accrediting Agency by veterans. Some of the applicants served as technicians while in the armed services.

The Accrediting Agency's objective is to provide the veteran with a program of competent instruction and practical work so that upon completion he will have received adequate training and experience in Technology.

The Committee on Medical Education and Hospitals is surveying the present requirements for technicians and will advise the Accrediting Agency as to its findings as an effort to help the Agency establish a training program that will be accreditable for the veteran.

VA PROVIDES LOCAL DENTAL CARE FOR VETERANS

Veterans with service-connected dental conditions now may choose among private, home-town dentists when Veterans Administration dental clinic service is not ''feasibly available'', it has been announced.

Under a new fee-schedule program, worked out in cooperation with the American Dental Association, the VA will pay for this service given by local dentists.

The dental program, similar to the plans for medical service in effect in 12 states and being negotiated by 20 other states, including Oklahoma, covers the entire country.

"HOW TO PICK YOUR DOCTOR"

The October issue of Coronet has a feature beginning on page 84 with the above title that suggests a number of rules for the public to follow in selecting a physician. The article excellently emphasizes the risk the average man takes by impromptu selection of a physician. As an example, the reader is advised to choose a family physician with broad clinical training who has graduated from a Class A medical school, followed with an internship in a moderate or large size hospital. The article contains simple but important instruction and it is recommended to our readers.

HOLDENVILLE GENERAL HOSPITAL NOW ST. FRANCIS

The Felician Sisters of Coraopolis, Pennsylvania, who have recently taken over the Holdenville General Hospital, announced through Sr. Mary Magdalen, R.N., B.S., Superintendent, that they anticipate opening their doors to the public around the last of October.

Holdenville General has been incorporated under the new name of St. Francis Hospital and has at present 27 beds and five basinets. Provision has been made for possible expansion to 40 beds in the future. St. Francis plans to have an open staff of physicians of the highest standing to insure the best possible service to the people of Hughes County as well as neighboring areas.

POLIOMYELITIS CONFERENCE

The University of Colorado School of Medicine is scheduling a Rocky Mountain Conference on Poliomyelitis for December 16 and 17, 1946. The Conference is to be held in Denver and will sponsor six guest speakers. Cordial invitation to attend the conference has been extended to all members of the Oklahoma State Medical Association by the Colorado University School of Medicine.

CREDIT SERVICE

330 American National Building

Oklahoma City, Oklahoma

(Operators of Medical-Dental Credit Bureau)

We offer a dignified and effective collection service for doctors and hospitals located anywhere in the State. Write for information.

28 YEARS

Experience In Credit and Collection Work

Robt. R. Sesline, Owner and Manager

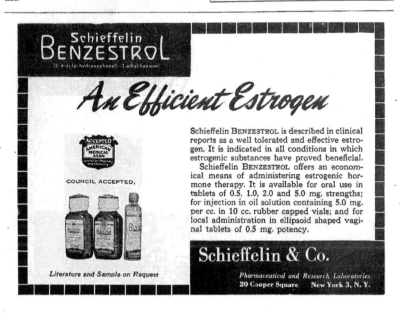

Schieffelin BENZESTROL
(2, 4-di-(p-hydroxyphenyl)-3-ethyl hexane)

An Efficient Estrogen

ACCEPTED AMERICAN MEDICAL ASSN
Council on Pharmacy and Chemistry

COUNCIL ACCEPTED

Schieffelin BENZESTROL is described in clinical reports as a well tolerated and effective estrogen. It is indicated in all conditions in which estrogenic substances have proved beneficial.

Schieffelin BENZESTROL offers an economical means of administering estrogenic hormone therapy. It is available for oral use in tablets of 0.5, 1.0, 2.0 and 5.0 mg. strengths; for injection in oil solution containing 5.0 mg. per cc. in 10 cc. rubber capped vials; and for local administration in ellipsoid shaped vaginal tablets of 0.5 mg. potency.

Literature and Sample on Request

Schieffelin & Co.

Pharmaceutical and Research Laboratories
20 Cooper Square   New York 3, N. Y.

SYMBOLS OF SIGNIFICANCE

DILANTIN SODIUM

The cry, the fall, the champing teeth, the tonic and clonic contractures, the incontinence—all may yield to

DILANTIN SODIUM. The E.E.G. can trace the pathologic brain wave, yet the epileptic may be spared his terrifying episodes. Powerfully anti-convulsant rather than dullingly hypnotic, DILANTIN SODIUM KAPSEALS* offer to the epileptic a sense of security and an opportunity to lead a more normal and useful life. DILANTIN SODIUM KAPSEALS — another product of revolutionary importance in the treatment of a specific disease; another of a long line of Parke-Davis preparations whose service to the profession created a dependable symbol of significance in medical therapeutics — MEDICAMENTA VERA.

DILANTIN SODIUM KAPSEALS
(diphenylhydantoin sodium), containing 0.03 Gm.
(½ grain) and 0.1 Gm. (1½ grains), are supplied in
bottles of 100, 500 and 1000. Individual dosage is
determined by the severity of the condition.
*Trademark Reg. U. S. Pat. Off.

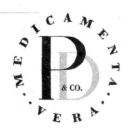

PARKE, DAVIS & COMPANY · DETROIT 32, MICHIGAN

Hits, Runs, Errors

SEPTEMBER 21: State Fair starts today and everyone is wondering how the "Life Show" will get over. Location not so good but many interesting exhibits are on hand.

SEPTEMBER 22: As anticipated "Life Show" position at Fair needs help and a broadcasting system is installed.

SEPTEMBER 23: Another check with Warren Humphries on the advertising campaign. Saw the first three ads and they are honeys. They will be presented at the Conference of Officers of County Medical Societies Sunday.

SEPTEMBER 24: To Rotary and a conference with Joe Hamilton on the Governor's appointments to the Crippled Children's Commission.

SEPTEMBER 25: Special train to Miami is set up by Frisco. Everything coming along nicely except hotel reservations in New Orleans on return trip. Looks as if as many will go to Southern Medical as to A. M. A. in San Francisco.

SEPTEMBER 26: To Enid with Dr. F. Redding Hood for a meeting with the Garfield County Society. Enjoyed President-Elect Champlin's hospitality and ended up talking to District Dental Society.

SEPTEMBER 27: To Cancer Meeting of the Women's Field Army and to hear the announcement that Governor Kerr will head the 1947 campaign. The medical profession can feel proud of the part it has played in making Oklahoma the Number One state in cancer education.

SEPTEMBER 28: Everyone working on program for the Secretaries Conference which will be tomorrow. Hope the officers of the county societies will be in in force.

SEPTEMBER 29: The Council, Committees and Conference held forth at the Skirvin and an excellent program was there for all to hear. Roast beef was served at the luncheon.

SEPTEMBER 30: A "flying" trip to Tulsa for a conference with the president of the Tulsa County Society, Dr. John Perry, and Dr. James Stevenson. The political pot is beginning to boil.

OCTOBER 1: To Holdenville to speak to the Rotary Club and an evening county medical meeting. Back to Wewoka with Dr. Shanholz to see his Seminole County Health Department set-up. Dr. Harry Daniels, who is the scientific paper, comes in on the Rock Island and gets a free ride back to the City.

OCTOBER 2: Dr. Tom Lowry of the V. A. in St. Louis arrives in town and tomorrow we will take on the problem of medical care for the veterans.

OCTOBER 3: Dr. John Burton gives his entire day to the V. A. program. As a chairman of a committee there is none finer. Looks as if the program will be ready to go in 30 to 60 days.

OCTOBER 4: To Norman to see about the Symposium on Compulsory Health Insurance that will be put on through the college and high school debate teams. We have an excellent chance to tell the story.

OCTOBER 5: Frankly, this is the day of the first football game at Norman and so we get the mail to date so our conscience will be clear for the weekend.

OCTOBER 7: The usual Monday morning mail. To Norman in the afternoon to see about the debate symposium for October 18. Dr. Stevenson and N. D. Helland of Tulsa will participate.

OCTOBER 8: Back to school at last. Appeared before the debate class of Central Highschool to discuss, of course, compulsory health insurance. Off for Durant at 10:00 o'clock for a county medical meeting. Meeting is in the fine clinic of Drs. Colwick, Baker, Hyde and Smith and Dr. Keiller Haynie provides a fine "steak" dinner.

OCTOBER 9: Morning conference with Mr. Harned of Tulsa, State Chairman for the Sister Kenney Fund. Seems to us that there should be a united front in the field of polio instead of several organizations doing the same work.

OCTOBER 10: Helped the K. U. Alumni honor Angelo C. Scott of Oklahoma City for his distinguished service as an Oklahoman. Worked the office force getting ready for a trip to Dallas tomorrow. Wonder why.

OCTOBER 11: Aggies 6-S. M. U. 15.

OCTOBER 12: O. U. 13-Texas 20 and what a battle.

OCTOBER 14: The special train to Southern Medical needed attention and we fought all day with Harry Kornbaum. Schedules of the trip will go out tomorrow. It looks like another wonderful trip.

OCTOBER 15: To Miami with Drs. John E. McDonald and E. Rankin Denny from Tulsa for a meeting of the Ottawa Society. Want to compliment Dr. Sayles on his excellent report to his society on the Conference of County Medical Officers, but found him in Chicago.

OCTOBER 16: Arrived home from Miami 5:15 A.M. It's a long story. The old Chevrolet has an ache and pain and has to go to the hospital so Fondren went to Pauls Valley for the medical meeting.

OCTOBER 17: The office is full of material for the socialized medicine debate at O. U. and Dr. Stevenson and N. D. Helland of Tulsa will be over tomorrow to give the 1-2 punch. Also have a session with Democratic and Republican headquarters concerning information they would like to have the membership receive.

OCTOBER 18: Drs. James Stevenson, N. D. Helland, W. R. Bethel, of Tulsa, in office early this A.M. Dick and the above going to Norman to appear on the Symposium sponsored by the Annual Oklahoma Debate and Discussion Institute at the University.

OCTOBER 19: The debate was a success and the material for the negative side is now in the hands of the debate teams. We still have some on hand for individuals. National Physicians Committee, A. M. A., and many other organizations are due thanks for their cooperation.

Money is character; money also is power. I have power not in proportion to the money I spend on myself, but in proportion to the money I can, if I please, give away to another.—*Bulwer-Lytton.*

MID-WEST SURGICAL SUPPLY CO., INC.

216 S. Market   Phone 3-3562   Wichita, Kansas

SALES AND SERVICE

FRED R. COZART
2437 N.W. 36th Terrace
Oklahoma City, Oklahoma
Phone 8-2561

N. W. COZART
Commerce Building
Okmulgee, Oklahoma
Phone 2403-W

"Soliciting The Medical Profession Exclusively"

NO. 5 In Schenley Laboratories' continuing summary of penicillin therapy

FURUNCULOSIS:

treatment with

PENICILLIN

SCHENLEY

The efficacy of penicillin in overcoming infections caused by the pyogenic cocci associated with furunculosis and carbuncles was established from the first clinical reports of the original Oxford investigators. Today penicillin is acknowledged to be the drug of choice in the treatment of pyogenic dermatoses.

Rapidly successful results are secured by following the dictum of clinicians widely experienced in penicillin therapy:

give enough—soon enough—long enough

1. PENICILLIN SCHENLEY (PARENTERAL) Initial injection of 25,000 units to establish an effective blood level—followed by injections of 25,000 units every 3 hours—are suggested.

2. THE VALUE OF PENICILLIN OINTMENT SCHENLEY for topical application is quickly demonstrable where lesions are on the surface or readily accessible. Each gram of ointment contains 1,000 units of calcium penicillin incorporated in an anhydrous base.

3. THE VALUE OF PENICILLIN TABLETS SCHENLEY administered orally as a supplement to parenteral therapy is well established. They are particularly useful when continuing penicillin therapy is desirable. Each tablet supplies 50,000 units of calcium penicillin buffered with calcium carbonate, specially coated to overcome penicillin taste.

EXECUTIVE OFFICES: 350 FIFTH AVENUE • NEW YORK CITY **SCHENLEY LABORATORIES, INC.**

Copyright 1947, Schenley Laboratories, Inc., N.Y.C.

Medical School Notes

Dean J. P. Gray of the University of Oklahoma Medical School and Dr. John Lamb of Oklahoma City were guest speakers at a meeting of the Duncan Rotary club, which district Governor Joe McBride of Anadarko also attended.

The Oklahoma Medical Research Foundation and proposed research institute were discussed by Dr. Lamb, while Dean Gray discussed further development of medical science in Oklahoma and the Wagner-Murray-Dingle bill.

"The need is for medical care, as well as hospital care, on a prepayment basis," Dean Gray said, "but what we need is a plan for prepayment upon which medical men could agree as feasible. We don't want someone in Washington setting up that plan for us."

Dr. Lamb discussed need for research in medicine in Oklahoma and said the profession has received considerable encouragement from private citizens for establishment of the proposed research institute.

Dr. Clifford Gastineau, Class '43 (Med), was a recent visitor to the School. Dr. Gastineau is serving a fellowship in Internal Medicine at the Mayo Clinic.

T. J. Barb, Jr., M.D., Class '33 (Med), has been released from military service and is now located with the Veteran's Administration Office at Oklahoma City.

The National Board Examinations were given at the School of Medicine, September 30th, October 1st and 2nd.

Dr. J. P. Gray, Dean, and Dr. J. F. Hackler, Professor of Preventive Medicine and Public Health, attended a conference on Preventive Medicine and Health Economics the week of September 30th at the University of Michigan, School of Public Health. At this conference sponsored by the Conference of Professors of Preventive Medicine, Association of Schools of Public Health, the University of Michigan, and Rockefeller Foundation, Dr. Gray presented a paper entitled "Who Should Teach Health Economics?"

PUBLIC HEALTH APPOINTMENTS

Appointment of the following physicians as health officers has been announced by the State Department of Health: *George Winn, M.D.*, Lawton, county superintendent of health of Comanche County; *James K. Gray, M.D.*, acting director of Kay County Health Department; *J. Walter Hough, M.D.*, acting director of the Ottawa County Health Department; *J. M. Gordon, M.D.*, Ardmore, county superintendent of health of Carter County, *W. W. Cotton, M.D.*, Atoka, county superintendent of health of Atoka County; *Alfred R. Sugg, M.D.*, of Ada, county superintendent of health of Pontotoc County. *Dr. J. R. Hinshaw* has resumed his post as director of the Pittsburg County Health Department. *Dr. Paul Powell* has resigned as the director of the Kay County Health Unit.

One half of the world must sweat and groan that the other half may dream.—*Longfellow.*

Your real influence is measured by your treatment of yourself.—*A. Bronson Alcott.*

There is more self love than love in jealousy.—*La Rochefoucauld.*

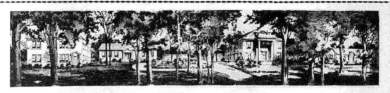

TIMBERLAWN SANITARIUM

for

Nervous and Mental Diseases

Phone Tenison 3-6333   DALLAS 1, TEXAS   P. O. Box 1769

Fifty private rooms. Complete modern facilities for Insulin shock and electro-shock therapy, under constant medical supervision. Psychotherapy. Occupational therapy. All other accepted methods of psychiatric treatment.

NARCOTIC CASES NOT ADMITTED

The Staff

Dr. Guy F. Witt
Dr. Perry C. Talkington, | Medical Directors
Major Perry C. Talkington, Associate Psychiatrist,
   (On leave for army duty.)
Dr. F. T. Harrington, Resident Psychiatrist.
Dr. Chas. F. Bullion, Associate Psychiatrist.

Mrs. Nellie Cooper, R. N., Supt. of Nurses.
J. E. Buford, C. P. A., Business Manager.
Mrs. Bess C. West, Record Librarian.
Miss Eura Gross, O. T. R., Director Occupational Therapy.

Have You Heard That...

Dr. *Henry Turner* will appear on the program of the Omaha Midwest Clinical Society at its 14th Annual Assembly in Omaha, Nebraska, October 27 to November 1. Dr. Turner will present a paper entitled "Present Limitations of Pituitary Therapy".

Dr. *Robert O. Ryan*, formerly of Fairview, Oklahoma, has joined the staff of the Oklahoma A & M College Infirmary, bringing the total of physicians to five. This includes another newcomer, *Dr. Betty Conrad*, of Sapulpa; *Dr. Roxie A. Webber*, assistant director; *Dr. John F. Reardon*; and *Dr. J. O. Thomson*, director of the student health service.

Dr. *J. R. Taylor* has become permanently associated with *Dr. F. C. Lattimore* in Kingfisher, following his discharge from the Army.

Dr. *John Y. Battenfield* has arrived in Liberia, West Africa, and has joined the staff of a Firestone Plantation Company. Dr. Battenfield was director of the University of Oklahoma student health service last year and has been succeeded by *Dr. James O. Hood*, president of the Cleveland County Medical Society.

Dr. *D. W. McCauley* has become associated with *Drs. C. H. McBurney and Hugh Hays* at the Clinton Clinic. Formerly of Okmulgee, Dr. McCauley was grauated from the University of Oklahoma School of Medicine and took his internship at the University of Colorado Hospital in Denver and practiced in Tulsa before serving in the Armed Forces.

Forty-seven years of service at the Central State Hospital, Norman, have been completed by *Dr. D. W. Griffin*. October 8 marked the beginning of his 48th year as superintendent.

Two members of the Anadarko hospital staff attended postgraduate courses in October. *Dr. Edward T. Cook, Jr.*, attended a course in internal medicine at the Cook County School of Medicine in Chicago and *Dr. J. B. Miles* attended the International College of Surgeons convention in Detroit, Michigan.

Appointment of *Dr. Herbert Howard* as house physician at Southwestern Hospital at Lawton has been announced. Dr. Howard served in the Army for three years and was relieved from active duty in March with the rank of Major.

Dr. *H. M. McClure*, Chickasha, has purchased *Dr. D. S. Downey's* interest in the Chickasha Hospital and Clinic. Dr. Downey, one of the founders, will continue his association with the hospital.

Dr. *Roy L. Fisher* of Frederick, formerly Col. Fisher of the United States Army Air Forces, has concluded his tour of duty and will resume private practice in Frederick on November 1, continuing his association with *Dr. O. G. Bacon* at the Frederick Clinic Hospital.

At the present time *Dr. O. E. Templin*, Alva, is vacationing in California.

Dr. *O. C. Newman* of Shattuck has recently visited the Mayo Clinic and attended a postgraduate course at the Cook County Graduate School in Chicago.

Dean of the Medical School, *Dr. J. P. Gray*, will address the Lions Club of Guthrie on November 29 as the guest of *Dr. J. L. LeHew*.

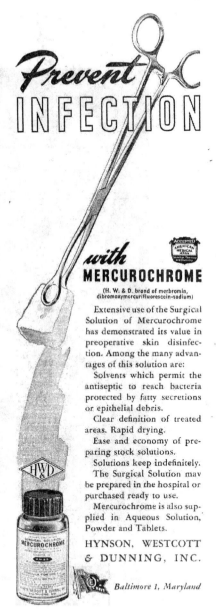

Prevent INFECTION

with MERCUROCHROME

(H. W. & D. brand of merbromin, dibromoxymercurifluorescein-sodium)

Extensive use of the Surgical Solution of Mercurochrome has demonstrated its value in preoperative skin disinfection. Among the many advantages of this solution are:

Solvents which permit the antiseptic to reach bacteria protected by fatty secretions or epithelial debris.

Clear definition of treated areas. Rapid drying.

Ease and economy of preparing stock solutions.

Solutions keep indefinitely.

The Surgical Solution may be prepared in the hospital or purchased ready to use.

Mercurochrome is also supplied in Aqueous Solution, Powder and Tablets.

HYNSON, WESTCOTT & DUNNING, INC.

Baltimore 1, Maryland

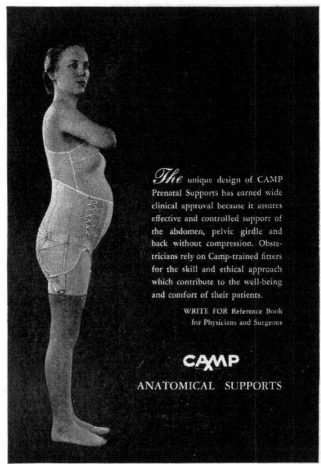

The unique design of CAMP Prenatal Supports has earned wide clinical approval because it assures effective and controlled support of the abdomen, pelvic girdle and back without compression. Obstetricians rely on Camp-trained fitters for the skill and ethical approach which contribute to the well-being and comfort of their patients.

WRITE FOR Reference Book for Physicians and Surgeons

CAMP

ANATOMICAL SUPPORTS

S. H. CAMP AND COMPANY • Jackson, Michigan
World's Largest Manufacturers of Scientific Supports
Offices in New York • Chicago • Windsor, Ontario • London, England

Book Review

PNEUMOPERITONEUM TREATMENT. Andrew Ladislaus Banyai, M.D. 366 pages. St. Louis: C. V. Mosby Company. Price $6.50.

Pneumoperitoneum Treatment provides us with the first complete treatise of this mode of therapy by one who is well qualified for the task.

The basic principles of artificial pneumoperitoneum are covered in considerable detail. The physiologic changes following pneumoperitoneum are well presented. In discussing intraperitoneal pressure Banyai points out how the subdiaphragmatic region differs from other parts of the abdominal cavity in that the intrapleural negative pressure is transmitted to this area. This is apparent when the subdiaphragmatic route is used in giving pneumoperitoneum. Here the manometer readings coincide with the intrapleural pressures.

In the section on the therapeutic application of pneumoperitoneum, all the possible uses of pneumoperitoneum are explored. In this section the various possible uses of pneumoperitoneum are given. The rational and the results of its use in tuberculous enterocolitis and peritonitis are presented in detail. Considerable discussion is given to tuberculous enterocolitis with many authors and their results cited.

As for its use in pulmonary tuberculosis, to quote Banyai: "In properly selected cases, pneumoperitoneum when given at regular intervals is capable of introducing a degree of relaxation of the lung that is known to be sufficient to improve the resistance, defense and repair of the pulmonary tissues and thus to bring about a condition which is favorable to the healing process of tuberculous lesions."

While we don't share Dr. Banyai's enthusiasm for pneumoperitoneum, particularly in entercolitis, all methods of therapy are presented so as to give the reader a good prospective of the entire subject of phthisiotherapy. We believe this book can be read with great profit by all interested in the management of the tuberculous.—Richard M. Burke, M.D.

Medical Abstracts

BILATERAL PARALYSIS OF THE ABDUCTOR MUSCLES OF THE LARYNX: ARYTENOIDECTOMY. Joseph Kelly. The Surgical Clinics of North America. Volume 26, pp. 464-476. April, 1946.

Until about 1939, all surgical attempt to correct the stenosis caused by bilateral muscular paralysis of the larynx had been directed at the interior of the larynx. Byron T. King was the first who tried to correct this condition by an extralaryngeal surgical procedure. However, even his operation met with but little success.

The author worked out a new procedure which gave satisfactory results. His technic of arytenoidectomy is outlined as follows.

A horizontal incision is made near the lower border of the thyroid cartilage, extending from the median line of the neck to the anterior border of the sternocleidomastoid muscle. The skin, the platysma and the pretracheal fascia are cut and the pretracheal muscles exposed, separated and cut according to the method of thyroidectomy. Then, the thyroid muscle is cut and elevated, and a window is made in the lower posterior third of the thyroid cartilage below the level of the thyroid notch; the size of the window varies with the size of the larynx; ordinarily, a ⅜ inch-square window is sufficient.

Then, the internal perichondrium is incised and removed, and by careful dissection the arytenoid cartilage and the cricoarytenoid articulation are exposed. The capsule of this articulation is severed, and the cartilage tumbled from its joint, lifted and freed of its remaining attachments. A vitallium wire suture is placed in the mucosa covering the vocal process of the arytenoid; this suture goes through the thyroid and the external perichondrium. This will pull the vocal cord away from the median line. Then, the external wound is closed layer after layer. It is sufficient to perform the operation on one side of the larynx only.—M.D.H.

DIAGNOSTIC CLINIC OF INTERNAL MEDICINE AND ALLERGY

Philip M. McNeill, M. D., F. A. C. P.

General Diagnosis

CONSULTATION BY APPOINTMENT

Special Attention to Cardiac, Pulmonary and Allergic Diseases

Electrocardiograph, X-Ray, Laboratory and Complete Allergic Surveys Available.

1107 Medical Arts Bldg.
Oklahoma City, Okla.   Phone 2-0277

In the Dietary
of Diabetes Mellitus

Prior to the advent of insulin, excessive protein breakdown was a frequent occurrence in the uncontrolled diabetic patient. This protein waste manifested itself in the excretion of large amounts of nitrogen in the urine, a situation encountered even today when long standing diabetes mellitus is first detected in a patient.

The basis underlying this faulty protein metabolism is an increased conversion of protein to carbohydrate, derived from the glycogenic amino acids. Consequently, restriction of protein intake was justified, even at the expense of negative nitrogen balance.

Through the use of adequate amounts of insulin, protein breakdown for glycogenesis is largely preventable. Based on the modern concept of the vital role of protein in the body economy, the prescribed dietary initially provides at least 1.5 Gm. of protein per Kg. of body weight* to compensate for past negative nitrogen balance. After the first few weeks of treatment, the protein intake is dropped to not less than 70 Gm. daily.

This liberal protein allowance, readily "covered" by insulin, has the additional advantages of providing generous amounts of B complex vitamins, and of exerting a beneficial influence upon hepatic function, derangement of which is considered by some investigators to be a factor in the pathogenesis of diabetes mellitus.

Among the protein foods of man, meat ranks high as a source of biologically adequate protein, capable of satisfying all protein needs. It provides generous amounts of B complex vitamins, and enhances the biologic quality of less complete proteins derived from other foods.

*Stare, F. J., and Thorn, G. W.: Protein Nutrition in Problems of Medical Interest, J. A. M. A. 127:1120 (April 28) 1945.

The Seal of Acceptance denotes that the nutritional statements made in this advertisement are acceptable to the Council on Foods and Nutrition of the American Medical Association.

AMERICAN MEAT INSTITUTE
MAIN OFFICE, CHICAGO . . . MEMBERS THROUGHOUT THE UNITED STATES

THE ROLE OF THE OTOLOGIST IN A HEARING CONSERVATION PROGRAM. W. E. Grove. The Annals of Otology, Rhinology and Laryngology, Volume 54, pp. 458-465. September, 1945.

Loss of hearing, as loss of vision or interference with any of the other body functions, is distinctly a medical problem. Yet, there was not much that the otologist did for the conservation of the hearing of the nation. In recent years, however, much more can be done, and is done for prevention of hearing defects than formerly when even our diagnostic tools were inaccurate.

Most of the hearing defects of adults are irreversible in character. They may be conductive in type, due to chronic adhesive processes or to the hereditary otosclerosis; they may be perceptive in type due to a great variety of causes, including even syphilis, endocrine and metabolic disorders, exposure to excessive noise or to blast concussions, excessive use of salicylic acid, salol, etc. Only a few of these fixed hearing changes are amenable to surgical treatment by the fenestration operation. For the remainder, one has to call in the help of lip-reading and the hearing aid.

Lip-reading is a science itself and belongs to specially trained teachers. The otologist should mobilize all the lip-reading facilities in his particular area so that he could intelligently direct his patients to the proper teacher. In regard to hearing aids, the modern radio-tube aid has made a great development. Many of these instruments now meet the minimum requirements set up by the Council of Physical Medicine of the American Medical Association. The list of approved instruments can be obtained from the Council.

In general, better performance can be expected from an air conduction than from a bone conduction instrument since it takes many times the electrical energy to make an individual hear by bone conduction than by air conduction. Fitting of these instruments must be made by trial and error. A hearing aid cannot be fitted to an audiometric curve; it must be fitted to the individual patient. Fitting is again a highly specialized job, and the otologist should only supervise the work of an expert fitter.

Hearing aids are still not perfect, especially for patients with a high degree of perceptive deafness. They can expect only a little boost from the hearing aids, and they must piece out the consonant pattern of speech by lip reading. The fenestration operation is still in its experimental stage, though great improvement can be expected in the properly selected cases.

Conservation of hearing finds its widest field among children who have hearing defects. Only in approximately 10 to 20 per cent of children is the hearing loss permanent. The remainder can be helped by proper attention to enlarged tonsils and adenoids, nasopharyngeal infections, repeated colds or repeated attacks of otitis media. Unfortunately, the adenoid operation is the most poorly performed operation in present day surgery.—M.D.H.

LIPIODOL INTRAVASATION DURING UTEROSALPINGOGRAPHY WITH PULMONARY COMPLICATIONS. D. Eisen, M.D., and J. Goldstein, M.D. Radiology, Vol. 45, p. 603. 1945.

The accidental intravasation of lipiodol into the venous system of the uterus during uterosalpingography has been repeatedly described in the literature. As a rule there were no ill effects, except perhaps slight temporary leucocytosis. In rare cases, pulmonary and cerebral embolism and pulmonary infarction were noted.

In an attempt to study the mechanism of lipiodol embolism in the lungs, Sicard and Forestier injected from two to four c.c. into the cubital vein. The lipiodol reached the lungs in five or six seconds, remained there for from six to eight minutes and then suddenly disappeared. The only effect in the patient was a slight cough. Walther

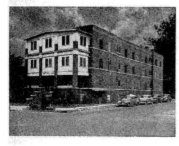

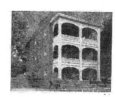

The Coyne Campbell Sanitarium, Inc.

Oklahoma City 4, Oklahoma

This is to announce that for convenience and because of the difficulty of working out a satisfactory schedule to fit into being at both places at the same time, we have moved our offices out of the Medical Arts Bldg. back to the sanitarium at

131 N. E. 4th
Oklahoma City 4, Oklahoma

Coyne H. Campbell, M.D., F.A.C.P.
Ben Bell, M.D.
Sybil Lane, R.N.
Margaret Byrd, R.N.
J. H. Barthold, Business Manager

injected lipiodol into the ear vein of rabbits. He found that practically all of the oil became arrested in the lungs where it underwent two processes. The major part was broken up into iodine and fat, the iodine being excreted through the kidneys during the first eight days as potassium iodide, and the fat being saponified and carried away by the circulation. A smaller part of the lipiodol became phagocytosed. Walther also suggested that an inflammation may develop around fat droplets because of bacteria carried along by the lipiodol from the uterus.

A review of the literature revealed that the various authors attributed the intravasation to trauma of the endometrium during the injection, to excessive pressure, and to an increased permeability of the receiving sinuses, such as is observed in idiopathic uterine bleedings or immediately after menstruation.

The authors themselves noted intravasation of lipiodol during uterosalpingography in a woman 28 years of age. The case is briefly described: The afternoon after the injection the patient developed a dry cough with a temperature of 102 degrees. The next day her cough increased and she brought up bloody sputum. The tem-

perature remained high until the fourth day when it dropped to normal. The cough persisted, however, and a roentgenogram of the chest on the ninth day revealed a dense patchy opacity involving the lower two-thirds of both lungs. Another roentgenogram one month later showed practically a normal appearance.

In conjunction with this case the authors recommended the following precautions: (1) uterosalpingography should not be performed sooner than from eight to ten days after the menstrual period or any operation on the uterus; (2) the position of the uterus should be determined preliminarily by the use of a sound and in case of angulation the injection should be done by properly circumventing the angulation so as to avoid trauma to the endometrium; (3) the pressure of the injection should not exceed from 180 to 200 mm. of mercury, a manometer being used for control; and (4) the amount of lipiodol injected should be no more than is necessary to fill the uterus and tubes, with a slight spill.

COMMENT: Lipiodol injection and gas insufflation into the uterus may be hazardous. Simple vaginal insufflation may also be dangerous. Gas embolism may occur.—G.P.

SPRINGER CLINIC
Tulsa, Oklahoma

Medicine
D. O. SMITH, M.D.
H. A. RUPRECHT, M.D.
E. G. HYATT, M.D.
ALBERT W. WALLACE, M.D.

Neurology and Psychiatry
TOM R. TURNER, M.D

Surgery
CARL HOTZ, M.D.

604 South Cincinnati

Urology
BERGET H. BLOCKSOM, M.D.

Eye, Ear, Nose and Throat
D. L. MISHLER, M.D.

Obstetrics
F. D. SINCLAIR, M.D.

Pediatrics
G. R. RUSSELL, M.D.
LUVERN HAYS, M.D.

Anesthesia
M. R. STEEL, M.D.

Phone 7156

C. A. GALLAGHER, M. D.
CURT VON WEDEL, M. D.
(Consultant)

PLASTIC and RECONSTRUCTION SURGERY

610 N. W. Ninth Street
Oklahoma City, Oklahoma

Office 2-3108

The Menninger Sanitarium

For the Diagnosis and Treatment
of Nervous and Mental Illness.

The Southard School

For the Education and Psychiatric
Treatment of Children of Average
and Superior Intelligence.

Boarding Home Facilities.

Topeka, Kansas

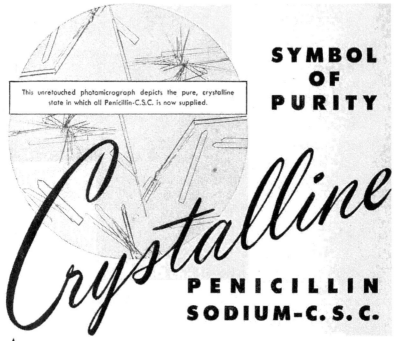

This unretouched photomicrograph depicts the pure, crystalline state in which all Penicillin-C.S.C. is now supplied.

SYMBOL OF PURITY

Crystalline PENICILLIN SODIUM-C. S. C.

As a result of special processes of purification and crystallization, all Penicillin-C.S.C. is now supplied in the form of the highly purified, heat-stable Crystalline Sodium Salt of Penicillin-C.S.C.

Well Tolerated Subcutaneously
In the crystalline state Penicillin Sodium-C.S.C. is so pure that it can be administered subcutaneously even in large doses with virtually no pain or danger of untoward reactions due to impurities.

No Refrigeration Required
Crystalline Penicillin Sodium-C.S.C. is so heat-stable that it can be kept at room temperatures, virtually indefinitely without losing its potency.* It can now be carried in the physician's bag or stored on the pharmacy shelf. No longer need the physician wait until the patient can be hospitalized or until refrigerated penicillin can be obtained from the nearest depot.

*CAUTION: Once in solution, however, penicillin still requires refrigeration.

Optimal Therapeutic Activity
Because of its high potency per milligram, Crystalline Penicillin Sodium-C.S.C. exerts optimal therapeutic activity. A recent report shows the advantage of highly potent preparations.[1]

Potency Clearly Stated on Label
The high state of purification achieved in Crystalline Penicillin Sodium-C.S.C. is indicated by *its high potency per milligram*. The number of units per milligram is stated on each vial, thus enabling the physician to know the degree of purification of the penicillin he is using.

[1] "The potency of the penicillin undoubtedly affected the results. The first 15 patients, all treated with the same batch of penicillin, were cured. The next 7 patients were treated with the same dosage of a different batch of penicillin. Five of these 7 were not cured. Assays of penicillin used for these 7 patients showed it to be of reduced potency." Trumper, M., and Thompson, G. J.: Prolonging the Effects of Penicillin by Chilling, J A M A. 130: 628 (March 9) 1946.

Crystalline Penicillin Sodium-C.S.C. is available in serum-type vials containing 100,000, 200,000, or 500,000 units.

PHARMACEUTICAL DIVISION
COMMERCIAL SOLVENTS Corporation
CSC

Penicillin-C.S.C. is accepted by the Council on Pharmacy and Chemistry of the American Medical Association

17 East 42nd Street   New York 17, N. Y.

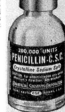

"HITS, STRIKES AND OUTS" IN THE USE OF PEDICLE FLAPS FOR NASAL RESTORATION OR CORREC-TION. Vilray P. Blair and Louis T. Byars. Surgery. Gynecology and Obstetrics. Vol. 82. No. 4. pp. 367-385; April, 1946.

"The purpose of this paper is to illustrate some of the underlying factors that can make either for success or for failure in the substitution of skin bearing flaps for lost or lacking nasal tissue. Such flaps may be used alone or supplemented with cartilage implants or free skin grafts. The need for nasal restorations or corrections might come from (1) congenital absence (total or partial), (2) post natal growth irregularities, (3) tissue loss through disease, accident or surgical destruction."

This is a most excellent paper in that it is highly technical, but at the same time is so richly illustrated with photographs that it can be read with profit by any surgeon. The presentation is refreshing because cases are shown and discussed in which the final results were not one hundred per cent perfect.

Lastly, it shows in a striking, graphic manner the enormous amount of work involved in reconstructive surgery.—J.F.B.

SOME INTERESTING LESIONS OF THE TONGUE. Russell A. Sage. Archives of Otolaryngology. Volume 43. pp. 122-133. February, 1946.

Observation and study of the tongue were once an important part of every general physical examination. The tongue contributes many signs for establishing a diagnosis, and it is easy to examine, always ready to give the evidence without elaborate clinical facilities.

The pathologic conditions of the tongue may result from metabolic diseases, infections, tumors, congenital abnormalities, and mechanical causes. Anemia is indicated by a pale tongue, while a slick tongue means vitamin deficiency. Coating may be due to lack of oral clean-

liness, or it may be the result of some general illness. Edema is the result of infection or allergy; it may occur after eating a food to which a person is sensitive, and may be relieved by epinephrine.

Inflammation of the folium linguae may be caused by a jagged tooth or by infection of the taste buds in the area. The so-called burning tongue results either from anemia, or vitamin deficiency, or an ill fitting and improperly vulcanized denture; it occurs also in excessive smokers. Various vitamin deficiencies may cause the pebbled tongue. The geographic tongue is a series of bare spots on the organ, surrounded by rings of whitish fur; it is also called wandering rash, a relatively harmless condition.

Leukoplakia is due to proliferation of the superficial layers of mucosa; its cause is not known, but it is aggravated by such irritants as alcohol, tobacco, and spices; the condition is considered as an introduction to cancer. Purpura occasionally is seen in serious general conditions. The furrowed, grooved or scrotal tongue is a congenital familial condition of little pathological significance. Ulcers may develop from various causes, from infection and chronic irritation; they are to be treated by chemical cautery. The variety of ulcer called canker sore is often due to food allergy, and may be relieved by light cauterization with Bonain's solution. One type of canker sore appears in young women at the menstrual period; this is probably due to a virus infection.

Syphilis may cause chancre, mucous patches and gummata in the tongue all of which need specific treatment by means of arsenical preparations. The most common tumors are papilloma, keloid, fibroma, carcinoma, and, on the under side of the tongue, cyst of salivary glands.

Pyogenic granuloma is a mushroom-shaped growth attached to the tongue by a pedicle. It is composed of simple granulation tissue, and contains staphylococci. It usually starts from an infected site of injury. It needs

ALCOHOL—MORPHINE—BARBITAL

ADDICTIONS Successfully Treated Since 1897—
Founded by B. B. Ralph, M.D.

Write for descriptive booklet

The Ralph Sanitarium

529 Highland Ave.   Kansas City. Mo.

Telephone—Victor 4850

Registered by the Council on Medical Education and Hospitals of the A. M. A.

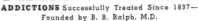
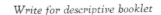
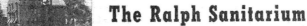

A COLLECTION SERVICE DEDICATED TO . . .
The Medical Profession . . . Hospitals
ALL MONEY IS PAID DIRECT TO THE CREDITOR

A record of twenty-eight years service to Doctors, Clinics and Hospitals insures a kindly and understanding service to your debtors. . . . Since all money is paid to you, you are still guardian of your accounts and all monies. . . . You pay us commission only on such amounts as are paid to you. . . . Won't you please write for a list of our Doctor and Clinic clients in Oklahoma, and enlist our help, while the time for collections is opportune?

READING & SMITH SERVICE BUREAU

COMMERCE BUILDING   KANSAS CITY 6, MISSOURI complete removal, with cauterization of its base, otherwise recurrence is possible.

Black tongue or hairy tongue is a condition in which the filiform papillae in the rhomboid area of the tongue become elongated and overgrown with the aspergillus niger fungus. The long papillae usually set up an irritation and tickling of the throat. Treatment consists in shaving off the growth with a dull knife and applying a 2 per cent solution of salicylic acid.—M.D.H.

HYPERTROPHY OF THE UTERUS. A. H. Curtis, M.D. American Journal of Obstetrics and Gynecology. Vol. 50, p. 748. 1945.

The usual symptoms of hypertrophy of the uterus are prolonged and/or excessive menstruation, pelvic pressure with more or less sensation of weight and pressure in the pelvis and usually a considerable increase in the vaginal discharge.

Examination reveals a large uterus, usually heavy, usually retrodisplaced, either movable or fixed and sometimes difficult to differentiate from adenomyosis, deeply buried myoma and carcinoma of the body. The differentiation of the latter may be difficult even after D & C, since there is usually a very active hypertrophy and hyperplasia of the endometrium.

The author then discusses various stains to be used in studying the myometrium to determine the proportion of muscle cells to connective tissue cells.

It seems evident that incomplete involution (subinvolution) of the uterus following delivery, associated with a low grade metritis (possibly following cervical lacerations) are the two causes which work synergistically to produce the condition, but the author thinks that possibly abnormal hormonal balance may be a factor.

The treatment is surgical; the D & C done for diagnosis may stop the abnormal bleeding for months. If abdominal surgery is necessary, the operation of choice is hysterectomy, either complete or supravaginal, depending on the condition of the cervix.—G.P.

THROMBIN TECHNIQUE IN OPHTHALMIC SURGERY. T. G. W. Parry and G. C. Laszlo. The British Journal of Ophthalmology. Vol 30, pp. 176-178. March, 1946.

The use of thrombin is well established in plastic surgery. It is an extract of blood platelets and its action is to reduce the bleeding time at any raw surface, thus securing quick and firm adhesion between two raw areas of tissue. Thrombin is capable of reducing the bleeding time from the normal 6-8 minutes to 15 seconds.

Plastic surgeons apply thrombin to the actual surfaces of the graft and bed, and it is generally agreed that the adhesion of such a graft becomes firm enough in many cases to dispense with sutures. The authors thought that thrombin might be of great value in cataract surgery and in conjunctival plastics and operations involving the conjuctiva in general.

In cataract cases the section was made in the usual manner with a large conjunctival flap. After completing the removal of the lens, the flap was grasped and turned with its inner surface upwards; previously prepared thrombin was instilled on the everted surface and on the raw area of the globe, and the flap placed back and ironed out. In cases of squint, catgut was used for suturing the muscle, and thrombin was instilled over the whole area of operation; then the edges of the conjunctival wound were immediately brought into apposition and held in this position for approximately one minute.

Though the number of operations carried out with the above technique is not large enough, it is possible to say that the authors managed to get well sealed wounds in cataract operations in which the sealing effect lasted through the danger period of rupture of the wound. In squint operations they obtained well healing wounds with good cosmetic results and with little local reaction, owing to the absence of conjunctival suture. —M.D.H.

J. E. HANGER, Inc.

ARTIFICIAL LIMBS, BRACES, AND CRUTCHES

Phone: 2-8500   612 N. Hudson

L. T. Lewis, Mgr.   BRANCHES AND AGENCIES IN PRINCIPAL CITIES   Oklahoma City 3, Okla.

FREE SAMPLE

DR. _____
ADDRESS _____
CITY _____
STATE _____

AR-EX COSMETICS, INC.,

ROUGH HANDS
FROM TOO MUCH SCRUBBING?

Soften dry skin with AR-EX CHAP CREAM! Contains carbonyl diamide, shown in hospital test to make skin softer, smoother, and even whiter! Archives of Derm. and S., July, 1943. FREE SAMPLE.

AR-EX CHAP CREAM

1036 W. VAN BUREN ST., CHICAGO 7, ILL.

WOODCROFT HOSPITAL

A modern institution for the scientific care and treatment of those nervously and mentally ill, the senile and addicts.

Pueblo, Colorado   Crum Epler, M.D.
Phone 84   Superintendent

Write for information

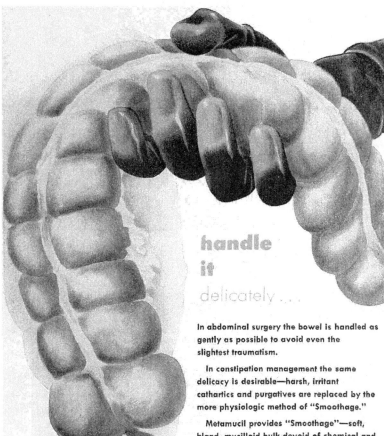

handle it delicately ...

In abdominal surgery the bowel is handled as gently as possible to avoid even the slightest traumatism.

In constipation management the same delicacy is desirable—harsh, irritant cathartics and purgatives are replaced by the more physiologic method of "Smoothage."

Metamucil provides "Smoothage"—soft, bland, mucilloid bulk devoid of chemical and physical irritants.

Metamucil is the highly refined mucilloid of a seed of the psyllium group, **Plantago ovata (50%), combined with dextrose (50%).**

Metamucil is the registered trademark of
G. D. Searle & Co., Chicago 80, Illinois

SEARLE

RESEARCH IN THE SERVICE OF MEDICINE

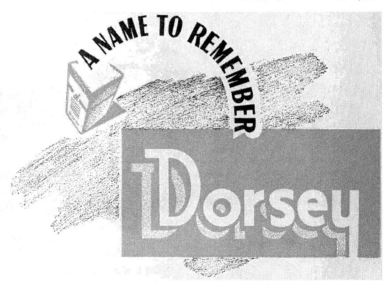

IT'S no trouble to remember the name of a friend . . . the street where you live . . . a favorite restaurant, clothier, druggist. These names are important; YOU DEPEND UPON THEM.

In professional life, also, a man remembers the names which play an important role: interesting patients, colleagues of consequence, medications you rely upon day after day—AND THE NAMES OF THEIR MANUFACTURERS.

Dorsey is one of the names you can count upon—a name to remember. For Dorsey (until recently Smith-Dorsey) has been making reliable pharmaceuticals for the medical profession since 1908. Dorsey products are backed by the Dorsey laboratories—fully equipped, capably staffed, following rigidly standardized testing procedures throughout.

Dorsey is a name you can depend upon . . .

THE SMITH-DORSEY COMPANY
LINCOLN, NEBRASKA
DALLAS, TEXAS　　　LOS ANGELES, CALIF.

MANUFACTURERS OF
PURIFIED SOLUTION OF LIVER-DORSEY
SOLUTION OF ESTROGENIC SUBSTANCES-DORSEY

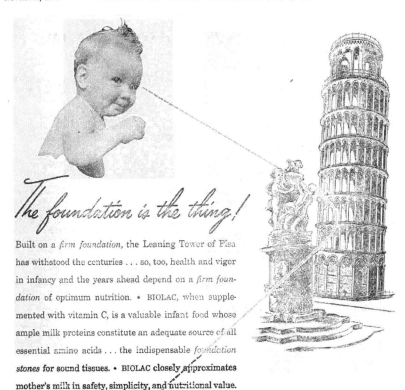

The foundation is the thing!

Built on a *firm foundation*, the Leaning Tower of Pisa
has withstood the centuries ... so, too, health and vigor
in infancy and the years ahead depend on a *firm foundation* of optimum nutrition. • BIOLAC, when supplemented with vitamin C, is a valuable infant food whose
ample milk proteins constitute an adequate source of all
essential amino acids ... the indispensable *foundation*
stones for sound tissues. • BIOLAC closely approximates
mother's milk in safety, simplicity, and nutritional value.

BORDEN'S PRESCRIPTION PRODUCTS DIVISION 350 MADISON AVENUE, NEW YORK 17, N. Y.

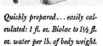

Biolac

"BABY TALK" FOR A GOOD SQUARE MEAL

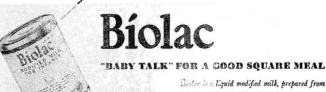

*Biolac is a liquid modified milk, prepared from
whole and skim milk with added lactose, and
fortified with vitamin B_1, concentrate of vitamins
A and D from cod liver oil, and iron citrate.
Evaporated, homogenized and sterilized, Biolac
is available in 13 fl. oz. cans at all drug stores.*

*Quickly prepared ... easily cal-
culated: 1 fl. oz. Biolac to 1½ fl.
oz. water per lb. of body weight.*

OFFICERS OF COUNTY SOCIETIES, 1946

★

COUNTY	PRESIDENT	SECRETARY	MEETING TIME
Alfalfa	W. G. Dunnington, Cherokee	L. T. Lancaster, Cherokee	Last Tues. each Second Month
Atoka-Coal	J. B. Clark, Coalgate	J. S. Fulton, Atoka	
Beckham	P. J. DeVanney, Sayre	J. E. Levick, Elk City	Second Tuesday
Blaine	W. F. Bohlman, Watonga	Virginia Curtin, Watonga	Third Thursday
Bryan	W. K. Haynie, Durant	Jonah Nichols, Durant	Second Tuesday
Caddo	P. H. Anderson, Anadarko	Edward T. Cook, Jr., Anadarko	Third Thursday
Canadian	G. L. Goodman, Yukon	W. P. Lawton, El Reno	Subject to call
Carter	J. Hobson Veazey, Ardmore	H. A. Higgins, Ardmore	Second Tuesday
Cherokee	P. H. Medearis, Tahlequah	R. K. McIntosh, Jr., Tahlequah	First Tuesday
Choctaw	Floyd L. Waters, Hugo	O. R. Gregg, Hugo	
Cleveland	James O. Hood, Norman	Phil Haddock, Norman	Thursday nights
Comanche	Wm. Cole, Lawton	E. P. Hathaway, Lawton	
Cotton	G. W. Baker, Walters	Mollie Sciam, Walters	Third Friday
Craig	Lloyd H. McPike, Vinita	J. M. McMillan, Vinita	
Creek	W. P. Longmire, Sapulpa	Philip Joseph, Sapulpa	Second Tuesday
Custer	Ross Deputy, Clinton	C. J. Alexander, Clinton	Third Thursday
Garfield	Bruce Hinson, Enid	John R. Walker, Enid	Fourth Thursday
Garvin	M. E. Robberson, Jr., Wynnewood	John R. Callaway, Pauls Valley	Wednesday before Third Thursday
Grady	Roy Emanuel, Chickasha	Rebecca H. Mason, Chickasha	Third Thursday
Grant	I. V. Hardy, Medford	F. P. Robinson, Pond Creek	
Greer	J. B. Lansden, Granite	J. B. Hollis, Mangum	
Harmon	W. G. Husband, Hollis	R. H. Lynch, Hollis	First Wednesday
Haskell	Wm. S. Carson, Keota	N. K. Williams, McCurtain	
Hughes	Victor W. Pryor, Holdenville	L. A. S. Johnston, Holdenville	First Friday
Jackson	E. W. Mabry, Altus	J. P. Irby, Altus	Last Monday
Jefferson	F. M. Edwards, Ringling	J. A. Dillard, Waurika	Second Monday
Kay	L. G. Neal, Ponca City	J. C. Wagner, Ponca City	Second Thursday
Kingfisher	John W. Pendleton, Kingfisher	H. Violet Sturgeon, Hennessey	
Kiowa	Wm. Bernell, Hobart	J. Wm. Finch, Hobart	
LeFlore	S. D. Bevill, Poteau	Rush L. Wright, Poteau	
Lincoln	J. S. Rollins, Prague	Ned Burleson, Prague	First Wednesday
Logan	James Petty, Guthrie	J. E. Souter, Guthrie	Last Tuesday
Mayes	L. C. White, Adair	V. D. Herrington, Pryor	
McClain	S. C. Davis, Blanchard	W. C. McCurdy, Purcell	
McCurtain	J. T. Moreland, Idabel	R. H. Sherrill, Broken Bow	Fourth Tuesday
McIntosh	F. R. First, Checotah	W. A. Tolleson, Eufaula	First Thursday
Muskogee-Sequoyah			
Wagoner	R. N. Holcombe, Muskogee	William N. Weaver, Muskogee	First Tuesday
Noble	A. M. Evans, Perry	Jesse W. Driver, Perry	
Okfuskee	W. P. Jenkins, Okemah	M. L. Whitney, Okemah	Second Monday
Oklahoma	W. F. Keller, Okla. City	John H. Lamb, Okla. City	Fourth Tuesday
Okmulgee	F. S. Watson, Okmulgee	C. E. Smith, Henryetta	Second Monday
Osage	E. C. Keyes, Hominy	Vincent Mazzurella, Hominy	Third Monday
Ottawa	C. F. Walker, Grove	W. Jackson Sayles, Miami	Second Thursday
Pawnee	H. B. Spaulding, Ralston	R. L. Browning, Pawnee	
Payne	F. Keith Oehlschlager, Yale	C. W. Moore, Stillwater	Third Thursday
Pittsburg	Millard L. Henry, McAlester	Edward D. Greenberger, McAlester	Third Friday
Pontotoc-Murray	John Morey, Ada	Ollie McBride, Ada	First Wednesday
Pottawatomie	F. P. Newlin, Shawnee	Clinton Gallaher, Shawnee	First and Third Saturday
Pushmataha	John S. Lawson, Clayton	B. M. Huckabay, Antlers	
Rogers	W. A. Howard, Chelsea	P. S. Anderson, Claremore	Third Wednesday
Seminole	Clifton Felts, Seminole	Mack I. Shanholz, Wewoka	Third Wednesday
Stephens	Everett King, Duncan	Fred L. Patterson, Duncan	
Texas	Daniel S. Lee, Guymon	E. L. Buford, Guymon	
Tillman	H. A. Culvert, Frederick	O. G. Bacon, Frederick	
Tulsa	John C. Perry, Tulsa	John E. McDonald, Tulsa	Second and Fourth Monday
Washington-Nowata	Ralph W. Rucker, Bartlesville	L. B. Word, Bartlesville	Second Wednesday
Washita	L. G. Livingston, Cordell	Roy W. Anderson, Cordell	
Woods	John F. Simon, Alva	O. E. Templin, Alva	Last Tuesday Odd Months
Woodward	T. C. Leachman, Woodward	C. W. Tedrowe, Woodward	Second Thursday

THE JOURNAL
of the
OKLAHOMA STATE MEDICAL ASSOCIATION

EDITORIALS

GIVING

In the November Atlantic Monthly, F. Emerson Andrews, in a discussion of "The New Era of Giving" says, "In 1941, which may be regarded as the last pre-war year if we forget December, reported charitable contributions totaled just a billion dollars. More than half this billion — 554 million — came from families whose income was estimated at less than $3000. To this 554 million dollars needs to be added the unknown but considerable contribution of those many other families with income below $3000 who used the short income tax form, 1040A, which does not list charitable contributions."

The author tells the following story which we should ponder. The old Scotsman who was dying said to his minister, "Will I be placed among the elect if I leave 10 thousand for Free Kirk Sustentation." The minister replied, "It's an experiment well worth trying."

The fact that much more than half the charitable contributions come from people with incomes of $3000 or less should make physicians ashamed of themselves.

Now that the Alumni or our own School of Medicine are striving to establish a creditable research fund, opportunity is knocking at the door of each member of the State Medical Association. If there is one physician whose income is not over $3000 he should give something to help maintain the reputation of that great dependable class which makes the United States the most wonderful country in the world. The physicians who have a good income and live in comfort should heed the call. Even though opportunity knocks more than once, there is never as much time as we think. It is sad to be too late. Those who live after us may deplore our procrastination. Physicians who are endowed with a wealth of worldly goods should give generously, not alone to save taxes, but for the sake of humanity. People who are well-to-do should give until they match the poor.

Again quoting from the Atlantic, Andrews says, "I have private information that the Recording Angel enters in the gift column only those dollars we have kept for ourselves. By such an accounting the poor give out of their poverty a larger part of each dollar than any other income class." While this opportunity is knocking why should not the physicians in Oklahoma, as an income class, save their faces by breaking this record.

The physicians of Oklahoma in the period of five and a half decades have made remarkable progress in clinical observation and practical therapy, but the time has arrived for concerted effort in the field of scientific research if we would continue to go forward.

The physician who thinks he should be exempt because of the charity work he does should remember that there is no such thing as a full, well rounded life in the field of medicine without a generous share in the care of the poor. More than he can realize, the physician's financial success is dependent upon grateful charity patients who have influence with the well-to-do. Physicians who are willing to lay down their lives for their patients should find it easy to lay down a few dollars for the advancement of medical knowledge.

INFLUENZA

The Commission on Acute Respiratory Diseases[1] has stressed the periodicity of influenza, and based upon the accepted interval between epidemics, the Commission anticipates such an epidemic this winter. In view of this probability the use of protective vaccines is to be considered. The available data is insufficient to truly establish the vaccines' effectiveness, but statistical studies on a limited scale is encouraging.[2][3]

The available vaccines are prepared from fertile hens' eggs and they contain both A and B viruses. But it is important to remember that the vaccine also contains egg protein. Considering the composition of the vaccine, two types of reaction may be expected: that due to the egg protein, and that related to the influenza virus. The latter stimulates the symptoms of influenza and are not considered of great importance. The former may vary from the mildest with carial manifestations to profound anaphylactic shock. When vaccination is contemplated, sensitivity to eggs should be investigated and, regardless of the history obtained, the advisability of skin tests with diluted vaccine should be considered.

Th optimal time for vaccination is at least two weeks before exposure or at least as soon as indications of an epidemic arise. The minimum duration of protective immunity is three to four months.

The danger of an epidemic this winter is rendered more emminent by certain areas and centers subjected to continuous overcrowding. Under present conditions there is great danger in colleges and universities.

BIBLIOGRAPHY

1. Commission on Acute Respiratory Diseases. Periodicity of Influenza. American Journal of Hygiene. Vol. 43; pp. 29-37. 1946.

2. T. Francis, Jr.; J. E. Salk; William Brace. Protective Effect of Vaccination Against Influenza. Journal of the American Medical Association. Vol 113; p. 275. 1946.

3. Come on Influenza et al. Clinical Evaluation Against Influenza: Preliminary Report Journal of the American Medical Association. Vol. 124; p. 987. 144.

COMPULSORY HEALTH INSURANCE AND THE TAX SITUATION

In the United States News of October 18 there is a table showing how family incomes must be increased to meet the pre-war standards of living for a family of four. With one or two exceptions, medical care shows the lowest advance in cost among all the important services. Food costs for 1941 were $935.00 as compared to $1,606.00 in 1946; clothing was $352.00 as against $528.00;

medical care $90.00 as compared to $107.00; taxes $66.00 in 1941 now estimated at $440.00.

According to the tabulation, government costs through taxation tower above all others. In view of the fact that most of the experts, including Colin Starn, America's greatest authority, believe there is little prospect of over-all tax reductions. How can the American people look with favor upon the Administration's proposal of compulsory health insurance?

Twelve billion in withholding taxes added to the present load, plus the possible necessity of making up deficits in the medical program would break the Nation's back economically and lead to a thin, anemic patriotism.

MASS MEDICAL MURDER

Only Hitler's physician and his associates who have suffered the professional degeneracy of compulsory health insurance could sink so low as to make use of medical knowledge in the willful pursuit of mass murder. Bismark, the pro-genitor of our so-called social security and the originator of compulsory health insurance in Germany, must be uneasy in his grave. Less powerful individuals, active in American politics, should sit up and take notice. Most of all, the American people should wake up and sock all such individuals. Only government controlled doctors could "murder hundreds of thousands of human beings". Private physicians never take orders from politicians or self-apointed dictators.

THE VETERANS ADMINISTRATION OUR OBLIGATION

The proposed cooperation between the Oklahoma State Medical Association and the Veterans Administration in the care of our boys should have the hearty cooperation of every member of the State Medical Association. Since the present policies of the Veterans Administration are so definitely in line with the practices of civilian medicine as a free enterprise, it would not only be short-sighted on our part to withhold cooperation, but it would be un-American. Our ex-servicemen are entitled to the best available medical and surgical care with maximum speed and a minimum of paper work and red tape.

THE OBSTETRICIAN'S RESPONSIBILITY TO THE NEW-BORN WITH ESPECIAL CONSIDERATION OF ASPHYXIA*

Roy E. Emanuel, B.S., M.D.

CHICKASHA, OKLAHOMA

Recently I heard Dr. Donovan J. McCune, while discussing abnormal children, state that the pertinent question was: "How was the child born?" His implication that the obstetrician often had the responsibility of the final outcome of the individual in his hands set me to pondering. Just how great is the obstetrician's responsibility to the new-born? I have set down some of these birth factors and have chosen to discuss them in some detail hoping that such a presentation will prove both interesting and stimulating, and bring about a keener appreciation of our responsibility in this field. We have a tremendous responsibility to the new-born; its future welfare may hinge on our skill and ability as obstetricians.

I wish to present some of the factors in outline and draw from certain of these conclusions of especial obstetric importance.

Factors influencing the condition of the infant at birth:

FIRST—Vitality of the germ plasm and hereditary influences. Over these we can have little influence other than through our study of genetic factors. I should like to call your attention to the recent studies of Dr. Clemens E. Benda on Mongolion idiocy and the frequency of its occurrence in pregnancies of late life. This is a fertile field for sound advice in presentative obstetric medicine.

SECOND—Maternal abnormalities: Anemia, infections, dietary deficiencies and metabolic disturbances, heart disease, toxemia, etc. These factors are of paramount consideration in the giving of good and adequate prenatal care.

THIRD—Fetal disease:
Syphilis and erythroblastoses
FORTH—Fetal maturity at birth:
  (a) Prematurity
  (b) Post maturity
(a) I wish to discuss prematurity at some length, because improved obstetrics

*Presented before the Section on Obstetrics and Gynecology, Oklahoma State Medical Association Annual Meeting, May 2, 1946.

management has achieved a marked reduction in the percentage of stillborn and neonatal deaths. In a statistical study of all deaths under one year of age in a large industrial town in England, it was found that 61 per cent of these death occurred in the new-born due either to birth injury or to prematurity; 34 per cent of all deaths under one year were due to prematurity. Formerly over 80 per cent of the premature infant deaths were taking place within the first 48 hours after birth. This large percentage presented a serious challenge to obstetricians. The challenge has been met with gratifying results through improved management.

Stage of prematurity: The weight of the premature infant at delivery is the most important single factor influencing its viability. With each 8 ounce increase in body weight there is a striking reduction in mortality. Evidence indicates that the foetus in utero gains weight at the rate of four ounces per week during the seventh lunar month, six ounces during the eighth and from eight to twelve ounces per week during the ninth lunar month. A three pound premature infant has a 25 per cent chance of survival, a four pound infant has a 75 per cent chance. It is clear that even a week's delay in preventing premature labor or termination by section may determine the viability of the baby.

Influence of drugs upon the premature infant: The premature infants of mothers who have received morphine or one of its derivatives have been found to encounter *twice* the death rate of infants whose mothers have not received the drug. Morphine must not be given to the mother expecting to deliver a premature infant. Other factors contributing to high mortality previously noted were type and character of anesthesia. I shall discuss these later. Also the obstetrician must choose the method of delivery which carries with it the least risk to the premature infant. Once premature labor is established the membranes should be left intact and oxytoxics withheld.

An analysis of a series of 958 premature deliveries gave the following results:

Method of Delivery	Mortality
Breech extraction	55 per cent
Caesarean section	54 per cent
Normal vertex	33 per cent
Low forceps with episiotomy	15 per cent

The unfavorable showing of caesarean section is believed due, not to the method of choice, but to its manner of execution. The faults have been the pre-operative medication and the type of anesthesia, which have exerted their unfavorable effects upon the infant. It is the asphyxia and atelectases which are productive of the high caesarean mortality. The avoidance of pre-operative medication known to depress the infant, such as nembutal and morphine and the selection of a type of anesthesia not adversely affecting the infant such as, local, spinal or caudal will favorably influence the results. Instead of a limp infant, in whom resuscitation is difficult or impossible, the delivery results in an infant that usually breathes and cries spontaneously.

The favorable showing of vertex delivery assisted by low forceps and wide episiotomy is understandable. The forceps tend to protect the head and the episiotomy reduces the resistance of the soft parts, thus minimizing the possibility of birth trauma.

(b) Post maturity presents a problem in the border line contracted pelvis, the elderly primipara with mild toxemia, not showing the desired response to indicated therapy. It is most difficult to ascertain with certainty the existence of post maturity, however, repeated and careful palpation of the abdomen and careful measurements of the height of the fundus give valuable information on the increasing size of the rapidly growing fetus. If the diagnosis of post maturity is adequately established and the indications clear, labor should be induced. The judicious employment of such a procedure may lessen the degree of birth trauma and in consequence reduce the possibility of the subsequent spastic child.

FIFTH—Anesthesia and analgesia and its production of asphyxia and atelectases:

Asphyxia is by far the most important cause of disease of the new-born. Some degree of asphyxia attends every normal birth. Until the past five or six years no one has ever paid a great deal of attention to asphyxia of the new-born infant. It has been found

to be the chief cause of death in 58 per cent of the infants autopsied at the Boston-Lying-In Hospital since 1931.

As the severity or duration of anoxemia increases physiologic and pathologic changes take place. These changes may involve every organ and tissue in the body and result in a wide variety of clinical symptoms at or following birth. Chief of these may be the permanent damage to the nervous system. Seldom is any correlation made between asphyxia at birth and abnormal conditions, which might later appear in the individual; hence the challenge from Dr. McCune as to the circumstances of the child's birth. So the justifiability of a review of the subject of asphyxia, its causes and treatment, hoping to lower its incidence. The term "Neonatal Asphyxia", should perhaps be more clearly designated as "Neonatal Apnea" and the old classification of Asphyxia lavida and pallida should give way to clinical classification of mild, moderate and severe asphyxia.

In *mild* asphyxia, muscle tone is present and pharyngeal and corneal reflexes are present. The infant is livid and has the appearance of simple breath holding.

In *moderate* asphyxia, muscle tone is present to a limited degree, but pharyngeal and corneal reflexes are lost. The infant is livid.

In *severe* asphyxia, all muscle tone is lost. The respiratory tract is a collapsed tube. No reflexes are present. The heart beat is slow and weak, the infant is either livid or pallid.

The causative asphyxiating factors may be produced in utero, during delivery and immediate post partum or during the neonatal period.

Asphyxia in utero has received careful study and though difficult to ascertain, certain facts are clearly established. Clinical observation has shown that when the fetus suffers sufficient disturbance of its utero-placental oxygenation its heart beat is altered, tonic movements resulting in the expulsion of neconicum and gasping movements indicative of attempts at respiratory functions may occur. Such violent muscular, gasping movements as occur on interruption of the cord circulation indicate that the fetus does not meet anoxemia below a certain level without signs of trouble, so anoxemia in utero may produce a living infant able to breathe, but with considerable inefficiency. As pointed out a moment ago, the mechanism of respiration is established long before birth; hence there is little difference between intrauterine respiration and extra-uterine except that of the time of onset of function of the lung as a factor in the gaseous exchange.

It seems therefore that extra-uterine respiration should begin at the instant of birth as a continuation of an already established function and not as the inauguration of a new function.

This places a new significance upon the baby that does not breathe immediately. Any baby that does not breathe within a half minute after birth may be regarded as abnormal and in danger of asphyxia. It is important to remember that about four minutes is the maximum time that brain cells can survive without some oxygen and in many cases irreversible changes may occur in a much shorter time.

We have long recognized "birth injury" as the cause of a variety of degenerative lesions of the nervous system and always thought of it as resulting from trauma or hemorrhage. We now have learned from the study of tissues from anoxemic infants, that the damage has resulted not so frequently from trauma and hemorrhage, but rather from the effects of anoxic changes associated with asphyxia at birth.

Dr. Frederic Schrieber has collected well over a thousand cases of children with spastic diplegia, cerebral atrophy, epilepsy, mental deficiency and other nervous lesions in which the only apparent causative factor was severe asphyxia at birth.

A great many factors contribute to the production of asphyxia, and in many cases several of them operate together. Over some of these we have little control such as over the factors relating to the mother. The incidence of asphyxia is twice as great in elderly primipara as in the presence of toxemia·and heart disease.

Other factors may be favorably influenced by modern obstetric skills as shown by the following·table:

Delivery	Per Cent of Deaths	Per Cent of Asphyxia
Version Extraction	25-35	75-85
High Forceps	20-30	75-85
Breech Delivery	12-15	50-60
Mid Forceps	9-12	40-50
Ceasarean Section	5- 9	90-95
Low Forceps	2- 4	15-20
Spontaneous	1-2.3	10-15
Low Forceps with Episiotomy	1-1.5	10-15

The primary cause of death in section babies is asphyxia, often diagnosed as congenital persistant atelectases. Post mortem examination of the lungs of these infants show in the alveoli a lining pseudo-membrane composed of amniotoic fluid, mucus, blood and meconium. Death appears to occur from the asphyxia resulting from the aspiration of this material lying in the upper respiratory passageway. This is born out by the findings of a much larger amount of such material when section babies are sucked out by intertrachael catheter, than is found on similar aspiration of babies born from below. It seems likely therefore that the mechanical squeezing incident to normal birth is the one factor accounting for the difference. Another factor already discussed is that of asphyxia in utero resulting from the type of pre-operative medication and type of anesthetic administered. When general anesthetics are given, the higher the percentage of asphyxiated babies. Three and five tenths per cent are reported as being stillborn, twenty-three per cent severely asphyxiated and only fifty-eight per cent breathed immediately. In comparison, when spinal anesthesia was used, which of course does not affect the baby, there were no stillbirths, only four per cent were severely asphyxiated and ninety-two per cent breathed at once. In this series all factors were the same except the type anesthesia used.

Routine intratrachael catherization may be a life saving measure for an infant delivered by ceasarean section. Of ninety-five cases delivered in a New Orleans Hospital without intratrachael catheterization nine died. Of 102 deliveries followed by routine intratrachael catheterization two died.

Over the factors of asphyxia of central origin, that is those directly interfering with the function of the baby's respiratory center, we as obstetricians have a great deal of control. This type of asphyxia may, and most frequently does, arise as a result of narcotics and anesthetics administered to the mother during labor. The greatest interest has centered around the influence of sedatives and analgesics and anesthetics administered to the mother for pain relief in child birth. It has been shown that every additional dose of sedative or analgesic increases the incidence of asphyxia in direct proportion to the amounts given. Some of these, acting through direct depression of the respiratory center, are more powerful than others. Chief of these are morphine and phenobarbital sodium.

In many large clinics the use of morphine in obstetric amnesia and analgesia has practically been discontinued. The newer drug

Demerol has many advantages. So much has appeared in recent literature on the use of this "wonder drug" in obstetrics that I shall pass by, simply commending it to you for serious study.

Careful study by a large southern obstetric service has pointed to the effects of phenobarbital sodium in the production of serious and re-occurring asphyxia. In consequence the use of large doses of such drug for obstetric analgesia is likely to result in a seriously asphyxiated infant. Less depressing drugs are recommended, and a combination of sodium amytol and seconal seems to fulfill this requirement.

Perhaps even more important than sedatives in producing asphyxia are the various anesthetics used in obstetrics. It is obvious that no general anesthetic can be given to a mother without also giving it to her baby if the placenta remains attached. All fetus have a normally low oxygen concentration in their blood, are highly sensitive to anesthetic agents and hence possess a very narrow margin of safety. It has been repeatedly shown that the longer an anesthetic was given the higher the percentage of asphyxiated babies. However, not alone the duration, but the degree of anesthesia used determines the degree of asphyxia. The greater the degree of anoxemia in the mother the more profound the asphyxia in the infant. It seems obvious therefore that nitrous oxide which produces its full anesthetic effect through the anoxemic state is definitely contraindicated.

I have previously mentioned the effects of blending of these factors in the production of severe asphyxiation. The worst results occur when a combination of all of them are present, as for example, a toxic elderly primipara with some mid pelvic contracture, a prolonged labor, repeated doses of analgesic and amnesic drugs and a fairly difficult delivery under surgical anesthesia. The chances of getting a normal baby are practically nil. It may be a live baby and we may feel proud of the achievement. Later the pediatrician examines the spastic hopeless bit of humanity and justly asks, "How was it born?"

Treatment of Asphyxia: Rarely can one be fortunate enough to have available the much coveted and all important assistance of the pediatrician to assume the responsibility of the care of the new-born. Consequently the obstetrician must assume this responsibility and must be prepared to care for the asphyxiated baby. Prompt recognition of the condi-

tion and the institution of correct procedures are all important.

The mildly asphyxiated infant will require a minimum of attention. This will consist of the aspiration of the oro-pharyngeal secretions, the application of a warmed blanket, a bit of friction, stimulation by rubbing along the spine, producing a vigorous cry. If slight cyanosis persists a few minutes of oxygen from a funnel and a pink healthy baby results.

Should a more moderate degree of asphyxia be present the same gentleness of procedure is followed carrying out the three requisities for resuscitation of a baby such as:

First and most important, keep the baby warm. In a warm delivery room the difference in its temperature and that of the preceding environment is about fifteen degrees. One of the outstanding characteristics of shock is a sub-normal temperature and associated circulatory collapse. The asphyxiated baby must be covered immediately with a warm blanket.

Second, remove foreign material from the air passageway. The folly of attempting artificial respiration before this is accomplished is obvious. The use of the trachael catheter should be learned and such should be in readiness for every delivery where some degree of asphyxia may be anticipated. Through the catheter oxygen or air may subsequently be introduced.

Third, get oxygen into the baby's lungs. This may be accomplished by several ways; however, should oxygen or a mixture of oxygen and carbondioxide not be available, mouth-to-mouth breathing should be employed. Infant resuscitators seldom are available when needed most, or when frantically searched for and found they may not be in perfect mechanical order. The controversy over pure oxygen or oxygen-carbondioxide still is unsettled, but from the point of view of ready availability and the chemical composition of the gaseous mixtures, the method of mouth-to-mouth breathing probably is as scientific and as readily available and practical as any.

It must be remembered that the infant is in a severe state of shock collapse and gentleness in treatment must be pursued. The old methods of hot and cold tubbings, vigorous swinging of the baby through the air, jack-knifing it for artificial respiration and so forth, are mentioned only to condemn. One would not think of treating an adult, in grave and profound shock by such methods.

Something may also be said about the use of various drugs widely employed as respiratory stimulants. Their usefulness seems questionable. Admittedly they produce a sudden stimulus to respiration, their action is almost immediately followed by a corresponding or even greater depression. The dose used must then be carefully selected to avoid the following toxic depression. The previously mentioned methods should be the procedure of choice rather than a "shot" of respiratory stimulant into the umbilical vein.

CONCLUSION

I think we can meet this challenge of the new-born through the improved methods presented above. I should like to urge a more careful and continuous effort toward the giving of adequate pre-natal care, thus preventing and ameliorating the medical complications which result in abnormal babies. I refer to syphilis, heart disease, metabolic and glandular disturbances, Rh negative mothers, etc.

Also the prevention of prematurity and the proper conduct of labor in case it occurs.

Again I stress the proper and judicious use of amnesic and analgesic drugs; and the

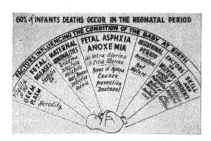

avoidance of anoxemic states in the mother at all times. Fetal asphyxia is serious and its consequences devastating.

I should like to urgently recommend that whenever operative obstetrics are necessary, low spinal anesthesia, pudendal block or local anesthesia be used is possible. This is very important in case of premature delivery. It is equally important to avoid morphine.

BIBLIOGRAPHY

1. Wymon C. Cole, M.D.: Journal of Pediatrics, Vol. No. 19-2; August, 1941.

PERENNIAL NASAL ALLERGY IN CHILDREN*

C. W. ARRENDELL, M.D.

PONCA CITY, OKLAHOMA

Perennial nasal allergy is a chronic, recurrent inflammation of the mucous membrane of the nose. It is also known as perennial vasomotor rhinitis, non-seasonal allergic rhinitis, perennial hay fever, and atopic coryza. It is caused by specific sensitization to inhalant factors and to various foods and is present in two or three per cent of children of all ages and too often is overlooked entirely or mistaken for some other condition.

Inhalant factors will be found more or less constantly in the patient's environment, the most frequent offenders being house dust, feathers and kapok dust, orris root, pyrethrum, and animal danders. The more common food factors are those contained in the everyday diet, namely: milk, wheat, eggs, orange juice, corn, potatoes, chocolate, beans, etc.

*Presented before the Section on Pediatrics of the Oklahoma State Medical Association, at the Annual Meeting, May 3, 1946.

Clinically, there are several diseases which are likely to be confused with perennial nasal allergy, such as the common cold, acute or chronic para-nasal sinusitis of virus or bacterial etiology, infected tonsils, hypertrophied adenoids, and deformities of the nose or throat. Moreover, the child with nasal allergy may, at the same time, be afflicted with one or more of these diseases. The presence of constitutional diseases, such as rheumatic fever, hypothyroidism, secondary anemia, and nutritional deficiencies, may be a further cause of confusion. The effect of such diseases is to lower the resistance of the child to bacterial infection anywhere in the body, but more particularly in the nose.

It is obviously important to differentiate bacterial infections from allergic inflammation. This often calls for a thorough and painstaking investigation, and a period of careful observation may be required to make an accurate appraisal.

In considering some of the more important clinical characteristics of perennial nasal allergy it may be observed that the hereditary factor is always present — at least theoretically — and upon investigation, the history of an atopic background is a common finding.

Either the history or physical examination of a child with perennial nasal allergy will usually reveal the presence of other allergic manifestations such as asthma, eczema, or seasonal hay fever. A common example of this is the occurrence of asthma a few days following the onset of a so-called "head cold". While at times the "cold" may be due to virus or bacterial invasion, concomitant allergic sensitization is the causative factor of the asthma. Also bacterial infection of the upper or lower respiratory tract often complicates a primary allergic manifestation.

Perennial nasal allergy exists more or less constantly, with variations of intensity from season to season, from month to month, or from day to day and is characterized by occasional or frequent acute episodes which resemble the common cold. However, the chronicity and the recurrent tendency of nasal allergy, especially when sinus infection can be ruled out, is definitely more marked than in the common cold or chronic bacterial rhinitis. It has been said that nasal allergy should be strongly suspected in any child who has more than three colds in a year.

Sneezing, while not indigenous to nasal allergy, becomes an important symptom when correlated with exposure to inhalant factors or when occurring at certain regular times during the day or night and in relation to the ingestion of a specific food.

Nasal blocking, usually on one side or the other, exists in a varying degree at all times. Also, itching of the nose will be indicated by rubbing or picking with the fingers. This symptom is a common one and is considered pathognomonic of nasal allergy due to food sensitivity.

Sniffling, caused by mucus or watery discharge, and known as "wet nose" is also a common feature. This discharge often suddenly becomes copious in amount, usually lasting only a few minutes, and often follows an attack of sneezing.

Physical examination may show four characteristic findings indicative of perennial nasal allergy. The first is the pale, somewhat bluish, boggy, water-logged, swollen appearance of the turbanates on either or both sides; however, in the acute flares, the mucous membrane covering the turbanates may be hyperemic. Second, the presence of phlyc-

tenular conjunctivitis is noted, almost without exception, while it is seldom or rarely seen in the non-allergic child. The third condition is the presence of islands of lymphoid tissue on the posterior wall of the pharynx. Allergic children are quite prone to have lymphoid tissue grow in the tonsillar fossae after tonsillectomy and also to have their "adenoids grow back". It should be noted too, that removal of tonsils and adenoids often gives little or no relief from nasal discharge, blocking, and other symptoms. The fourth pathological condition is the presence of nasal polypi. These are not found in the younger children, but in those above six years of age they are fairly common and in themselves are pathognomonic of nasal allergy.

There are four laboratory and clinical procedures which are valuable in the differential diagnosis, though unfortunately they are not helpful to physicians other than those with special training and experience.

One procedure is a microscopic examination of the nasal discharge to determine the percentage of eosinophilic cells present. While a low eosinophile count does not rule out nasal allergy, a count above fifteen or twenty per cent is definitely in favor of its presence.

The second procedure is skin testing. The value of this procedure depends on many factors, such as the type of technic and materials used, and above all, on proper interpretation and translation in terms of correct clinical application. The procedure should not be used to determine if an individual is allergic, but should be reserved for those in whom allergic sensitization has been recognized by other methods. Skin testing in seasonal hay fever which is due to pollen sensitization is invaluable. Especially is this true when it is used in proper dilutions and intervals during the active pollen season. Skin testing for the inhalant factors in perennial nasal allergy is also quite accurate if the testing is properly done and correlated with specific exposure and clinical signs and symptoms. Unfortunately no method of skin testing for foods is dependable and cannot be used satisfactorily as a guide to diagnosis or management.

The third laboratory and clinical procedure is the deliberate trial ingestion of a single food. This procedure was first introduced by Vaughan and later modified and refined by Rinkel. Omitting details of the test, the patient is given the food which is under study and then closely observed for the appearance of allergic phenomena such as sneezing, itching, coughing, blocking of nose, headache, etc. During the period of observation a series of leucocyte counts are made. In the non-allergic individual the normal response to feeding is an increase in the leucocyte count while in the allergic child there is a definite and progressive drop in the total count when such a child is given a food to which he is sensitive. The degree and type of leucocytic response in the allergic patient is known as the leucopenic index. When the leucopenic index is correlated with the appearance of characteristic signs and symptoms of nasal allergy it is undoubtedly the most valuable procedure in the field of allergy to determine sensitivity to a specific food. .

The fourth diagnostic procedure, and the one which is also of great value in the treatment of nasal allergy, is the use of elimination diets and food diaries. These are for the primary purpose of making clinical studies of the effects of ingesting certain foods. There are several variations and types of this procedure since most original workers in the field have devised their own methods.

In conclusion, it may be stated catergorically that the diagnosis of any allergic disturbance is not certain until all of the etiologic factors have been found and proved. This proof is complete when two effects are obtained: first, the relief or cure of the patient resulting from the elimination of all causative factors which it has been possible to eliminate, or by the desensitization to those allergens capable of such response, or by the development of tolerance by known clinical methods. The other effect which proves the specificity of an allergen is the reproduction of a definite allergic response by exposure to the specific causative factor.

Summarizing, inflammations of the nasal tract may be divided into three groups: 1. Allergic; 2. Non-Allergic; 3. Combination of the first two. The allergic group is caused by specific sensitization to inhalant factors and foods. The non-allergic group is made up of primary nasal infections and secondary infections complicating constitutional diseases. The clinical characteristics of perennial nasal allergy are atopic background, frequent presence of other allergic manifestations, chronicity, and recurrent acute episodes.

Symptoms are sneezing, nasal blocking, itching of nose, sniffling, and watery discharge, all of which occur in certain patterns and may be correlated with exposures to a specific allergen by the trained observer.

The signs of perennial nasal allergy are a characteristic appearance of the turbanates, phlyctenular conjunctivitis, islands of lymphoid tissue in the pharyngeal wall, and the presence of nasal polypi.

Four laboratory or clinical procedures are microscopic examination of the nasal smear, skin testing, deliberate trial ingestion of a food correlated with leucopenic index determination, and the use of elimination diets and food diaries.

FOR COURAGE AND DEVOTION BEYOND THE CALL OF DUTY*

*From the book of the same name being published by Mead Johnson and Company, Evansville, Ind.

CAPT. CHARLES DONOVAN TOOL. M. C.

Capt. Charles Donovan Tool of Edmond, Oklahoma, is the recipient of the Distinguished Service Cross, awarded him ''for extraordinary heroism in action on March 18, 1944, in the vicinity of Cassino, Italy''. The citation states: ''An urgent call for aid was received from a battery that was suffering many casualties during a heavy enemy counter-battery barrage. Captain Tool drove his ambulance into a position in the midst of the shelling in order to attend to the wounded. After treating some of the more seriously wounded who had been moved to a stone culvert for protection, he made his way through flying shell fragments to care for men in a gun pit where many hits were being sustained. Finding a survivor who was seriously wounded, he immediately set to work to save him, oblivious to the crash of incoming rounds. Fragments from a shell bursting nearby struck Captain Tool and pierced his spine. Captain Tool calmly continued working to save the wounded man and only after being certain that all casualties had received treat-ment did he allow his own wound to be dressed. By his courageous performance under fire, Captain Tool saved the lives of eleven men. His fearless calm gave comfort to the wounded and contributed to the high morale of the troops under fire.'' Captain Tool also wears the Purple Heart. He graduated from the University of Oklahoma School of Medicine, Oklahoma City, in 1931.

CAPT. ROBERT L. KENDALL. M. C., U.S.A.

Capt. Robert L. Kendall (Okmulgee), formerly of Ardmore, Oklahoma, was awarded the Bronze Star ''for meritorious service in direct support of combat operations from August 15, 1944 to January 15, 1945 in France. During this period Captain Kendall's station has operated under a variety of conditions ranging from rapid advances requiring a high degree of mobility to static conditions with a large number of casualties. Despite adverse circumstances, Captain Kendall obtained a high state of efficiency and standard of medical care. The problem of serving two additional regiments was handled promptly and efficiently under his direction.'' Dr. Kendall graduated from the University of Oklahoma School of Medicine, Oklahoma City, in 1940 and entered the service January 6, 1942.

TYPHOID VACCINE FOR INDUCTION OF FEVER IN NEUROSYPHILIS [*]

PHYLLIS JONES, M.D. AND
JOHN H. LAMB, M.D.

OKLAHOMA CITY, OKLAHOMA

Fever therapy as a therapeutic agent in neurosyphilis has been used for many years. The value of the various methods of producing fever has been discussed by many authors. This paper is concerned only with a discussion of the use of typhoid vaccine for producing fever and the technique of its administration. Nelson in 1931 demonstrated that he could produce any desired temperature rise with typhoid vaccine by a method of divided dosage. This work has been substantiated by a number of investigators since then and in the last few years foreign protein fever therapy is being used more widely with satisfying results. Both the multiple injection technique and the method of continuous intravenous infusion of typhoid vaccine have been shown to produce fever comparable to that produced by malaria.

The mechanism involved in fever protein therapy is not clearly understood but we feel that the physiologic effects of high temperature increase resistence and metabolic activities of the body resulting in accelerated tissue immunity formation and altered sensitivity of cells. Fever also increases the permeability of the capillary walls and tissue cells to antibodies and most chemicals. With this method of producing fever mapharsen and bismuth can be given in conjunction with the fever thus reducing the total amount of drug ordinarily required and having the added advantage of combined fever and chemotherapy.

*Presented before the Section on Dermatology and Radiology, Annual Meeting, Oklahoma State Medical Association, May 3, 1946.

Typhoid vaccine as a thermal agent has certain advantages over malaria. It is a safe method with a low mortality rate. It is available to any hospital at a minimal cost while the average institution has difficulty in keeping an active strain of malaria on hand. Fever produced by typhoid vaccine is controllable. If any complication should arise, fever can be withheld for as long a period as is necessary or it may be discontinued without delay if this is desirable. Some individuals have a natural immunity to malaria which prevents successful treatment but this is not true with typhoid vaccine which can be given to any person if there are no contraindications to fever. It does not have the debilitating effect on the patient that malaria produces. Most patients are up and about the ward between fever bouts and many even gain weight during the treatment.

Contraindications to foreign protein fever therapy are cardiovascular disease, active pulmonary disease, advanced renal disease, debility and advanced age. Kemp and Stokes stated that "careful individual adjustment of dosage and the avoidance of treatment in the face of definite contraindications make this a very safe and controllable form of therapy."

Duration of fever following a single intravenous injection of typhoid vaccine is relatively short. A rapid increase in the dosage is necessary to produce a satisfactory hyperpyrexia. With improved methods of administration by divided dosage and improvement of technique by use of blankets, hot water bottles or heat cradle, a satisfactory prolonged fever comparable to that produced by malaria is obtainable with decreased dosage.

We feel that fever therapy should be followed by regular chemotherapy with arsenicals, bismuth and penicillin for a long period in order to prevent relapses and to obtain optimal results.

PROCEDURE

Careful study of the patient is necessary before fever therapy is administered. A complete physical examination includes electrocardiographic studies and fluoroscopy of the chest, heart and aorta; necessary laboratory tests consisting of complete blood count, urinalysis, serological studies of the blood and spinal fluid, blood urea or N.P.N., plasma proteins and chlorides. Any abnormal findings should be thoroughly investigated and corrected if possible before proceeding.

In our cases the patients were prepared by covering with several blankets and hot water bottles were applied to help maintain the fever. The method described by Smith and associates of placing the patient under a large light cradle well insulated with blankets is a definite advancement and aids in producing prolonged high temperatures. The equipment is simple consisting of a light metal cradle from which is suspended a 100 watt light bulb protected by a screen. The bed is protected by a large rubber sheet covered with a cotton sheet. The cradle is placed on the bed and covered with a large rubber sheet and several blankets large enough to tuck in at the sides and foot of the bed and extending over the patient's shoulders. The head is also covered with several layers of blankets leaving the face the only exposed part. With this arrangement the patient is comfortable and free to move about in the bed without the annoying weight of heavy wet blankets. This also makes nursing care during the fever easier.

Typhoid—paratyphoid vaccine—"Parke-Davis"—(2000 million organisms per cc) is used as the thermal agent. This is properly diluted with normal saline solution and an initial dose of 50,000,000 organisms is given intravenously for an average size male. Dosage will necessarily vary according to the size of the patient and his general physical condition. It is better to use a single injection dosage for the first two or three fevers in order to determine the patient's sensitivity and response to the vaccine. Some patients are very sensitive to the vaccine and may have prolonged fever from the initial dose

requiring a rest period until the temperature becomes stabilized.

If the febrile response on the initial dose is satisfactory, the number of organisms can be doubled for the next fever. After the second or third fever divided dosage schedule may be started using much smaller doses. This may be calculated by giving $\frac{1}{4}$ to $\frac{1}{2}$ the amount of the last dose and repeating in one and one-half to two hours. The first dose may produce a slight chill or none at all and the temperature will usually rise between 99° and 101°. The second or booster dose given about two hours later will produce a hard shaking chill lasting twenty to forty-five minutes and the temperature rises rapidly to 104°, 105°, or 106° and is maintained by the insulated cradle and radiant light. This double dosage schedule will reduce the total amount of vaccine necessary by 50 per cent. The dosage is increased with each fever from 25 to 50 million organisms or more according to the response. Often only a small increase in dosage is necessary and some patients will have a satisfactory response to the same dosage repeated on several occasions. If larger doses are necessary, they should be used without hesitation.

The temperature should be taken each morning preceding the injection of vaccine since a slight elevation of 99° to 100° may act as a trigger and have the same effect as doubling the dose.

The chill may be aborted without affecting the febrile response by giving calcium thiosulfate or calcium gluconate intravenously at the first sign of chilling.

The temperature is taken at 15 minute intervals and the pulse and blood pressure are checked frequently. If the temperature rises above the desired level, the light bulb can be turned off and the pack loosened to allow the temperature to fall. This procedure should be carried out cautiously to prevent a rapid fall in temperature. The patient can be covered again when the desired temperature is reached and maintained at this level. If the temperature continues to rise after the covers are loosened, a cool sponge and intravenous glucose solution may be used. Proper observation and nursing care will usually obviate this difficulty and a fairly constant temperature can be maintained four to six hours if desired.

Breakfast is served on the morning of the fever treatment but lunch is omitted. If vomiting occurs, it is occasionally necessary to omit breakfast. An additional feeding may be offered at bedtime. Fluids should be limited to 30 to 60 cc of water or saline solution every thirty minutes during the fever but should be given freely before and following the fever. At the termination of each bout of fever 1,000 cc of 5 per cent glucose in normal saline solution with added vitamin B complex and ascorbic acid may be given intravenously to speed recovery. A high protein, high vitamin diet and additional sodium chloride is desirable.

To obtain cooperation from the patient and allay pain and restlessness codeine or morphine and barbiturates are given as needed during the day, the first dose being administered before the chill. Minor reactions such as headache, nausea, vomiting, muscle soreness and aching are occasionally present but are usually controlled by sedation.

If there is evidence of impending vasomotor collapse during the fever, recognized by falling blood pressure and rapidly rising pulse rate 25 to 50 mg. of ephedrine sulfate should be given. If it is not controlled by this, intravenous glucose solution should be given and the fever bout terminated.

Mapharsen and bismuth may be administered during the fever if desired. Penicillin has been given in conjunction with fever but in two of our cases where it was used there was an exacerbation of symptoms which subsided as soon as the drug was discontinued. We feel it is better to follow the fever therapy with the administration of penicillin than to give penicillin along with the fever therapy.

We prefer to give three bouts of fever each week on alternating days. If there is a prolonged fever lasting through the night, a rest period is given until the temperature becomes stabilized. The patient is permitted to be up on rest days and is encouraged to eat heartily during this time.

We have tried the administration of the vaccine by continuous intravenous infusion but we found no advantage in this method. It requires the constant attention of a competent attendant to maintain the temperature at a constant level. The patients complained of the presence of the needle in the arm during the fever. The fever curves were about the same as those obtained by the divided dosage method.

There is considerable variation in the response to typhoid vaccine in different individuals, some being very sensitive to a slight increase in dosage. A very unusual response occurred in the case of a woman, 30 years old, who had meningovascular syphilis with symptoms of headache, vertigo, diploplia, and episodes of loss of consciousness of a few weeks duration. This patient was given fifteen million typhoid organisms intravenously on the first dose and received five hours of fever above 103° (R). The dosage was increased five to ten million organisms each treatment giving a satisfactory response (105° to 106° (R)) each time. She was given eight fever bouts receiving a total of thirty-six hours of fever above 103° (R). It was never necessary to give a booster dose and only eighty million organisms were required for the eighth treatment. This is an unusual case and we have had no other patients who responded to small single injections of the vaccine.

CHART 1

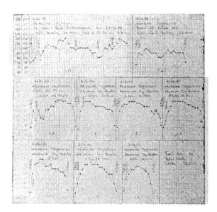

Chart 1 is presented as an illustration of the prolonged fever which may result from the initial dose. This occurred in a 34 year old man who complained of lightning pains in the feet and legs. An initial dose of 50 million killed typhoid organisms was given intravenously in the morning but the patient did not have a chill until 8 p.m. He had fever for the next twenty-four hours including three other slight chills. Temperature remained above 102° for 9 hours and 15 minutes. After a suitable rest period therapy was continued and he had a normal response receiving 30 hours of fever above 102° in nine fever bouts.

Charts 2 and 3 illustrate a dosage schedule in an average case:

CHART 2

Date	First Dose	Second Dose	Temperature Peak	Hours of Fever Above 102°
10-30-43	50,000,000	No Booster	102.8	2 hrs. 35 min.
11- 1-43	50,000,000	No Booster	103.6	3 hrs.
11- 3-43	100,000,000	No Booster	102.4	2 hrs.
11- 5-43	100,000,000	100,000,000	104	3 hrs. 15 min.
11- 8-43	150,000,000	150,000,000	105	4 hrs.
11-10-43	200,000,000	200,000,000	105	4 hrs.
11-12-43	250,000,000	250,000,000	106.2	4 hrs. 15 min.
11-14-43	280,000,000	280,000,000	105.2	4 hrs. 15 min.
11-16-43	300,000,000	300,000,000	105.8	3 hrs. 45 min.
11-18-43	350,000,000	350,000,000	104	3 hrs. 30 min.
11-20-43	400,000,000	400,000,000	105.6	4 hrs.

CHART 3.

Date	First Dose	Second Dose	Temperature Peak	Hours of Fever Above 102°
6-24-44	50,000,000	No Booster	102.2	15 min.
6-26-44	100,000,000	No Booster	103.6	3 hrs. 30 min.
6-28-44	25,000,000	25,000,000	104.2	2 hrs. 30 min.
6-30-44	25,000,000	25,000,000	104.6	2 hrs. 45 min.
7- 3-44	35,000,000	35,000,000	103.6	2 hrs. 15 min.
7- 5-44	50,000,000	50,000,000	104	2 hrs. 15 min.
7- 7-44	60,000,000	60,000,000	104.4	2 hrs. 15 min.
7-10-44	80,000,000	80,000,000	104.2	2 hrs. 30 min.
7-12-44	110,000,000	110,000,000	104.2	2 hrs. 30 min.
7-14-44	120,000,000	120,000,000	104	3 hrs.
7-17-44	130,000,000	130,000,000	104.2	2 hrs. 30 min.

ILLUSTRATIVE TEMPERATURE GRAPHS

CHART 4   CHART 5

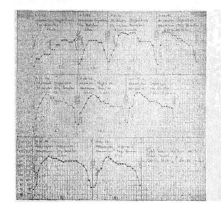
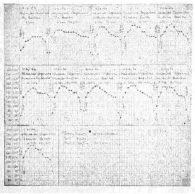

Case 1: A white female, aged 40, complained of nervousness and daily fever of 100° to 101° first appearing in 1942. A diagnosis of syphilis was made and routine anti-syphilitic treatment for 18 months controlled the symptoms until she had a severe reaction to neoarsaphenamine when treatment was discontinued. Symptoms recurred and in August, 1944, spinal fluid was reported: Cells 18; Globulin negative; Kolmer: 4 4 4 4 4; Col. Gold: 5-5-5-4-3-2-1-1-0-0. Four million units of penicillin, followed by 13 bouts of fever with typhoid vaccine (25 hours above 102°) was given. Two more courses of penicillin were given later and symptoms were controlled. Patient has gained weight and has been feeling fine. In the last few weeks, however, she has had a recurrence of the daily fever. Spinal fluid on February 27, 1946: Globulin 2 plus; Kolmer: 4 4 4 2; Col. Gold: 0-1-2-3-2-1-0-0-0-0.

Case 2: A white male, aged 35, was seen in January, 1944, with symptoms of mild euphoria and nervousness. Examination revealed irregular pupils which reacted sluggishly to light and absent knee and ankle jerks and uncertain gait. Spinal fluid: Cells 4; Globulin positive; Kolmer: 4 4 4 4 4; Col. Gold: 5-5-4-3-3-2-1-1-0-0. Five bouts of fever with typhoid vaccine (20 hours above 102°) were given but treatment was discontinued because of shock and convulsions followed with temperature of 107.4° (axillary). Regular treatment, including 3 million units of penicillin was given after fever therapy. Spinal fluid on April 27, 1946: Cells 0; Globulin trace; Total protein 32 mgs per cent; Kolmer: 4 4 4 4 3; Col. Gold: 1-1-2-2-2-1-0-0-0-0. The patient is greatly improved clinically has no symptoms and is working at his former job. He has gained 15 to 20 pounds weight.

Case 3: A white male, aged 37, was examined in October, 1943, complaining of nervousness and 50 pounds weight loss. He had had 18 months routine treatment. Examination revealed Argyl-Robertson pupils and hyperactive reflexes. Spinal fluid: Cells 9; Globulin positive; Kolmer: 4 4 4 4 4; Col. Gold: 1-1-2-2-1-0-0-0-0-0. Eleven bouts of fever with typhoid vaccine totaling 38 hours above 102° were given followed by bismuth, tryparsamide and penicillin. There was clinical improvement until January, 1945, when he developed diploplia and paralysis of the right lateral rectus muscle. Spinal fluid January, 1945: Globulin 2 plus; Kolmer: 4 4 4 3; Col. Gold: 0-0-1-1-0-0-0-0-0-0. Patient has

not been seen for one year, but was unimproved at last examination.

Case 4: A white male, aged 44, developed sharp shooting pains in the back with weakness in the hips, resulting in lameness in 1937. Routine anti-syphilitic treatment was administered for 18 months. Spinal fluid was positive in 1940 and tryparsamide was given until 1943, at which time he complained of muscle tenderness and examination revealed slurring of the speech, pinpoint pupils which reacted sluggishly to light and hypoactive reflexes. Spinal fluid on October, 1943: Cells 1; Globulin negative; Kolmer: 4 4 4 4 0. Ten bouts of fever with typhoid vaccine (27 hours above 102°) were given in December, 1943, and followed with routine therapy. The patient is greatly improved clinically and is working in the oil fields. He has gained weight and feels fine. Spinal fluid April 10, 1946: Cells 0; Total protein 36 mgs per cent; Kolmer: 4 4 4 2 1; Col. Gold: 0-1-2-2-1-0-0-0-0-0.

Case 5: A white male, aged 39, complained of pain in the right shoulder and inability to raise the right arm. In 1937 spinal fluid Wassermann was 4 plus; Col. Gold: 0-0-1-2-2-2-1-0-0. He took treatment irregularly for about 3 years when he began to complain of headaches and loss of libido. In 1939 he received six fevers in the hypotherm at weekly intervals. In 1940 he received six fevers with typhoid vaccine (11 hours above 102°). Routine treatment was continued until 1945. Spinal fluid on April, 1946: Cells 2; Globulin trace; Total protein 34 mgs per cent; Kolmer: 4 2 1 0 0; Col. Gold: 0-1-2-2-2-1-0-0-0-0. The patient is greatly improved clinically, showing a gain in weight of 20 pounds. He has no symptoms and is holding a responsible position.

Case 6: A white male, aged 35, was seen in February, 1945. He showed loss of memory, slurring of speech, disorientation and emotional instability. He walked with a broad slapping gait. Babinski was positive. Spinal fluid: Cells 0; Globulin positive; Kolmer: 4 4 4 4 4; Col. Gold: 5-5-4-4-3-2-1-0-0. Thirteen bouts of fever with typhoid vaccine (34 hours above 102°) were given, followed by 4 million units of penicillin and later routine therapy. Eight months later penicillin was repeated. Spinal fluid October, 1945: Cells 2; Globulin trace; Kolmer: 4 4 4 4 0; Col. Gold: 1-1-2-2-1-0-0-0-0-0. There is marked clinical improvement. The patient is working steadily and has no complaints. He has gained 20 pounds in weight.

Case 7: A white female, aged 39, was seen in 1942 complaining of tinnitus in the right ear, sensations of falling forward and walking in air and paresthesia of the right forearm. Reflexes were hyperactive and Babinski and Rhomberg tests were positive. Spinal fluid: Cells 3; Globulin 2 plus; Kolmer: 4 4 4 4 4. Fever therapy with typhoid vaccine (33 hours above 102°) was given followed by tryparsamide, bismuth, and two courses of penicillin. Spinal fluid on December, 1945: Cells 1; Globulin trace; Kolmer: 1 1 0 0 0; Col. Gold: 1-1-2-2-1-0-0-0-0-0. The patient has gained weight and has no symptoms. She is working regularly.

~ Case 8: A white male, aged 47, complained of dizziness and a dermatitis over the body due to arsenicals and bismuth. He had had treatment for 2½ years. Spinal fluid September, 1944: Cells 1; Globulin negative; Kolmer 4 4 4 3 1; Col. Gold: 0-1-2-2-1-0-0-0-0-0. Eleven bouts of fever with typhoid vaccine (28 hours above 102°) were given, followed by penicillin and a small amount of bismuth. Patient is greatly improved clinically and serologically. He is working regularly ten or twelve hours daily as a radio mechanic. Spinal fluid on April, 1946: Cells 0; Total protein 39 mgs per cent; Kolmer: 0 0 0 0 0; Col. Gold: 0-0-1-1-0-0-0-0-0-0.

Case 9: A white male, aged 34, complained of lightning pains in the feet and legs. He gave a history of previous anti-syphilitic treatment and was found to have a positive spinal fluid while in the army. Spinal fluid on January, 1945: Cells 6; Globulin 2 plus; Kolmer: 4 4 4 4 4; Col Gold: 1-2-3-3-3-2-1-0-0-0. Nine bouts of fever with typhoid vaccine (36 hours above 102°) were given, followed by penicillin, tryparsamide, and bismuth. The patient is greatly improved clinically, feels fine, has gained 30 pounds and is working daily. He has had no lightning pains for over two months. Spinal fluid April, 1946: Cells 2; Globulin trace, total protein 43 mgs per cent; Kolmer 4 4 4 4 2; Col. Gold: 0-1-2-2-0-0-0-0-0-0.

Case 10: A white woman, aged 39, complained of headaches, diplopia and vertigo of two or three months duration. When seen in March, 1940, she had on three occasions lost consciousness and fallen on the stove injuring herself. Examination revealed a loss of pain sensation over the entire body. She had received anti-syphilitic treatment at intervals for thirteen years. Spinal fluid: Cells 3; Globulin trace; Wasserman 1 plus with 0.1 cc; Col. Gold: 1-1-1-1-0-0-0-0-0-0. Eight bouts of

fever were given (36 hours above 102°) and patient showed marked improvement during this time. Regular treatment was continued after her fever and she reports that she is feeling fine and has no symptoms. There has been no recheck on the spinal fluid.

Case 11: A white male, aged 34, received anti-syphilitic treatment for three and a half years. He had no symptoms, but serology remained positive and spinal fluid in November, 1944 was reported: Cells 1; Globulin negative; Kolmer: 4 4 3 0 0; Col. Gold: 1-2-2-2-2-1-1-0-0-0. Nine bouts of fever with typhoid vaccine (32 hours above 102°) were given followed by tryparsamide, bismuth and 4 million units of penicillin in January, 1945. He has continued to work and feels fine. Spinal fluid October, 1945: Cells 1; Globulin negative; Kolmer 3 2 1 0 0; Col. Gold. 1-2-3-3-1-0-0-0-0.

Case 12: A white female, aged 30, had a syphilitic child who died from an arsenical injection. She was nervous but had no other symptoms. Spinal fluid September, 1943: Cells 0; Globulin negative; Kolmer: 4 4 4 2 0; Col. Gold: 2-1-1-0-0-0-0-0-0-0. Eight bouts of fever with typhoid vaccine (31 hours above 102°) were followed by regular chemotherapy. Spinal fluid September, 1944: Cells 1; Globulin negative; Kolmer: 0 0 0 0 0; Col. Gold: 0-0-0-0-0-0-0-0-0, The patient feels fine, has gained weight and delivered a normal, healthy child in April, 1945.

Case 13: A white female, aged 39, was found to have syphilis in 1944. There were no clinical symptoms. Spinal fluid was reported: Cells 42; Globulin trace; total protein 52 mgs per cent; Kolmer: 4 4 4 4 0. Chemotherapy was given for one year, followed by eleven fever bouts with typhoid vaccine (25 hours above 102°). Routine treatment was continued after the fever. Spinal fluid January, 1946: Cells 1; Globulin 1 plus; Kolmer: 4 4 2 0 0; Col. Gold: 0-1-2-2-1-1-0-0-0-0. The patient is well and continues to work regularly.

Case 14: A white female, age 21, acquired syphilis at the age of 16. She took treatment for three years. Serology remained positive. Spinal fluid May, 1944: Cells 42; Total protein 26 mgs per cent; Kolmer: 4 4 4 3 0; Col. Gold: 1-2-3-1-0-0-0-0-0-0. She received eleven bouts of fever with typhoid vaccine (27 hours above 102°), followed by routine chemotherapy. She has had no symptoms. She has been well and working regularly. Spinal fluid March, 1946: Cells 4; Globulin negative; Kolmer: 4 4 4 3 1; Col. Gold: 0-0-1-1-1-0-0-0-0-0.

Case 15: A white male, aged 43, developed

a sensitivity to arsenicals after one year's treatment. He had no symptoms except for arthritis of the knees and elbows. Spinal fluid on January 7, 1944: Globulin trace; Cells 0; Total protein 42 mgs per cent; Kolmer: 3 2 0 0 0; Col. Gold: 1-1-1-0-0-0-0-0-0-0. Eight bouts of fever with typhoid vaccine (21 hours above 102°) were given, followed by penicillin. During fever there was an exaggeration of the arthritic pains but the arthritis improved later. He gained 15 pounds and is feeling fine. Spinal fluid on August, 1944; Cells 0; Total protein 33 mgs per cent; Kolmer: 2 1 0 0 0; Col. Gold: 0-0-0-0-0-0-0-0-0-0.

Of twenty-one cases treated by foreign protein fever with typhoid vaccine, we have a follow up on sixteen cases. Two cases of the total twenty-one have been treated less than three months and two other cases have not been heard from since they received fever therapy. One case of primary optic atrophy with inability to read regained his sight after a few bouts of fever and reports that he is now working at his old job with the Railway Express Company. We have not included this case, however, since he has not reported for a check up. Six cases of the total sixteen were asymptomatic, the diagnosis being made on the basis of a positive spinal fluid. Of the remaining cases, three were diagnosed paresis, five taboparesis, one tabes dorsalis and one meningovascular syphilis.

The patients received from twenty to thirty-eight hours of fever above 102° F. with the exception of one case which has only eleven hours of fever above 102° F.

Of the sixteen patients that we have treated and followed from six months to six years all but one show clinical improvement. There has been no progression of symptoms in the one case which is unimproved. All the patients are working at jobs equivalent to or better than those held previous to treatment. Serologically seven or 43 per cent of the patients show negative or inactive spinal fluid while eight cases show very little change in the spinal fluid findings and one case has not been rechecked.

Examination of the spinal fluid must be depended upon as the most accurate guide for determining activity of the disease. The cell count, globulin, protein and colloidal gold curve show improvement earlier than the Wassermann reaction. Five or six years may be required after treatment is discontinued for the Wassermann reaction to become completely negative. Dattner states that if the

cell count is below four or five and there is a diminution of the protein six months after treatment is discontinued, in all probability the activity of the syphilitic infection in the nervous system is permanently controlled. The follow-up on several of our cases has been less than one year which may account for the slight change in the spinal fluid findings.

CONCLUSIONS

Typhoid vaccine as an agent for producing foreign protein fever is a safe, simple and effective method of fever therapy in neurosyphilis. With the use of multiple injections combined with external heat to maintain the temperature at the desired level for several hours, fevers comparable to those obtained with malaria or the hypertherm can be produced. This method of fever therapy is controllable and can be combined with chemotherapy. Relatively small amounts of vaccine are required to produce the desired fever when the dose is divided and only a small increase in dosage for each succeeding treatment is usually necessary. In addition to the fever the shock protein reaction is believed to be of therapeutic importance. This method of fever therapy is recommended because of its safety and freedom from severe reactions, ease of administration and therapeutic results.

SUMMARY

A method of administering foreign protein fever therapy with typhoid vaccine using single and multiple dosage technique is described.

A small series of cases are reported showing results obtained with this method of therapy.

BIBLIOGRAPHY

1. M. O. Nelson: An Improved Method of Protein Fever Treatment in Neurosyphilis. American Journal of Syphilis. Vol. 15; pp. 185-189. 1931.
2. M. O. Nelson: An Effective Method of Protein Fever Treatment in Neurosyphilis. Southern Medical Journal. Vol. 26; pp. 424-427. May, 1933.
3. D. C. Smith, J. C. Shafer, A. J. Crutchfield: Fever Therapy with Intravenous Foreign Protein in Neurosyphilis. Southern Medical Journal Vol. 38; pp. 194-203. March, 1945.
4. B. Dattner, Evan W. Thomas: The Management of Neurosyphilis. American Journal of Syphilis, Gonorrhea and Venereal Disease. Vol. 26; pp. 21-31. 1942.
5. J. E. Kemp, J. H. Stokes: Fever Induced by Bacterial Proteins in the Treatment of Syphilis. Journal of American Medical Association. Vol. 92; pp. 1737-1741. May 25, 1929.
6. H. C. Knight, M. L. Emory, L. D. Flint: A Method of Introducing Therapeutic Fever with Typhoid Vaccine Using the Intravenous Drip Technique. Venereal Disease Information. Vol. 42; No. 11; pp. 323. November, 1943.
7. H. Lawrence: Induction of Fever by the Intravenous Infusion of Triple Typhoid Vaccine in the Treatment of Syphilis. American Journal of Syphilis, Gonorrhea and Venereal Disease. Vol. 28; pp. 289-304. May, 1944.
8. A. Heyman: Treatment of Neurosyphilis by Continuous Infusion of Typhoid Vaccine. Venereal Disease Information. Vol. 26; No. 3. March, 1945.
9. E. W. Thomas: Fever As An Adjuvant to Specific Therapy in Syphilis. New York State Journal of Medicine. Vol. 44; pp. 157-161. January 15, 1944.

CLINICAL PATHOLOGICAL CONFERENCE

University of Oklahoma School of Medicine

Presented by the Departments of Pathology and Surgery

HARRY WILKINS, M.D. AND BELA HALPERT, M.D.

DR. HALPERT: An injury to a specific portion of the brain, regardless of the cause, produces certain clinical manifestations which may be similar or identical. A neoplasm which arises within the cranial cavity does not usually metastasize outside. Because of this, if there is known to be a malignant neoplasm in the body (outside the central nervous system) and clinical signs and symptoms of central nervous system involvement are found, the lesion in the brain is usually considered to be metastatic. A notable exception to this generalization is the case that we are going to discuss this morning. Dr. Wilkins, Professor of Surgery, will present and analyze the clinical data.

PROTOCOL

Patient: T. P., white female, age 25; admitted November 8, 1945; died November 30, 1945.

Chief Complaint: Headache for two and .one-half years; nausea and vomiting for five months.

Present Illness: The patient was well until the Spring of 1943, at which time there was insidious onset of recurrent headaches which were especially prone to occur in the mornings. She was seen by a physician in May, 1945, and was told that she had "stomach ulcer and nervousness". In June, 1945, nausea and vomiting began to accompany the headaches and she was admitted to St. Anthony's Hospital where a tumor of the left lung along with signs and symptoms of increased intracranial pressure were noted. On June 12, 1945, ventriculography and right parietal craniotomy were performed. Within the substance of the parietal lobe there was found a "black" tumor and this was removed. She was discharged improved following an uneventful postoperative course during which

time she received x-ray therapy. After a few days at home, she again developed headaches and malaise with fever of 105° to 108° F., and was readmitted to St. Anthony's Hospital where she was treated medically for about three weeks. She remained relatively asymptomatic until September 29, 1945, when she again developed malaise and headache. In the course of the next few days she became unable to walk or to take nourishment, and was admitted to University Hospital.

Past and Family History: Noncontributory.

Physical Examination: On admission, the patient was well developed, poorly nourished and in a state of semicoma. The temperature was 99° F., pulse 120 and respirations 18 per minute. The blood pressure was 120/80. There was dullness at the left lung base. The heart was within normal limits and no murmurs were heard. Scars of recent operations were seen on the head and the healed craniotomy incision was bulging. The right eye exhibited an internal squint. There were bilateral choked discs without impairment of extra-ocular movements. There was a left facial paresis of the central type. The neck was stiff and there was pain on movement. No sensory changes were demonstrated. There was a left hemiplegia with hyperactive deep reflexes. Brudzinski, Chaddock, Gordon and Oppenheim signs were positive.

Laboratory Data: On November 8, 1945, the urine was brown, clear and acid. Specific gravity was 1.039 with a trace of albumin, but no glucose. The urine contained an occasional white and red blood cell. Hemoglobin was 15 Gm., the red blood cell count was 4,680,000, and the white blood count 9,600 with 72 per cent neutrophils (1 per cent stabs), 1 per cent eosinophils, 24 per cent lymphocytes and 3 per cent monocytes. On November 9, 1945, the hemoglobin was 15.5 Gm., red blood cells numbered 4,650,000/cu. mm. and white blood cells 6,900 with 82 per cent neutrophils and 18 per cent lymphocytes. On November 11, 1945, the urine was negative for melanin. X-ray plates showed a large single round area of increased density in the left lung base.

Clinical Course: The patient received general supportive therapy including gastric gavage of high caloric diet, and fluids, intravenously. The course was rapidly downhill with a terminal fever of 105.8° F. She died on November 30, 1945.

CLINICAL DIAGNOSIS

DR. WILKINS: Since you all have copies of this case report, I shall bring out only the more pertinent facts for our further consideration. This patient was particularly interesting from a diagnostic standpoint. When she was first seen by me in St. Anthony's Hospital in June, 1945, the question of whether the primary lesion was intracranial or intrathoracic seemed to be still before us. She was admitted to the medical service, but shortly thereafter there was a request for neurosurgical consultation. This was prompted by the findings of choked disc along with nausea and weakness. These completed the triad indicative of increased intracranial pressure. There was a lesion in the chest observed upon x-ray examination and I believe that originally the roentgenologist thought this was a benign growth. With the finding of a tumor mass somewhere in the body which is associated with symptoms and signs of increased intracranial pressure, one must always consider the possiblity of a malignant neoplasm which has metastasized to the brain. It becomes routine to examine the chest by x-ray because carcinoma of the lung is one of the most common causes of intracerebral metastasis. At least one explanation for this lies with the fact that if tumor emboli are discharged into the blood stream, they are set free into the systemic *arterial* circulation and there is no intermediary mechanical filter bed to restrict their passage directly to the brain. In this instance we were dealing with a woman 25 years old who had no pulmonic symptoms, whereas ordinarily patients with carcinoma of the lung are 40 to 60 years of age. Experience has shown that these patients do not necessarily manifest pulmonic signs or symptoms however. Notwithstanding, a pulmonic mass was vis-

ualized by x-ray and of course we had to consider the possible relationships between this silent chest lesion and the obvious intracerebral disease. We had practically nothing of localizing value to tell us the position of the intracranial lesion. After the routine x-ray of the skull we inserted air into the ventricles and found a defect in the ventricular system accounted for by a process in the right parietal lobe. Despite the lesion in the lung and the probability that this was a *metastatic* lesion, we felt that we should give this woman the benefit of the doubt and so we performed a craniotomy. This mass appeared on the surface as a dark, almost coalblack circumscribed lesion. Beneath the surface it was approximately four to five cm. in diameter. We had the impression, as we exposed and looked at it, that it was black because of melanin pigment. It was my impression that this was a metastic malignant melanoma and that somewhere there was a primary lesion which we had overlooked. This tumor mass shelled out with ease and the postoperative course was rather uneventful. There was some question as to whether or not the black color was from blood pigment, but our clinical impression of malignant melanoma remained unchanged. We thought that the lesion in the lung was of similar nature. The patient was discharged, but readmitted when symptoms recurred. She was treated with general supportive therapy and again discharged. She was admitted next to the University Hospital. On admission she had a temperature of 99° F. and her pulse was rapid. Blood pressure was at a normal level. Dullness was detected over the lung base on the left. Scars of recent operation were seen on the head. At the base of this horseshoe shaped scar, there was left a bony defect and the dura was also left open. Removal of bone alone is inadequate for releasing intracranial pressure — the dura is so resistant to stretch that an opening in the dura must also be maintained. This point of decompression was bulging markedly. There was an internal squint of the right eye. This failure of function of the lateral rectus is a sign of *generalized* intracranial pressure. The nerve which supplies this muscle goes a long way along the base of the brain before it leaves the cranium so that when you see a patient presenting other signs of intracranial pressure, internal squint, is an added indication of generalized pressure rather than a sign of localization. There were bilateral choked discs and a left facial paresis of the central type. Only the lower half of the face was paralyzed, i.e., the patient was able to wrinkle her forehead and close her eyes. The neck was stiff and there was pain on move- ment. No sensory changes were noted. Re- flexes were hyperactive. The stiff neck and positive Brudzinski speak for meningeal ir- ritation. For the most part there is nothing of particular interest in the laboratory work with the exception that the urinary specific gravity was rather high; this can be related to the patient's vomiting and attendant de- hydration. The urine was examined for melanin and none was found. The patient received general supportive care but did not respond. Her terminal temperature was 105.8° F. The fact that spinal fluid was not examined in this case deserves comment. We are aware of the fact that examination of the spinal fluid in cases of malignant melanoma may reveal large cells filled with melanin and thus firmly establish the diagnosis. It was unnecessary here to examine the spinal fluid because we were fairly sure of the diagnosis. There was contraindication to spinal punc- ture because of the great amount of intra- cranial pressure. Under such conditions, a release of spinal fluid pressure from spinal puncture will cause herniation of the brain stem into the foramen magnum and will oft- en result in sudden death.

CLINICAL DISCUSSION

DR. BENDER: The chest plate shows a cir- cumscribed area of increased density in the base of the left lung. Our impression was that this was a metastatic neoplasm.

DR. HALPERT: Would you think the lesion was primary in the lung or in the brain?

DR. WILKINS: In such cases as these we examine our patients carefully from head to foot and sometimes we encounter a pigment- ed "mole" which has recently increased in size and this gives away the diagnosis. On the other hand, one may get the history that the patient has had a black mole which might have been bleeding and painful, but that it was surgically removed several months or so ago. This woman did not have one sign of a dermal lesion which we could find. The retina was considered as a possible primary site, but excluded because no tumor was present. This lesion may have been primary in the brain but such would be very rare; I have never encountered a primary malignant melanoma in this region.

ANATOMIC DIAGNOSIS

DR. HALPERT: The nature of the growth in the lungs and the growth in the brain seem to be the main questions that were left for the pathologist to answer. The patient was

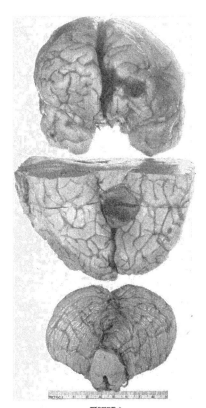

FIGURE 1
External surfaces of the brain revealing several foci of malignant melanoma. That nodule 3 cm. in diameter on the medial surface of the left cerebral hemisphere is the primary site of origin. Note the area of depression in the subjacent cerebellum.

quite emaciated and she had decubital ulcera- tions over the sacrum and over the left thigh, suggesting that she probably had been lying on the left side. There was pitting on pressure about the ankles. Both lungs were increased in weight. The left lung, which contained neoplasm, weighed 750 Gm., three times the normal. The right lung weighed 500 Gm. There was a patchy pneumonic pro- cess, but there was no neoplastic involvement. A regional lymph node (tracheobronchial) contained similar dark neoplastic tissue with- in its substance. In the brain there were three morphologic changes indicative of in- creased intracranial pressure: the brain bulged from the operative defect, the convolutions were flattened and the sulci narrowed, and there was a moderate cerebellar pressure cone. The original lesion was apparently on the right side and it is stated that the major tumor mass was completely removed. At necropsy five distinct nodules of black tumor tissue were apparent. These measured from one to three cm. in diameter. Two of these were within the right frontal lobe and three within the left. No undue pigmentation was seen in the leptomeninx. A frontal section at about the level of the optic chiasm revealed considerable deformity in that the longitudinal fissure and septum pellucidum were pushed considerably to the right, and the left anterior horn was compressed. The primary neoplasm was probably that nodule three by four cm. which seemed to arise from the left cerebral hemisphere on the medial surface adjacent to the cerebral peduncles. This caused a depression of the adjacent cerebellar hemisphere over an area three by three cm. No direct connection could be traced to the choroid plexus. We were forced to conclude that the primary site of origin of the malignant melanoma was the brain itself.

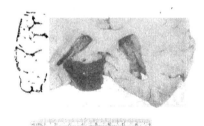

FIGURE 2
Frontal section of the brain illustrating the site of origin of the primary malignant melanoma and the extent of local involvement

The most common site of such a neoplasm is the skin. There are other possible sites, but these are quite limited in number and include only the retina of the eye, the rectum, the suprarenal glands and the brain. Since this particular neoplasm is of melanoblastic cells, it may arise only from those areas in which these cells exist. Actually, melanoblasts are present wherever ectodermal or entodermal tissue joins mesodermal tissue.

DISCUSSION

DR. WILKINS: Is it your opinion that the primary site was the medial surface of the left cerebral hemisphere?

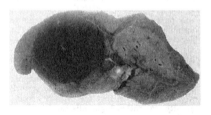

FIGURE 3
Cut surface of the left lung which reveals a large metastatic nodule — malignant melanoma, primary in the brain.

DR. HALPERT: Yes. The only other sites of tumor involvement were the lung and tracheobronchial lymph nodes. These must have been metastatic lesions because melanoblasts, — the cells of origin of this tumor, — do not occur in the lungs or lymph nodes.

DR. WILKINS: This is certainly a unique brain tumor. Apparently from all we can learn its origin was within the brain. It is most unusual for a neoplasm to arise in the brain and then pass outward to other structures. We have had only one other tumor here in the University Hospitals in the last 15 years that manifested a similar ability to pass out of the brain and into other tissues and its extension was limited to the head and neck. In reviewing in my mind the experience we have had with this type of tumor, two patients who were of the personnel of the hospital and medical school stand out. One, a young man with what appeared to be a benign melanoma, had this lesion excised widely. A few months later, this young man struck his head and was admitted to the hospital because of what appeared to be concussion and contusion related to the trauma. To everyone's surprise he soon developed more than 100 black metastatic nodules of the skin, all over the body. This patient actually had a silent cerebral metastasis at the time of his head injury and the injury precipitated hemorrhage within the tumor. In addition it brought about widespread hematogenous dissemination of the neoplasm. Another patient, a young lady, had what appeared to be an innocent mole removed from the neck. A rather short time later there developed an acute cerebral episode similar to a stroke. She had a fatal intracranial hemorrhage which began within the substance of the metastatic tumor.

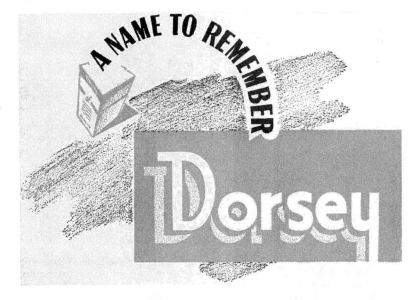

IT'S no trouble to remember the name of a friend . . . the street where you live . . . a favorite restaurant, clothier, druggist. These names are important; YOU DEPEND UPON THEM.

In professional life, also, a man remembers the names which play an important role: interesting patients, colleagues of consequence, medications you rely upon day after day—AND THE NAMES OF THEIR MANUFACTURERS.

Dorsey is one of the names you can count upon—a name to remember. For Dorsey (until recently Smith-Dorsey) has been making reliable pharmaceuticals for the medical profession since 1908. Dorsey products are backed by the Dorsey laboratories—fully equipped, capably staffed, following rigidly standardized testing procedures throughout.

Dorsey is a name you can depend upon . . .

THE SMITH-DORSEY COMPANY
LINCOLN, NEBRASKA
DALLAS, TEXAS   LOS ANGELES, CALIF.

MANUFACTURERS OF
PURIFIED SOLUTION OF LIVER-DORSEY
SOLUTION OF ESTROGENIC SUBSTANCES-DORSEY

President's Page

THE LAMP LIGHTER

There is an old nursery rhyme which runs something like "Christmas is a'coming and the geese are getting fat, please to put a penny in an old man's hat. If you haven't got a penny, half a cent will do, etc." While this may be the Christmas spirit, it is not the spirit of giving that will accomplish the tremendous work being done by the National Tuberculosis Association campaign to stamp out tuberculosis.

On the cover of the Journal is the Lamplighter, illuminating the darkness with a spark of light to bring good cheer and happiness to the world. When he arrives on your desk, with cheer and happiness as his background for those who are suffering from tuberculosis, give him a royal welcome, more liberal than ever before.

No other cause can be any more worthy and your Christmas spirit will have received a decided lift and the holiday season will be a little more real, because it is still more blessed to give than to receive.

Merry Christmas!

L. E. Fuymkendall

President.

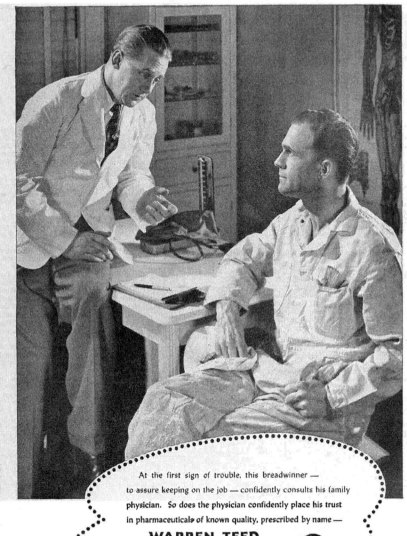

At the first sign of trouble, this breadwinner —
to assure keeping on the job — confidently consults his family
physician. So does the physician confidently place his trust
in pharmaceuticals of known quality, prescribed by name —

WARREN-TEED

Medicaments of Exacting Quality Since 1920

THE WARREN-TEED PRODUCTS COMPANY, COLUMBUS 8, OHIO

*Warren-Teed Ethical Pharmaceuticals: capsules, elixirs, ointments, sterilized solutions,
syrups, tablets. Write for literature.*

ASSOCIATION ACTIVITIES

ASSOCIATION MEMBERSHIP AT FIFTEEN YEAR HIGH

1947 Dues To Be Twenty-Two Dollars

Membership in the Oklahoma State Medical Association is now larger than at any time in the past fifteen years. Membership in the Association as of November 1st was fifteen hundred and forty-one, exclusive of honorary members, and which during the year representd one hundred and fifty service members. This latter figure has now been reduced to seventy-six.

By unanimous action of the 1946 House of Delegates, dues in the Association have been increased from twelve to twenty-two dollars. The House of Delegates, recognizing the extent to which the business and activities of the Association have increased, met the issue by authorizing an increase in the operating budget. All activities of the Association, such as post-graduate courses, will be continued and in many instances intensified.

Members are urged to cooperate with the secretaries of their county societies in remitting their dues for 1947.

POSTGRADUATE COURSE IN GYNECOLOGY

Arrangements are rapidly being completed for the coming postgraduate course in Gynecology. This course will be taught by J. R. Bromwell Branch, A.B., M.D., F.A.C.S., who has been enthusiastically received and highly recommended in another state where he has been teaching the past four years.

Dr. Branch has an excellent background, considerable teaching experience and has completed many years of active practice. Following a clinical trip in January, at which time he will visit medical centers and obtain the newest information on his teaching subject, he will initiate a course in Gynecology in Northeastern Oklahoma.

The Committee is in no sense hesitant to urge every doctor in the state of Oklahoma to take advantage of this course. Every practicing physician solves, or attempts to solve, gynecological problems almost daily in his practice.

On Monday, February 3, 1947, the lectures will begin in the Northeastern circuit which will include the counties of Ottawa, Delaware, Craig, Mayes, Rogers, Nowata and Washington. The teaching centers will be: Miami, Vinita, Pryor, Claremore and Bartlesville. Announcement letters will be mailed in the near future.

FREE PLASMA NOW AVAILABLE

The Commissioner of Health has announced that Normal Human Plasma is now available to all physicians having need for it. Distribution is being made through hospitals and county health units throughout the State, with a reserve supply to be kept on hand at the State Department of Health in Oklahoma City. Plasma will be supplied upon request, without cost, except for transportation costs. No charge shall be made for the plasma itself, although a charge for its administration is permissible.

The Oklahoma Highway Patrol has volunteered to transport additional plasma in cases of emergency or distress.

A.M.A. COMMITTEE TO SURVEY MEDICAL OFFICERS

Dr. V. C. Tisdal Member of Committee

Former Medical Officers from the State of Oklahoma will soon be mailed questionnaires relative to their military service, Edward L. Bortz, M.D., of Philadelphia, Chairman of the Committee on National Emergency Medical Service of the American Medical Association announced.

"Since the results of the questionnaire will serve as a useful guide in preparing for any new national emergency" Dr. Bortz said, "the committee urges all the returned medical officers to express frankly, fully and completely their reaction to military service."

The questionnaire will be mailed from A.M.A. headquarters during November and should be returned within a month. The results will be tabulated and analyzed in detail.

Dr. George F. Lull, Secretary and General Manager of the A.M.A., has sent an accompanying letter with each questionnaire in which he states that the House of Delegates of the American Medical Association in December, 1945, created a committee to study the over-all needs and utilization of medical skills and resources of the nation in the case of an emergency. The House passed a resolution to undertake a critical study of the duties of medical officers during the war just passed, with special reference to (1) opportunities for study, research and actual treatment of the sick; (2) rotation of medical assignments; (3) quasi-medical duties for which technicians and specially trained enlisted personnel might replace physicians. Also, a resolution was passed to appoint a special committee to study by means of these questionnaires.

The Committee is a fact finding board and hopes to make recommendations that will lead to better utilization of medical skills and resources in a future emergency.

In discussing the questionnaire, Dr. Bortz stressed the desirability of deliberation on the part of every physician in answering the questions. "The objective sought," he said, "can be best attained by careful consideration of each and every question."

DIRECTORY CORRECTIONS

Dr. C. P. Gillespie, now located in Miami, Oklahoma, has been erroneously listed as a non-member of the Oklahoma State Medical Association in the Oklahoma County roster. This is an error as Dr. Gillespie is a member in good standing of the Oklahoma State Medical Association.

Dr. M. O. Hart of Tulsa is incorrectly listed at 2529 S. Boston. His correct mailing address is 1228 S. Boulder.

Dr. Onis G. Hazel's correct address is Medical Arts Building, Oklahoma City, and not 1200 N. Walker as listed in the alphabetical list of members.

Our apologies to Dr. Gillespie, Dr. Hart and Dr. Hazel.

DIAGNOSTIC CLINIC OF INTERNAL MEDICINE AND ALLERGY

Philip M. McNeill, M. D., F. A. C. P.

General Diagnosis

CONSULTATION BY APPOINTMENT

Special Attention to Cardiac, Pulmonary and Allergic Diseases

Electrocardiograph, X-Ray, Laboratory
and Complete Allergic Surveys Available.

1107 Medical Arts Bldg.
Oklahoma City, Okla.   Phone 2-0277

SPRINGER CLINIC
Tulsa, Oklahoma

Medicine
D. O. SMITH, M.D.
H. A. RUPRECHT, M.D.
E. G. HYATT, M.D.
ALBERT W. WALLACE, M.D.

Neurology and Psychiatry
TOM R. TURNER, M.D.

Surgery
CARL HOTZ, M.D.

604 South Cincinnati

Urology
BERGET H. BLOCKSOM, M.D.

Eye, Ear, Nose and Throat
D. L. MISHLER, M.D.

Obstetrics
F. D. SINCLAIR, M.D.

Pediatrics
G. R. RUSSELL, M.D.
LUVERN HAYS, M.D.

Anesthesia
M. R. STEEL, M.D.

Phone 7156

WILLIAM E. EASTLAND, M.D.
F. A. C. R.

RADIUM AND X-RAY THERAPY
DERMATOLOGY

405 Medical Arts Bldg.

Oklahoma City, Oklahoma   Phone 3-1446

NEWS   HAVE YOU HEARD THAT

DR. MOORMAN TO BROADCAST ON A.M.A. PROGRAM IN DECEMBER

"Doctors — Then and Now" and "A Century of Progress by American Medicine" are title and theme respectively of the AMA-NBC "Centennial Year" series of dramatized radio programs to begin over a nation-wide hook-up during the month of December.

Dr. L. J. Moorman, Editor of the Journal, and Secretary-Treasurer of the Oklahoma State Medical Association will broadcast from WKY in Oklahoma City on one of these series of radio programs scheduled for 3:00 P.M., Saturday, December 14. The program originates in Chicago with Dr. Moorman's portion to be picked up through WKY. The broadcast is in two parts. The first is a dramatization dealing with historic physicians and medical events in th Kansas-Oklahoma area. The second part, to be presented by Dr. Moorman, will cover a summary of the present status of medicine in this region by reference to medical practice, hospital developments, medical schools, post-graduate education, public health, medical progress, and other significant features of the medical situation in this geographic area. The A. M. A. has segregated the nation into twenty-five regions, having in view the grouping together of states that have similar history and other general characteristics, hence the Oklahoma-Kansas combination.

The radio program represents one of the twelve annual series of broadcasts by the AMA-NBC as a special feature celebration of this, the centennial year of the A. M. A. The dramatized broadcasts will be devoted to features of medical progress throughout the uited States during the 100 years of the existence of the A. M. A.

RADIOLOGICAL SOCIETY ORGANIZED IN OKLAHOMA

The Oklahoma State Radiological Society was organized on October 28, 1946. The following officers were elected: Dr. J. E. Heatley, Oklahoma City, President; Dr. W. E. Brown, Tulsa, Vice-President; Dr. P. E. Russo, Oklahoma City, Secretary-Treasurer. The Society plans to hold three regular meetings during each year.

STATE PHARMACEUTICAL ASSOCIATION TO PARTICIPATE IN VETERANS CARE PROGRAM

The Oklahoma Pharmaceutical Association has announced through its secretary, Mr. E. R. (Pete) Weaver, that 933 drug stores throughout the State have been mailed agreements on the State Pharmaceutical Association's plan of pharmaceutical service to eligible veterans. The program is in addition to the Oklahoma State Medical Association's plan of medical care and takes up the program when the physician completes his portion. Drugs and supplies prescribed by the physician will be taken by the veteran to a pharmacist participating in the State Pharmaceutical Association's Agreement with the Veterans Administration. The entire program is to make available complete medical service to eligib'e veterans. The Veterans Administration will require that physicians' prescriptions for veterans be made in duplicate. One copy is for the pharmacist for his submittal to the Veterans Administration for his payment for products and services rendered. The other copy is to be retained

(Continued on Page 520)

Dr. G. H. Stagner, formerly of Erick, is taking some special work in Chicago at the Eye, Ear, Nose and Throat College and after a visit to the Mayo Clinic he will return to Edmond, Oklahoma, to practice.

Dr. D. H. Miller, Manager of the Veterans Administration in Muskogee, and his wife, Dr. Evelyn Miller, recently attended the 48th Annual Convention of the American Hospital Association. Combining business with pleasure, they enjoyed a vacation in New York City, Washington, D. C., Virginia and Kentucky after attending the meeting in Philadelphia.

Dr. R. H. Mayes, the former secretary of the Pontotoc-Murray County Medical Society, has resigned his post as county public health unit director and gone into private practice in Lindsey. Dr. E. C. Keys succeeds Dr. Mayes as secretary of the county society.

Wedding bells sounded on October 17 for Dr. Richard F. Shriner, of Hobart, when he and Miss Jimmie Nell Peters, also of Hobart, were married in Vernon, Texas.

Former director of the Kay County Health Department, Dr. Paul T. Powell, who recently resigned to enter private practice, has opened offices in the Royalty Building in Ponca City.

Lt. Col. Clifford Bassett is back "home" in Cushing where he was a practicing physician and surgeon before serving fifty months with the U. S. Army in the European theatre. Welcome home, Dr. Bassett.

Dr. A. B. Leeds, who actively practiced medicine in Chickasha since 1902, is now associated with the Albuquerque Medical Center. Dr. Leeds will be missed in civic and youth activities in Chickasha, as well as medical circles.

Dr. and Mrs. George Niemann of Ponca City have recently been notified by the President of the University of Oklahoma that four new student apartments at the University have been named the Niemann apartments in memory of their son, Hal Niemann, who was killed in a polo accident in 1936 while a student at the University. Dr. and Mrs. Niemann will be guests of honor at the dedication ceremony. The apartments are located adjacent to the Hal Niemann Polo Field, dedicated to him in 1938.

Dr. Joseph G. Breco of Ada is retiring after 45 years of practice in Ada.

The Legion of Merit was recently awarded to Lt. Col. Fratis L. Duff, M. C., A. N. S. (Med '39) for outstanding work from April, 1944 to April, 1946, during which period he served as director of training, chief, department of tropical medicine, and assistant commandant, Army Air School of Aviation Medicine. He was responsible for many advancements in the administration of the school and contributed greatly to medical research.

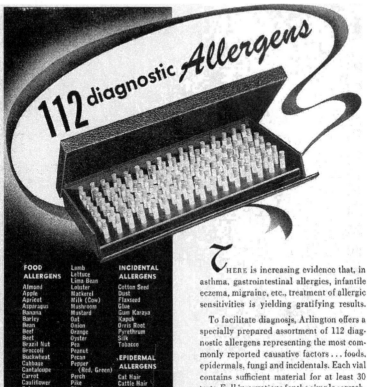

112 diagnostic Allergens

FOOD ALLERGENS	Lamb	INCIDENTAL ALLERGENS
	Lettuce	
	Lima Bean	
Almond	Lobster	Cotton Seed
Apple	Mackerel	Dust
Apricot	Milk (Cow)	Flaxseed
Asparagus	Mushroom	Glue
Banana	Mustard	Gum Karaya
Barley	Oat	Kapok
Bean	Onion	Orris Root
Beef	Orange	Pyrethrum
Beet	Oyster	Silk
Brazil Nut	Pea	Tobacco
Broccoli	Peanut	
Buckwheat	Pecan	EPIDERMAL
Cabbage	Pepper	ALLERGENS
Cantaloupe	(Red, Green)	
Carrot	Perch	Cat Hair
Cauliflower	Pike	Cattle Hair
Celery	Pineapple	Dog Hair
Cheese, American	Pork	Goat Hair
Cheese, Swiss	Potato	Feathers, mixed
Cherry	Prune (Plum)	Hog Hair
Chicken	Pumpkin	Horse Dander
Clam, Hard	Quince Seed	Rabbit Hair
Cocoa	Radish	Sheep Wool
Cocoanut	Rice	
Codfish	Rye	FUNGUS
Coffee	Salmon	ALLERGENS
Corn	Sardine	
Crab	Scallop	Alternaria sp.
Cucumber	Shrimp	Aspergillus
Duck	Soy Bean	fumigatus
Eggwhite	Spinach	Chaetomium sp.
Eggyolk	Strawberry	Cladosporium
Flounder	Sweet Potato	Epidermophyton
Gelatin	Tomato	inguinale
Ginger	Tuna Fish	Hormodendron
Grape (Raisin)	Veal	Monilia sitophila
Grapefruit	Walnut	Mucor plumbeus
Halibut	(English)	Penicillium
Herring	Wheat	digitatum
Honeydew	Whitefish (Lake)	Trichophyton
Lactalbumin	Yeast	interdigitale

𝒯HERE is increasing evidence that, in asthma, gastrointestinal allergies, infantile eczema, migraine, etc., treatment of allergic sensitivities is yielding gratifying results.

To facilitate diagnosis, Arlington offers a specially prepared assortment of 112 diagnostic allergens representing the most commonly reported causative factors ... foods, epidermals, fungi and incidentals. Each vial contains sufficient material for at least 30 tests. Full instructions for the simple scratch-test technique and a supply of N/20 NaOH are included.

These dry allergens remain active indefinitely at room temperature. The allergens listed represent the standard Arlington selection. If preferred you may make your own selection of 112 allergens from our current list, available upon request.

$35.00 ALLERGY DIAGNOSTIC SET

Biological Division

THE ARLINGTON CHEMICAL COMPANY

YONKERS 1   NEW YORK

Arlington

SYMBOLS OF SIGNIFICANCE

Tyrothricin

Parke-Davis

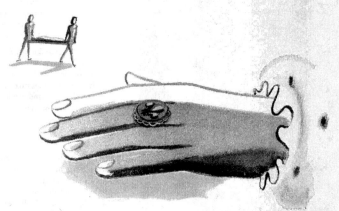

The King's Touch

• Man's longing for a simple, topical cure for disease, symbolized in the
King's Touch, now approaches reality with the development of TYROTHRICIN
and topical antibiotic therapy.

Many gram-positive microorganisms now yield to the bactericidal potency of
TYROTHRICIN in infected wounds, various types of ulcers, abscesses, osteomyelitis,
and certain infections of eye, nasal sinus and pleural cavity.

Whenever streptococci, staphylococci and pneumococci are present
and directly accessible, TYROTHRICIN may be called upon for purely topical
therapeusis by irrigation, instillation and wet packs.

TYROTHRICIN is one of a long line of Parke-Davis preparations
whose service to the profession created a dependable
symbol of significance in medical therapeutics—MEDICAMENTA VERA.

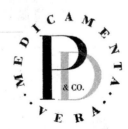

TYROTHRICIN is available in 10 cc. and 50 cc. vials,
as a 2 per cent solution, to be diluted with sterile distilled
water before use.

PARKE, DAVIS & COMPANY · DETROIT 32, MICHIGAN

HITS, RUNS, ERRORS

OCTOBER 21: Final session on newspaper ads. They will run during the week of October 27-November 2. President Kurykendall called and there will be a session during the Clinical Society.

OCTOBER 22: A visit from the representatives of the Bureau of Narcotics. They were excited over the use being made of Demerol. Dr. Moorman will write an editorial.

OCTOBER 23: Everyone working on the letters to membership covering the stand of the various candidates. Hope everyone votes November 5.

OCTOBER 24: Dr. John Burton gave his afternoon to the Veterans Medical Care fee schedule and the meeting of the Committee Sunday should complete the program.

OCTOBER 25: Trip to Mangum for tomorrow to talk about hospital construction called off. County Society will give further study.

OCTOBER 26: Final arrangements made for Veterans Medical Care Committee meeting tomorrow. It has been a big job and the Committee is to be congratulated.

OCTOBER 27: Medical Board of Examiners met in session along with Veterans Medical Care Committee. It was a long day, but over 900 fee schedule items were approved and will be sent to St. Louis and on to Washington.

OCTOBER 28-31: Oklahoma City Clinical Society had their usual outstanding meeting. Visited with more members than can be listed. Also accomplished some work with the President and Dr. McLain Rogers, Chairman of Public Policy Committee.

NOVEMBER 1: Long conference with Erwin-Wassey on next series of ads for papers. They are doing wonderful work.

NOVEMBER 2: The usual Saturday, but a lot of correspondence is dictated and out.

NOVEMBER 3: For the first time in weeks there is no Sunday meeting, but a busy week ahead.

NOVEMBER 4: To Chamber of Commerce for Policy Committee Meeting and preparation of material for meeting of Muskogee County Medical Society tomorrow.

NOVEMBER 5: Off early for Muskogee. Stopped to see Drs. Haynes and Bollinger in Henryetta on business and finally arrived in Muskogee in a nice rain strom, but President Holcombe takes the chill off guests. Had a fine meeting on veterans medical care program. How I wish all county societies were as aggressive as Muskogee-Sequoyah-Wagner. Dr. First up from Checotah for the meeting. Tomorrow, on way home, will stop to see the new Congressman in Okemah, Glen Johnson, and as many of the M.D.'s as possible.

NOVEMBER 6: Today was inventory day, detailed count of all office supplies. Conference with engraver on plates for new Journal cover. Young veteran in office to inquire about male nurse training — we shall try to help him contribute his services to this needful field.

NOVEMBER 7: President Kuyrkendall came through town and Jane met the train and brought him to date. Lunched with Dr. Rountree to discuss A. M. A. matters. Editorial Board met at the Beacon Club. Be prepared for a new Journal. Dr. Rice was called home for a doctor's wife's baby. Timing bad for the office, will speak to the father.

NOVEMBER 8: Another session on the advertising and, oh, how the correspondence got worked over. For the first time in several weeks a military M. C. officer was in looking for a location. As usual, he got the works.

NOVEMBER 9-10: With Dr. Moorman to Enid to meet Dr. Champlin and then a duck hunt. No ducks, but the steaks and apple pie were wonderful.

NOVEMBER 11: Another session with Erwin-Wassey on the ad schedule. Hope next time the members see the ads in the paper.

NOVEMBER 12: To Hugo for a meeting with Mc-Curtain, Choctaw and Pushmataha County Medical Societies. A wonderful meeting and a replay scheduled for December. Mrs. Switzer and Mrs. Woods are fine cooks.

NOVEMBER 13: A busy evening. First to the Cancer meeting of Dr. McHenry's and then to the Oklahoma Medical Research Foundation. Both excellent meetings. The Research Foundation now has an office, 208 Braniff Building.

NOVEMBER 14: The correspondence got some attention and then came the shock. Fondren called from Tulsa that plans for annual meeting are up in the air. Time will tell the outcome.

NOVEMBER 15: To Sentinel to talk to the 4th District Federated Women's Club and a visit with Drs. McMurry and Stowers. Have you ever met their wives? Seen their hospital?

NOVEMBER 16: Oklahoma takes Missouri, 27-6. Cotton Bowl, here we come.

NOVEMBER 18: N.P.C. called from Chicago and they would like to have Governor Kerr for a meeting in December. Now to see if it's possible. Mike Monroney called about medicine and it was interesting.

NOVEMBER 19: First editorial comment was received on ads run in the papers. Comment is excellent and will be sent on to the county societies. Rotary and Research Foundation clash on a luncheon. Research wins. Let's get it under way.

NOVEMBER 20: Attended Oklahoma County Medical Society's Board of Trustees Meeting to discuss possible change of state meeting. Board was willing to accept the responsibilities only upon assurance that meeting would return to Tulsa the following year.

CLASSIFIED AD

FOR SALE. Small, well equipped hospital in Oklahoma. Key N, care of the Journal.

THE COYNE CAMPBELL SANITARIUM, INC.

131 N. E. 4th Street

Oklahoma City, Oklahoma

Coyne H. Campbell, M.D., F.A.C.P.   Helen Callaway, Lab. Tech.

Ben Bell, M.D.   Lucille Dunn, R.N.

J. H. Barthold, Business Manager

C. A. GALLAGHER, M. D.
CURT VON WEDEL, M. D.
(Consultant)

PLASTIC and RECONSTRUCTION
SURGERY

610 N. W. Ninth Street
Oklahoma City, Oklahoma

Office 2-3108

THE MEDICAL SCHOOL

MEDICAL SCHOOL EXTENDS INVITATION TO STATE PHYSICIANS

The Journal is indeed pleased to cooperate with the suggestion of J. P. Gray, M.D., Dean of the Oklahoma School of Medicine, that the Journal keep the members of the Association informed of the various scientific offerings available each month to all physicians who might be in a position to attend.

The invitation Dr. Gray wishes to extend to the members of the Association is as follows:

TO THE READERS OF THE JOURNAL:

The University of Oklahoma School of Medicine extends a sincere invitation to the physicians of Oklahoma when in the vicinity of Oklahoma City to attend clinics, conferences and other meetings as they are scheduled from time to time. We should be very glad to see in attendance at these several offerings planned for students and for staff our colleagues of the communities of the State of Oklahoma.

J. P. Gray, M.D., Dean
University of Oklahoma School of Medicine

CALENDAR — DECEMBER, 1946

SURGICAL PATHOLOGIC CONFERENCES — Each Tuesday 12:00 Noon to 1:00 P.M.
MEDICAL CONFERENCES — Each Wednesday 9:00 A.M. to 10:00 A.M.
CLINICAL PATHOLOGICAL CONFERENCE — Each Thursday 12:00 Noon to 1:00 P.M.
TUMOR CLINIC — Tuesday, December 3 and December 17 8:00 A.M. to 9:00 A.M.
UROLOGIC-PATHOLOGIC CONFERENCE — Tuesday, December 10 8:00 A.M. to 9:00 A.M.
MONTHLY STAFF MEETING — Friday, December 13. Dinner, 6:15 P.M.
RADIOLOGIC CONFERENCE — Monday, December 23 6:45 P.M. to 7:30 P.M.

Dr. H. A. Shoemaker, Assistant Dean, represented the University of Oklahoma School of Medicine at the annual meeting of the Association of the American Medical Colleges held at Edgewater Park, Mississippi, October 28 to November 1.

Dr. Vernon C. Merrifield (Med '45), recently released from Medical Service, is serving a residency at St. Anthony's Hospital, Oklahoma City.

Dr. Mark Everett and Dr. A. A. Hellbaum attended the meeting of the Society of Experimental Biology and Medicine held at the University of Texas Medical School at Galveston, Texas, October 25 and 26. Dr. Hellbaum visited the Andrews Cancer Institution and Baylor Medical School at Houston, Texas, enroute.

Dr. Polk Fry (Med. '36), recently discharged from the Army Medical Corps, has returned to Frederick, Oklahoma, for private practice.

Dr. Howard C. Hopps, Professor of Pathology and Dr. Willard Thompson, instructor in Legal Medicine, attended the Post-graduate course in Legal Medicine given at Harvard University in October. In the course specific information was obtained relating to the proposed Medical Examiner Bill which is to be introduced at the next meeting of the State Legislature. Dr. Thompson remained in Boston for one month's intensive study which is specifically related to the function and methods

of operation of the Medical Examiner System in effect in Boston. The Department of Legal Medicine at Harvard University is one of the outstanding ones in the world, and since the Medical Examiner is in use there, is considered one of the best in the United States. It is felt that considerable information of value to the School of Medicine and to the State of Oklahoma will result from this trip. Enroute, Dr. Hopps spent one day at the Army Institute of Pathology in Washington, D. C., and visited also the Rockefeller Institute and Schools of Medicine at Cordell and Columbia in New York City.

Dr. J. P. Gray, Dean, attended the local medical society meeting at Hugo on Friday, October 25th. He was accompanied by Dr. Lamb and Mr. Hugh Payne, Executive Secretary of the Oklahoma Division of the American Cancer Society.

Dr. Leonard James Ellis (Med '42) has located in Oklahoma City, following release from the Army.

Dr. Charles L. Brown (Med '21) Dean of Hahnemann Medical College, Philadelphia, Pennsylvania, was a guest lecturer at the recent meeting of the Oklahoma City Clinical Society.

Dr. Martin D. Edwards (Med '45), is on terminal leave from the Navy Medical Corps and was a recent visitor to the School. He plans to locate in Oklahoma in the near future.

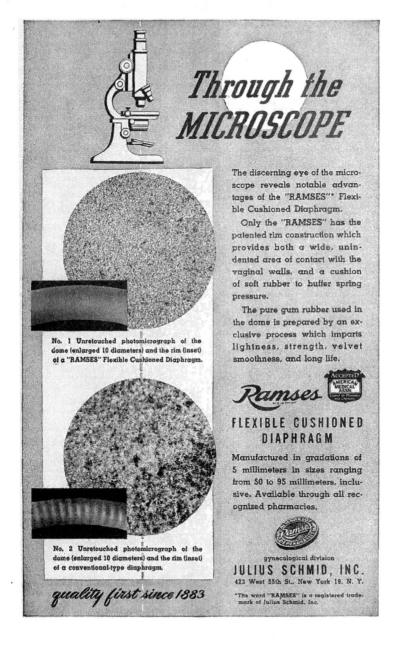

Through the MICROSCOPE

No. 1 Unretouched photomicrograph of the dome (enlarged 10 diameters) and the rim (inset) of a "RAMSES" Flexible Cushioned Diaphragm.

No. 2 Unretouched photomicrograph of the dome (enlarged 10 diameters) and the rim (inset) of a conventional-type diaphragm.

quality first since 1883

The discerning eye of the microscope reveals notable advantages of the "RAMSES"* Flexible Cushioned Diaphragm.

Only the "RAMSES" has the patented rim construction which provides both a wide, unindented area of contact with the vaginal walls, and a cushion of soft rubber to buffer spring pressure.

The pure gum rubber used in the dome is prepared by an exclusive process which imparts lightness, strength, velvet smoothness, and long life.

Ramses

FLEXIBLE CUSHIONED DIAPHRAGM

Manufactured in gradations of 5 millimeters in sizes ranging from 50 to 95 millimeters, inclusive. Available through all recognized pharmacies.

gynecological division

JULIUS SCHMID, INC.
423 West 55th St., New York 19, N. Y.

*The word "RAMSES" is a registered trademark of Julius Schmid, Inc.

BOOK REVIEWS

PRACTICAL MALARIOLOGY. Paul F. Russell, M.D., M.P.H., Colonel, M.C., Parasitology Division, Army Medical School, Field Staff, International Health Division, Rockefeller Foundation; Luther S. West, Ph.D., Major, Sn.C., Entomologist, Parasitology Division, Army Medical School, Head of Biology Department, Northern Michigan College of Education; and Reginald D. Manwell, Sc.D., Captain, Su.C., Protozoology Section, Parasitology Division, Army Medical School, Professor of Zoology, Syracuse University. 684 pages, with 208 illustrations, Philadelphia and London: W. B. Saunders Company (National Research Council), 1946.

Under one of the chapter headings in this book is the following quotation, ''The most hazardous of human tendencies is the drawing of general conclusions from limited experience.'' The authors cover all phases of malariology in their wide experience and are certainly not open to the above criticism. One has long been interested in all of the clinical and preventive aspects of the problem, another approaches it from the viewpoint of the medical entomologist, and the other has done a great deal of basic research on the plasmodia causing malaria. Impetus was given to the study of malaria during World War II. All three of the authors were actively engaged in this work. Their book is timely because it not only evaluates the older material but brings the reader the results of much of the work that was done under the cloak of censorship during the war years.

The book is very well written and illustrated. The color plates are exceptionally good. There is probably no disease that has more complicated relationships than malaria. They involve human habits, physiology, geography, economics, temperature, vegetation, moisture, shade, mosquito habits, etc. Here the clinical, pathological, morphological, laboratory, field and control aspects of the disease are brought together in a logical and revealing manner. Too often books by experts on medical problems tend to leave the impression that all is known that is worth knowing on the subject. This book is refreshing and stimulating because it points out the wide gaps in our knowledge of this disease, the greatest single threat to human health. It is stated that under endemic conditions 30-50 per cent, and under epidemic conditions nearly 100 per cent of the cases relapse regardless of the treatment used. With veterans returning from malarious areas, added to our native cases, the clinician will be interested in getting the rationale for treating and following up these patients. It is unusual to find a book of equal interest to all who are working on malaria. This book is of value to the clinician, the technician, the sanitary engineer, and the medical entomologist. Practical malariology is a cooperative endeavor and this book not only brings the latest developments to

each of the above, but it should impress the readers with the importance of the part played by others.—Donald B. McMullen, Sc.D.

MEDICAL USES OF SOAP. Edited by Morris Fishbein, M.D. J. B. Lippincott Company: Philadelphia. 195 pages. $3.00.

This book is a composite of varied articles by different specialists on the subject of soap. Beginning with a definition of soap and an elaborate discussion of the chemistry of saponification, they very glibly explain what makes the ring on the bath tub surface after a bath in soapy water. Detergents are described.

Chapters on the following are found: Unusual or Abnormal Effects of Soap on the ''Normal'' Skin; the Effects of Soap on the Abnormal or Diseased Skin; the Effects of Soap on the Hair; Soaps for Industry and the Industrial Worker; Surgical Uses of Soap; Medical Uses of Soap.

The entire thought of the book is fairly well summed in the following quotation, ''The most important function of soap is to remove dirt from dirty objects. Simple as this action appears, it is in reality complex, partially because of the varied nature of both dirt and objects. Largely because of its capacity to remove great numbers of micro-organisms from the skin surface, from the crypts, folds, and fissures of the skin, from the hairs, from beneath the nail edges and from around the nails and perhaps also because of its direct antiseptic action, soap and water washing is a very real and valuable medical and sanitary procedure.''—John F. Burton, M.D.

DISEASES OF THE RETINA. Herman Elwyn, M.D. Senior Assistant Surgeon, New York Eye and Ear Infirmary. First Edition. 587 pages with 170 illustrations (217 Figures), 18 in color. The Blakiston Company: Philadelphia. 1946. Price $10.00.

This is the first complete and systematic book on retinal diseases since the great work of Leber in 1915 and 1916.

There is a real need for such a book and this ably supplies that need to both practitioners and students.

The author is eminently qualified, and is indebted to the late Dr. Sanford R. Gifford for his encouragement and for his readings and criticism.

This book is clearly written, systematic, complete, up-to-date, and has excellent illustrations and bibliography.

It will be welcomed by opthalmologists, neurologists, internists and general practitioners.—James R. Reed, M.D.

STATE PHARMACEUTICAL ASSOCIATION
(Continued from Page 512)

by the pharmacist for a special veterans prescription file. Physicians' prescriptions for veterans must bear two specific statements: First, ''I am authorized to treat and prescribe for the above named Veteran Administration patient, ...''. The blank carries the physician's name. The other statement, ''I acknowledge receipt of prescription No. .... on .... (date)..........'' carries the signature of the veteran.

The pharmaceutical service program is an agreement between the Veterans Administration and the Pharmaceutical Association. Each participating drug store must

sign an individual agreement, which includes an established fee schedule to serve as a basis for charges. The agreement does not allow refilling of prescriptions — each prescription must be an original. At the present time specific provisions have not been established for the physician.

The adoption of the Pharmaceutical program by the Pharmaceutical Association is a very important phase of the veterans care program for veterans having service-connected disabilities. Working in alignment with the Oklahoma State Medical Association's veteran care program, it will greatly aid in the completion and insurance of the successful program designed for the ex-servicemen of our State.

The BROWN SCHOOL

For Exceptional Children

Four distinct units. Tiny Tots through the Teens. Ranch for older boys. Special attention given to educational and emotional difficulties. Speech, Music, Arts and Crafts. A staff of 12 teachers. Full time Psychologist. Under the daily supervision of a Certified Psychiatrist. Registered Nurses. Private swimming pool, fireprof building. View book. Approved by State Division of Special Education.

•

BERT P. BROWN, Director
PAUL L. WHITE, M.D., F.A.P.A.,
Medical Director
Box 3028, South Austin 13, Texas

ACCIDENT • HOSPITAL • SICKNESS

INSURANCE

For Physicians, Surgeons, Dentists Exclusively

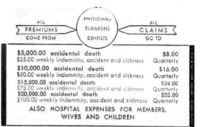

ALL PREMIUMS COME FROM	PHYSICIANS SURGEONS DENTISTS	ALL CLAIMS GO TO

$5,000.00 accidental death $8.00
$25.00 weekly indemnity, accident and sickness   Quarterly
$10,000.00 accidental death $16.00
$50.00 weekly indemnity, accident and sickness   Quarterly
$15,000.00 accidental death $24.00
$75.00 weekly indemnity, accident and sickness   Quarterly
$20,000.00 accidental death $32.00
$100.00 weekly indemnity, accident and sickness   Quarterly

ALSO HOSPITAL EXPENSES FOR MEMBERS, WIVES AND CHILDREN

86c out of each $1.00 gross income used for members' benefit

$2,900,000.00 INVESTED ASSETS $13,500,000.00 PAID FOR CLAIMS

$200,000.00 deposited with State of Nebraska for protection of our members.

Disability need not be incurred in line of duty—benefits from the beginning day of disability

PHYSICIANS CASULTY ASSOCIATION
PHYSICIANS HEALTH ASSOCIATION
44 years under the same management
400 FIRST NATIONAL BANK BUILDING - OMAHA 2, NEBRASKA

THE MAJOR CLINIC AND HOSPITAL

3100 Euclid Avenue   Kansas City, Missouri

A Well Equipped Institution for the Treatment of Nervous and Mental Diseases and Alcohol, Drug and Tobacco Addictions

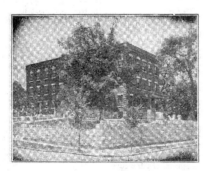

Beautiful Location Large, Well Shaded Grounds. Spacious Porches. All Modern Methods for Restoring Patients to a Normal Condition

HERMON S. MAJOR. M.D.   HERMON S. MAJOR. JR.
Medical Director   Business Manager

OBITUARIES

MEDICAL ABSTRACTS

Ivo Amazon Nelson, M.D.
1894-1946

Ivo Amazon Nelson, M.D., of Tulsa died October 21, 1946, following an illness of two years. Death was attributed to a cardiac ailment.

Born in Para, Brazil, in 1894, Dr. Nelson was the son of a Baptist Missionary. He was educated at Oklahoma A. & M. College and the University of Oklahoma, being graduated from the Medical School in 1925. After practicing for a short time at Enid, he went to Tulsa in 1927 as staff pathologist at St. John's Hospital, a position which he held for many years. In 1943 he was appointed visiting lecturer in the Department of Pathology at the University of Oklahoma School of Medicine. On September 1, 1946, he was appointed Associate Professor of Pathology on a half-time basis. Dr. Nelson's research studies gained wide attention in national medical circles.

William E. Van Cleave, M.D.
1877-1946

William E. Van Cleave, M.D., 68, died suddenly on October 23 in McAlester.

Dr. Van Cleave was born November 3, 1877, at New Market, Indiana. He was graduated from the University of Kentucky Medical School in 1903. After serving as superintendent and medical director of the Indian Hospital at Talihina for more than twenty years, he retired in 1942 when he moved to McAlester and opened an office as an optician.

Dr. Van Cleave was affiliated with the First Christian Church and the Lions Club, as well as the Pittsburg County Medical Society and the Oklahoma State Medical Association. Survivors include Mrs. Van Cleave, a daughter, Miss Maurine Van Cleave, two brothers and a sister.

RESOLUTION
W. E. Van Cleave, M.D.

Through the days we come to the realization of the uncertainty of human life and as in the present instance, we are shocked by the sudden death of a friend and colleague and we are poorly prepared to meet the irreparable loss.

Dr. Van Cleave has been an intimate friend of the Medical Profession of Pittsburg County for many years, even before he moved to McAlester, while he was associated with the Indian Service at Talihina. Since coming here, he has endeared himself to the local profession. His stand as a physician and a Christian gentleman is recognized and appreciated by us all and in his passing we feel very keenly our loss.

THEREFORE, BE IT RESOLVED that we, The Pittsburg County Medical Society, note with deep regret the death of Dr. Van Cleave and extend to his bereaved family our most sincere sympathy.

BE IT FURTHER RESOLVED that a copy of this resolution be made a part of the minutes of this society, a copy sent for publication to the Journal of the Oklahoma State Medical Association, and a copy sent to the family of the deceased.

Signed this 25th day of October, 1946.

COMMITTEE
L. S. Willour, M.D.
E. D. Greenberger, M.D.
T. H. McCarley, M.D.

METATARSAL FRACTURES. E. J. Morrissey, Jr. Bone & Joint Surgery, Vol. 28, No. 3, p. 594, July, 1946.

The author prefaces the article by stating that, "foot trauma, both in industry and in the Armed Forces, is probably one of the most frequent contributors to the loss of vitally needed man-hours". The author then describes a method to minimize the period of disability and discomfort, yet produce the desired end result. He reviews the current method of treatment by means of a plaster cast and the old method of a flexed wooden splint, etc.

His treatment consists of the application to the foot of a simple molded leather arch which may be with or without a metatarsal pad of sponge rubber. Leather arches are strapped to the foot by mean of adhesive type. It includes only the foot but does not encircle the foot, but rather comes up either side of the foot. The arch support is placed carefully in position and held there after careful cleansing and application of tincture of benzoin. The strapping is usually changed once a week for an average period of four weeks. Strapping is removed at the end of four weeks and the patient wears the arch support for an additional month. Cases in which there is marked swelling, with or without abrasions and lacerations of the skin, the leather arch is held in place by means of an elastic bandage and physiotherapy in the form of whirl pool is used until the swelling has subsided and the skin is in condition to permit adhesive strapping.

With a total of 61 cases, 35 began weight-bearing immediately; seven in one to five days after injury; six in six to ten days after injury, and 13 resumed weight bearing more than eleven days after injury. These 61 cases included practically all types of fractures and included single and multiple fractures of the metatarsals. He prefers weight bearing as soon as possible, and prefers the patient to be kept on his job, either at his regular work or at selected work. Many cases in industry would do better if they were allowed to do selected work but this is sometimes difficult due to the fact that many companies will not allow the men to go back to work.

Factors that also influence return to work are: type of injury to soft tissue, where severe soft tissue contusion, laceration or maceration; type of fracture, whether simple transverse fracture of one metatarsal, with no displacement, to complicated comminuted fractures of many metatarsals; there were also two compound fractures. Also, the age of the individual and the type of work performed, whether office work, skilled light work or heavy manual labor.

Follow up study was made on these 61 cases and the author states that from an anatomical, economic, and functional point of view, the end results were excellent. The author highly recommends this type of treatment, which certainly seems a bit radical since while the fractures are reduced it is possible that no traction is applied to an oblique fracture and no effort is made to mold the arch of the foot as has been previously recommended.

His x-ray studies are certainly convincing and it should be an excellent addition to treatment of so-called "minor fractures" which in reality are serious injuries in selected cases.—E.D.M.

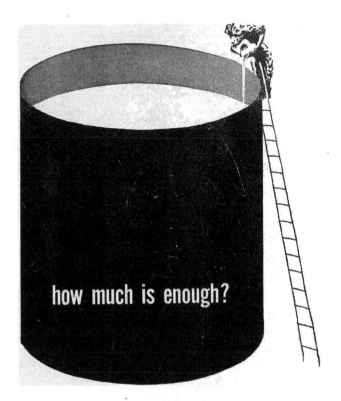

how much is enough?

"How much is enough?" is a pertinent question in vitamin administration. Heretofore, vitamins were most extensively used for supplementation. Today therapeutic requirements are clearly recognized and differentiated from maintenance needs. Vitamins in therapeutic potencies are now recommended for the multiple deficiencies so frequently associated with certain acute and chronic illnesses. Upjohn provides vitamins in economical, effective forms and in potencies to meet therapeutic needs as well as maintenance requirements.

Upjohn
KALAMAZOO 99, MICHIGAN

FINE PHARMACEUTICALS SINCE 1886

UPJOHN   VITAMINS

VOL. XXXIX   INDEX TO CONTENTS   1946

PAGES INCLUDED IN EACH ISSUE

The use of the index will be greatly facilitated by remembering that articles are often listed under more than one heading. Scientific articles may be found under both the name of the author and the various phases of the subject discussed. Editorials, Book Reviews and Obituaries are listed under the special headings as well as alphabetically.

KEY TO ABBREVIATIONS

(S)—Scientific Articles
(E)—Editorial
(SP)—Special Article
(A)—Association Activities

(BR)—Book Review
(Abs)—Abstract
(O)—Obituary
(Pic)—Picture

RADIUM

(Including Radium Applicators)
FOR ALL MEDICAL PURPOSES

Est. 1919

Quincy X-Ray and Radium Laboratories
(Owned and directed by a Physician-
Radiologist)

HAROLD SWANBERG, B.S., M.D., Director
W.C.U. Bldg.   Quincy, Illinois

NEUROLOGICAL
HOSPITAL

Twenty-Seventh and The Paseo
Kansas City, Missouri

Modern Hospitalization of
Nervous and Mental Ill-
nesses, Alcoholism and Drug
Addiction.

THE ROBINSON CLINIC
G. WILSE ROBINSON, M.D.
G. WILSE ROBINSON, Jr., M.D.

MID-WEST SURGICAL SUPPLY CO., INC.

216 S. Market   Phone 3-3562   Wichita, Kansas

SALES AND SERVICE

FRED R. COZART
2437 N.W. 36th Terrace
Oklahoma City, Oklahoma
Phone 8-2561

N. W. COZART
Commerce Building
Okmulgee, Oklahoma
Phone 2403-W

"Soliciting The Medical Profession Exclusively"

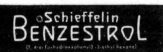

the Preferred Estrogen

COUNCIL ACCEPTED

Schieffelin BENZESTROL is rapidly becoming the therapeutic agent of choice where estrogen therapy is indicated.
Clinical potency, marked tolerance and economy are the
features to recommend its use.

Available in tablets, potencies of 0.5, 0.1, 2.0 and 5.0 mg.;
in 10 cc. vials containing 5.0 mg. per cc., and in ellipsoid
shaped vaginal tablets of 0.5 mg. strength, the physician
has a choice of three modes of administration.

Literature and Sample on Request

Schieffelin & Co.
Pharmaceutical and Research Laboratories
20 Cooper Square   New York 3, N. Y.

A balanced formula

basis for general

infant feeding

FORMULAC Infant Food provides a flexible formula basis for general infant feeding, whether normal or difficult diet cases.

Developed by E. V. McCollum, FORMULAC is a concentrated milk in liquid form, fortified with all vitamins known to be necessary for adequate infant nutrition. No supplementary vitamin administration is necessary. No carbohydrate has been added to FORMULAC. This permits you to prescribe both the amount and type of carbohydrate supplementation.

An increase in the vitamin D content of FORMULAC from 500 to 800 U.S.P. units not only broadens the margin of safety for normal, healthy babies—but provides additional protection for unusual cases, such as prematures.

Priced within range of even low-income groups, FORMULAC is available at most grocery and drug stores from coast to coast.

• For further information about FORMULAC, and for professional samples, mail a card to National Dairy Products Company, Inc., 230 Park Avenue, New York 17, N. Y.

Distributed by KRAFT FOODS COMPANY

NATIONAL DAIRY PRODUCTS COMPANY, INC.

New York, N.Y.

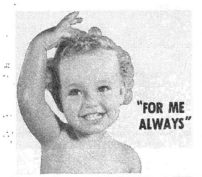

"FOR ME ALWAYS"

Because DARICRAFT

1. is EASILY DIGESTED
2. has 400 U. S. P. Units of VITAMIN D per pint of evaporated milk.
3. has HIGH FOOD VALUE
4. has an IMPROVED FLAVOR
5. is HOMOGENIZED
6. is STERILIZED
7. is from INSPECTED HERDS
8. is SPECIALLY PROCESSED
9. is UNIFORM
10. will WHIP QUICKLY

PRESCRIBED BY MANY DOCTORS
. . . You also may want to utilize Daricraft as a solution to your infant feeding problems, as well as in special diets for convalescents.

PRODUCERS CREAMERY CO., SPRINGFIELD, MISSOURI

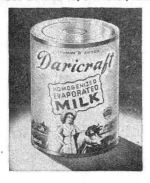

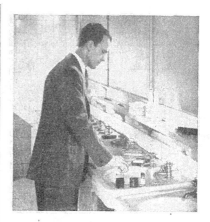

In Any Place
At Any Time

Routine testing of the urine for sugar becomes a vital procedure in the daily life of many diabetic patients.

Clinitest is so simple, so convenient, so speedy, that it can be used indoors or outdoors, in the washroom of a train, service station or elsewhere, with no more inconvenience than in the privacy of a home.

CLINITEST

Tablet — No Heating — Urine-Sugar Test

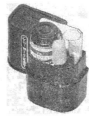

PLASTIC POCKET-SIZE SET (NO. 2106) Includes all essentials for testing.

Complete information upon request. Distributed through regular drug and medical supply channels.

AMES COMPANY, Inc., Elkhart, Ind.

A valuable intranasal agent "... for the patient to use, between treatments or when it is not convenient to take one, is the Benzedrine Inhaler."

Wier, F. A.: Clin. Med. & Surg. 43:217.

Between office treatments... your

head-cold patients will be grateful for the relief of nasal congestion afforded by Benzedrine Inhaler, N.N.R. The Inhaler produces a shrinkage of the nasal mucosa equal to, or greater than, that produced by ephedrine—and approximately 17% more lasting.

Each Benzedrine Inhaler is packed with racemic amphetamine, S. K. F., 250 mg.; menthol, 12.5 mg.; and aromatics.

Benzedrine Inhaler
a better means of nasal medication

Smith, Kline & French Laboratories, Philadelphia, Pa.

"don't smoke"...

IS ADVICE HARD FOR PATIENTS TO SWALLOW!

May we suggest, instead, SMOKE "PHILIP MORRIS"? Tests* showed 3 out of every 4 cases of smokers' cough cleared on changing to PHILIP MORRIS. Why not observe the results for yourself?

*Laryngoscope, Feb. 1935, Vol. XLV, No. 2, 149-154

TO THE PHYSICIAN WHO SMOKES A PIPE: We suggest an unusually fine new blend—COUNTRY DOCTOR PIPE MIXTURE. Made by the same process as used in the manufacture of Philip Morris Cigarettes.

There is no substitute for ACCURACY in manufacturing and standardizing
PHARMACEUTICALS

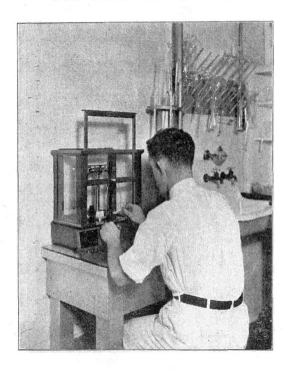

We Have Supplied The Profession With *Ethical Products* For More Than 46 Years.

"We Appreciate Your Preference"

FIRST TEXAS CHEMICAL MFG. CO.

Dallas, Texas

CREDIT SERVICE

330 American National Building

Oklahoma City, Oklahoma

(Operators of Medical-Dental Credit Bureau)

We offer a dignified and effective collection service for doctors and hospitals located anywhere in the State. Write for information.

28 YEARS
Experience In Credit and Collection Work

Robt. R. Sesline, Owner and Manager

THE
MARY E. POGUE
SCHOOL

For Retarded Children and Epileptic Children

Children are grouped according to type and have their own separate departments. Separate buildings for girls and boys.

Large beautiful grounds. Five school rooms. Teachers are all college trained and have Teachers' Certificates. Occupational Therapy. Speech Corrective Work. The School is only 26 miles west of Chicago. All west highways out of Chicago pass through or near Wheaton. Referring physicians may continue to supervise care and treatment of children placed in the School. You are invited to visit the School or send for catalogue.

30 Geneva Road, Wheaton, Ill.

Phone: Wheaton 319

Metrazol - *Powerful, Quick Acting Central Stimulant*
COUNCIL ACCEPTED

ORALLY - for respiratory and circulatory support
BY INJECTION - for resuscitation in the emergency

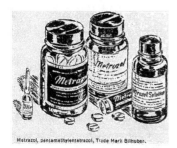

Metrazol, pentamethylentetrazol, Trade Mark Bilhuber.

INJECT 1 to 3 cc. Metrazol as a restorative in circulatory and respiratory failure, in barbiturate or morphine poisoning and in asphyxia. PRESCRIBE 1 or 2 Metrazol tablets for a stimulating-tonic effect to supplement symptomatic treatment of chronic cardiac disease and fatigue states.

AMPULES - 1 and 3 cc. (each cc. contains 1½ grains.)
TABLETS - 1½ grains.
ORAL SOLUTION - (10% aqueous solution.)

Bilhuber-Knoll Corp. Orange, N. J.

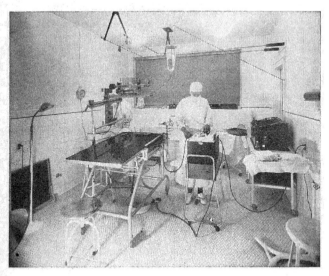

One of Polyclinic's three modern operating rooms.

EFFICIENTLY EQUIPPED
OPERATING ROOMS

Correct equipment complements the surgeon's skill at Polyclinic. One example of thoughtful planning is a modern sterilizing plant, accessible to all operating rooms. Another is a special cabinet for warming blankets. There is new and specialized equipment for the study and care of urological cases.

At Polyclinic, operating room service is maintained on a 24-hour basis with a staff of anaesthetists and specially trained graduate nurses on duty at all times.

POLYCLINIC HOSPITAL

THIRTEENTH and ROBINSON   OKLAHOMA CITY

MARVIN E. STOUT, M.D.
Owner

Antirabic Vaccine

SEMPLE METHOD

U. S. Government License No. 98

1. Patients bitten by suspected rabid animals, on any part of body other than Face and Wrist, usually require only 14 doses of Antirabic Vaccine.

      Ampoule Package.....................$15.00

2. Patients bitten about Face or Wrist, or when treatment has been delayed, should receive at least 21 doses of Antirabic Vaccine. (Special instructions with each treatment.)

      Ampoule Package.....................$22.50

Special Discounts to Doctors, Druggists, Hospitals and to County Health Officers for Indigent Cases.

Medical Arts Laboratory

1115 Medical Arts Building
Oklahoma City, Oklahoma

SHOULD VITAMIN D BE
GIVEN ONLY TO INFANTS?

VITAMIN D has been so successful in preventing rickets during infancy that there has been little emphasis on continuing its use after the second year.

But now a careful histologic study has been made which reveals a startlingly high incidence of rickets in children 2 to 14 years old. Follis, Jackson, Eliot, and Park* report that postmortem examination of 230 children of this age group showed the total prevalence of rickets to be 46.5%.

Rachitic changes were present as late as the fourteenth year, and the incidence was higher among children dying from acute disease than in those dying of chronic disease.

The authors conclude, "We doubt if slight degrees of rickets, such as we found in many of our children, interfere with health and development, but our studies as a whole afford reason to prolong administration of vitamin D to the age limit of our study, the fourteenth year, and especially indicate the necessity to suspect and to take the necessary measures to guard against rickets in sick children."

*R. H. Follis, D. Jackson, M. M. Eliot, and E. A. Park: Prevalence of rickets in children between two and fourteen years of age, Am. J. Dis. Child. 66:1-11, July 1943.

MEAD'S Oleum Percomorphum With Other Fish-Liver Oils and Viosterol is a potent source of vitamins A and D, which is well taken by older children because it can be given in small dosage or capsule form. This ease of administration favors continued year-round use, including periods of illness.

MEAD'S Oleum Percomorphum furnishes 60,000 vitamin A units and 8,500 vitamin D units per gram. Supplied in 10- and 50-cc. bottles and bottles of 50 and 250 capsules. Ethically marketed.

MEAD JOHNSON & COMPANY, Evansville 21, Ind., U.S.A.

Ind.

The
JOURNAL
OF THE OKLAHOMA STATE MEDICAL ASSOCIATION

Christmas Seals

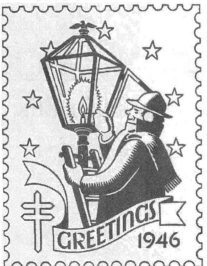

GREETINGS 1946

. . . Your Protection
Against Tuberculosis

| Volume 39 | DECEMBER, 1946 | Number 12 |

PUBLISHED MONTHLY AT OKLAHOMA CITY, OKLAHOMA UNDER DIRECTION OF THE COUNCIL

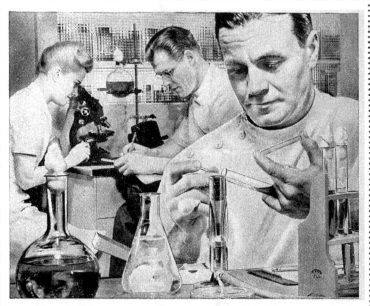

The Doctors behind the Doctor

● Magical penicillin . . . the amazing "sulfas" . . . and now the new streptomycin . . . Thank the men of research medicine for those . . . and for all the other valuable aids they have placed in the doctor's "little black bag."

Biochemists and bacteriologists . . . pathologists and physiologists . . . whatever the field of research . . . they are, first and foremost, *doctors!* And, like all doctors, they are tirelessly devoting their lives to the cause of human health and happiness.

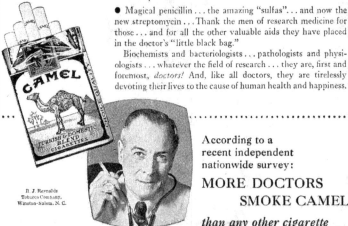

R. J. Reynolds Tobacco Company, Winston-Salem, N. C.

According to a recent independent nationwide survey:

MORE DOCTORS SMOKE CAMELS

than any other cigarette

Antirabic Vaccine

SEMPLE METHOD

U. S. Government License No. 98

1. Patients bitten by suspected rabid animals, on any part of body other than Face and Wrist, usually require only 14 doses of Antirabic Vaccine.

Ampoule Package.....................$15.00

2. Patients bitten about Face or Wrist, or when treatment has been delayed, should receive at least 21 doses of Antirabic Vaccine. (Special instructions with each treatment.)

Ampoule Package.....................$22.50

Special Discounts to Doctors, Druggists, Hospitals and to
County Health Officers for Indigent Cases.

Medical Arts Laboratory

1115 Medical Arts Building
Oklahoma City, Oklahoma

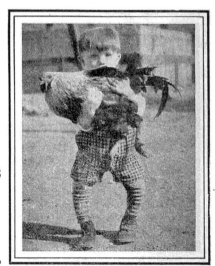

The rooster's legs
are straight.

The boy's are not.

The rooster got plenty of vitamin D.

Fortunately, extreme cases of rickets such as the one above illustrated
are comparatively rare nowadays, due to the widespread prophylactic use of vitamin D recommended by the medical profession.

One of the surest and easiest means of routinely administering vitamin D (and vitamin A)
to children is MEAD'S OLEUM PERCOMORPHUM WITH OTHER FISH-LIVER
OILS AND VIOSTEROL. Supplied in 10-cc. and 50-cc. bottles. Also supplied in bottles
of 50 and 250 capsules. Council Accepted. All Mead Products Are Council Accepted. Mead
Johnson & Company, Evansville 21, Ind., U.S.A.

LIBRARY OF THE
COLLEGE OF PHYSICIANS
OF PHILADELPHIA

This Book is due on the last date stamped
below.   No further preliminary notice
will be sent.   Requests for renewals must
be made on or before the date of expiration.

DUE	RETURNED
FEB 15 1954	FEB 15 1954

A fine of twenty-five cents will be charged for
each week or fraction of a week the book is
retained without the Library's authorization.

www.ingramcontent.com/pod-product-compliance
Lightning Source LLC
Chambersburg PA
CBHW071354050326
40689CB00010B/1642

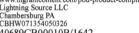